Viral Diseases in South-East Asia and the Western Pacific

Patron

Sir Macfarlane Burnet O.M., A.K., K.B.E., M.D., F.A.A., F.R.S., Nobel Laureate

Programme and Organizing Committee

Chairman
David O. White

Organizing Secretary
John S. Mackenzie

Gordon L. Ada
Michael P. Alpers
Ralph L. Doherty
Frank J. Fenner
Eric L. French
Ian D. Gust
Ian H. Holmes
Ian D. Marshall
Gustav J. V. Nossal
Neville F. Stanley

Representing the Australian Academy of Science
Jacques F. A. P. Miller

Representing the Australian Development Assistance Bureau
Margaret Phillips

Proceedings of a Research for Development Seminar
of the Australian Development Assistance Bureau

Co-sponsored by:
World Health Organization
Australian Academy of Science
Australian Society for Microbiology, Inc.

Viral Diseases in South-East Asia and the Western Pacific

Proceedings of an International Seminar on Viral Diseases
in South-East Asia and the Western Pacific
held in Canberra, Australia, 8–12 February 1982

Edited by

John S. Mackenzie
Department of Microbiology
University of Western Australia

ACADEMIC PRESS
A Subsidiary of Harcourt Brace Jovanovich, Publishers
Sydney New York London
Paris San Diego San Francisco São Paulo Tokyo Toronto
1982

ACADEMIC PRESS AUSTRALIA
Centrecourt, 25–27 Paul Street North
North Ryde, N.S.W. 2113

United States Edition published by
ACADEMIC PRESS INC.
111 Fifth Avenue
New York, New York 10003

United Kingdom Edition published by
ACADEMIC PRESS, INC. (LONDON) LTD.
24/28 Oval Road, London NW1 7DX

Printed in Australia

National Library of Australia Cataloguing-in-Publication Data

---

Viral diseases in South-East Asia and the Western Pacific.

Bibliography.
Includes index.
ISBN 0 12 484820 6.

1. Virus diseases — Congresses. 2. Communicable diseases — Asia, Southeastern — Congresses. 3. Communicable diseases — Islands of the Pacific — Congresses. I. Mackenzie, John S.

616.9'25

Library of Congress Catalog Card Number: 82-71823

Academic Press Rapid Manuscript Reproduction

Contents

Part VI Specific Viral Diseases

A. Respiratory Viruses

B. Hepatitis Viruses

D. Arboviruses

Preface

Virus diseases continue to represent a major cause of death and debility in tropical areas of the world. Of the three equatorial regions, Central and South America, Africa, and Southern Asia and the Western Pacific, most attention has been focussed on viral diseases of the Americas and Africa through international collaborative research and development programmes within the two regions, established in association with the World Health Organization, the Pan-American Health Organization, United States and European government agencies and private foundations, and through international meetings which have provided an opportunity for dialogue and for the discussion of common problems in diagnosis and control. The viral diseases of Southern Asia and the Western Pacific, however, have been relatively neglected in comparison to those of the Americas and Africa, yet half of the population of this planet lives in those countries spanning the area from India to the People's Republic of China. Many of the problems in this region are similar to those in other tropical areas, such as malnutrition, the ubiquity of intercurrent parasitic and bacterial infections, the dearth of trained personnel, the lack of adequate water and sewerage facilities, and economic problems in providing health care services, whereas others are significantly different, especially those associated with high rural population densities, the island nature of many nations, and the large inland water masses resulting from irrigated agriculture and monsoonal weather conditions.

The past decade has witnessed a remarkable increase in the quantity and excellence of virological studies in the region. These have been accomplished through the abilities of a growing number of virologists in different countries and through the assistance of both the World Health Organization's Regional Offices and international collaborative research and health programmes. Not only has the complete eradication of smallpox been achieved in the region (and indeed elsewhere), but the marked success of immunization programmes in China, the eradication of foot-and-mouth disease from most of Indonesia, and the considerable body of knowledge that has accrued concerning the incidence, epidemiology and pathogenesis of viral diseases in many countries of the region all bear testament to the extensive work being carried out.

With this increasing wealth of knowledge and expertise, it was felt that a forum should be established to allow greater dialogue and exchange of information between virologists of different nations in the region, and to provide them with the opportunity to hold discussions with their colleagues from developed nations.

Moreover, it was hoped that such discussions might help in furthering regional control objectives and might delineate those areas needing more specific assistance and collaboration.

It was with this background that an international seminar on viral diseases in South-East Asia and the Western Pacific was initiated. The seminar was funded principally by the Australian Government's Department of Foreign Affairs as a Research for Development Seminar of The Australian Development Assistance Bureau, with the collaboration and support of the World Health Organization's Regional Offices for South-East Asia and the Western Pacific. The seminar was also co-sponsored by the Australian Academy of Science and the Australian Society for Microbiology, Inc. More than 40 virologists were invited to participate, representing most nations in the region, although unfortunately invitees from Vietnam and Kampuchea were unable to attend. The seminar was held at the Australian National University, Canberra, from 8–12 February 1982.

The seminar was dedicated to Professor Frank Fenner in honour of his many achievements in virology and the biomedical sciences and to mark his retirement from the Australian National University. Professor Fenner was the Foundation Professor of Microbiology at the John Curtin School of Medical Research of the Australian National University from 1949 to 1967, then Director of the John Curtin School of Medical Research, and finally Foundation Professor of Environmental Studies and Director of the Centre for Resource and Environmental Studies, from 1973. More recently, Professor Fenner was Chairman of the World Health Organization's Global Commission for Certification of Smallpox Eradication, and in May 1980 he presented the final report of the Commission to the General Assembly of the World Health Organization in which it was concluded that smallpox had indeed been eradicated. A significant number of the participants at the seminar, coming from India, Malaysia, America, Europe and Australia, were colleagues or postgraduate students in his Department at the John Curtin School of Medical Research. Others had a still earlier association, being colleagues of his at the Walter and Eliza Hall Institute of Medical Research in Melbourne. All of us owe Frank much for his help, guidance, enthusiasm and generosity over many years. Indeed virologists everywhere have been influenced and stimulated by his extensive contributions to virology. It is therefore fitting that this seminar should pay tribute to his inspiration and his achievements.

This volume brings together the papers presented at the international seminar of Viral Diseases in South-East Asia and the Western Pacific, with the addition of four extra papers which were unable to be delivered. The volume has been organized into seven sections with a final appendix. The first section contains the opening addresses and the keynote lecture by Professor Frank Fenner. The next three sections contain a number of reviews on more general aspects of virology and on the diagnosis and control of viral diseases. The topics discussed in those sections include geographic and sociologic factors in viral epidemiology, pathogenesis of viral infections, immune responses to viral infections, the problems associated with malnutrition and intercurrent infections, rapid diagnostic techniques, the difficulties in providing diagnostic services in developing nations, the newer approaches using monoclonal antibodies and recombinant DNA technology, priority programmes of the World Health Organization, viral vaccines and viral chemotherapy.

2

OPENING REMARKS

F.M. Burnet

'Kenilworth'
48 Monomeath Avenue
Canterbury, Victoria

I am happy to have the opportunity and the honour of opening this Conference on Viral Diseases in South-east Asia and the Western Pacific, for three very good reasons.

In the first place the whole occasion is designed to honour the work and achievement of the most distinguished virologist Australia has produced, in the person of Frank Fenner.

Secondly it is a conference concerned primarily with those aspects of human viral disease that were my own major interest for some 30 years - the clinical, pathological and epidemiological aspects of viral disease in man. This approach has of course never ceased but it tends nowadays to be relegated to second place by the molecular biologists.

My third reason is the fine response to our invitation to workers in the region we are concerned with from India, China and South-East Asia to the islands of the Pacific - as well as distinguished workers from Europe and America.

First I should like to pay a brief tribute to the man that the Conference honours - Frank Fenner. When a scientist of my age looks back on his professional career, I fancy that what he cherishes most are the achievements of those who in one way or another he has initiated into the field of their research. Fenner had the genes and the background that would have made him a fine scientist however he had come into the fold. But I take a special pleasure in remembering that in late 1945 (while he was an Australian Army Medical Officer then stationed in the Moluccas), he received a letter from me inviting him to come to the Hall Institute to work on ectromelia of mice.

VIRAL DISEASES IN SOUTH-EAST ASIA
AND THE WESTERN PACIFIC
ISBN 0 12 484820 6

We had recently found that the virus was immunologically closely related to vaccinia and it seemed likely that this resemblance might have many interesting implications. Two of his findings with ectromelia (mousepox) that have become classics are his use of the experimental disease as a model of the pathology of the human exanthemata, and for immunization of experimental mouse stocks against ectromelia with vaccinia virus. Incidentally it says a lot for Fenner's capacity as a highly self-disciplined experimenter that for two years he carried out large scale experiments with ectromelia without ever letting it escape into stock mice or the experimental animals in other parts of the Hall Institute.

As we all know, Fenner later collaborated with Ratcliffe and others in a masterly study of the Australian epizootic of myxomatosis of rabbits, another poxvirus. Today we find him completing something no other human being has ever done, the production of a complete history of one of the classic plagues of the human species. Smallpox killed its millions from antiquity until October 1977 when the last case of naturally transmitted smallpox was recognized in Somalia. Fenner had an important part in the work, chaired the W.H.O. committee that certified global freedom from smallpox and was commissioned with Henderson and Arita to write the history of the now extinct disease. No-one could possibly wish for a more satisfying or appropriate culmination of a splendid professional career.

On my second point I shall say only that despite all the recent exciting advances of molecular virology I still believe that the old fashioned way we approached the problems of virus disease between 1930 and 1950 was immensely fruitful. There have been many technical improvements since then but the same broad pattern of epidemiological and laboratory study will almost certainly be equally effective against any dangerous viral agents that may emerge in the future.

This Conference will provide a series of papers on general aspects of virus disease as well as a comprehensive coverage of the local situation and its control, in most of the significant areas of the geographical region being considered. On behalf of the organizing committee I offer a warm welcome to our visitors from overseas. I hope and believe that they and their Australian colleagues will find this Conference a very rewarding experience.

I have much pleasure in declaring the Conference open!

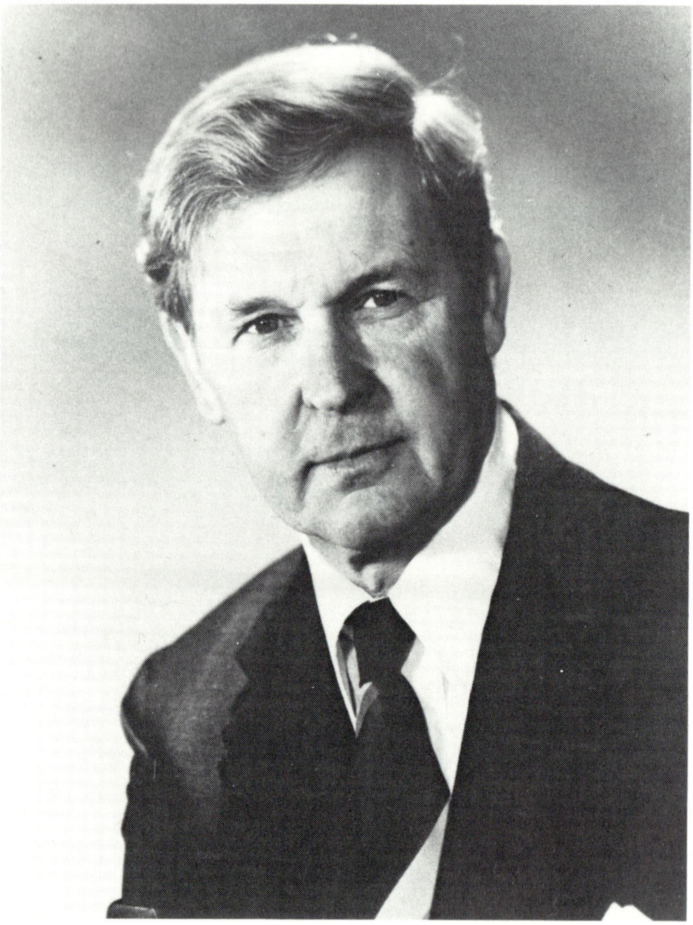

Professor Frank J. Fenner, CMG, MBE, MD(*Adel.*), DTM(*Syd.*), Hon.MD(*Monash*), FRACP, FRCP, FAA, FRS

3

VIRAL DISEASES IN SOUTH-EAST ASIA AND THE WESTERN PACIFIC : AN OVERVIEW

Frank Fenner

John Curtin School of Medical Research
The Australian National University
Canberra

THE BIOGEOGRAPHY OF THE REGION

The most striking thing about the geography of the region with which we will be concerned this week, South-East Asia and the Pacific, is that it is mainly ocean. We are interested in viral diseases of man, so that we are concerned with the vast areas of ocean only as barriers to the movement, or the rapid movement, of animals, insects and man. The land areas of the region comprise four distinct biogeographical entities, which have very different biotas and different histories of human occupation. These are (a) South-East Asia, which for our purposes comprises the archipelagos of Indonesia and the Philippine Islands, Malaysia, Thailand, and Indochina, stretching across to India in the west and up to China in the north, (b) Australia, (c) New Zealand and (d) the oceanic islands of Micronesia and Polynesia. New Guinea occupies an intermediate position; its biota derives from both southern Gondwanic stocks (i.e., those of the Australian region) and from South-East Asian immigrants, all of which have speciated abundantly in the geologically recent past.

South-East Asia is a peripheral but integral part of the great Eurasian land-mass, a home of mankind for more than a million years, during which there have been large-scale movements of man from Eurasia to the peripheral regions for tens of thousands of years. Australia and New Zealand are associated with another tectonic plate that was part of Gondwanaland until Cretaceous times, joined with Antarctica,

VIRAL DISEASES IN SOUTH-EAST ASIA
AND THE WESTERN PACIFIC
ISBN 0 12 484820 6

India, southern Africa and southern South America. I have called Australia and New Zealand different biogeographic sub-regions because they are large land-masses compared with other islands in the western Pacific, and they separated from each other long enough ago to have developed quite different fauna and flora. Australia was invaded by man, coming from the north, more than 50,000 years ago; New Zealand from the Central Pacific a little over 1,000 years ago. Finally, there are the oceanic islands of the south Pacific, not parts of any tectonic plate but excrescences on the floor of the Pacific basin, volcanic in origin and often with a coral growth above or on the fringes. Their fauna and flora, prior to human occupation, which first occurred less than four thousand years ago, consisted of what had flown or blown or floated there, and the evolutionary products of these immigrants.

HUMAN MOVEMENTS IN THE REGION

Pithecanthropus and other forms of early man had moved to the Indonesian islands upwards of a million years ago. The first migration of modern man from the continental landmass to the south and east appears to have been the Austro-Melanesian movement, which reached Australia and Papua New Guinea some 50,000 years ago and by 10,000 B.P. had settled in the Bismark Archipelago. The sea-going communities to whom the conquest of the Pacific is due, speakers of languages of the Austronesian family, to which the modern Indonesian and Filipino languages belong, probably settled the islands of South-East Asia some 6,000 years ago. By 4,000 B.P. speakers of related languages were moving into the Pacific proper (western Micronesia and the Melanesian chain) and about 3,000 years ago people were beginning to settle the scattered island groups which today we call Polynesia. This process was completed by the discovery of New Zealand 1,000 years ago.

Human movement between South-East Asia and Australia, New Zealand and the islands of the Pacific Ocean was a rare event until the fifteenth century, but long before this there was extensive movement from India, China and the Arab world into South-East Asia. This situation changed when the sailing ships of European navigators entered the Pacific Ocean late in the fifteenth century, after which travel and migration increased, at first rather slowly but with quantum leaps in volume and speed with the introduction of steamships in the nineteenth century and aircraft some forty years ago.

VIRAL DISEASES IN FOUR BIOGEOGRAPHICAL SUB-REGIONS

I have mentioned the biogeographical diversity of South-East Asia and the Western Pacific because the viral diseases of man in every part of the world are the consequence of the interactions of humans with each other and with their environment, which includes especially other animals, vertebrate and invertebrate, which may be reservoirs and/or vectors of diseases that can affect man. The speed and volume of human movement between different parts of the world is a major determinant of the pattern of viral diseases, which can be conveniently subdivided into those that are cosmopolitan, which are mostly the specifically human viral infections, and those that have a more limited geographical distribution.

South-East Asian Sub-region

As part of the Eurasian land-mass and the islands adjacent to this, people in this sub-region have long been subject to all the cosmopolitan viral diseases, as we can learn from the ancient Chinese and Indian writings. Further, because the population of humans in the great river valleys of the Yangtse and Yellow Rivers has been very large for so long, and because people there have been living close to their domestic animals for thousands of years, mainland China was probably the site of origin of many of the serotypes of viruses that now primarily affect man. From these river valleys the viruses were spread by human movement to south China and eventually to other parts of South-East Asia. It is likely that this process is still going on; at least two recent types of human influenza A virus, H2N2 and H3N2, appear to have originated in China in 1957 and 1968 respectively.

The region also has a rich fauna of vertebrate animals that could serve as reservoirs of viruses transmissible to man and invertebrate animals that could act as vectors. We think immediately of various arboviruses; the dengue viruses, whose reservoir hosts are probably canopy-dwelling primates in Malaysia and other parts of South-East Asia, and Japanese encephalitis, which finds a reservoir host in the waterbirds of the sub-region and is amplified in the very large populations of pigs. For these, and a host of other arbovirus infections which only rarely cause human disease, the rich fauna of mosquitoes of the Oriental region provides a wealth of vectors.

Australian Sub-region

Australia stands in sharp contrast to the South-East Asian sub-region. Separating from the ancient land-mass of Gondwanaland before the evolution of placental mammals, it developed a very different mammalian fauna, dominated by marsupials but with several indigenous species of bats and rats that evolved from ancestors that flew or floated in subsequent to the separation. It has been occupied by man for tens of thousands of years, but in contrast to the great river valleys of China, Australia never saw the development of indigenous agriculture. Its peoples remained hunter-gatherers, albeit skilled in the encouragement of production by some native plants and animals. In consequence the population, even in the hospitable river valleys and along the sea shores, was always relatively sparse.

Despite the fact that during the period of human occupation of South-East Asia sea-barriers were usually narrower than they are today, Australia remained isolated from cultural developments of the kind that flourished in Asia. Although agriculture was established in New Guinea more than 6,000 years ago, the narrow Torres Strait, or the physical or cultural environments of Australia, prevented its spread into that continent. Except for limited incursions along the north coast, Australia remained isolated from the rest of the world until the European invasion some 200 years ago.

Not only did the aboriginal invaders not develop agriculture, they could not become intensive pastoralists, for marsupials provide poor starting material, compared with the ungulates available in Asia. The dingo was introduced over 3,000 years ago, but fortunately none of the founder stock was incubating rabies.

In consequence of his isolation and the relative sparsity of the population, Australian aboriginal man was probably free of most of the specifically human viral diseases except those associated with chronic or recurrent infectivity, such as various herpesviruses and hepatitis B. Further, although many arboviruses, belonging to several viral families, have been recovered from Australian mosquitoes, midges, ticks, birds and mammals, there appear to be only four that affect man adversely: Murray Valley encephalitis and more rarely Kunjin flaviviruses and Ross River and more rarely Sindbis alphaviruses.

The European invasion brought some of the cosmopolitan viruses to Australia and the first outbreak of smallpox began near Sydney in 1789. However, the long sea voyage still provided an effective barrier to many viruses, and the sparse population of colonists did not maintain most of those which were introduced. Even during this century, quarantine measures had partial success in delaying the spread of pandemic influenza into the civilian population of Australia until early 1919 and were very effective in excluding smallpox.

New Zealand

Much smaller in size than Australia, lacking indigenous mammals except a few migrant rodents, and with a much smaller indigenous mosquito fauna, New Zealand supported only one indigenous mosquito-borne virus, Whataroa alphavirus, and a few tick-borne viruses of birds. The small scale and long travel times of the early Polynesian migrations ensured that only viruses that would remain latent or produce chronic infectivity could be introduced, so that the early inhabitants of New Zealand, like those of Australia, were by and large free of viral infections. After the European occupation and with the development of rapid trans-oceanic travel, New Zealand became part of the global ecosystem as far as human viral infections are concerned.

The Oceanic Islands

The oceanic islands, except perhaps for New Caledonia, differ biogeographically from all the other sub-regions, in that they have never formed part of a large land-mass on which a substantial fauna and flora could evolve. The volcanoes that constitute the larger islands of the Hawaiian group, Fiji and Tahiti, and the coral atolls that developed on submerged volcanic peaks, were at first devoid of land animals and plants. They were populated by chance landfalls of seeds, birds and other animals and eventually by similar chance landfalls of man. The poverty of the indigenous fauna, the isolation of the islands in a vast ocean and the small size of the founder populations combined to render the human inhabitants of these islands, before the "fatal impact" of the European explorations in the late eighteenth century, less subject to infectious diseases of any sort than any other population on earth, except perhaps for some Eskimo tribes. Of course this made them highly vulnerable to such diseases, as the disastrous history of infectious diseases in the islands during the nineteenth century well demonstrates.

SOME HISTORICAL INCIDENTS

Clearly, in this introductory address, I cannot hope to traverse the full range of viral diseases that occur in the region. But I thought that it would be appropriate to present vignettes describing some aspects of the history of some of these diseases.

Smallpox

I hope you will forgive me if I start with this extinct disease, but it now dominates my thoughts. Further, because of its severity and the pathognomonic clinical picture, we can recognize descriptions of the disease in ancient writings. Smallpox was first accurately described by the Chinese physician Ko Hung in the fourth century AD. By the tenth century variolation was probably practised in China as a mode of protection, although the rite was protected by secrecy.

Coming to more recent times, an outbreak of what appears to have been smallpox started among aborigines near Sydney in 1789, but died out in a year or so. The disease did not reach Hawaii until 1853, when a case imported by a steamship from California caused an outbreak in which 10,000 persons died.

Smallpox was long endemic throughout South-East Asia, but not in Australia, New Zealand or the oceanic islands. Country-wide eradication was achieved in Indonesia in 1937, using air-dried vaccine which retained potency under tropical conditions, but with the disorders of war smallpox was reintroduced and spread widely throughout the archipelago, being again eliminated in 1972.

Finally, it is worth acknowledging the splendid achievement of the then newly established Peoples Republic of China in interrupting the transmission of smallpox in all but a few southern and western border areas by 1954, and in the whole country by 1960, without assistance from WHO.

Measles

The initial impact of measles on the peoples of Polynesia was as catastrophic as that of smallpox. Introduced into Fiji in 1875 it killed 30% of the population, partly because of the social disruption caused by the impact of this highly infectious disease on a virgin population. Indentured labour was introduced from India to make good the loss of plantation workers, with the result that Fiji now has as many Indian as Austronesian inhabitants. The islands of the Pacific and the Caribbean provided the raw material for a short but important paper by Dr Black, in which he described the relation of population size and dispersion to the endemicity of measles.

Influenza

I have already mentioned that the vast country on the northern fringes of our region, China, was the birthplace of the two recent pandemic strains of influenza A virus, H2N2 and H3N2; a topic on which we will hear more later this week.

The dispersion of the islands of the Pacific Ocean also provided good evidence for the ship-borne spread of influenza. The 1918 pandemic strain was probably brought to New Zealand by the s.s. *Niagara*, which berthed in Auckland on October 12, 1918, and in 1964 a Trust Territory supply ship spread influenza A2 virus to three of the eleven inhabited islands and atolls of the Western Caroline islands, which had been free of influenza for some 20 years. Overt disease occurred in virtually all inhabitants and the mortality was 7% on the most severely affected atoll.

Poliomyelitis

The three types of polioviruses circulated readily but did not produce disease amongst the infants in densely populated parts of the region, especially in the areas and the days before sanitation lowered the rate of faecal-oral transfer. As sanitation developed, the deferment of infection from infancy to childhood, and the absence of particular serotypes from the population for some years, led to epidemics of infantile paralysis; Australia and New Zealand were among the first countries in the world to experience such epidemics. None of the isolated islands of the Pacific had populations large enough to maintain these viruses endemically, but severe outbreaks sometimes occurred following an introduction. In the Marshall Islands, for example, a very severe outbreak of poliovirus type 1 occurred in 1963, resulting in 196 cases and an attack rate for paralytic disease of 2%. Finally, just at the time that vaccination began to alter the epidemiological pattern of poliomyelitis, the emerging affluence and improving sanitation of places like Singapore were manifested by the development of epidemic infantile paralysis.

Dengue Haemorrhagic Fever

The four serotypes of dengue appear to have a sylvan cycle amongst canopy dwelling primates and canopy mosquitoes in Malaysia and adjacent parts of South-East Asia, comparable to that of yellow fever in Africa. As populations of *Aedes aegypti* developed in the villages and towns of South-East Asia, dengue became endemic there and in the Second World War it caused severe epidemics in the Allied and Japanese soldiers and the indigenous inhabitants of New Guinea, transmitted by the coconut-breeding mosquitoes, *Aedes albopictus* and *Aedes scutellaris*.

The post-war development of air travel has spread all four dengue serotypes throughout South-East Asia, with occasional extensions into the Pacific islands. About thirty years ago what appeared to be a new syndrome, or at least its much more frequent occurrence, became apparent in the Philippines and Thailand - dengue haemorrhagic fever or dengue shock syndrome. We shall hear more about this later in the symposium.

Australian X Disease

What was called Australian X disease in 1917 was later shown to be the same as Murray Valley encephalitis. I mention it here to note that the virus that caused this disease was the first arbovirus to be passed in an experimental animal, by the late Sir John Cleland, in 1918.

The zoogeographic distributions of different arboviruses are intriguing. The dengue viruses are cosmopolitan but yellow fever virus has never reached Asia. Within the region, Murray Valley encephalitis and Kunjin viruses appear to be restricted to Australia and New Guinea while Japanese encephalitis virus occurs north and west of Weber's line. Possible explanations include the distributions of the major mosquito vectors and/or those of the species of heron that constitute a major vertebrate reservoir.

Ross River Disease

This disease was first recognized as a polyarthritis occurring in southern New South Wales in 1928, and subsequently among Army personnel stationed in the Northern Territory of Australia during the Second World War. There was a large epidemic in the Murray Valley in 1956, and the probable etiological role of an alphavirus was recognized in 1960. The causative virus was finally recovered from mosquitoes in 1963. I mention it here to foreshadow discussion of the remarkable spread of this virus outside its original endemic zone (Australia and New Guinea), which started in 1979, when it spread to Fiji and then to outlying Polynesian islands. The feature of especial interest is that this spread was probably due to the movement by air of viraemic humans. Several virologists working in the islands have shown that virus could be readily recovered from the blood of Polynesians suffering from the disease, although Australian virologists have consistently failed to recover the virus from humans in Australia. Perhaps the virus has undergone a change in its pathogenicity, following its introduction into new populations of humans and mosquitoes.

Australia Antigen

Although the official committee on viral taxonomy has yet to pronounce on its classification, more is known of hepatitis B virus than of most other human viruses; even to the sequence of its unique double-stranded DNA with a single-stranded "tail". Discussions of hepatitis B will loom large in the regional reports and in the special half-day session on hepatitis viruses, because it is one of the most important viruses for which control measures have yet to be developed. It is interesting to recall that all this knowledge has developed since 1965, when Dr Kirk of ANU sent specimens of Australian aboriginal serum to Dr Blumberg in Philadelphia, both being interested in blood group polymorphisms. Dr Blumberg found that the aboriginal serum, alone of a panel of 24 sera, gave a precipitin line with serum from a haemophilic patient in New York, and by skilful detective work the Australia antigen was eventually identified with hepatitis B virus surface antigen. It is of interest that its occurrence is unusually high in some populations of the Pacific islands and in the Philippines.

Kuru

Finally, we should recall that a remarkable new group of viruses was recognized as human pathogens after Dr Gajdusek had passaged brain material from patients from the Fore region of New Guinea in chimpanzees. Subsequently Gajdusek grouped together several disease entities as the subacute spongiform viral encephalopathies, which includes two human diseases: the geographically localized disease, kuru, and the cosmopolitan Creutzfeld-Jakob syndrome. In spite of intensive efforts, we are still not certain whether these diseases are caused by true viruses or by free nucleic acid molecules, analogous to the well-characterized "viroids" of plants.

WHAT OF THE FUTURE?

I have surveyed very broadly the biogeographical environment in which our conference is set and in which the viral diseases with which we are concerned occur. Many of these diseases are cosmopolitan, but are unusual in some parts of the region like the Pacific islands, because of their geographical isolation; other cosmopolitan diseases like hepatitis B have an unusually high incidence in some parts of the region. Other diseases, like Japanese and Murray Valley encephalitis, are widespread, with non-overlapping distributions covering wide areas within the region, whereas kuru is uniquely localized to a small region of Papua New Guinea and to a narrow segment of time.

During this conference we shall hear from virologists working in all corners of South-East Asia and the Pacific islands about peculiar and interesting features of viral diseases in various countries in the region. We shall also hear more general accounts of the advancing edge of virology in aspects that range from molecular biology to epidemiology. The future, in terms of research and the prevention and control of these diseases, is largely in your hands, as the active practitioners of virology in this part of the world. I hope that the work of all of us who are participating in this conference may be enriched and stimulated by the activities of the week ahead, both in the formal sessions and during the coffee and luncheon breaks and in the evenings. I am sure that all of us will benefit by the presence at our conference of so many virologists from different countries of the Region, and the world renowned experts from Europe and north America who have joined the conference as contributors and discussants.

ACKNOWLEDGMENTS

I am indebted to Professors Jack Golson and Donald Walker for commenting critically on my excursions into prehistory and biogeography and to Dr I.D. Marshall for tempering my speculations about arboviruses.

Part II
General Overviews

Chairman D. O. White
Co-Chairman N. F. Stanley

4

GEOGRAPHIC AND SOCIOLOGIC FACTORS IN THE EPIDEMIOLOGY OF VIRUS DISEASES

Francis L. Black

Department of Epidemiology and Public Health
Yale University, New Haven, CT

Like a cake, epidemiology can be sliced in many ways. When we are concerned with geographic differences in disease distribution, as we will be at this symposium, I find it useful to slice the cake along the planes which separate virus diseases whose agents differ with respect to their reservoirs. The first cut separates off those viruses which have no significant reservoir, viruses which must constantly circulate seeking new human hosts. The second basic cut is between those viruses whose reservoir is in man and those persisting in a non-human host. This classification permits that type of ecological and zoological study which has proven so useful in the epidemiology of arboviruses to be extended to the full spectrum of virus disease. Indeed, this approach can be used equally well in studying non-viral diseases. With them, however, one must recognize a fourth segment incorporating disease agents which can remain latent in an inanimate reservoir. In making this extension of environmental considerations to the full range of virus disease in man, we will find that demographic and sociologic characteristics of the human population are often more important than climate or natural fauna.

VIRUSES WHICH POSSESS NO RESERVOIR

I would define a "reservoir" not just as any place where live virus can persist for extended periods, but also as a place from which virus is released in the natural course of

VIRAL DISEASES IN SOUTH-EAST ASIA AND THE WESTERN PACIFIC
ISBN 0 12 484820 6

events. Then, virus diseases which have no reservoir include all those diseases caused by paramyxoviruses which have been adequately studied - parainfluenza, measles, mumps and respiratory syncytial disease. Smallpox fell into this group; at least some rotaviruses probably belong here; and, with respect to the whole virus genome, the influenzas are part of this group. The fact that measles virus may persist in one person for long periods, as evidenced in subacute panencephalitis, does not mean that it has a reservoir, because the virus in SSPE cases never escapes naturally and, therefore, it plays no role in spread of disease. Perhaps because viruses without reservoirs must be very efficient in infecting their host, they are highly host specific and agents of human disease are usually confined in nature to humans and higher primates.

Viruses of this group only remain endemic in areas where they can constantly find adequate numbers of susceptible persons. Some, as for example, RSV, induce poor local immunity and can reinfect the same person on more than one occasion. This increases the number of potential hosts and reduces the size of the population needed to sustain them. Others, such as measles and mumps viruses, are dependent on the number of children who enter the pool by birth. The problem of finding a new host during a brief period of infectiousness is the same for all viruses without reservoirs, but they are most acute for, and best illustrated by measles, mumps and smallpox which infect each person only once.

To me the greatest achievement of medicine in the past decade and perhaps of the century has been the eradication of smallpox. A key to the success of that campaign was recognition of the fact that smallpox required a large number of susceptible persons to maintain itself (1). Mass vaccination programs never succeeded in immunizing everyone, but they could reduce the number of susceptible persons in any one village below that needed to maintain the virus. The persistent pools of circulating virus were then confined to larger cities. Concentration of effort on controlling urban outbreaks eliminated the virus from West Africa and set the pattern for attacking the great endemic area of South Asia. Because of this historic significance, it would be appropriate to stay with smallpox as our model for consideration of quantitative aspects of endemicity without a reservoir. However, smallpox is finished, while measles remains a problem. Moreover, we have more data on measles, and I am personally more familiar with measles.

Measles does not persist in small or even medium sized populations. It can persist in a single individual in infectious form for only two weeks, on the average. This means that it needs to find, at the very least, 26 new susceptible persons a year. Production of this number of new susceptibles might require a total population of about 1000. That estimate, however, presumes that the infections are evenly spaced, a requirement which is never fulfilled. As a result of seasonal differences in the ability of the virus to spread, as well as for stochastic reasons, measles virus consumes available subjects rapidly at one time of the year and then has difficulty surviving in the off-season. Because of this, the actual number of new susceptibles required for endemicity is very much greater. Bartlett (2) has shown that in a Western urban setting about 300,000 persons are needed to maintain measles endemicity.

Two other factors influence the number of persons needed to maintain a virus. If a population is dispersed over a large area, as for example in pre-1950 Iceland, the speed of virus spread is reduced and an epidemic will last longer. The number of persons needed to maintain endemicity is then decreased (3). An inverse relationship can be shown between population density and duration of epidemics. On the other hand, when a large proportion of the population is initially susceptible, the intensity of the epidemic builds very quickly; by the second or third cycle, half the population may be sick at one time and it becomes very difficult for any susceptible person to escape infection. The establishment of an endemic situation is then, less probable. I like to think of this as epidemic momentum. If an epidemic gets going very quickly because transmission is not damped by a pre-existing proportion of immune persons in the population, then the epidemic will carry the residual proportion susceptible to a very low level. The probability of establishing endemicity is then substantially reduced.

The best documented example of this phenomenon was during the 1951 epidemic in South-west Greenland. There Christensen *et al.* (4) found that after the epidemic, only 5 of more than 4000 inhabitants were left without a history of measles. It would have taken more than four years, even with the extraordinarily high Greenland birth rate, until the proportion susceptible again reached the level Hedrick found necessary to sustain an epidemic in Baltimore, MD (5).

The geographic patterns of endemicity of viruses without reservoirs depend much more on demographic factors than on climate or flora and fauna. Spread of these viruses may be temporarily inhibited by provision of greater living space around each person as when school lets out for the holiday season. Persons living in developed countries generally have

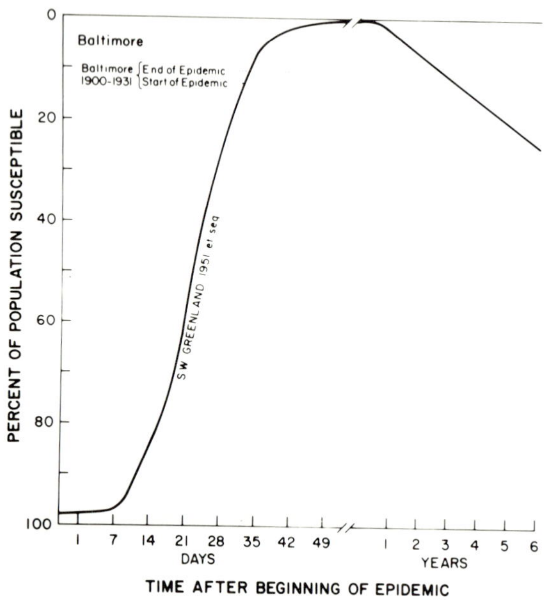

FIGURE 1. Proportion of the population with measles immunity during the course of a virgin soil epidemic compared to a population with endemic measles.

more personal space and, therefore, are not usually infected as early in life as persons living in less developed areas. This lowered contact rate in developed countries is soon balanced by an increase in proportion of the population susceptible. The virus then infects essentially the same percentage of the population as in developing countries, but hits an older age group.

The effect of vaccination is essentially to reduce the number of susceptible persons entering the pool; this was shown by Griffiths (6) in 1973. For an epidemic to occur after a vaccination campaign, the number of persons remaining unprotected must be essentially the same as the number which remain susceptible at epidemic equilibrium in an unprotected population. If a vaccination program is 90% effective,

Griffiths would predict that the interval between epidemics would be prolonged ten-fold. There are, however, some differences: on the one hand circulation is slowed by the fact that the reduced number of susceptible persons are scattered over the original area, while, on the other hand, as the susceptible population becomes older, it often tends to associate in larger groups and thus, to become more accessible to the virus. In developed countries, children are brought together in progressively larger groups as they move from the home to nursery school, through elementary and high schools, until they reach military age. As the number of unvaccinated persons has decreased, the age at which numbers, sufficient to support an epidemic, come together in one place has moved steadily upward, and the age specific incidence has shifted dramatically. In less developed countries where the number of persons in the lowest age strata is relatively large, where houses are open and where infants are frequently carried out of the home, there are frequent contacts at an early age. This has made effective immunization very difficult and, as I will discuss in a later session, changed measles from a nearly universal disease to one which might well be termed "Tropical."

Because viruses without reservoirs cannot persist in small populations they are dependent on large social organizations. Even today there are small isolated populations in the Amazon which have never been infected with many of these diseases. In as much as we believe that, until a few millenia ago, all mankind lived in small population groups, it is probable that these diseases, in their present form, are new. Indeed, McNeil (7) has found historical references to events which he interprets as the first virgin soil epidemics of measles in China in 162 AD and of smallpox in the Roman empire in 165 AD. If we consider the slow evolution of the Australian rabbits toward resistance to myxomatosis virus in terms of biological generations, it becomes clear that human evolution toward accommodation to measles and smallpox may still be far from equilibrium.

Not only are these diseases relatively new, they are also not irreversibly established in their ecological niches. The absence of a reservoir made eradication of smallpox possible. The recent US experience with measles indicates that eradication of this disease is at least a theoretical possibility. There are no known reasons why mumps would not also be vulnerable. Those viruses which infect the same person more than once are better adapted to their unique host, and more secure in their ecological niches.

VIRUSES WITH A RESERVOIR IN HUMANS

The *Herpesviridae* are the largest important group of viruses with the ability to use man as a reservoir, but several other taxonomically distinct viruses also fall into this class. Hepatitis B virus and the Papova viruses belong here; the Adenoviruses probably belong here, but we lack specific data on many types. If we were dealing with zootic diseases, the Retroviruses would be the ultimate example of this type of endemicity, but Retroviruses are strangely rare in human populations. Many important non-viral diseases also have human reservoirs and share key epidemiological characteristics.

The original work in this area was done by Hope-Simpson (8), who showed in 1954 that varicella could persist in the small, 2000 person, population of the island of Yell in the Shetlands. He found that new epidemics of chickenpox were initiated with no outside contribution, but in association with a case of herpes zoster. As most of this audience knows, varicella virus persists in nerve ganglia after primary infection and may occasionally be reactivated to cause the localized, semi-chronic, lesions of herpes zoster. We have observed similar endogenous initiation of a varicella epidemic in the Xikrin Indians of Brazil, a tribe sufficiently isolated to be free of measles, mumps, rubella and two types of poliomyelitis. On the other hand, when varicella virus was introduced to the 700 Trio Indians along the Surinam-Brazil border it caused a virgin soil outbreak affecting all age groups. Thus, although it seems likely that varicella virus can persist in groups of as few as 100 persons it is not ubiquitous in mankind. Incidentally, many of the Trio Indians were under treatment for malaria at that time with doses of 600mg chloroquine per week. The varicella was particularly severe in those on this drug and six died with confluent vesicular lesions (9).

Blumberg's finding of a high incidence of hepatitis B surface antigen in Australian Aborigines identified the reservoir of a new virus (10). The prevalence of hepatitis B is strongly influenced by social factors, some of which are not yet well understood. In Western societies, its spread has been fostered by drug abuse and by faulty medical practices, but in less developed countries there is another and even more widespread mechanism of transmission in the family. Grayston *et al.* (11) have studied this in Taiwan. While this does not seem to be true vertical transmission prior to birth, there is transmission from mother to child during the period of intimate contact in early life. It is a very effective means of virus perpetuation, and this virus has been found, I believe, in every population where it has been sought with a single exception. Kaplan (12) found a village of Waorani Indians in the Ecuadorian Amazon to be free of this disease.

BK, the human polyoma virus, is another agent which is capable of persisting in man for very long periods with occasional reactivation. Brown *et al.* (13) have found antibody to this virus in sera from many small isolated populations, including the islands of the South Pacific, but it was missing from sera of South American Indian isolates. Apparently the virus was lost at some point in the long tenuous migration route from Asia to South America.

The only reasonably well studied viruses to which antibody has been found in every population examined are *Herpesvirus hominis* and Epstein-Barr virus. To the best of my knowledge these viruses may be truly ubiquitous in human populations.

In general, viruses which can use man as a reservoir are more widely distributed geographically than those without a reservoir. The minimum population needed to sustain them may be very small, certainly less than a few hundred persons. Not only are these viruses extremely well adapted to following mankind wherever they go, they are also generally well adapted in the sense that they cause little harm to their host, if the infection occurs early in life, as is usual in primitive society. We've never seen a case of labial herpes, of infectious mononucleosis or of Hepatitis B in examining more than 1000 South American Indians in whom the prevalence of the relevant viruses is very high. Neither have we seen any evidence of hepatoma which might have been caused by the hepatitis virus. Here, however, because most of the older age group had been killed by epidemic diseases, the numbers examined may have been inadequate. Most of the sympotomatic diseases caused by these viruses seem to occur in societies of developed countries where hygenic precautions have delayed the age of infection, but not prevented.

Vaccines against these viruses have been slow to appear and our methods for controlling them are very limited. This does not seem to be due to any consistent immunogenic characteristic; there is a live varicella vaccine which seems to work well (14), and the new inactivated Hepatitis B vaccine is very promising (15). More likely, the paucity of vaccines is due to the reluctance of the medical community to administer an agent which is likely to persist in the body for the life of the recipient, often in close association with cellular DNA.

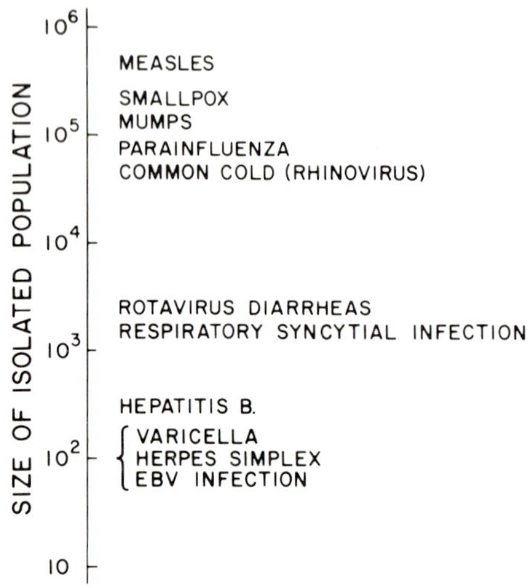

FIGURE 2. Approximate maximal population in which specific diseases would fail to persist.

When dealing with these first two groups of viruses we can place each one on a scale of "endemogenicity" based on the size of population needed to maintain it. Populations greater than that designated will maintain endemic virus, smaller ones may experience epidemics when the virus is introduced from outside. The position of a virus on this scale is not fixed, but influenced by sociologic characteristics. Measles and smallpox are near the top of this scale requiring between 200,000 and a million persons for endemicity. Chickenpox seems to need a population of about 100. In favorable demographic circumstances, Hepatitis B may persist in a still smaller population and herpes simplex and EBV may, in favorable sociologic situations, be able to persist in minimal human breeding units.

VIRUSES WITH NON-HUMAN RESERVOIRS

We are most accustomed to think of the importance of a virus reservoir when concerned with the arboviruses and the zoonoses which, by definition, have a non-human vector or animal reservoir. Sometimes the reservoir is a species which replicates fast enough to provide an adequate supply of new susceptible individuals to maintain active virus transmission; sometimes the virus persists in a single host for the normal life span of that host or even passes through the germ cells to succeeding generations. The vector may, or may not, be the reservoir species. Several papers in this symposium will discuss the specifics of these diseases and it is neither practical nor necessary to deal with them here.

These are the diseases which show the most pronounced geographic limitations. Whether the reservoir is a tick, or an Apodemus field mouse, its distribution in the world is likely to be much more limited than that of mankind. Although host specificity of these viruses is important in determining the identity of the reservoir or vector, the viruses can by definition pass from one host species to another and are thus, not as restricted as most members of the other two groups. Except for dengue, they are not dependent on the availability of humans for their persistence and their evolution may have been quite independent of our species.

MARGINAL CASES

Biology rarely divides into as neatly separate layers as a cake and any system of classification will produce marginal cases. Poliovirus sits near the dividing line between viruses with and without an effective reservoir in man. Although it may persist in one person several months and reinfect repeatedly, it does not persist in Arctic (16) or Amazon (17) populations composed of a few hundred people. It fits with the first group in that a reduction, by vaccination, of the number of persons susceptible has interfered with continuity of transmission of wild virus (18), but it is like the second in that infection at an early age does little harm.

Yellow fever used to persist without an effective reservoir by circulating in urban populations. It did not persist in Northern countries where there was a break in transmission in winter in spite of its capacity for transovarial passage in mosquitoes, but neither did the forest reservoir play a significant role. Now, of course, like most arboviruses it is dependent on an extra-human reservoir.

APPLICATIONS

If we can determine in which of these reservoir categories a virus best fits we can predict:

1. Whether it will be essentially universal, endemic only in large human populations, or endemic only in limited geographic areas.
2. Whether immunization of less than the entire human population will interrupt virus spread. If so, we can make some estimate of the fraction which must be immunized to obtain this effect.
3. Whether control of a non-human animal species offers potential for control of the disease.
4. Whether sociological factors, such as crowding and personal hygiene are likely to be important in determining distribution of the disease.

REFERENCES

1. Foege, W.H., Mullar, J.D., and Lane, M., *Am. J. Epid. 94,* 311 (1971).
2. Bartlett, M.S., *J.R. Stat. Soc. Ser. A 123,* 37 (1960).
3. Black, F.L., *J. Theor. Biol. 11,* 207 (1965).
4. Christensen, P.E., Henning, S., Bang, H.O., Anderson, V., Jordal, B., and Jensen, O., *Acta. Med. Scand. 144,* 430 (1952).
5. Hedrick, A.W., *Am. J. Hyg. 17,* 636 (1933).
6. Griffiths, D.A., *J.R. Stat. Ser. A 136,* 441 (1973).
7. McNeil, W.H., "Plaques and Peoples. A Natural History of Infectious Diseases." Doubleday, New York (1976).
8. Hope-Simpson, R.E., *Lancet ii,* 1299 (1954).
9. van Mazijk, J., Personal communication.
10. Blumberg, B.S., Alter, J.H., and Vinich, S., *J. Am. Med. Assoc. 191,* 541 (1965).
11. Beasley, R.P., Trepoc, C., Stevens, C.E., and Szmuness, W., *Am. J. Epid. 105,* 94 (1977).
12. Kaplan, J.E., Larrick, J.W., Yost, J., Farrell, L., Greenberg, H.B., Herrmann, K.L., Sulzer, A.J., Walls, K.W., and Pederson, L., *Am. J. Trop. Med. Hyg. 29,* 298 (1980).
13. Brown, P., Tsai, T., and Gajdusek, D.C., *Am. J. Epid. 102,* 331 (1975).
14. Asano, Y., and Takahashi, M., *Pediat. 60,* 810 (1977).

15. Szmuness, W., Stevens, C.E., Harley, E.J., Zang, E.A., Oleszko, W.R., William, D.C., Sadovsky, R., Morrison, J.M., and Keller, A., *New Engl. J. Med. 303,* 833 (1980).
16. Paul, J.R., Riordan, J.T., Melnick, J.L., *Am. J. Hyg. 54,* 275 (1951).
17. Black, F.L., Hierholzer, W.J., Pinheiro, F.P., Evans, A.S., Woodall, J.P., Opton, E.M., Emmons, J.E., West, B.S., Edsell, G., Downs, W.G., and Wallace, G.D., *Am. J. Epid. 100,* 230 (1974).
18. U.S. Public Health Service. Poliomyelitis Surveillance Summary. *Morb. Mort. Wkly Rpts. 28,* 483 (1979).

5

IMMUNE RESPONSES TO VIRAL INFECTIONS

Robert V. Blanden

Department of Microbiology
The John Curtin School of Medical Research
Australian National University
Canberra, A.C.T.

I. THE EVOLUTION OF THE IMMUNE SYSTEM IN RELATION TO VIRAL INFECTION

The immune system of higher vertebrates is a very complex multicellular system that has evolved to detect and eliminate threats to the health and life of the host animal, thus enabling the animal to survive, mature, and reproduce. Viral infections early in life are clearly a major threat that has shaped the evolution of the immune system. Although the prime purpose of the immune system is to recognize, respond to, attack and eliminate all "non-self" material, it is obvious that normal "self" components should not be harmed (1). Therefore, the antigen-sensitive cells in the developing immune system of each individual embryo must undergo rigorous processes of selection and control so that the system "learns" not to respond to inherited, polymorphic, self antigens, e.g., blood group or major histocompatibility (MHC) antigens, while ideally retaining the ability to respond to all foreign antigens.

This ideal situation is not always achieved, as we shall see below. Furthermore, as the immune system has evolved, viruses have concurrently evolved strategies to enable them to reproduce and spread despite the immunological capabilities of their hosts. It is evident that unbalanced host-parasite combinations would not persist in nature (2). Highly pathogenic infections would either kill all

VIRAL DISEASES IN SOUTH-EAST ASIA
AND THE WESTERN PACIFIC
ISBN 0 12 484820 6

susceptible hosts, or disappear because they killed the infected hosts so rapidly that transmission to a new susceptible host was infrequent. Similarly, hosts with a highly effective mechanism for eliminating infection would reduce the frequency of transmission. It is also evident that unbalanced combinations of host and virus are usually poor models for the study of immune responses to viral infection, because such studies require the host to survive for a week or more to allow the immune response to develop, and the effective stimulation of a full range of immune responses requires a substantial antigenic load, both in the form of virus-infected cells, and virus-coded antigenic molecules.

II. IMMUNE RESPONSES TO VIRAL ANTIGENS

An effective immune response to viral antigens can be a crucial determinant of recovery from primary viral infection, or resistance to reinfection, though the mechanisms involved in recovery may be quite different from those conferring resistance. It is beyond the scope of this paper to deal with all of these mechanisms in detail. Many appropriate reviews and books are available. As a generalization, mechanisms mediated by thymus-derived (T) lymphocytes are often important in the early recovery process, whereas antibodies may be produced too late or in insufficient amounts to be a major factor in recovery. In any case, antibody-mediated mechanisms may not effectively counter established infection in solid tissues through which the virus can spread from infected cell to contiguous uninfected cell. However, pre-existing antibodies can prevent reinfection eg. IgA may neutralize virus on mucosal surfaces before the initiation of infection of epithelial cells. Antibodies can also prevent spread of infection from the point of entry to target organs eg. IgM or IgG may neutralize viremia. Once these barriers are breached, T cell-mediated mechanisms would be important during reinfection, just as they were during primary infection. Long-lived memory T cells would be important in this context.

In the remainder of this paper I will focus on two related aspects of the immune response to viral infections. First, I will discuss the cellular and subcellular factors that may influence the class and magnitude of immune responses to viral antigens, and then outline the T cell-triggered mechanisms that can eliminate viral infections from host tissues. The unifying element in these two discussions is that both of them illustrate the fundamental role of MHC antigens in T cell function.

A. The Major Histocompatibility Complex (MHC)

In mice the major histocompatibility gene complex (MHC) is designated the *H-2* complex and the antigens it controls, H-2 antigens. In humans the MHC is called the *HLA* complex. The *H-2* complex is the main experimental prototype because of the speed with which new inbred, congenic, recombinant, or mutant mouse strains can be produced and analysed, but all of its main features have a counterpart in the *HLA* complex. Furthermore, the amino acid sequences of H-2 and HLA glycoprotein antigens are very similar, implying that they must have evolved from a common ancestral molecule. Therefore, the basic structural and functional features of the *H-2* complex are likely to be shared by the *MHC* of all higher vertebrates (3).

A number of different genetic loci have been defined within the *H-2* gene complex. Three of them, *K*, *D* and *L*, are known to code for the polypeptide chains of H-2 glycoprotein antigens of about 45,000 MW. The *I*-region contains genes which code for at least 2 other smaller polypeptide chains giving glycoproteins of 20,000 and 33,000 MW. The *H-2* complex may also control glycolipid antigens (4).

B. MHC Restriction

In the context of antiviral immune responses, probably the single most important observation in the last decade has been the discovery in late 1973 by Zinkernagel and Doherty (5) of "H-2 restriction" in connection with the recognition and lysis *in vitro* of virus-infected target cells by murine cytotoxic T lymphocytes (Tc cells). Together with related evidence already published, this discovery provided a working hypothesis concerning the induction and genetic control of T cell responses, viz. that resting, precursor T cells are optimally activated to become effector cells when they encounter a cell surface displaying a combination of foreign antigen and a self marker controlled by the MHC. In turn, this has led to a rationalization of the evolution and "raison d'etre" for the MHC, viz. that the role of its gene products as a "guidance system" for T cells arose from a simple cell-to- cell communication system and evolved to its present complex state because of the life-saving qualities of T cell responses against viruses and other infectious agents (6-8).

Although the nature of T cell antigen-receptors is not yet known, the last 8 years have provided much new information about the factors that control T cell induction, regulation and effector activity in viral infections. It became apparent that murine antiviral Tc cells recognized infected self cells through cell surface antigenic moieties dependent upon the *K*, *D* and sometimes *L* regions of the *H-2* gene complex together with viral antigens (9-11). The use of *H-2K* mutants identified a locus required for infected-self recognition by Tc cells as the same locus that codes for the 45,000 MW glycoprotein antigens that are responsible for allograft rejection (12,13). While the *I* region of the *H-2* complex also contains genes that control graft rejection antigens, and that act as targets for alloreactive Tc cells, *I*-region-restriction has not been observed for antiviral Tc cells.

Considerable evidence now supports the idea that self-recognition by antiviral Tc cells is "learned" and not genetically determined. Zinkernagel and Doherty first showed that (P1xP2)F1 hybrid antiviral Tc cells were of two broad classes, (a) those that recognized P1 + virus, (b) those that recognized P2 + virus (14). Later it was shown that within each broad class there were subsets of antiviral Tc cells that recognized either self H-2K or H-2D antigens on virus-infected target cells, not both, although the Tc cells expressed both H-2K and H-2D antigens on their own cell surface (15,16). In irradiation chimeras the antigens recognized by antiviral Tc cells as "self" H-2 restriction antigens can be those of the thymus phenotype in which the T cells differentiate; they are not automatically determined by the genotype of the Tc cell (17,18). Thus Tc cells originating from stem cells of "low responder" *H-2* genotype to a given virus can become Tc cells of "high responder" phenotype if allowed to differentiate and respond in a "high responder" environment (18,19).

The need for self tolerance affects the repertoire of T cell antigen-receptors that is expressed by an individual animal. Thus, the diverse array of T cells with the capacity for both self and foreign recognition that may arise from germline and somatic variation of the genes controlling T cell antigen-receptors would need to be modified by deletion or suppression of those T cells that react with normal antigens (20,21). The experiments of Müllbacher using irradiation chimeras and neonatally tolerant mice clearly point to the possibility that this mechanism is a major factor in "MHC-linked" immune response gene effects (22,23). Thus, self-tolerance to a particular self antigen requires deletion or suppression of T cells that cross-react with a particular combination of another self antigen and foreign antigen; this results in a gap in the repertoire of T cells capable of reacting with that foreign antigen.

Another possible mechanism accounting for "low responders" is that certain combinations of self MHC and foreign antigen molecules are incapable of physically associating in antigen-presenting cell surface membranes in the manner required for T cell activation (24).

C. T Cell Activation and Regulation

Although advances in the relevant biochemistry and cell biology will undoubtedly lead to future revision, we can now postulate that contact with any infected cell surface that displays an appropriate combination of self MHC antigens plus viral antigens, together with a sufficient concentration of interleukin 1 and/or interleukin 2 (25,26) from macrophages and T cells respectively in the local environment, would activate a precursor T cell with antigen-receptors that can bind to that combination of self MHC and viral antigens (Fig. 1). The pathways by which viral antigens are expressed on antigen-presenting cell surfaces apparently determine the nature of the self MHC plus viral antigen moiety that is formed, and ultimately the class of T cell response. This area is under active investigation, and a great deal more remains to be learned, but some general rules can be proposed at this time.

First, there are two pathways to the H-2K, D, L class of MHC-restriction exhibited by Tc cells, (a) fusion of the viral envelope with a cell surface membrane as occurs with paramyxoviruses (27) and certain myxoviruses (28) and poxviruses (29) and (b) new protein synthesis specified by the viral genome within infected cells (30). Both of these mechanisms result in viral glycoproteins being inserted in cell surface membranes, from without or within the cell respectively, so that the combination of self-MHC plus viral antigen essential for Tc cell activation is displayed on the infected cell surface.

Second, it seems possible that only phagocytosis of viral antigens by some class of mononuclear phagocyte leads to an appropriate combination of Ia plus viral antigen being displayed and a resulting response of Ia-restricted Th or Td

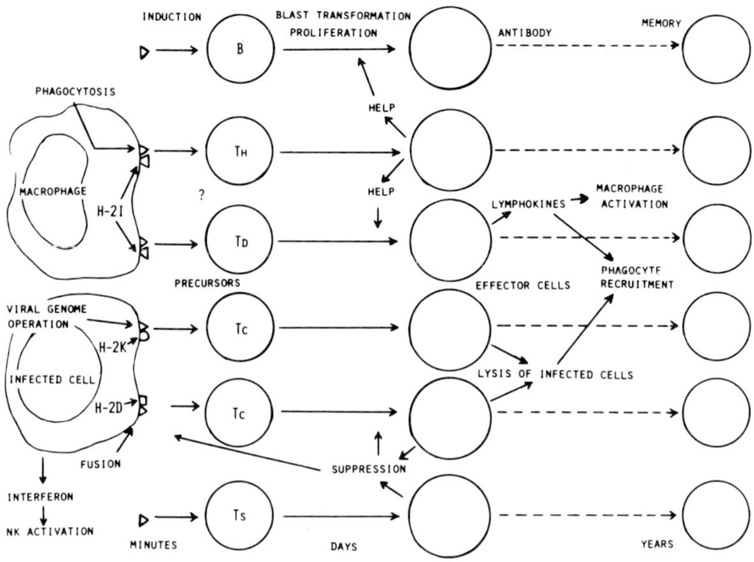

FIGURE 1. A simplified scheme of the cells and factors involved in immune responses to viral antigens (triangles).

cells (31). A demonstration of this point is in the work of Ertl using Sendai virus (32). Activation of Ia-restricted Td cells occurred only when T cells were exposed to adherent cells, presumably mononuclear phagocytes, which had been allowed to interact with UV-inactivated virus with an uncleaved, inactive fusion protein (31,32). Presumably, such virus particles, being incapable of either fusion or direction of new protein synthesis, were phagocytosed and processed by mononuclear phagocytes. In contrast, when fusion-active virus particles were permitted to fuse with LPS-induced, Ia-positive B cell blasts, these cells could not present antigen for Ia-restricted Td cell activation, but could do so for H-2K, D restricted Tc cells (31,32). The reasons necessitating phagocytosis of virus for Ia-restricted T cell activation remain a subject for speculation, but one possible explanation comes from the observation of Beller and Unanue that phagocytosis provokes a burst of Ia antigen synthesis and cell surface display in macrophages (33). The role of other Ia-positive cells such as dendritic cells in antigen presentation for antiviral T cell responses requires investigation.

Superimposed on the primary determination of class of T cell response by the mode of viral antigen presentation, is a potentially complex web of T cell interaction that has been studied and reviewed extensively by Ada and coworkers using influenza and Sendai viruses (31). Injection of UV-inactivated, fusion negative virus which induces Ia-restricted Td or Th cells suppresses the later induction of H-2K, D restricted Tc cells after injection of fusion-positive or infectious virus (31,34). Conversely, a first injection of fusion-positive infectious virus that induces H-2K, D restricted Tc cells suppresses the later induction of Ia-restricted Td cells by an injection of UV-inactivated fusion-negative virus (31,35). In each case, the suppressive effects could be transferred by T cells (34,35), but the precise mechanisms of suppression are not yet clear.

One other important point to be resolved concerns the induction of Th versus Td cells. Both have the Ly $1^{+}2^{-}3^{-}$ phenotype, are apparently Ia-restricted, and are induced by inactivated virus, but are functionally distinct (31).

A number of quantitative and qualitative factors make it probably that antiviral T cells are stimulated to proliferate most efficiently by virus-infected cells in secondary lymphoid tissues such as spleen and lymph nodes. First, virus particles or effete, infected cells are cleared from the blood or lymph by mononuclear phagocytes lining vessels in these tissues. Second, T cells of the recirculating pool migrate through thymus-dependent areas of the spleen and lymph nodes (36,37). Third, lymphoid cells and mononuclear phagocytes particularly, display higher concentrations of MHC antigens on their surface membranes than do other cell types (38,39) and O'Neill and Blanden have shown that MHC antigen concentration quantitatively influences the efficiency of T cell activation (40). Third, in the murine example, H-2K, D and L antigens that are recognized by Tc cells are present on most cell types in the body, but the Ia antigens recognized by T cells that mediate help (Th) and delayed hypersensitivity (Td) are almost exclusive to lymphoid tissues (39). Fourth, an inhibitor of interleukin 2 is present in normal serum (41). Thus, continued T cell proliferation, which requires both antigen and interleukin 2, would occur most efficiently in lymphoid tissues where both of these factors are most abundant. Fifth, Ashman and Müllbacher have shown that virus-specific Th cells can facilitate the response of antiviral Tc cells (42). Such Th cells seem to be restricted to Ia antigen recognition for their activation (43,44), but the delivery of their help to Tc cells is genetically unrestricted (42).

Pang and Blanden showed that Tc cell responses to viral infection *in vivo* can be regulated by simple feedback (45). Thus as effector Tc cells are produced in increasing numbers and then progressively destroy virus-infected cells, the antigen presentation necessary for their continued stimulation is progressively reduced, and the primary effector Tc response wanes and is replaced by memory (46). In most acute viral infections in mice, the primary Tc response reaches a peak from 5-9 days after infection and wanes to a low level by 12-14 days (47,48). Memory antiviral Tc cells persist for the total lifespan of a mouse (2 years or so) in the absence of continued stimulation by reinfection (46,49).

D. Elimination of Viral Infection

T cells and mononuclear phagocytes acting in concert are responsible for acquired antiviral effector mechanisms. Clearance of ectromelia virus infection from the spleen and liver, and influenza infection from the lungs of mice are examples (50-54). Transfer of virus-immune T cells can trigger viral clearance in infected recipient mice but only when H-2K or D antigens are shared between donor and recipient (54-57). This H-2K, D restriction and the finding that the kinetics of generation of cytotoxic (assayed *in vitro*) and effector (assayed *in vivo*) T cell activities are similar (47) suggest that Tc cells trigger viral clearance.

What is known about Tc cell-target cell interaction is consistent with this role. Antiviral Tc cells recognize infected self cells that display H-2K, D, L antigens plus viral antigens, the latter being present immediately after infection in the case of virus-cell fusion (27-29) or within a few hours after infection and resulting virus-specified protein synthesis (30,58). Therefore, infected cells are vulnerable to Tc cell-mediated lysis hours before assembly of progeny virus occurs. Since almost all cells in the body display H-2K, D, L type antigens (3), Tc cells acting alone are theoretically capable of preventing the spread of infection. This is what is observed in ectromelia-infected tissues of irradiated recipient mice (lacking accessory antiviral mechanisms such as blood monocytes) that are given intravenous injections of ectromelia-immune T cells (51).

During the course of acute viral infection in a normal animal, effector Tc cells are produced within secondary lymphoid tissues and migrate via blood to sites of infection (52,53). Both specific antigen-recognition, and a nonspecific propensity for localizing in inflamed areas could contribute to the accumulation of effector Tc within virus-infected foci (53,59). While some viruses nonspecifically produce inflammation at sites of infection others, such as ectromelia in mouse liver, do not (52). However, after virus-specific effector Tc cells enter the lesions, there follows a short-lived accumulation of polymorphs and a more lasting accumulation of mononuclear phagocytes (52). The latter are derived from blood-borne monocytes that originate from dividing precursors in bone marrow (60,61). Mononuclear phagocytes actively invade and ingest cell debris containing infectious virus particles (52).

Once virus-specific Tc cells and mononuclear phagocytes are present in virus-infected lesions, and continue to accumulate in them via the blood, the complete clearance of infection can result through a combination of mechanisms. First, virus infection of mononuclear phagocytes may not produce infectious progeny (62). Second, even if productive infection of either mononuclear phagocytes or T cells is possible, infected cells of either type can be lysed very efficiently by other Tc cells (9,16) before assembly of progeny virus. Thus, provided the production and migration of effector Tc cells and monocytes is sustained at an adequate level the processes outlined above can eliminate infection within 24 to 48 hours (51).

There has been a consistent failure to demonstrate a role for Ia-restricted Td cells in viral clearance in the ectromelia and influenza systems, in which Tc cells are dramatically effective (31,54,57). Furthermore, Leung and Ada (31) have shown that infleunza-immune Td cells can trigger such a large influx of mononuclear phagocytes into the lungs of influenza-infected mice, that consolidation and death may be caused. Such phenomena emphasize the need for careful evaluation of viral vaccine strategy.

It seems to be appropriate to sound a note of caution concerning the potential of "synthetic" vaccines. While it is feasible to produce large amounts of pure viral proteins using recombinant DNA techniques, and while these proteins may carry the antigenic determinants that are recognized by the lymphocytes mediating the processes of recovery from primary infection or resistance to reinfection, there is reason to believe that they may be quite inadequate in terms of stimulating such lymphocytes to respond. Tc cell responses are often important for recovery, and memory Tc can contribute to resistance to reinfection, but there is no evidence that purified viral proteins can induce either primary Tc cell responses or the production of memory Tc cells. IgA on mucosal surfaces is the only means of totally preventing the entry of certain viruses into the body, but there is no evidence that purified viral proteins can induce IgA responses. At best, such proteins seem to be weakly immunogenic for serum antibodies (IgM and IgG), and it is imperative to study their ability to induce potentially dangerous responses of Ts cells of various classes, or Td cells.

The scheme in Fig. 1 is greatly oversimplified. A great deal more needs to be learned about the cells required for antigen presentation to certain classes of T cells, the appropriate form for antigen preparations to achieve the desired interaction with antigen presenting cells, and the interactions between the various lymphocyte subsets.

REFERENCES

1. Burnet, F.M., and Fenner, F., "The Production of Antibodies". 2nd Ed. Macmillan, Melbourne, (1949).
2. Fenner, F., and Ratcliffe, F.N., "Myxomatosis". Cambridge Univ. Press, London and New York, (1965).
3. Klein, J., "Biology of the Mouse Histocompatibility-2 Complex". Springer-Verlag, Berlin, Heidelberg, New York, (1975).
4. O'Neill, H.C., Parish, C.R., and Higgins, T.J., *Mol. Immunol. 18,* 663 (1981).
5. Zinkernagel, R.M., and Doherty, P.C., *Nature, 248,* 701 (1974).
6. Doherty, P.C., and Zinkernagel, R.M., *Lancet i,* 1406 (1975).
7. Blanden, R.V., Hapel, A.J., and Jackson, D.C., *Immunochemistry, 13,* 179 (1976).
8. Langman, R.E., *Rev. Physiol. Biochem. Pharmacol., 81,* 1 (1978).
9. Blanden, R.V., Doherty, P.C., Dunlop, M.B.C., Gardner, I.D., Zinkernagel, R.M., and David, C.S., *Nature, 254,* 269 (1975).
10. Blanden, R.V., McKenzie, I.F.C., Kees, U., Melvold, R.W., and Kohn, H.I., *J. Exp. Med., 146,* 869 (1977).
11. Biddison, W.E., Hansen, T.H., Levy, R.B., and Doherty, P.C., *J. Exp. Med., 148,* 1678 (1978).
12. Blanden, R.V., Dunlop, M.B.C., Doherty, P.C., Kohn, H.I., and McKenzie, I.F.C., *Immunogenetics, 3,* 541 (1976).
13. Zinkernagel, R.M., *J. Exp. Med., 143,* 437 (1976).
14. Zinkernagel, R.M., and Doherty, P.C., *Nature, 251,* 547 (1974).

15. Zinkernagel, R.M., and Doherty, P.C., *J. Exp. Med., 141,* 1427 (1975).
16. Davidson, W.F., Pang, T., Blanden, R.V., and Doherty, P.C., *Aust. J. Exp. Biol. Med. Sci., 54,* 413 (1976).
17. Zinkernagel, R.M., Callahan, G.N., Althage, A., Cooper, S., Klein, P.A., and Klein, J., *J. Exp. Med., 147,* 882 (1978).
18. Zinkernagel, R.M., and Doherty, P.C., *Adv. Immunol., 27,* 51 (1979).
19. Müllbacher, A., and Blanden, R.V., *J. Exp. Med., 149,* 786 (1979).
20. Jerne, N.K., *Eur. J. Immunol., 1,* 1 (1971).
21. Blanden, R.V., Ashman, R.B., O'Neill, H.C., Woodhams, C.E., Kees, U.R., and Andrew, M.E., *Immunol. Rev., 58,* 25 (1981).
22. Müllbacher, A., *Proc. Natl. Acad. Sci. U.S.A.,* in press (1981).
23. Müllbacher, A., *Transplantation, 32,* 58 (1981).
24. Blanden, R.V., *Immunology Today, 1,* 33 (1980).
25. Möller, G., (ed) *Immunol. Rev., 51,* (1980).
26. Andrus, L., and Lafferty, K.J., *Scand. J. Immunol.,* in press (1981).
27. Schrader, J.W., and Edelman, G.M., *J. Exp. Med., 145,* 523 (1977).
28. Kurrle, R.A., Wagner, H., Rollinghöff, H., and Rott, R., *Eur. J. Immunol., 9,* 127 (1979).
29. Hapel, A.J., Bablanian, R., and Cole, G.A., *J. Immunol., 124,* 1990 (1980).
30. Ada, G.L., Jackson, D.C., Blanden, R.V., Tha Hla, R., and Bowern, N.A., *Scand. J. Immunol., 5,* 23 (1976).
31. Ada, G.L., Leung, K-N., and Ertl, H., *Immunol. Rev. 58,* in press (1981).
32. Ertl, H., submitted (1981).
33. Beller, D.I., and Unanue, E.R., Naito Foundation Symposium, in press (1981).
34. Leung, K.N., Ashman, R.B., Ertl, H.C.J., and Ada, G.L., *Eur. J. Immunol., 10,* 801 (1980).
35. Liew, F.Y., and Russell, S.M., *J. Exp. Med., 151,* 799 (1980).
36. Gowans, J.L., *J. Physiol., 146,* 54 (1959).
37. Parrott, D.H.V., de Sousa, M.A.B., and East, J., *J. Exp. Med., 123,* 191 (1966).
38. Parr, E.L., *Transplantation, 27,* 45 (1979).
39. McKenzie, I.F.C., and Potter, T.J., *Adv. Immunol., 27,* 181 (1979).
40. O'Neill, H.C., and Blanden, R.V., *J. Exp. Med., 149,* 724 (1979).

41. Wagner, H., Hardt, C., Heeg, K., Pfizenmaier, K., Solbach, W., Bartlett, R., Stockinger, H., and Röllinghoff, M., *Immunol. Rev., 51,* 215 (1980).
42. Ashman, R.B., and Müllbacher, A., *J. Exp. Med., 150,* 1277 (1979).
43. Pang, T., McKenzie, I.F.C., and Blanden, R.V., *Cell. Immunol., 26,* 153 (1979).
44. Pang, T., and Blanden, R.V., *Aust. J. Exp. Biol. Med. Sci., 55,* 549 (1977).
45. Pang, T., and Blanden, R.V., *J. Exp. Med., 143,* 469 (1976).
46. Gardner, I.D., and Blanden, R.V., *Cell. Immunol., 22,* 283 (1976).
47. Gardner, I.D., and Blanden, R.V., *Cell. Immunol., 22,* 271 (1976).
48. Blanden, R.V., Progress in Immunology III, 463 (1977).
49. Ashman, R.B., *Immunology,* in press (1982).
50. Blanden, R.V., *J. Exp. Med., 132,* 1035 (1970).
51. Blanden, R.V., *J. Exp. Med., 133,* 1074 (1971).
52. Blanden, R.V., *J. Exp. Med., 133,* 1090 (1971).
53. Blanden, R.V., *Transplant. Rev., 19,* 56 (1974).
54. Yap, K.L., Ada, G.L., and McKenzie, I.F.C., *Nature, 273,* 238 (1978).
55. Blanden, R.V., Progress in Immunology II, 117 (1974).
56. Blanden, R.V., Bowern, N.A., Pang, T.E., Gardner, I.D., and Parish, C.R., *Aust. J. Exp. Biol. Med. Sci., 53,* 187 (1975).
57. Kees, U., and Blanden, R.V., *J. Exp. Med., 143,* 450 (1976).
58. Jackson, D.C., Ada, G.L., and Tha Hla, R., *Aust. J. Exp. Biol. Med. Sci., 54,* 349 (1976).
59. Koster, F.T., McGregor, D.D., and Mackaness, G.B., *J. Exp. Med., 133,* 400 (1971).
60. Volkman, A., and Gowans, J.L., *Brit. J. Exp. Pathol., 46,* 62 (1965).
61. van Furth, R., and Cohn, Z.A., *J. Exp. Med., 128,* 415 (1968).
62. Mims, C.A., *Bacteriol. Rev., 28,* 30 (1964).

6

IMMUNOPATHOLOGY OF VIRAL INFECTION

C.A. Mims

Department of Microbiology
Guy's Hospital Medical School
London Bridge

I think I have been a bit disappointed with my title of viral immunopathology. I thought there would be a lot to talk about but when I got down to it I realized how little progress there had been in this subject over the past ten years. The immunologists keep providing us with powerful mechanisms for tissue damage and I never cease to wonder at their ability to draw boxes and arrows in a diagram and spell out the pathways to damage and disaster. But as often as not the role of these things in the infected host have remained unclear.

CIRCULATING IMMUNE COMPLEXES

Take circulating immune complexes. The really good examples of their pathogenicity come from a few animal virus diseases such as the chronic glomerulonephritis in LCM carrier mice, and arteritis and glomerulonephritis in aleutian disease of mink. Admittedly immune complexes have an accepted role in one or two virus infections in man, such as the arthralgia, vasculitis, and sometimes chronic membranous glomerulonephritis seen in hepatitis B. But as the tests for circulating complexes increased in sensitivity, it became clear that they are a more or less normal phenomenon during a wide variety of infections. Indeed, circulating IgA immune complexes are present in the serum of normal individuals after a meal! We have now been forced to ask the more important questions about immune complexes. What

VIRAL DISEASES IN SOUTH-EAST ASIA
AND THE WESTERN PACIFIC
ISBN 0 12 484820 6

determines their localisation in joints, glomeruli, choroid plexus? Is it due to the presence of Fc and C3b receptors in endothelial cells in these regions? Also, we still need to know more about the normal mechanisms for the disposal of circulating complexes and how these can be overloaded.

NK CELLS

NK cells are interesting not only for their possible role in recovery from virus infection, but also for their theoretical ability to cause tissue damage. Unfortunately there is still no clear evidence that NK cells matter in recovery from infection. Some of the best work, such as that from Geoff Shellam and his colleagues on mouse cytomegalovirus infections (1) still leaves open the question as to whether interferon is important because it increases NK activity, or whether interferon itself is the antiviral force, acting directly on virus replication in susceptible cells. Until recently I had high hopes for NK cells in immunopathology. In several virus infections, including LCM in the mouse, Lassa fever in man, and CMV in the mouse, there is a striking necrosis in the spleen (2). In the case of CMV it begins only a few days after infection, initially affects the perifollicular region, and is unaffected by immunosuppression with either cyclophosphamide or antilymphocyte serum. Although it depends on virus replication in the spleen it soon becomes so massive and involves so many uninfected cells, that I wondered whether it was due to activated NK cells running wild in the spleen. So we tried preventing the NK cell activation by giving CMV-infected mice a sheep anti-interferon serum supplied by Ion Gresser. Far from reducing necrosis, this increased it, showing that the interferon response either directly or via NK activation, protected against spleen necrosis.

CYTOTOXIC T CELLS

For many years it has been the custom to talk about immunopathology and cytotoxic T cells almost in the same breath. Classic examples have been the disease caused by infection of adult mice intracerebrally with LCM virus. It seems logical that an infiltration of cytotoxic T cells into the infected meninges could cause tissue destruction and inflammation and give rise to a fatal disease with convulsions. When Peter Doherty took cerebrospinal fluid from an infected mouse and showed that it contained Tc cells that killed LCM-infected target cells, the matter seemed settled. But doubts have arisen, which I know will also be aired by Fritz Lehman-Grube at a later stage in this meeting. For instance, there is almost no cell damage detectable by electron microscopy in the brains, meninges, ependyma, choroid plexus of infected mice (3). Evidently the immunopathological mechanism must be reconsidered. We are now coming to realize that the old T cell subsets are not so clearly or so irrevocably defined as had been thought. Dr. Askonas and her colleagues have produced a cloned line of cytotoxic T cells that react specifically with, and kill H_2 compatible target cells infected with influenza A virus. When transferred to infected mice, these cells protect against the virus infection. But the same cells also transfer dth responses to the recipient mice, as elicited in the footpad test. Very recently Dr. Askonas' group have made the important observation that the same cloned and specifically reactive cytotoxic T cells produce γ interferon when exposed to influenza A-infected cells (4). In other words cytotoxic T cells can also have an antiviral action by releasing interferon.

To go back to LCM, the CSF of infected mice presumably contains T cells mediating dth as well as cytotoxicity. These cells could liberate lymphokines which caused oedema, or in some way interfered with neuronal function without actually destroying the cells. One candidate lymphokine would be gamma interferon, now known to be produced by cytotoxic T cells. Highly purified alpha interferon has been shown to cause malaise, headache and myalgia in normal individuals when administered extraneurally (5), although few, if any, side effects were seen when rather less pure β interferon was administered intrathecally (6). There is evidence that interferon production is associated with the intracerebral virulence of LCM virus (7). When non-lethal strains of LCM are injected intracerebrally they can be rendered lethal by giving various types of interferon inducer extraneurally. It may be noted that interferon is also associated with the virulence of LCM virus for newborn mice (8), but this is less relevant to my discussion because the immunopathological events are different in neonatally infected mice. It is not known how interferon acts to increase the adult mouse intracerebral lethality of LCM virus strains. LCM virus is sensitive to interferon and one possibility would be that it restricts the extraneural growth of the less lethal virus strains. If growth in the brain was unaffected it would mean that the T cell response could then be focused more exclusively into the brain to cause greater immunopathology, rather than weakened by distribution also to numerous extraneural sites of virus growth. Interferon itself does not appear to cause illness when present in the cerebrospinal fluid of mice. I have injected up to 500 U purified Type I interferon intracerebrally into adult mouse without ill effect, but I have not tried γ interferon. It is worth pointing out that the characteristic LCM type of disease is not exclusive to LCM virus infection. A clinically indistinguishable hyperexcitability, with convulsions and death inducible on tail twirling, can also be induced by intracerebral injection of other viruses such as influenza A and ectromelia (9,10). This is often present within a day or so of infection, before immune events have an opportunity to play a part. Evidently in LCM infection of mice, that classic of viral immunopathology, we still have a lot to learn.

HAEMORRHAGIC FEVERS

A meeting about viral diseases in South East Asia would be incomplete without discussion of the immunopathology of haemorrhagic fevers, especially dengue haemorrhagic fever. In this particular disease it at one time seemed likely that circulating immune complexes were of major importance in pathogenesis. Patients with antibodies to one strain of dengue virus can be affected with a different strain of virus and when the circulating viral antigens produced during this infection reacted with pre-existing antibody to the original strain of virus, immune complexes were formed. Blood levels of C4 and Clq were shown to be inversely proportional to disease severity (11). It was suggested that complement components were activated and by a series of acceptable steps, the patient developed shock, haemorrhages, and collapse. The pre-existing viral antibodies, far from protecting, could even increase the extent of infection of susceptible mononuclear cells, so that plenty of viral antigen was produced. These enhancing antibodies, originally discovered in bird serum by Hawkes and Lafferty (12) in Professor Fenner's laboratory, were described in dengue virus infection and extensively studied by Dr. Scott Halstead. Now that this phenomenon is being analysed with monoclonal antibodies, a clearer picture is emerging. Evidently the entry of virus into a macrophage via a virus receptor gives a different result from entry (of antibody-coated but infectious virus) via an Fc receptor. These and related studies will provide a better understanding of the fate of virus in the phagosome, and matters such as the rate of fusion of virus envelope with phagosome wall in relation to the rate of lysosomal fusion.

But there have been doubts as to the role of circulating immune complexes in dengue haemorrhaging fever. Evidence for complement activation has not always been obtained. Scott Halstead has suggested that infected macrophages release vasoactive mediators (13) but he has always been aware of one other interesting possible pathogenic mechanism (14). I refer to the growth of virus in vascular endothelial cells. Without attempting to pass judgement on the question of dengue haemorrhagic fever pathogenesis, I would like to stray from immunopathology and say a few words about vascular endothelium in virus infections.

VIRUSES IN VASCULAR ENDOTHELIUM

When a virus in the blood infects distant organs, whether it is mumps in the parotid gland, poliovirus in the central nervous system, or Coxsackie B viruses in striated muscle, the first barrier to be passed is the endothelium in the capillaries and venules of that organ. Viruses that grow in these cells and are discharged from their external surface are seeded into extravascular tissues. If a particular organ is infected, we can ask why the virus localised there. Did it pass passively through small blood vessels in many organs and tissues, but then found susceptible cells only in this site? Or alternatively is it only in this particular organ that the endothelial cells are susceptible to infection, perhaps because they have virus receptors? A great many interesting problems in pathogenesis could be studied at the level of the vascular endothelial cell. For instance, can a virus-infected endothelial cell serve as an initiation site for an atherosclerotic lesion? Involvement of Marek's disease virus in the genesis of atheroarteriosclerotic lesions in chickens was suggested by Minick *et al.* (15), but the evidence was not very convincing. Nevertheless, important pathological events can be caused by a virus behaving in an unusual fashion in a very small proportion of infected individuals. Viruses that do not regularly spread via the blood might have to be considered. In experimental animals for instance, parainfluenza viruses are known to infect vascular endothelial cells (16).

Viruses infecting endothelial cells can also be discharged back into the circulation again, making a contribution to the viraemia, and substantial viraemias are especially important in arthropod-born virus infections. The pathogenesis and thus the virulence of these infections may well depend on which side of the endothelial cell the virus is released from. Work on epithelial cells *in vitro* has given intriguing information about these matters. Although certain viruses are released from all surfaces of a fibroblast, they are released in a more restricted fashion from epithelial cells (17). Influenza virus, for instance, buds exclusively from the surface of the epithelial cell facing the outside world, as befits a virus that is discharged from the respiratory tract. Vesicular stomatitis virus on the other hand is released from the inner surface of the cell, adjacent to the basement membrane, and has the opportunity to spread to underlying tissues. This polarity of budding can be correlated with the fact that epithelial cells also have a polarity at the biochemical and functional level. It would be of great interest to have this sort of information for virus infections of vascular endothelial cells.

If an endothelial cell is infected it may die, and this would contribute to the tissue lesion. Alternatively, it may undergo functional impairment, but recover from infection. Finally it may suffer no ill effects. Independent of the direct effect of the virus on the cell, viral antigens expressed on the surface would render it vulnerable to immune damage. So far I have considered the localization of viruses in endothelial cells in specific organs or tissues, but if vascular endothelium throughout the body is susceptible to infection, then the exact nature of the changes in infected cells become more important. Extensive disruption of endothelial cells in small vessels would clearly have a catastrophic effect on the circulation. Functional impairment could be serious if infected cells showed for instance the *in situ* equivalent of "rounding up" or early cpe seen in cell culture. Changes in the junction between endothelial cells might have serious consequences if widespread, and an increase in capillary fragility could be of critical importance (18). Damaged endothelial cells could make various other contributions to pathology (19).

Dengue virus grows in human and rabbit endothelial cells *in vitro* (18). Does it also grow in endothelial cells in the infected human being? Many years ago Sabin (20) biopsied the

TABLE. Virus Infection of Vascular Endothelium in Vivo

Virus	Host*	Method used	Reference
K virus	Mouse	FA	21
Feline panleucopenia	Cat	FA	22
Mouse Adenovirus	Mouse	EM	23
Equine viral arteritis	Horse	EM	24
Varicella	Man	H	25
Cowpox	Mouse	FA	26
Cytomegalovirus	Mouse	FA	27
Epizootic Haemorrhagic disease of deer	Deer	EM	28
Distemper	Dog	FA	29
Canine hepatitis	Dog	FA	30
Measles	Man	EM	31
Vesicular stomatitis	Mouse	FA	32
Influenza	Chick	FA	33
Parainfluenza I	Mouse	FA	16
LCM	Mouse	FA	34
West Nile	Mouse	FA	35
Sindbis	Mouse	FA	36
Hog cholera	Pig	H	37
Reovirus 1	Mouse	FA	38

* FA - Immunofluorescence
EM - Electron microscopy
H - Routine histology

rash appearing in volunteers infected with dengue virus and found endothelial swelling, but so far there is no evidence for virus replication in endothelial cells. I have made a table of virus infections in which endothelial cell infection has been demonstrated *in vivo* (Table). Techniques for *in vitro* culture of endothelial cells were described long ago (39). So far in man it has been possible to study vascular endothelium from umbilical veins, and in animals from large vessels such as the aorta and vena cava (18). Varicose veins will provide another source of differentiated human endothelial cells, but we need to improve on the rabbit ear chamber or its mouse equivalent and develop a system for *in situ* studies of capillaries and venules. The best we can do at present is to prepare and culture capillary endothelium from individual organs.

Endothelial cells are important not only in viral pathogenesis as mentioned above but also in immunology. In certain organs, and for unknown reasons, they bear IgG Fc receptors or Clq receptors (40). The high endothelium in post-capillary venules has lymphocyte-binding receptors (41) which may function in lymphocyte recirculation, and circulating IgA plasmablasts from the intestine somehow localise in vessels in parotid, mammary etc. glands, migrate to the submucosa and secrete antibody in these organs. We know that endothelial cells can function as antigen-presenting cells (42), and I wonder whether antigens from the tissues in which they are located are present on their lumenal surface. This could give a basis for organ-specific virus receptors as well as for the specific localisation of the IgA plasmablasts. It could also enable a circulating lymphocyte primed to a tissue antigen to localise in the relevant tissue and initiate pathological changes, as seen for instance in experimental allergic neuritis.

CONCLUSIONS

In conclusion, and to return to my original subject, immunopathology inevitably makes a contribution to most virus infections. The exact mechanisms, however, are generally obscure even in classical examples such as LCM virus infection of mice. It may be noted that in this instance the intracerebrally injected adult mouse is a laboratory artefact. Furthermore, I believe that the carrier mouse in the laboratory suffering from glomerulonephritis and uraemia is another type of artefact, and that naturally infected wild mice are less likely to develop these immunopathological complications. Indeed, it can be argued that whereas laboratory mice can be coerced into telling us a great deal about infectious diseases, it is wild mice that are the natural survivors and they generally behave differently (43). A recent analysis of mitochondrial DNA of mice shows that 15 out of 20 wild mice from different localities had distinct mt DNA, whereas all the older (more than 40 years old) strains of laboratory mice had the same mt DNA (although different nuclear genomes). From the history of domesticated mice, it was concluded that the old laboratory strains are descended from a single female who lived at some time between 1200 BC when mice were first domesticated in China, and about 1920 AD when laboratory colonies were established in the U.S.A. (44).

REFERENCES

1. Bancroft, G.J., Shellam, G.R., and Chalmer, J.E., *J. Immunol. 126,* 988 (1981).
2. Mims, C.A., and Gould, J., *J. Inf. Dis. 137,* 587 (1978).
3. Walker, D.H., Murphy, F.A., Whitfield, S.G., and Bauer, S.P., *Exp. Molec. Pathol. 23,* 245 (1975).
4. Morris, A.G., Lin, Y.L., and Askonas, B.A., *Nature 295,* 150 (1982).
5. Scott, G.M., Secher, D.S., Flowers, D., Bate, J., Cantell, K., and Tyrrell, D.A.J., *Brit. Med. J. Apr 25,* 1345 (1981).
6. Jacobs, L., O'Malley, J., Freeman, A., and Ekes, R., *Science 214,* 1026 (1981).
7. Jacobson, S., Friedman, R.M., and Pfau, C.J., *J. Gen. Virol. 57,* 275 (1981).
8. Riviere, Y., *et al., J. Exp. Med. 152,* 633 (1980).
9. Mims, C.A., *Brit. J. Exp. Path. 41,* 586 (1960).
10. Mims, C.A., *Brit. J. Exp. Path. 41,* 52 (1960).
11. Bokisch, V.A., Top, F.H., Russell, P.K., Dixon, F.J., and Muller-Eberhard, H.J., *New Engl. J. Med. 289,* 996 (1973).
12. Hawkes, R.A., and Lafferty, K.J., *Virology 33,* 250 (1967).
13. Halstead, S.B., Marchette, N.J., and O'Rourke, E., *Asian J. Inf. Dis. 2,* 85 (1978).
14. Halstead, S.B., *J. Inf. Dis. 143,* 127 (1981).
15. Minick, C.R., Fabricant, C.G., Fabricant, J., and Litrenta, M.M., *Am. J. Path. 96,* 693 (1979).
16. Mims, C.A., and Murphy, F.M., *Am. J. Path. 70,* 315 (1973).
17. Boulan, E.R., and Sabatini, D.D., *Proc. Nat. Acad. Sci. USA 75,* 5071 (1978).
18. Andrews, B.S., *et al., Infect. Immunity 20,* 776 (1978).
19. Thorgeirsson, G., and Robertson, A.L., *Am. J. Pathol. 93,* 801 (1978).
20. Sabin, A.B., *Am. J. Trop. Med. Hyg. 1,* 30 (1952).
21. Greenlee, J.E., *Infect. Immunity 26,* 705 (1979).
22. Csiza, C.K., de Lahunta, A., Scott, F.W., and Gillespie, J.H., *Infect. Immunity 3,* 838 (1971).
23. Blailock, Z.R., Rabin, E.R., and Melnick, J.L., *Science 157,* 69 (1967).
24. Estes, P.C., and Cheville, N.F., *Am. J. Pathol. 58,* 235 (1970).
25. Tyzzer, E.E., *J. Med. Res. 14,* 361 (1906).
26. Mims, C.A., *Brit. J. Exp. Path. 49,* 24 (1968).

27. Mims, C.A., and Gould, J., *J. Med. Microbiol. 12,* 113 (1978).
28. Tsai, K., and Karstad, L., *Am. J. Path. 70,* 379 (1973).
29. Coffin, D.L., and Liu, C., *Virology 3,* 132 (1957).
30. Coffin, D.L., Coons, A.H., and Cabasso, U.J., *J. Exp. Med. 98,* 13 (1953).
31. Kimura, A., *et al., Arch. Virol. 47,* 205 (1975).
32. Bruno-Lobo, M., Peralta, P.H., Bruno-Lobo, G.G., and Pada, D., *Annals de Microb. 15,* 53 (1968).
33. Hook, E.W., Luttrell, C.N., Slaten, K., and Wagner, R.R., *Am. J. Pathol. 41,* 593 (1962).
34. Tosolini, F.A., *Aust. J. Exp. Biol. Med. Sci. 48,* 445 (1970).
35. Kundin, W.D., Liu, C., Hysell, P., and Hamachige, S., *Arch. ges. virus. forsch. 12,* 514 (1963).
36. Johnson, R.T., *Am. J. Path. 46,* 929 (1965).
37. Siefried, O., and Cain, C.B., *J. Exp. Med. 56,* 345 (1932).
38. Kundin, W.D., Liu, C., and Gigstad, J., *J. Immunol. 97,* 393 (1966).
39. Pomerat, C.M., and Slick, W.C., *Nature 198,* 859 (1963).
40. Andrews, B.S., Shadforth, M., Cunningham, P., and Davis, J.S., *J. Immunol. 127,* 1075 (1981).
41. Carey, G.D., Chin, Y.H., and Woodruff, J.J., *J. Immunol. 127,* 976 (1981).
42. Hirschberg, H., Bergh, D.J., and Thorsby, E., *J. Exp. Med. 152,* 249s (1980).
43. Gardner, M.B., *Int. Rev. Exp. Path. 23,* (1981).
44. Ferris, S.D., Sage, R.D., and Wilson, A.C., *Nature 295,* 163 (1982).

7

MALNUTRITION AND CONCURRENT INFECTIONS. COMPARISON OF TWO POPULATIONS WITH DIFFERENT INFECTION RATES[1]

Leonardo Mata

Instituto de Investigaciones en Salud (INISA)
University of Costa Rica,
Ciudad Universitaria Rodrigo Facio
Costa Rica

Repetitive infections induce malnutrition and growth retardation in children living in impoverished environments, even if food is available. Infection precipitates severe malnutrition in individuals already undernourished. Mechanisms include anorexia, nutrient losses, abnormal synthesis, and diversion from usual metabolic pathways. Infectious diarrheas, malaria, measles, and respiratory infections, all may cause malnutrition, disability, growth retardation, and death.

In two different rural populations of Central America, differences in infant nutrition, health, and survival were more related to the infectious environment than to amount and quality of food consumed.

Exposure to infection was related to living conditions. Thus, the public health goal should be to raise the quality of life in order to diminish the force of infection. Measures recommended are: improvement of environmental sanitation, expansion of primary health care (including oral rehydration therapy and immunoprophylaxis), and promotion of maternal technology (breast-feeding and child-care practice), family planning, and health education. The approach should be holistic.

[1]*Supported by: USAID Loan 515-T-026, the University of Costa Rica, the Ministry of Health and Social Security Bureau (Costa Rica), CONICIT (Costa Rica), and the British ODA.*

VIRAL DISEASES IN SOUTH-EAST ASIA
AND THE WESTERN PACIFIC
ISBN 0 12 484820 6

I. INTRODUCTION

Epidemiologic studies in tropical and subtropical regions highlighted the interaction between malnutrition and infectious disease, and its contribution to determining much of the morbidity and mortality in developing countries. There is no doubt that infectious diseases cause physiologic and biochemical alterations leading to malnutrition, while a deficient nutritional status worsens the outcome of infection (1). However, the argument persists as to whether concurrent infections or deficient diets are the main contributors to the malnutrition, growth retardation and premature death so commonly observed among children in impoverished societies (2). Clarification of this question is fundamental for establishing priorities and policies aimed at prevention and control of infection and malnutrition.

Prospective observations in different parts of the developing world revealed that growth faltering invariably begins at about 3 to 6 months among infants at the breast in traditional societies, or even earlier if infants are prematurely weaned as is the case of populations in transition that adopt bottle-feeding (3). It is not yet clear if onset of stunting is primarily related to supplementation with inadequate foods when mothers' milk becomes insufficient; or to infectious disease; or to an interaction of both. An inadequate milk supply without proper supplementation is commonly the case in developing societies, but the striking even during weaning is the occurrence of infectious diseases (4).

Among the communicable diseases of childhood, infectious diarrhea ranks first in incidence and implications for nutrition and health, followed by acute respiratory disease which is very important as a cause of morbidity and death primarily in infancy. In the third place rank communicable diseases like measles, whooping-cough, chickenpox, rubella, and tuberculosis. Still, malaria, kala-azar, many viral fevers, and other ailments occur in particular ecosystems.

II. FIELD STUDIES ON NUTRITION AND INFECTION

The long term prospective studies to be described here concern two indigenous populations in Central American highlands devoid of malaria, trypanosomiasis, jungle fevers, and other "tropical diseases". In one of them, Santa María Cauqué, the burden of infection is overwhelming because crowding, poverty, and underdevelopment favor its perpetuation (4). In the other, Puriscal, improved home environment and maternal technology, health services, and scattering of the population result in a very low incidence of infectious disease (5).

At the time of the study most homes in Cauqué had only one room and families slept in one or two beds or mats on the floor; preparation and cooking of food was on a hearth on the dirt floor; water had to be carried from public faucets and reservoirs; few families had intradomiciliary water and only a third use latrines. These factors potentiate transmission of infectious agents, especially enteric and respiratory, a condition favored by poverty, iliteracy, cohabitation with domestic animals, and crowding of families within the limited space of dwellings, and of homes within the compact village structure (4), Table I.

In rural Puriscal, living conditions are better as homes are larger; there is greater availability of intradomiciliary water, latrines and water toilets, and widespread use of electricity. This condition, together with a high literacy rate, greater income and availability of health services, improved maternal technology, and ruralism (marked separation of homes from each other), result in a very low incidence of infectious disease (5), Table I.

TABLE I. Differences in Host and Environment between Cauqué (Guatemala) and Puriscal (Costa Rica)

Variable	Cauqué, 1967	Puriscal, 1981
Population	1000	24000
Type of population	Rural, crowded	Rural, sparse
% literate	56	85
% use latrine or toilet	32	95
% has private piped water	7.4	84
Human milk intake, ml, 1-3 mo.	674	652
Energy intake, kcal, 6 mo.	400	480
Protein intake, g, 6 mo.	7	9
Energy intake, kcal, lactation	2078	2111
Protein intake, g, lactation	59	53
Weight, kg, 6 mo.	6.3	7.1
Height, cm, 6 mo.	60.5	66.0
Height, cm, pregnant women	143	153
% low birth weight infants	42	6
% vaccinated: measles, DPT	0	95
Infant mortality per 1000 l.b.	93	10

TABLE II. Infection in Cauqué and Puriscal

Infection	Cauqué, 1965-72	Puriscal, 1980-81
Mothers		
Ascaris, *%prevalence*	83	10
Shigella, *%prevalence*	9	<1
Bacteriuria, %incidence	27	6
Neonates		
Shigella, *%incidence*	3.6	0
Intestinal protozoa, %incidence	4.7	0

In both field studies the ecosystem and characteristics of the population remained undisturbed, although in Puriscal interventions were established to improve incidence and duration of breast-feeding, making them similar to those in Cauqué, at least during the first six months of life (6). Food consumption by pregnant and lactating women in Puriscal was equal or less than for women of Cauqué. Food consumption by children in both settings was similar during healthy periods.

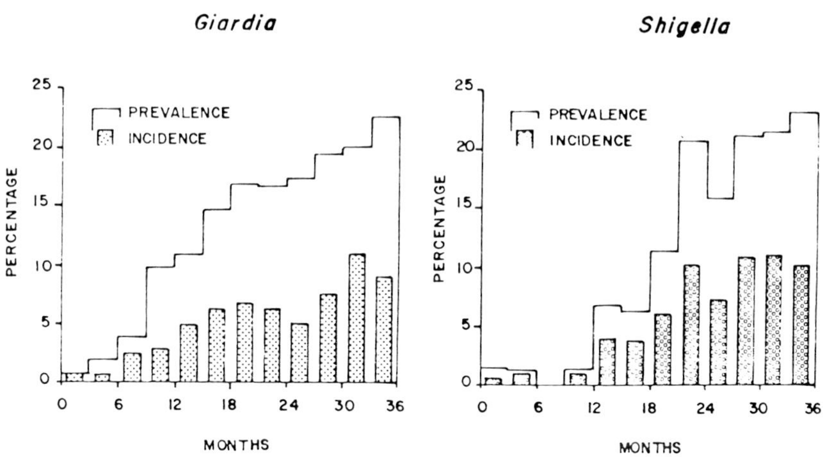

Fig. 1. Infection in a cohort of 45 Cauqué children, from birth to three years of age. Rates were calculated from weekly examination or culture of feces (7).

While similar dietary conditions prevailed in both rural settings, marked differences were noted in children in both studies regarding incidence of infectious disease, occurrence of malnutrition, and growth retardation and mortality, all of which were markedly greater in Cauqué.

III. INFECTION AND INFECTIOUS DISEASE

Cauqué mothers are common carriers of enteric organisms, and are a source of infection for their infants from birth onwards, Table II. This is favored by traditional delivery in the home in the squatting or kneeling position, and by exposure of neonates to maternal feces (7). Infections occur as early as the first few days or weeks of life, and usually are asymptomatic, probably as a result of protection afforded by human colostrum and milk (8).

By contrast, intestinal infection in Puriscal neonates is virtually absent since mothers are relatively free of infection and almost all deliveries are in clinics or hospitals which thereby reduces the opportunity for fecal contamination at delivery (6).

Customarily, Cauqué infants are exclusively breast-fed until 4 to 9 months. The burden of infection in the environment is so large, however, that diarrheal disease begins in the early months of life, increasing with age as breast milk and transplacental immunities fade away and infants begin consuming contaminated foods (7). Infants are progressively infected with enteric viruses, pathogenic bacteria and parasites, and by one year of age most had been exposed to a wide variety of pathogenic agents, as revealed by weekly examination of feces of cohort children for at least the first three years of life (4). By the third year, more than 50% carry enteroviruses, and more than 25% excrete *Shigella* and *Giardia*. Figure 1 illustrates incidence and prevalence of *Giardia* and *Shigella* in a cohort of children examined weekly during the first three years of life (7). Prevalences are larger than incidences because some infections last for several weeks. Undernourished children also show abnormalities in intestinal flora and colonization of the upper intestine (9).

Puriscal infants also are exclusively breast-fed, although for a shorter interval than Cauqué infants, but the rate of infection is markedly lower.

Diarrhea among Cauqué children averaged seven or eight episodes per child per year in the first three years of life, a contrasting figure with the low rates for Puriscal children,

Table III. The maximum incidence and severity of diarrhea and other infections in Cauqué were observed during and after weaning (4). The etiology of diarrhea is similar in both settings with rotaviruses being predominant, followed by enterotoxigenic *Enterobacteriaceae, Shigella, Campylobacter, Giardia,* and other parasites.

The enormous infection burden observed in Cauqué can be accounted for by deficient sanitary conditions and traditional practices which potentiate communicability of enteric and respiratory agents. Children excrete as many as 10^6-10^9 shigellae per gram of wet feces during bouts of diarrhea, and carriers may excrete bacilli for several months (4, 10). Thus, children in poor villages are at disadvantage when compared to their industrial counterparts, due to exposure to larger doses of virulent organisms. This might account for the greater severity of disease among children and adults in tropical areas regardless of their nutritional state, if sanitation and hygiene are deficient.

Few comprehensive studies on the etiology of respiratory disease in poor traditional societies have been conducted (11) but on clinical and epidemiological grounds, responsible viruses and bacteria are the same as described for industrial nations. Mortality due to respiratory disease is high among infants, especially if they are feeble or undernourished.

Measles, whooping-cough, chickenpox, rubella and mumps, induce severe manifestations among indigenous populations, and although they normally attack once in a lifetime, they are of great public health importance due to their malnourishing effect, disability, and mortality (4, 7, 9, 12).

TABLE III. Incidence of Infectious Diseases in Cauqué and Puriscal Infants, per 100 Person-Months

Age, months	*Number of infants*	*Person-months*	*Enteric*[a]	*Respiratory*[b]
		Cauqué, 1964-69		
0-5	*45*	*270*	*33.3*	*15.9*
6-11	*45*	*270*	*63.0*	*23.0*
		Puriscal, 1979-81		
0-5	*115*	*690*	*4.2*	*5.5*
6-11	*114*	*684*	*7.5*	*7.7*

[a]*Diarrhea and dysentery*
[b]*Laryngotracheobronchitis, bronchitis and bronchopneumonia*

IV. NUTRITIONAL IMPLICATIONS

The negative effects of infectious disease on the nutritional state are reduced food consumption, nutrient losses, metabolic alterations, hormonal imbalances, and alterations in immune function. They are manifested as wasting, stunting, reduced activity, acute malnutrition, and death.

A. Reduced food consumption

This is best illustrated by enteric disease, in which agents adhere, colonize or invade mucosal cells, initiating pathophysiologic processes in susceptible individuals. Anorexia, febrile infections, diarrhea, and vomiting were the main cause for reduced food consumption in Cauqué children. This was complicated by food withdrawal and inappropriate treatment and feeding during convalescence. Marked reduction in calorie intake ("dips") coincided with infectious diseases (13, 14) in all fully weaned two-year-old children, among a cohort of 45 studied by weekly surveys, Figure 2.

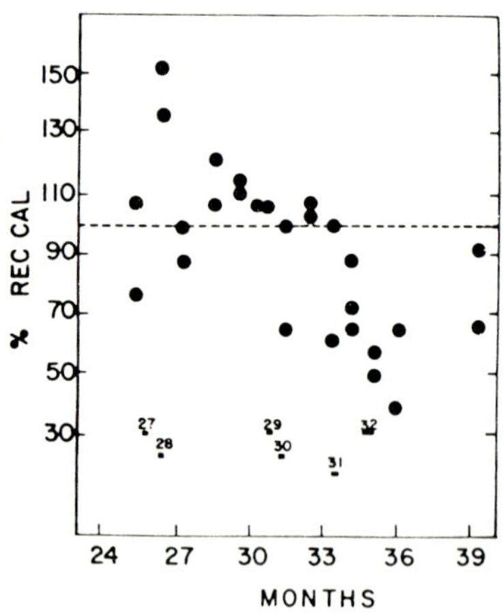

Fig. 2. Energy intake by Cauqué child 24, as % of recommendation by weight. Dots are daily means; numbers are illnesses; bars duration. Episodes 27, 29 (diarrheas), 30 (rubella), 31 (fever, respiratory disease), and 32 (cellulitis, bronchitis) were associated with reduced consumption (13).

Energy and protein consumption was measured during weeks of diarrhea and during healthy periods; convalescence weeks were excluded from the analysis. Energy consumption was reduced by 21% and protein by 24% during bouts of diarrhea, Table IV. It is estimated that as much as 16% of dietary calories and 18% of protein were not consumed by Cauqué children as a result of infections since children were ill during one fourth to one third of their entire first three years of life (4). The impact is considerable for children at risk of becoming malnourished or already undernourished, as food consumption is often below recommended levels (4, 13, 14). Similar results were obtained in other societies of different ethnic background (15-17). Anorexia also occurs in acute respiratory disease and it is noteworthy during attacks of whooping-cough and measles, but reduced food consumption is observed even with mild infections (7, 14, 17, 18).

B. *Altered digestive - absorptive processes*

Diarrhea accelerates transit through the intestinal tract, and this restricts consumption and interferes with digestion. The surface epithelium can be coated and altered by *Giardia* or bacteria or it may be damaged by invading viruses, bacteria and parasites. Microscopic mucosal lesions concurrent with bacterial colonization are seen in persons living in the tropics (9, 19); jejunitis and the accompaniying malabsorption of sugars, fats, and vitamins disappear spontaneously after the person settles in an environment with better sanitation (20). Enterotoxins stimulate formation of cAMP and cGMP impairing absorption of sodium and water. Certain bacteria split bile

TABLE IV. Food Consumption by 19 Cauqué Fully Weaned Preschool Children, 1964-1969

Health condition	*Weekly measurements*	*Mean daily consumption*	
		Energy, kcal(MJ)	*Protein, g*
Well	*105*	*914(3.82)*	*25*
Diarrhea	*84*	*721(3.02)*	*19*
% Difference Well-Diarrhea		*21*	*24*

salts reducing micelle formation and fat absorption, and increasing the bile acids pool which, in turn, irritates the mucosa. Bacteria and parasites are capable of sequestering nutrients that are needed by the host.

The intestine can be regarded as a secreting organ, diarrhea being an abnormal hypersecretory state, with losses of fluid, electrolytes and protein. Hypersecretion is caused by imbalances in digestive-absorptive processes; changes in hydrostatic pressure; synthesis or increase in enterotoxins, bile and fatty acids, hormones and neurotransmitters; and greater calcium permeability (21).

C. Metabolic alterations

Practically all metabolic pathways become altered during the course of infection (22). Abnormalities also occur with mild or asymptomatic infections. The most important alterations are negative nitrogen balance, protein-losing enteropathy, and abnormal nutrient metabolism. The stress of fever, cramps, tenesmus, anxiety, and the need to satisfy gluconeogenesis, result in corticosteroids release and mobilization of aminoacids from muscle (1). Protein losses probably relate to thinning and alterations of the intestinal wall (18) and occur in diarrheas of various etiologies, as with *Shigella,* enterotoxigenic *E.coli* and rotaviruses (23). There are important losses of sodium, potassium, bicarbonate, chloride and phosphate during enteric and systemic infections. There is an increased synthesis of liver enzymes; of foreign protein, lipid, and carbohydrate (in viral replication); and of acute-phase reactant proteins (nutrient diversion). Also, there is a decrease of circulating trace elements (zinc, iron and copper) and concentration in hepatic cells (nutrient sequestration); and an increased expenditure of energy sources and vitamins (nutrient over-utilization) (22, 24).

D. Wasting and Stunting Effect

Repetitive infections and infectious processes, particularly in children who normally do not consume an optimal amount of food, conduce to progressive deterioration of the nutritional status, manifested as weight stagnation or weight loss, and impaired linear growth. These effects are evident in individual growth curves of Cauqué children observed prospectively throughout preschool age.

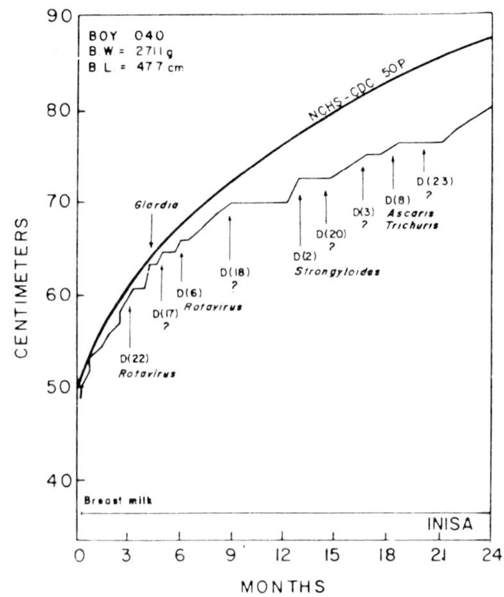

Fig. 3. *Growth of a Cauqué breast-fed child born with adequate weight. Periods of growth arrest were associated with diarrhea of various etiologies (5).*

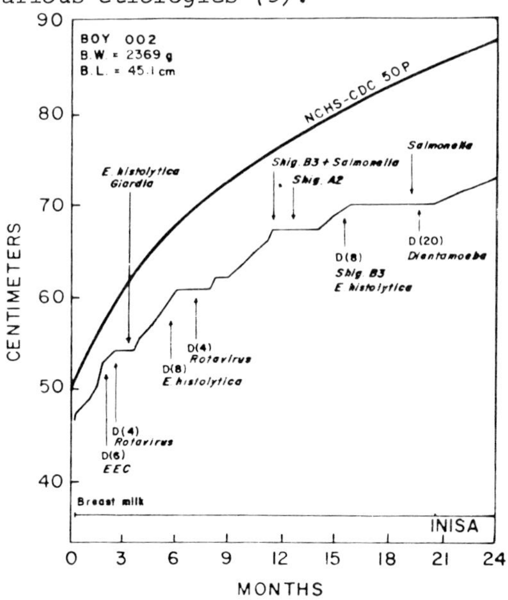

Fig. 4. *Growth of a Cauqué breast-fed child who had fetal growth retardation. Diarrheas were related to growth arrest. Marked stunting was evident at one year of age (5).*

In Cauqué there was about 40% low birth weight infants; breast-feeding was universal; and the association of diarrhea with weight faltering and stunting was clear. There was no adequate knowledge of oral rehydration, while other forms of handling severe dehydration were not accepted by the community during the study period, contributing to the severity of the disease (4).

In general, growth during exclusive breast-feeding exhibited a velocity comparable to that of the NCHS-CDC reference curves. At about 3 to 6 months there was a tendency to growth faltering with onset of supplementary feeding. Often, foods were poorly prepared, too bulky, and contaminated. Inadequate supplementation after mother's milk became insufficient (four to six months) resulted in subtle starvation of infants remaining at the breast. However, marked inflections in growth curves during weaning corresponded, more often than not, to concurrent infectious diseases, particularly diarrhea.

Figure 3 shows the growth curve (body length) and diarrheal episodes of a Cauqué child who had normal intrauterine growth. Diarrheas were associated with weight loss or weight stagnation regardless of their etiology. Obviously, losses of water, electrolytes, plasma, and cells during diarrhea had a negative effect on nutrition. Acute weight loss of the order of 5-10% or more was common. Furthermore, wasting (deficit of weight for height) persisted for weeks or months, contributing to the genesis of marasmus. This was complicated in many instances by inadequate feeding during convalescence.

The wasting and stunting phenomena ocurred also in conjunction with other diseases, very notoriously with measles and whooping-cough. The malnourishing capacity of illnesses that attack only once can be more pronounced that that of diarrhea.

In general, impaired growth was more evident if infants had fetal growth retardation, or were prematurely weaned (5). Figure 4 depicts the growth curve (body length) and diarrheal episodes of another Cauqué child who had fetal growth retardation. Several diarrheas associated with a variety of agents occurred concomitantly with periods of arrest in linear growth. One double infection with *Shigella* and *Salmonella* occurred without recognized diarrhea, and yet was concurrent with marked growth retardation lasting for more than two months. At the age of two years the child was, as the previous case, considerably stunted. Cauqué infants with normal fetal growth can also be affected by infection and become stunted, although not as severily.

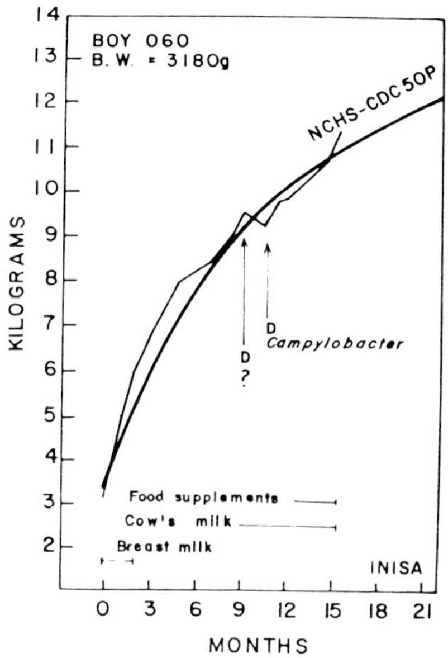

Fig. 5. Growth of a Puriscal weaned child born with adequate weight. A bout of diarrhea caused significant weight loss.

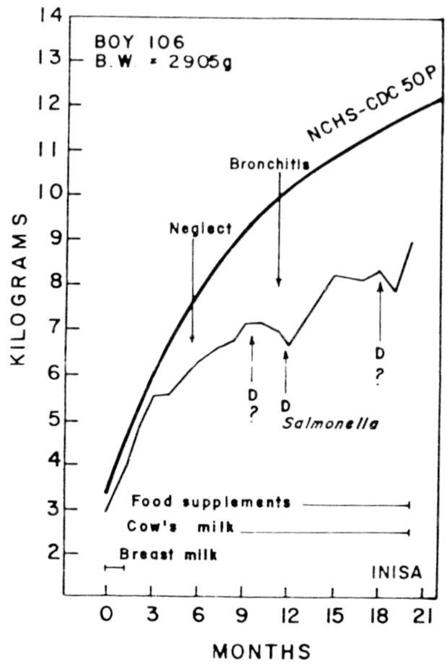

Fig. 6. Growth of a Puriscal weaned child who became undernourished due to neglect, and resulted very ill after bouts of diarrhea requiring hospitalization.

The situation of Puriscal children studied more recently (1979-81), was markedly different in that only 6% of them had low birth weight. Sanitary conditions, education, and hygiene were significantly better than those in Cauqué. There had been a deterioration of breast-feeding in Puriscal evident at the beginning of the study, but hospital and field interventions commencing in 1977 resulted in more than 90% or infants being breast-fed for at least one to two months (6). Puriscal infants usually had fewer infections which were also milder than in Cauqué, probably due to smaller inocula and fewer sources of infection resulting from improved hygiene, and from isolation of dwellings (ruralism).

Most Puriscal children are vaccinated against measles, whooping-cough and other communicable diseases. A very low rate of diarrhea was observed in Puriscal breast-fed infants (see Table III). Furthermore, diarrhea generally did not show a marked negative impact in breast-fed children as it did in Cauqué. However, weaned Puriscal children experienced weight loss and growth retardation as a result of infectious diseases, particularly diarrhea. To illustrate, Figure 5 depicts a prematurely weaned child with normal fetal growth who developed diarrhea associated with weight loss. Another child prematurely weaned and suffering from neglect and several bouts of diarrhea, exhibited marked weight loss and required hospitalization (Figure 6). No marked inflection in the growth curve of breast-fed infants could be attributed to infections.

Thus, the main environmental difference between the two settings is the considerably greater risk of infection and infectious morbidity in Cauqué as compared to Puriscal. The notorious biologic difference was the exceedingly higher frequency of prematurity and fetal growth retardation in Cauqué, as contrasted with Puriscal. No marked differences were evident regarding food consumption among mothers and children of the two populations. In fact, breast milk intake by Cauqué infants was slightly greater than in Puriscal. Because Cauqué women consume about one half kilogram of corn per day, their calorie and protein consumption is similar, or greater than those of Puriscal women.

If infection is an important determinant of malnutrition, marked differences in growth are to be expected among the two cohorts. To explore this possibility, mean weight curves were computed for 133 cohort Cauqué infants born in the period 1964-67 (4), and were compared with mean curves for 277 cohort Puriscal infants born during 1979-81. Children in both cohorts were consecutively born during the stated periods. Cohort infants were classified according to fetal maturity.

Term-adequate-for gestational age Cauqué infants were notoriously smaller than their Puriscal counterparts which matched the 50th P of the NCHS-CDC reference curve, Figure 7. Furthermore, term-small-for gestational age Cauqué infants exhibited an even greater growth retardation, while the comparable Puriscal infants followed the corresponding track of the reference curve. Also, it should be noted that no large-for-gestational age infants were observed in Cauqué, a reflection of the marked fetal growth retardation observed in this village (4). It is rather evident that in Cauqué, infection together with fetal growth retardation, appear as the main determinants of postnatal growth failure, both of body weight and length.

E. Severe malnutrition and death

Repetitive infectious diseases lead to chronic malnutrition. This is clearly evident in village children observed longitudinally, as progressive wasting and stunting develops. The marasmic state persists for months and it is similar to that resulting from food shortage, or child abuse. Marasmic children become critically ill under the stress of acute watery diarrhea, dysentery, measles and other infectious diseases,

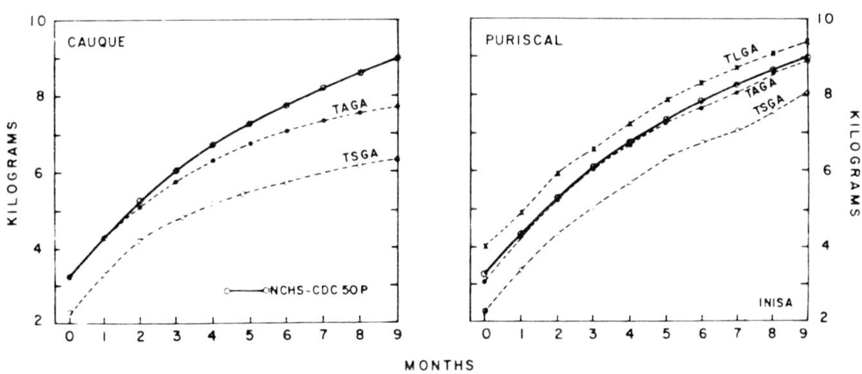

Fig. 7. Mean weight curves of Cauqué and Puriscal cohort infants observed prospectively from birth to nine months of age. TLGA= term-large, TAGA= term-adequate, and TSGA= term-small for gestational age.

as they do after episodes of social and psychologic perturbation of the home environment, for instance, the loss of a parent, violence in the family, or child neglect (25).

Sudden falls in serum albumin concurrent with infections (measles, hookworm, diarrhea) may precipitate kwashiokor. This possibility would explain the etiology of edematous malnutrition which could result from hypoproteinemia in marasmus after severe diarrhea (18). When serum albumin falls slowly and an attack of measles or diarrhea develops, kwashiorkor may occur. It has been known for decades that severe energy-protein malnutrition appears in the community a few weeks or months after outbreaks of diarrhea, measles, and malaria (26, 27), sometimes quite independent of the availability of food (4, 28).

Children in poor villages may suffer infectious diseases for a fourth to a third of their entire infancy and preschool age. Thus, they represent a main determinant of acute malnutrition, and are responsible for elimination of children who are weak, born premature of with fetal growth retardation, or suffering immunologic, biochemical or organic deficiencies. Figure 8 illustrates the life history of a Cauqué girl who grew well in the first two months of life until she developed mild respiratory infection and bronchitis with marked growth deceleration. After several weeks of weight stagnation, and

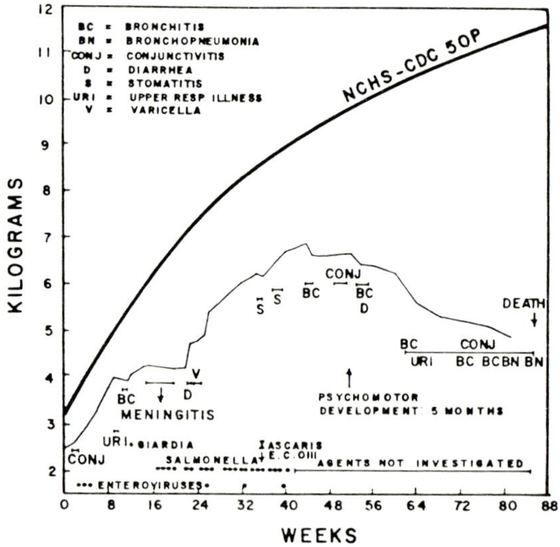

Fig. 8. Weight curve, enteric infections and morbidity of Cauqué female child 19. Two distinct episodes of malnutrition developed in connection with infectious diseases. The girl died from acute lower respiratory disease (4).

despite being at the breast, she developed meningitis due to *Streptococcus pneumoniae*. Although growth improved significantly thereafter, a series of mouth, respiratory, eye, and gastrointestinal infections, and malnutrition, ended in death (4).

In the absence of adequate family technology, health services, and oral rehydration, infectious diseases represent the main factor generating malnutrition and death in malnourished children in developing countries.

V. EFFECT OF NUTRITION ON RESISTANCE

The most important host factor curtailing or ameliorating infection is breast-feeding in the first months of life (3). Other mechanisms of host defense against infection are gastric acidity, intestinal motility, intestinal microflora, and specific immune response and its amplification. Adequately nourished individuals can cope better with dehydration, nutrient losses, and other consequences of infection; they also exhibit a competent cell-mediated immunity, a good amplification of the immune response, and an integrity of natural barriers (1).

Intrauterine growth retardation results in impaired immunocompetence, and small-for-gestational age infants exhibit a higher incidence of infection and mortality in the first years of life (4, 29). Postnatal undernutrition, whether of a nutritional origin (as in famine) or due to nutrition-infection interaction (the commonest form in Central America) is associated with alterations in resistance. Alterations in integrity of skin and mucosae, hypochlorhydria, and changes in intestinal microbiota, all favor infection. Furthermore, severely undernourished children may have a decreased lymphoid cell mass, an impaired function of T and B immunocytes, and diminished synthesis of complement and secretory IgA (30, 31).

Undernourished Cauqué children experienced a higher attack rate of diarrhea, a greater severity and mortality due to infectious diseases, and a greater difficulty in controlling infection and recovering from illness (4, 32, 33). In fact, duration of infectious disease and of the carrier state (as in shigellosis and measles) was generally longer in undernourished than in well nourished individuals (4). Severely malnourished children show an absent or diminished T cell response, and children may die of measles without manifestation of the exanthem.

Severe undernutrition observed under conditions of extreme food deprivation, may result in depletion of the immune system which may rather antagonize infection. Thus, starved individuals may develop acute infectious disease upon nutritional recuperation (34, 35). On the other hand, infection may alter immune function in a variety of ways including exacerbation of immune function, secondary immunodeficiency and immunological paralysis (36).

COMMENTS

It may be equivocal to assume that malnutrition predisposes to infection since infection rather depends on exposure of the host to the agent. This is subtantiated by the high acquisition rate of enteric infection and diarrhea among well-nourished travelers to tropical regions (37), thus incriminating the environment with its high potential for host contamination, much more than the nutritional status as the crucial factor for inducing infectious disease.

In traditional societies breast-feeding is a part of the culture, and nutrition and growth are adequate for the first three to six months of life. During this period, the child is much protected from infection and from its negative nutritional impact by maternally-derived nutrition and immunity. Also, dehydration is corrected or ameliorated by a continuous supply of breast milk. As weaning begins, continuous expossure to infection results in concurrent diseases and a deterioration or the nutritional state. In transitional societies, many infants are not breast-fed at all, or are weaned early in life, and the deleterious effects of infection may be evident shortly after birth if infants live in a deprived environment. If this is the case, recurrent disease episodes induce weight loss and growth arrest, leading to chronic or acute malnutrition.

The nutritional damage is worse if oral rehydration and other forms of treatment are not available, a common situation in villages throughout the world. Recurrency of diarrhea, anorexia, and fever, coupled with diets of low biological value and unhygienically prepared (38), induce marasmus, or precipitate kwashiorkor. Death is common among dehydrated children not receiving fluid therapy. The risk of death is greater for preterm and small-for-gestational age infants, or for those with chronic or severe malnutrition. Well nourished children, however, may also die from diarrhea, bronchopneumonia and other infectious diseases.

Prospective community studies emphasize the importance of environmental sanitation and home technologies (4, 14) for promotion of child nutrition and health, as opposed to food distribution programs and isolated nutritional interventions. However, populations suffering from acute food shortages constitute an exception in that food distribution should receive immediate consideration.

A practical way to know whether infection or diet should be the target for intervention is to examine community prevalence of undernutrition and mortality behavior. When food supply is limited, as a result of natural or man-made disasters or war, undernutrition and excess mortality appear in all ages and sometimes in all social classes. The usual situation in the developing world, however, does not seem to be a limitation in diet, as children in Asia, Africa and Latin America consume more than 80% of the calories and protein recommended by WHO/FAO; this level seems compatible with normal growth of children in industrial nations (39). Furthermore, undernutrition in most developing countries is circumscribed to infants and very young children and to the very old who live in isolation (4). Then, a logic explanation for the malnutrition observed in children of developing countries is the continuous stress resulting from infection and social pathology. In this regard, observations in Uganda and Costa Rica revealed that psychosocial factors lead to voluntary and involuntary child abuse and neglect, and precipitate severe undernutrition (25, 40). Deficient maternal technology (14) or maternal incompetence (41) in many cases promote infection and potentiate its sequelae.

Epidemiologic evidence indicates that prevention and control of infection, particularly enteric disease, correlate with improved nutrition. For instance, a decrease in diarrheal disease deaths in Costa Rica was highly correlated with a decline in infant mortality and a secular positive trend in height of children (42, 43). During the observation period, no drastic changes in individual food consumption were recorded that could account for the significant gains in nutrition and infant mortality. Nevertheless, there was a dramatic reduction in deaths due to diarrheal and respiratory diseases, measles, whooping-cough and other communicable diseases. These changes were concurrent with a marked increase in *per capita* income, sanitation, immunizations, and availability of health services.

It is then expected that widespread application of oral rehydration, and current trends in improved water supplies, primary health services (including immunizations, family planning), and education, will result in a generalized betterment of the world nutritional situation, without necessarily requiring an increase in food consumption. This comment, however, does not apply to areas where there is a proven limitation in food availability.

ACKNOWLEDGMENTS

Special recognition is given to the Governments of Guatemala and Costa Rica, and to the staffs of INCAP and INISA, especially Drs. Juan Urrutia, Patricia Jiménez and Bernardo Castro. Thanks are proffer to Ms. Giovanna Carrillo who typed the paper, and to Mrs. Ilse Blanco for the artwork.

REFERENCES

1. Scrimshaw, N. S., Taylor C. E., and Gordon, J. E., "Interaction of Nutritian and Infection". Monograph 57. World Health Organization, Geneva (1968).
2. Waterlow, J. C., *J. Human Nutr. 35*, 85 (1981).
3. Jelliffe, D. B., and Jelliffe, E. F. P., "Human Milk in the Modern World". Oxford Univ. Press, New York (1978).
4. Mata, L. J., "The Children of Santa María Cauqué". The MIT Press, Cambridge (1978).
5. Mata, L., Jiménez, P., Allen, M. A., Vargas, W., García, M. E., Urrutia, J. J., and Wyatt, R. G., in "Acute Enteric Infections in Children. New Prospects for Treatment and Prevention" (T. Holme, J. Holmgren, and M. H. Merson, eds.), p. . Elsevier/North Holland, Amsterdam (1981).
6. Mata, L., Allen, M. A., Jiménez, P., García, M. E., Vargas, W., Rodríguez, M. E., and Valerín, C., in "Diarrhea and Malnutrition. Interactions, Mechanisms and Interventions" (L. C. Chen, and N. S. Scrimshaw, eds.), p. . Plenum Pub. Co, New York (1982).
7. Mata, L. J., Urrutia, J. J., Cáceres, A., and Guzmán, M. A., in "Proc. Western Hemisph. Nutr. Congr. III" p. 257. Futura Pub. Co. Inc., New York (1972).
8. Mata, L. J., and Wyatt, R. G., *Am. J. Clin. Nutr. 24*, 976 (1971).
9. Mata, L. J., Jiménez, F., Gordón, M., Rosales, R., Prera, E., Scheneider, R. E., and Viteri, F., *Am. J. Clin. Nutr. 25*, 1118 (1972).
10. Dale, D. C., and Mata, L. J., *Am. J. Trop. Med. Hyg. 17*, 397 (1968).

11. Kloene, W., Bang, F. B., Chakraborty, S. M., Cooper, M. R., Kulemann, H., Ota, M., and Shah, K. V., *Am. J. Epidemiol. 92,* 307 (1970).
12. Mata, L. J., Urrutia, J. J., Albertazzi, C., Pellecer, O., and Arellano, E., *Am. J. Clin. Nutr. 25,* 1267 (1972).
13. Mata, L. J., Kronmal, R. A., Urrutia, J. J., and García, B., *Am. J. Clin. Nutr. 30,* 1215 (1977).
14. Mata, L., *Proc. Nutr. Soc. 38,* 19 (1979).
15. Cole, T. J., and Parkin, J. M., *Trans. Roy. Soc. Trop. Med. Hyg. 71,* 196 (1977).
16. Martorell, R., Lechtig, A., Yarbrough, C., Delgado, H., and Klein, R. E., *Ecol. Food Nutr. 7,* 147 (1978).
17. Molla, A., Molla, A. M., Sarker, S. A., Khatoon, M., and Rahaman, M. M., Working Paper 19. ICDDR,B, Dacca (1981).
18. Whitehead, R. G., in "The Impact of Malnutrition on Immune Defense in Parasitic Infestation" (H. Isliker, and B. Schurch, eds.), p. 15. Hans Huber Pub., Bern (1981).
19. Gracey, M., *Am. J. Clin. Nutr. 32,* 234 (1979).
20. Lindebaum, J., Gerson, C. D., and Kent, T. H., *Ann. Int. Med. 74,* 218 (1971).
21. Field, M., in "Etiology, Pathophysiology, and Treatment of Acute Gastroenteritis". 74th Ross Conf. Ped. Res., p. 57. Ross Lab. Columbus (1978).
22. Beisel, W. R., *Am. J. Clin. Nutr. 30,* 1236 (1977).
23. Wahed, M. A., Rahaman, M. M., Gilman, R. H., Greenough, W. B., and Sarker, S. A., Working Paper 22, ICDDR,B, Dacca (1981).
24. Beisel, W. R., *Med. Clin. N. Am. 60,* 831 (1976).
25. Goodall, J., *Proc. Nutr. Soc. 38,* 17 (1979).
26. Gordon, J. E., Chitkara, I. D., and Wyon, J. B., *Am. J. Med. Sci. 245,* 345 (1963).
27. McGregor, I. A., Rahman, A. K., Thompson, B., Billewicz, W. Z., and Thomson, A. M., *Trans. Roy. Soc. Trop. Med. Hyg. 62,* 341 (1968).
28. Longhurst, R. W., *Proc. Nutr. Soc. 38,* 11 (1979).
29. Chandra, R. K., *Am. J. Dis. Child. 129,* 450 (1975).
30. Faulk, W. P., Mata, L. J., and Edsall, G., *Trop. Dis. Bull. 72,* 89 (1975).
31. Chandra, R. K., and Newberne, P. M., "Nutrition, Immunity and Infection". Plenum Press, New York (1977).
32. Gordon, J. E. Wyon, J. B., and Ascoli, W., *Am. J. Med. Sci. 254,* 357 (1967).
33. Chen, L. C., Alaudin-Chowdhury, A. K. M. and Huffman, S. L., *Am. J. Clin. Nutr. 33,* 1836 (1980).
34. Murray, M. J., and Murray, A. B., *Lancet 1,* 123 (1977).

35. Murray, M. J., and Murray, A. B., *J. Roy. Coll. Phys. London 14,* 197 (1980).
36. Targett, G. A. T., in "The Impact of Malnutrition on Immune Defense in Parasitic Infestation". (H. Isliker, and B. Schurch, eds.), p. 158. Hans Huber Pub. Bern (1981).
37. Lee, J. A., and Kean, B. H., *J. Infect. Dis. 137,* 355 (1978).
38. Capparelli, E., and Mata, L., *Appl. Microbiol. 29,* 802 (1975).
39. Waterlow, J. C., and Thompson, A. M., *Lancet 2,* 238 (1979).
40. Mata, L., Quesada, A. V., Saborío, F., and Mohs, E., *Rev. Méd. Hosp. Nal. Ni;os, Costa Rica. 15,* 137 (1980).
41. Wray, J. D., and Aguirre, A., *J. Trop. Ped. 15,* 93 (1969).
42. Mata, L., Kronmal, R. A., and Villegas, H., in "Cholera and Related Diarrheas" (O. Ouchterlony, and J. Holmgren, eds.), p. 1. S. Karger, Basel (1980).
43. Mata, L. J., and Mohs, E., in "Progress in Human Nutrition". Vol. II (S. Margen, and R. A. Ogar, eds.), p. 254. Ari Pub. Co. Inc. Westport (1978).

8

VIRAL INFECTIONS IN CHILDHOOD IN SOUTH-EAST ASIA AND THE WESTERN PACIFIC

D. Carleton Gajdusek

National Institute of Neurological and
Communicative Disorders and Stroke
N.I.H.
Bethesda, U.S.A.

Child patients are often the principal subject of investigation and the key to the epidemiology of viral infection since first infection and lasting immunity are usually established in childhood. Interpretation of the pattern of occurrence, serology and natural cycle of the major viral plagues of the area, tick (RSSE), Jap B, and MVE, dengue haemorrhagic fever, Ross River infection, and haemorrhagic fever with renal syndrome have required study of child populations.

Child patients were critical in the elucidation of the first proved slow virus infection of man, kuru, in its remote focus in the highlands of New Guinea, and they are proving important in the study of a second probably viral slow infection Viliuisk encephalomyelitis in Iakut people in the Viliui River valley of Soviet Siberia. The first serologically proved virgin populations to influenza, measles, rubella and adenovirus infections were found in Micronesia and Melanesia, and some of these populations provided in the course of their immunization new data on vaccine response and, for influenza, on the serological characteristics of 1918-1922 pandemic influenza virus. CMV, EB and herpes simplex Type I virus infections are acquired in early infancy in all children in much of the area, and the related problem of low incidence of CMV-caused congenital disease requires investigation.

High incidence maxilofacial carcinoma and of Burkitt lymphoma (with highest incidence outside Africa in New

VIRAL DISEASES IN SOUTH-EAST ASIA
AND THE WESTERN PACIFIC
ISBN 0 12 484820 6

Guinea) and their relation to such EB infections are problems of the area as is high incidence primary hepatoma in populations with widespread hepatitis B infection in infancy and high Australian antigenemia. A distinct form of chronic molluscum contagiosum affects most infants and toddlers in the coastal areas of tropical Western Pacific Islands.

Part III
Diagnosis of Viral Diseases

Chairman F. Lehmann-Grube

Co-Chairman I. H. Holmes

9

RAPID VIRAL DIAGNOSIS BY ELECTRON MICROSCOPY, IMMUNOFLUORESCENCE AND IMMUNOASSAYS[1]

Pekka Halonen

Department of Virology
University of Turku
Turku, Finland

I. INTRODUCTION

In the development of new viral diagnostic techniques the most interest during recent years has been in the assays which result in specific diagnosis from a single specimen within the same day or at least within 24 hours after the specimen has arrived at the laboratory. This can be achieved either by detecting virus or viral antigens directly in the clinical specimen or by detecting IgM class viral antibodies in the serum or cerebrospinal fluid.

Detection of virus is traditionally done by electron microscopy and more recently by the modification of solid phase immune electron microscopy. Immunofluorescence has also been used for a long time for the detection of viral antigens in infected cells. The immunofluorescence method for the detection of respiratory virus antigens in nasopharyngeal specimens developed by Gardner and McQuillin (1), the pioneers of rapid virus diagnosis, is probably the most important development in this field. More recently highly sensitive immunoassays including radioimmunoassay (RIA) and enzyme-immunoassay (EIA), have been applied to virus

[1]Supported by grants from Sigrid Juselius Foundation and Academy of Finland, Medical Research Council.

VIRAL DISEASES IN SOUTH-EAST ASIA
AND THE WESTERN PACIFIC
ISBN 0 12 484820 6

antigen detection directly in clinical specimens. These techniques have been used earlier for the assay of hepatitis B surface antigen but they are also particularly useful in the assay of gastroenteritis viruses in stool and can be adapted to the assay of respiratory viruses in aspirates of nasopharyngeal secretions.

In IgM serology the most commonly used techniques include immunofluorescence by anti-human IgM conjugates and immunoglobulin class-specific immunoassays. The most promising modification is the reversed immunoassay where anti-human IgM is the capture antibody in solid phase. Rheumatoid factor does not interfere significantly with this assay.

Since 1976 our laboratory has developed radioimmunoassays and enzyme-immunoassays for the detection of a large variety of virus IgM antibodies (2-4) and later indirect immunoassays for the detection of gastroenteritis (5-8) and respiratory viruses (9-11). These antibody and antigen assays have been used in our routine diagnostic laboratory, some of them for several years. This experience together with the experience of the member laboratories of the European Group for Rapid Viral Diagnosis, form the basis of this presentation.

II. DETECTION OF VIRUSES OR VIRAL ANTIGENS DIRECTLY IN CLINICAL SPECIMENS

A. Electron microscopy in detection of viruses in stool specimens of patients with acute gastroenteritis

In our laboratory electron microscopy has not proven to be as reliable in the detection of rotavirus and adenovirus in stool as reported in Australia (12) and England (13). This may be partially due to the fact that our laboratory is a training center for clinical virologists and each trainee is responsible for electron microscopy for a certain period of time. When a more experienced electron microscopist re-examined the specimens routinely checked in electron microscope it was found that both false-positive and false-negative results had been obtained and these were further verified by the results of the indirect radioimmunoassay (5). We want to point out that electron microscopy is an important diagnostic method but requires expertise and reliable equipment.

With unconcentrated stool suspensions clarified by low-speed centrifugation the positive rate for rotavirus is 10 % less and for adenovirus 50 % less by electron microscopy than by the indirect radioimmunoassay. However, electron microscopy is the most valuable and the only method for the diagnosis of "new" viruses as reported in many studies and as clearly demonstrated in Paris by Chany, Moscovici et al. (14) during a severe epidemic of gastroenteritis in newborns caused by coronavirus.

B. Solid phase immune electron microscopy

A considerable improvement to diagnostic electron microscopy is the solid phase immune electron microscopy method first used by plant virologists and applied to rotavirus diagnosis by Obert et al. (15). In this technique grids are first coated by protein A followed by the optimal dilution of viral antibody. The specimen is incubated on the coated grids for 1 to 16 hours before staining. The sensitivity of rotavirus detection is increased 10 to 100 times when compared with standard electron microscopy and approaches the same sensitivity as the indirect immunoassay. In addition, an almost complete reduction of all contaminating material is seen on coated grids. This new method may further potentiate the usefulness of electron microscopy in diagnosis of many virus infections.

C. Detection of respiratory viruses by the indirect immunofluorescence in aspirates of nasopharyngeal secretion

We have used the indirect immunofluorescence method since 1978 and the results of this rapid diagnostic test have probably been more valued by the clinicians in pediatric clinics and in hospitals for infectious diseases than any other test in our diagnostic laboratory. In this test the cells contained in aspirates of nasopharyngeal secretion are carefully washed off from mucus and stained by the indirect immunofluorescence technique using reagents commercially available. The results obtained during a respiratory epidemic period are shown in Table I.

The test requires a well-trained technician for removing mucus from the cells and for making and staining the slides and the details of these procedures are difficult to

TABLE I. Results of the indirect immunofluorescence test on nasopharyngeal specimens (NPS) in the diagnosis of acute respiratory disease during October 1979 to June 1980

Month	No. of NPS tested	Positive no.	(%)	RSV	Infl. A	Parainfl. 1	Parainfl. 2	Parainfl. 3	Adeno
Oct 1979	25	0							
Nov 1979	47	7	(14)	7					
Dec 1979	34	11	(32)	11					
Jan 1980	195	97	(50)	46	44	1			6
Feb 1980	222	93	(42)	70	21		2		
Mar 1980	151	69	(46)	63	2			1	3
Apr 1980	79	23	(29)	17		2	1	2	1
May 1980	45	7	(16)	4				3	
Jun 1980	27	1	(4)						1
Total	825	308	(37)	218	67	3	3	6	11

learn from written instructions; special training courses are usually suggested. During a 1 day period a technician can make and stain for 5 antigens slides prepared from no more than about 10 specimens. The reading of the stained slides must be done by a very experienced virologist and it takes approximately two hours to read the slides made from 10 specimens. The aspirate specimens must be placed in ice water immediately after collection and the cells must be separated and fixed within a few hours. However, if clinical laboratories in hospitals are trained to make fixed slides, they can be mailed to virus laboratory for staining and examination.

D. Detection of rotavirus and adenovirus in stool specimens by the indirect radioimmunoassay or enzyme-immunoassay

We have used both radioimmunoassay and enzyme-immunoassay for the detection of rotavirus and adenovirus in stool specimens of patients with acute gastroenteritis. If the same immunoreagents are used there are no differences between these two tests in sensitivity and specificity (7). The RIA is mainly used in the diagnostic laboratory because of the availability of the iodinated indicator antibody and partially also because the RIA has one incubation and washing less than the EIA and the standardization of the RIA is better.

The principle of the indirect RIA we have used is shown in Fig. 1. Polystyrene beads (6.4 mm, Precision Plastic Ball Co., Chicago, Ill.) are used as the RIA solid phase and microtiter plates as the EIA solid phase. The primary catching antibody is the total immunoglobulin (Ig) fraction of guinea pig anti-virus hyperimmune serum and the optimal concentration is 0.25 ug/bead in the rotavirus assay and 0.5 ug/bead in the adenovirus assay. The secondary antibody is the Ig fraction of rabbit anti-virus hyperimmune serum and the optimal concentration is 0.8 ug/200 ul (rotavirus) and 1.6 ug/200 ul (adenovirus). The rotavirus hyperimmune sera were prepared by immunizing the animals with

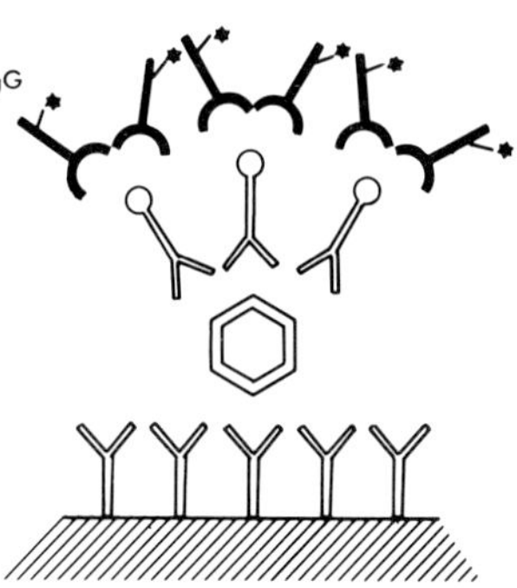

LAYER	IMMUNOREAGENT TYPE	IMMUNOREAGENT CONCENTRATION	INCUBATION AT 37 °C
^{125}I-LABELLED ANTI-RABBIT IgG ANTIBODY	IMMUNOSORBENT PURIFIED ANTIBODY	1–3 ug/200 ul (5000/LABEL COUNTER)	1 HOUR
RABBIT ANTI-VIRUS ANTIBODY	Ig FRACTION	0.8–3.2 ug/200 ul	1 HOUR
SPECIMEN	VIRUS	1 ug ⟶ 1 mg/ml	
GUINEA PIG ANTI-VIRUS ANTIBODY	Ig FRACTION	0.25–1.0/BEAD	1 HOUR (STOOL) 16 HOURS (NPS)
POLYSTYRENE BEAD			

Fig. 1. The indirect radioimmunoassay for the detection of rotavirus and adenovirus in stool specimens and adenovirus, respiratory syncytial virus, parainfluenza virus types 1, 2 and 3, and influenza types A and B in aspirates of nasopharyngeal secretion.

highly purified Nebraska calf diarrhea virus grown in cell cultures (8) and the immunizing antigen of adenovirus was crystallized hexon antigen of adenovirus type 2 (6). The sensitivity of these assays is 1 to 10 ng of viral protein/ml. In order to reach this high sensitivity level it is necessary to obtain low background values with the diluent controls and with the negative specimens and this is achieved by the use of 20 % fetal calf serum and 2 % Tween in the diluent.

In the test a 10 % stool suspension is clarified by low speed centrifugation and incubated with beads coated by guinea pig Ig. The beads are then washed and incubated with anti-viral rabbit Ig, washed again and finally incubated with the iodinated indicator antibody. Each incubation is for one hour at 37°C. After the final wash the beads are changed to clean tubes and counted in a LKB Wallac Rackgamma programmed for the test. The results of a representative test are shown in Table II. The test is standardized by diluting the label to give 5000 to 6000 cpm bound when incubated with a bead coated with 2 ug of purified rabbit IgG. The cut-off value for the estimation of the sensitivity of the test using the reference antigen is two times the cpm value of the diluent control (0 ng/ml) but in the test a better cut-off value for the positive specimens is two times the mean of the negative specimens. In our test the minimum cut-off value is 500 cpm.

About 7 % of the stool specimens are low positives (between 500 and 1000 cpm) and more than 70 % of these are non-specific (16). For this reason a confirmatory test is done with each low-positive by incubating the specimen before the rabbit Ig is added in triplicate tubes containing

a) dilution buffer
b) hyperimmune guinea pig serum
c) pre-immune (normal) guinea pig serum.

The binding of radioactivity is considered specific if the hyperimmune serum blocks 50 % or more of the binding. Non-specific reaction is indicated by no blocking, less than 50 % blocking or blocking also obtained by the pre-immune serum.

Additional reliability is obtained by always testing the specimens simultaneously in the rotavirus and adenovirus assays. The non-specific reactions are almost always obtained in both assays. True dual positive specimens have been obtained in only 5/2681 (0.2 %) of the stool specimens tested (16).

Comparison of the indirect radioimmunoassay and electron microscopy is shown in Table III.

TABLE II. Results of a representative indirect RIA test for rotavirus and adenovirus antigen in stool specimens of 8 patients with acute gastroenteritis

Controls and specimens		CPM			Conclusion
		Control	Rota	Adeno	
Equipment backround (mean automatically deducted)		145 159 148			
Label control[1]		6405			
Reference antigen[2]	100 ng/ml		2549	1942	
	10		1162	641	
	1		372	310	
	0		204	291	
Specimen no.	1		1633	309	rotavirus +
	2		349	375	negative
	3		282	407	negative
	4		2167	269	rotavirus +
	5		658	2723	adenovirus +
	6		312	450	negative
	7		2644	345	rotavirus +
	8		246	3397	adenovirus +

[1] Radioactivity bound with a bead coated with 2 ug of rabbit IgG

[2] Rotavirus antigen: semi-purified Nebraska calf diarrhea virus; adenovirus antigen: purified adenovirus type 2 hexon antigen.

The rotavirus and adenovirus assays were used in a prospective study which included 283 hospitalized children consecutively admitted during a one-year period because of acute diarrhea. Rotavirus was associated in 49 % and adenovirus in 11 % including, however, a few possible dual infections (17).

TABLE III. Comparison of the indirect radioimmunoassay and electron microscopy in the detection of rotavirus and adenovirus in stool specimens of patients with acute gastroenteritis

Electron microscopy	Virus	No. of specimens	Radioimmunoassay Positive	Radioimmunoassay Negative
Positive	Rota	89	89	0
Negative	Rota	58	6	52
		Positive rate:	EM 89/147	(61 %)
			RIA 95/147	(65 %)
Positive	Adeno	13	13	0
Negative	Adeno	200	14	186
		Positive rate:	EM 13/213	(6 %)
			RIA 27/213	(13 %)

E. Detection of respiratory viruses in nasopharyngeal secretion by the indirect radioimmunoassay

Immunoassays identical to those described above for the detection of gastroenteritis viruses have been developed in our laboratory for the detection of respiratory viruses in aspirates of nasopharyngeal secretion from patients with acute respiratory infections. These viruses include respiratory syncytial virus, influenza A and B viruses, parainfluenza virus types 1, 2, and 3 and adenovirus. The immunizing antigens for the production of guinea pig and rabbit hyperimmune sera were purified virus or viral nucleoproteins (9-11). The sensitivity of the assays is 1 to 30 ng of viral protein/ml and they are specific for influenza A and B and for parainfluenza types. The test specimens are aspirates of nasopharyngeal secretions taken in the same way as for immunofluorescence, diluted 1/5 in the RIA diluent and sonicated in a Branson Sonifier cell disrupter for two minutes to solubilize the mucus and to break the cells.

Many specimens are strong positives with the antigen titers up to 1/100 to 1/10.000. We are now testing the specimens in a single dilution of 1/5 or 1/10. A typical test is shown in Table IV. Beginning from November 1981 we have replaced the respiratory virus immunofluorescence test with radioimmunoassay and nearly 1000 specimens have now been tested, of these 36 % have been positive, 30 % to RSV and 5 % to adenovirus. The number of confirmatory tests required for testing the specificity of binding is considerably less than with stool specimens and the rate of specimens reacting nonspecifically is even less. Simultaneous testing for several antigens is again an additional control for a possible nonspecific reaction.

The indirect RIA test has clear advantages over the immunofluorescence. The storage and shipment of specimens is not critical, one technician can test at least twice as many specimens per day; the results are printed out on paper and the evaluation of the test is done in a few minutes and needs no great expertise.

F. Detection of viral antigens by time-resolved fluoroimmunoassay

A new type of non-isotopic immunoassay has been developed recently by LKB Wallac (Turku, Finland). It is based on a time-resolved fluorescence principle using chelates of Europium, a rare earth metal as a label (18). Obtained fluorescent has a long lifetime. A pulsed light excitation is used and the fluorescence intensity is measured after a selected, delay period which eliminates the short duration background fluorescence. The indirect time-resolved fluoroimmunoassay (TR-FIA) we have applied to the detection of viral antigens is identical with the indirect RIA except that the iodinated anti-rabbit IgG antibody is replaced by Eu-chelate labelled antibody. A comparison of the indirect TR-FIA and the indirect RIA for detection of purified rotavirus reference antigen is shown in Table V. The ratios are significantly higher in the TR-FIA than in the RIA but with the other viruses the ratios were almost identical. Also when more than 200 stool specimens were tested by the TR-FIA for rotavirus and adenovirus and about 300 nasopharyngeal specimens for respiratory viruses the ratios of positive specimens were almost identical. The agreement of the results between these two tests was higher than 95 % with each antigen. The advantages of the TR-FIA are nontoxicity and stability of the labels, short counting time of one second, the same or higher sensitivity as in the RIA

TABLE IV. Results of a representative indirect RIA test for respiratory syncytial virus (RSV), influenza A and B, parainfluenza types 1, 2, and 3, (Para-1, Para-2, Para-3) and adenovirus in sonicated aspirates of 8 patients with acute respiratory disease

Controls and specimens	RSV	Influenza A	Influenza B	Parainfluenza 1	Parainfluenza 2	Parainfluenza 3	Adeno	Conclusion
Reference								
1000 ng	982			2206	1897	3343		
100		3061	2782				1762	
0	418	136	133	115	157	268	133	
Specimen								
no. 1	445	280	316	136	268	415	337	Negat.
2	4765	154	403	160	298	448	400	RSV
3	514	262	238	133	184	388	259	Negat.
4	418	247	394	3643	169	346	217	Para-1
5	385	586	349	169	499	373	4756	Adeno
6	349	193	244	187	157	277	217	Negat.
7	526	256	307	157	211	394	316	Negat.
8	556	352	289	208	334	502	436	Negat.

TABLE V. Comparison of the indirect time-resolved fluoroimmunoassay (TR-FIA) and the indirect radioimmunoassay (RIA) in the detection of rotavirus reference antigen

Concentration of reference antigen (ng/ml)	RIA		TR-FIA	
	cpm	Ratio/ buffer blank	cps ($x10^3$)	Ratio/ buffer blank
100	1294[1]	7.5	39.3[2]	56.1
10	465	2.7	14.3	20.4
1	224	1.3	2.3	3.3
0	172		0.7	
Total activity	80.000		1.110,0	
Label control	5.000		468,0	
Per cent bound	6.3		42	

[1] Counts per minute
[2] Counts per second

and increased possibilities to standardize the test. We feel that the TR-FIA is a good candidate to replace the RIA in the detection of viral antigens and it has been also adapted to the antibody assays.

III. ASSAY OF IgM CLASS VIRAL ANTIBODIES

A. Assay of Epstein-Barr virus IgM antibodies by immunofluorescence

Since 1973 we have used indirect immunofluorescence in the assay of Epstein-Barr virus (EBV) IgG and IgM antibodies (19). The P3HR-1 line of Burkitt cells are used in the assay because they are negative for direct non-specific IgG and IgM fluorescence and there is a clear specific EBV fluorescence in 15 to 20 per cent of the cells. The fixed slides are overlaid by serum dilutions, incubated for 3 hours at 37°C, washed and overlaid with a 1/20 dilution of anti-human IgM conjugate (Dako, Denmark) for one hour. After washing the slides are mounted with glycerol PBS and examined in a Leitz Dialux 20 microscope with a 100 W Halogen lamp. The reading requires some training and high quality UV microscopy.

The non-specific reactions caused by rheumatoid factor are always a problem in the indirect IgM assays. We normally retest each specimen positive in EBV IgM after adsorbtion with heat aggregated human gamma globulin. EBV IgM antibodies can be regularly detected 3 to 4 days after onset of the disease and they remain at detectable levels for 3 to 8 weeks. The test has been valuable in the diagnosis of EBV infections negative for heterophil antibody. However, for practical reasons an immunoassay test, preferably a reversed type, would be better.

B. The indirect radioimmunoassay and enzyme-immunoassay in the detection of IgM specific viral antibodies

The principle of the test is shown in Fig. 2.
A semipurified or crude virus preparation is adsorbed on to the solid phase, the test serum specimen usually in serial dilutions, is incubated with the solid phase virus and finally the anti-human IgM labelled with ^{125}I or with

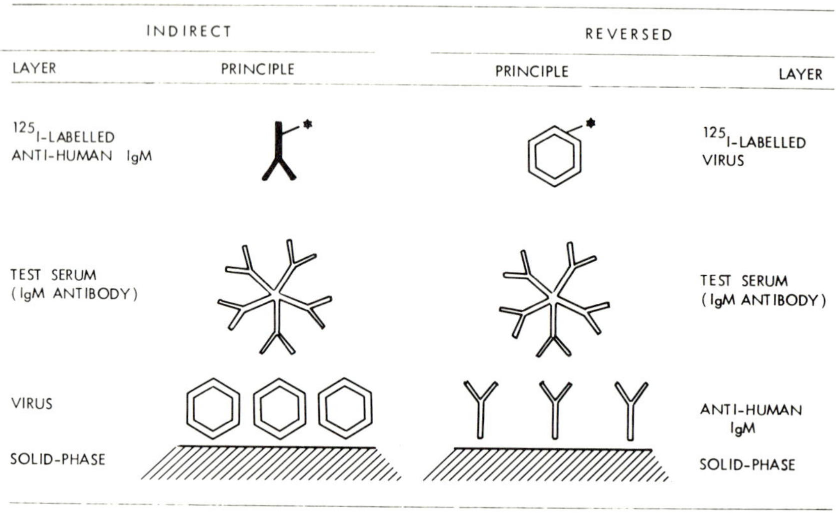

Fig. 2. Principles of the indirect radioimmunoassay and the reversed radioimmunoassay for the detection of IgM antibodies.

enzyme is added. We have used the indirect radioimmunoassay for the detection of rubella IgM since 1978 (20). The optimal incubation of the test serum with the beads coated by virus is for one hour at 37°C. The second incubation is overnight at 37°C. The antigen used for coating is rubella virus grown in Vero cells, concentrated by Amicon hollow fiber filtration and purified by ultracentrifugation through 15 % sucrose (21). The results of a typical test are shown in Table VI. As indicated by the cpm values obtained by the positive reference serum and the strong positive test serum an unexplained prozone is often found in lower serum dilutions. For this reason each test serum must be assayed in serial dilutions. Rheumatoid factor again causes non-specific binding in this IgM assay if the test serum also contains rubella IgG antibodies (21). However, we have found that this problem is not a major one although theoretically important. The non-specific binding is lower than the specific binding and after testing the suspected specimens by latex these specimens can be identified (specimen no. 99376 in Table VI). If necessary the specimen can also be adsorbed by heat aggregated human gamma globulin.

TABLE VI. Results of a representative test for rubella IgM by the indirect radioimmunoassay

Reference or test serum	Dilution	cpm	Conclusion
Reference negative serum	16	230	
	64	395	
	256	242	
	1000	109	
	4000	20	
Reference positive serum	16	1822	IgM titer $\geq$ 1/4000
	64	2620	
	256	2061	
	1000	959	
	4000	417	
Specimen no.99729	16	289	Negative
	64	353	
	256	206	
	1000	39	
Specimen no.99526	16	860	Strong positive; clear prozone
	64	1772	
	256	2267	
	1000	1420	
	4000	707	
Specimen no.99376	16	1228	Latex +; nonspecific binding
	64	992	
	256	194	
	1000	40	

IgM antibodies are detected in rubella in 12 % of patients on the day the rash appears, and in 45 %, 64 %, 84 % and 92 % on the consecutive days. Only on day 5 and thereafter are IgM antibodies detected in every patient (22).

In addition to rubella we are using the indirect radioimmunoassay or enzyme-immunoassay in the detection of IgM antibodies to herpes simplex, measles, mumps and tick-borne encephalitis. Purified virus is used in rubella and tick-borne encephalitis IgM assays and a crude cell-lysate antigen in the other assays.

C. The reversed radioimmunoassay and enzyme-immunoassay in the detection of IgM class viral antibodies

Another type of IgM immunoassay in which rheumatoid factor does not significantly interfere has been developed. In this reversed assay the IgM antibodies of the test specimen are captured by anti-human IgM on the solid phase and the specificity of the captured IgM is detected by a labelled virus antigen (Fig. 2) or with non-labelled virus followed by labelled IgG antibody to the virus. The reversed assay has been applied for IgM detection of many viruses, e.g. hepatitis A (23, 24), hepatitis B core antigen (25), tick-borne encephalitis (26), varizella-zoster (27) and cytomegalovirus (28).

IV. CONCLUSIONS AND FUTURE PROSPECTS

Diagnostic virus laboratories which directly serve hospitals and out-patient clinics should adapt rapid virus diagnostic techniques whenever possible. Detection of virus antigen directly in clinical specimens is the most straightforward way to diagnose virus infection and is least likely to cause difficulties in interpretation. Which are the best techniques for the detection of viral antigens? The most sensitive is to isolate the virus if highly sensitive cell cultures are available. Unfortunately, virus isolation and identification of the isolates usually takes many days, if not longer, and the procedure has many known inherent difficulties. Our experience with immunoassays demonstrates that a susprisingly large number of viruses can be consistently detected in secretions by these techniques.

Apparently high concentrations of structural virus proteins are excreted in addition to virions and they all are detectable by the immunoassays. The calculated concentrations of rotavirus and adenovirus (hexon) antigens are 100 to 1000 ug/gm of stool and in the nasopharyngeal secretions the concentrations of respiratory virus proteins are often 1 to 10 ug/ml. These concentrations are quite sufficient for the indirect immunoassays with sensitivities of 1 to 30 ng of virus protein /ml.

A serious limitation of the diagnostic methods based on antigen detection is the relatively short duration of antigen excretion. Adenovirus and rotavirus are apparently excreted for a relatively long time but many other viruses causing acute gastroenteritis may be excreted for a shorter period. In respiratory infections our relatively limited experience indicates a persistence of excretion for 2 to 4 days only after the first specimen has been collected at admission. Of course respiratory patients are usually ill for several days before they are admitted.

In the near future more sensitive immunoassays are likely to be developed and this will increase the possibilities for rapid virus diagnosis by antigen detection. At the same time the techniques will be more simple. Preliminary experience with the time-resolved fluoroimmunoassay indicates that a direct assay with two incubations and with a high sensitivity can be developed using monoclonal antibodies and even an assay with only one incubation may be possible.

In addition to gastroenteritis, respiratory infections and hepatitis B, the virus infections where antigen excretion may be sufficient enough for diagnosis include herpes simplex, possibly herpes encephalitis, varicella-zoster, cytomegalo and mumps. This leaves out many virus infections where the virus usually disappears at the same time as the clinical symptoms appear. In these cases IgM assay is the best choice if the response is consistent. Such virus infections include rubella, measles, hepatitis A, Epstein-Barr virus infections and many arbovirus infections. A simple reverse type of IgM assay or other assays not interfered with by rheumatoid factor should be developed for these viruses if they are not already available.

V. REFERENCES

1. Gardner, P., and McQuillin, J., "Rapid Virus Diagnosis Application of Immunofluorescence", Butterworths, 2nd ed., London, (1980).
2. Kalimo, K., Meurman, O., Halonen, P., Ziola, B., Viljanen, M., Granfors, K., and Toivanen, P., *J. Clin. Micro. 4*, 117 (1976).
3. Kalimo, K., Ziola, B., Viljanen, M., Granfors, K., and Toivanen, P., *J. Immunol. Methods 14*, 183 (1977).
4. Frisch-Niggemeyer, W., Halonen, P., Heinz, F., Kunz, C., and Ziola, B., *Immunität und Infection 6*, 110 (1978).
5. Sarkkinen, H., Halonen, P., and Arstila, P., *J. Med. Virol. 4*, 255 (1979).
6. Halonen, P., Sarkkinen, H., Arstila, P., Hjertsson, E., and Torfason, E., *J. Clin. Micro. 11*, 614, (1980).

7. Sarkkinen, H., Tuokko, H., and Halonen, P., *J. Virol. Methods 1*, 331 (1980).
8. Sarkkinen, H., *J. Clin. Path. 34*, 680 (1981).
9. Sarkkinen, H., Halonen, P., Arstila, P., and Salmi, A., *J. Clin. Micro. 13*, 258 (1981).
10. Sarkkinen, H., Halonen, P., and Salmi, A., *J. Med. Virol. 7*, 213 (1981).
11. Sarkkinen, H., Halonen, P., and Salmi, A., *J. Gen. Virol. 56*, 49 (1981).
12. Bishop, R., Davidson, G., Holmes, I., and Ruck, B., *Lancet 2*, 1281 (1973).
13. Flewett, T., Davies, H., Bryden, A., and Robertson, M., *J. Clin. Path. 27*, 608 (1974).
14. Chany, C., Moscovici, O., Lebon, P., and Rousset, S., *Pediatrics*, in press.
15. Obert, G., Gloeckler, R., Burckard, J., and van Regenmortel, M., *J. Virol. Methods 3*, 99 (1981).
16. Sarkkinen, H., "Viral Antigen Detection in Clinical Specimens by Solid-Phase Radioimmunoassay and Enzyme-immunoassay", Academic Dissertation, Turku, (1981).
17. Vesikari, T., Mäki, M., Sarkkinen, H., Arstila, P., and Halonen, P., *Arch. Dis. Childhood 56*, 264 (1981).
18. Soini, E., and Hemmilä, I., *Clin. Chem. 25*, 353 (1979).
19. Nikoskelainen, J., Leikola, J., and Klemola, E., *Brit. Med. J.*, 72 (1974).
20. Meurman, O., *J. Clin. Micro. 7*, 34 (1978).
21. Meurman, O., and Ziola, B., *J. Clin. Path. 31*, 483 (1978).
22. Meurman, O., Fifth International Congress of Virology Abstracts, 166, Strasbourg (1981).
23. Duermeyer, W., Wielard, F., and van der Veen, J., *J. Med. Virol. 4*, 25 (1979).
24. Meurman, O., Matter, L., Krishna, R., and Krech, U., *Acta Path. et Microbiol. Scand. Section C 89*, 79 (1981).
25. Gehrlich, W., and Lüer, W., *J. Med. Virol. 4*, 227 (1979).
26. Roggendorf, M., Heinz, F., Deinhardt, F., and Kunz, C., *J. Med. Virol. 7*, 41 (1981).
27. Tedder, R., Mortimer, P., and Bridget Lord, R., *J. Med. Virol. 8*, 81 (1981).
28. Van Loon, A., Heessen, J., van der Logt, J., and van der Veen, J., *J. Clin. Micro. 13*, 416 (1981).

10

PROBLEMS IN PROVIDING DIAGNOSTIC SERVICES IN DEVELOPING COUNTRIES

S. K. LAM

Department of Medical Microbiology
University of Malaya
Kuala Lumpur Malaysia

The WHO World List of Virus Laboratories (1979) lists 616 laboratories located in 89 countries. The distribution by WHO Regions is as follows:

Region	*No. of laboratories*	*No. of countries*
African	*17*	*12*
American	*163*	*19*
Eastern Mediterranean	*25*	*11*
European	*327*	*29*
South-East Asia	*27*	*7*
Western Pacific	*57*	*11*

It is evident from the above that in regions where virus diseases are still major problems, there are very few laboratories that can provide diagnostic services.

The major viral diseases in South-East Asia and the Western Pacific are:

Viral gastroenteritis
Acute respiratory diseases
Dengue and dengue haemorrhagic fever
Viral hepatitis
Poliomyelitis
Measles
Rubella
Rabies

VIRAL DISEASES IN SOUTH-EAST ASIA
AND THE WESTERN PACIFIC
ISBN 0 12 484820 6

Many of these diseases e.g. poliomyelitis and measles are seldom seen in developed countries because of effective immunization programmes. In developing countries these are still important health problems and contribute significantly to morbidity and mortality. Preventive measures through immunization are expensive and there are many local problems which hinder progress and wide acceptance of the expanded programme of immunization.

It is therefore important to provide diagnostic services for the differential diagnosis of viral infections in regions where the diseases exist. In 1966 the Department of Medical Microbiology in Kuala Lumpur was assigned the task of starting up a virus diagnostic unit to serve the 800-bed University Hospital. From a very modest beginning of providing diagnosis of enteroviruses and poxvirus infections, we have over a period of years, expanded our diagnostic services to cover all major viral infections in Malaysia. From 1967 to 1971 we were able to offer diagnostic services for hepatitis B, rubella, influenza and other respiratory viruses. Many of our efforts were aided by research grants and collaborative projects with international organizations. From 1971 to 1974 we consolidated our work and carried out basic research into epidemiological studies of acute respiratory infections, rubella and hepatitis B.

From 1975 onwards, we underwent another expansion programme in the field of viral diagnosis. At that time, there was interest in the rapid diagnosis of viral infections spurred on by the discovery of rotavirus by electron microscopy and the use of immunofluorescence in the diagnosis of respiratory syncytial virus infection. Realizing the importance of this development, we were able to introduce some of these new rapid techniques which proved to be well received by the clinicians. Our range of tests based on rapid techniques expanded to include the para-influenza virus, influenza virus, herpesvirus, rotavirus, adenovirus, measles virus and varicella-zoster virus. As a direct outcome of this, we were designated a WHO-recognized National Centre for the Rapid Diagnosis of Viral Infections in 1979.

We faced many problems during the development of the virus diagnostic units but none of them were insurmountable. When I undertook to talk on the problems associated with providing diagnostic services in developing countries, I sent out a questionnaire to a number of laboratories in South-East Asia and the Western Pacific to identify these problems and to offer solutions for them. Thirteen countries responded to the questionnaire and the problems were broadly divided into:

Finance
Equipment
Personnel
Supplies

Finance

Contrary to popular belief, it is not finance which is the most important problem in providing diagnostic service in developing countries. There are adequate funds for the day-to-day running of the service, although inflation and tight foreign exchange have caused some concern in recent years.

Equipment

All laboratories who responded to the questionnaire cited the problem of maintenance and repair of sophisticated machinery as a major problem. This is often due to inadequate or non-existent after-sales service. Much of the equipment is old and spares are no longer available. Often there is irregular power supplies which play havoc with ultracentrifuges and deep freezers.

Personnel

Labour is relatively cheap in developing countries so that there is no shortage of unskilled manpower. Some countries experience problems in the recruitment of science and medical graduates and this may be linked to a low-salary structure and the lack of motivation and incentive.

Supplies

This is a very important problem and often hinders and retards diagnostic services. There is not a great demand for viral reagents and consequently there are very few local suppliers. Often orders are allowed to accumulate over several months before being attended to. The service is slow and there is a long delay with deliveries. Reagents are not properly transported under ideal conditions.

SOLUTIONS

Finance

Giving cash grants may not, in many instances, be the answer. A better solution would be to provide a regular supply of reagents under collaborative projects that are of mutual interest. Such collaborative projects need not always involve international organizations.

Equipment

There should be regular training courses in the maintenance and repair of equipment to keep the machinery in good working order. The onus should be on the companies who market these machines. Adequate spares should also be ordered along with any piece of new machinery and generators provided for those that require a constant power supply.

Personnel

Advanced training courses are essential for senior technical staff which, while providing the added skill, will also prove to be a good incentive.

Supplies

This problem could be overcome if a collective effort was made by some international organizations to purchase viral reagents in bulk for a particular region for redistribution as and when the need arose. I feel strongly that this would help to overcome a very important problem in providing viral diagnoses to developing countries.

Encouragement should be given to produce reagents locally, but international organizations should help in the quality control of these locally produced reagents.

THE SETTING UP OF A VIRUS DIAGNOSTIC LABORATORY TODAY IN A DEVELOPING COUNTRY

For those developing countries who are contemplating setting up a virus diagnostic laboratory, I would like to offer a few suggestions for their consideration in the light of my own personal experience.

Classical laboratory techniques currently used in virology, although specific and sensitive, are often tedious, difficult, or in some laboratories, impossible to work. In recent years several new, simple and rapid methods for the diagnosis of virus infections have been devised and a WHO publication on this has just been issued (WHO Technical Report Series No. 661, 1980).[1] Rapid viral diagnosis is defined as a method that would provide acceptable results in a shorter time than classical methods would, and allow successful intervention into the treatment of patients and their contacts, or in the control of disease in communities.

Rapid viral diagnosis offers many advantages over conventional methods of virus isolation and virus serology. Its rapidity and simplicity make it easier to carry out surveys of infectious diseases in a certain area. The information obtained may lead to the implementation of individual or public health action. The early diagnosis of viral infections will help to prevent hospital cross-infection and their spread to contacts. The use of anti-viral drugs, both prophylactically and therapeutically, is increasing, although still very limited. Their successful application will depend on specific and early viral diagnosis.

THE APPLICATION OF RAPID TECHNIQUES IN THE DIAGNOSIS OF IMPORTANT VIRAL DISEASES IN SOUTH EAST ASIA AND THE WESTERN PACIFIC

Listed below are the diseases and the rapid techniques available for their laboratory diagnosis:

[1] *Report of a WHO Scientific Group. Technical Report Series No. 661: Rapid laboratory techniques for the diagnosis of viral infections (1981).*

Diseases	*Recommended methods*
Rotavirus diarrhoea	*ELISA, EM, IEOP*
Acute respiratory infection	*FAT*
Hepatitis B	*RPHA, ELISA, IEOP*
Hepatitis A	*RIA*
Rubella and Cytomegalovirus infection	*IgM detection*
Measles	*FAT*
Rabies	*FAT, ID*
Herpes simplex infection	*EM, FAT*

The successful and wide application of these new methods has been hampered by the lack of quality-controlled reagents, essential equipment and trained personnel. These problems will continue to be tackled by WHO during the next two years.

Although it is recognized that rapid techniques cannot fully replace conventional ones, they will contribute to the knowledge on viral infection as a cause of morbidity and mortality. They will help to improve primary health care and the control of viral diseases of public health importance.

11

PROBLEMS IN THE DIAGNOSIS OF CNS INVOLVEMENT IN VIRUS INFECTION IN INDONESIA

Soeprapti Thaib

Virus Department
Perum. Bio Farma
Bandung, Indonesia

PREVALENCE OF SUSPECTED CNS VIRUS INFECTIONS

Information from neurologists has revealed that suspected CNS virus infections occur throughout the year, occasionally showing variations in seasonal distribution, the incidence being higher in April, May and June, during the transition period from rainy to dry season. They include clinically diagnosed polyneuritis and polyradiculitis cases in Bandung.

A sudden high fever of 39°-40°C develops, with one or more neurological manifestations, frequently followed by various degrees of impaired consciousness resulting in death or otherwise leaving sequelae on survival.

A special study on suspected viral meningitides/ encephalitides in Bandung since 1980 up till now, has revealed a CFR of around 20-25% in children and adults.

Neurologists in Bandung have claimed that an increase of malignancy has recently occurred resulting from such high CFRs.

ATTEMPTS AT LABORATORY CONFIRMATION

According to Brown (1,2), if encephalitis is a complication of a disease, more characteristic features of the

VIRAL DISEASES IN SOUTH-EAST ASIA
AND THE WESTERN PACIFIC
ISBN 0 12 484820 6

illness become evident. However, if it is the major illness, minor influenza-like prodromal symptoms are present.

Usually CNS infections with clear CSF are diagnosed as suspect tuberculosis meningitis; and if bacterial examinations are negative, then the diagnosis will suggest a virus infection, considering also the clinical manifestations and CSF analysis, not supported by viro-serological examinations.

There have been reports of various types of viral meningitides and encephalitides, the majority being diagnosed without viro-serologic confirmation, such as cases of post-vaccinal encephalitis after smallpox (3) and nerve tissue rabies vaccination (4). Other reports supported by virus isolation and/or serologic tests, all undertaken in Bandung in 1972, 1977 and 1980 (5-9) have revealed that a variety of viruses may be incriminated such as polio and coxsackie viruses, mumps, herpes simplex, swine influenza, rubella, measles, JBE, etc.

THE PROBLEMS IN INDONESIA

The most reliable diagnosis in viral CNS infection has been the isolation of the virus from CSF and/or brain specimens, depending on the clinical symptoms and the suspected aetiological agent.

Serological tests are impracticable in terms of time and antigens, as many viruses may affect the CNS.

The main reasons for the scarcity of viro-serological confirmations in Indonesia have been:

(1) the high costs of laboratory examinations, particularly isolation procedures, in order to obtain local strains;

(2) the inability to do brain biopsies even in fatal cases, because of religious and other reasons;

(3) the difficulty in obtaining reagents for the new rapid virus diagnosis techniques which are usually very expensive;

(4) the high cost of imported semisynthetic media for certain stable cell lines, antigens, antisera, and the sera required for media preparation;

(5) the ignorance of physicians in selecting the proper specimens for laboratory confirmations and neglect in specimen storage before submission to the laboratory, and the method of packing specimens during transportation;

(6) the shortage of basic equipment for the preparation of antigens and antisera.

CONCLUSIONS AND SUGGESTIONS

With CFRs as high as 20-25%, non-bacterial CNS infection will become a health problem, more so if brain biopsies cannot be done to determine the most frequent aetiological virus and to determine its epidemiological pattern.

It is felt that more virus laboratories should be established, since Indonesia consists of more than 3,000 islands, yet only two laboratories (Jakarta and Bandung) are able to do virus work.

However, special funds should be available, not only for basic equipment, training, experimental animals and other requirements, but also to buy antigens, antisera, and conjugates.

It would also be useful if aid could be channeled into the upgrading of existing laboratories, and in providing various diagnostic kits, standard virus strains, and standardized antigens and antisera, etc.

Furthermore if certain laboratories could be appointed, by W.H.O. for instance, to support other virus laboratories in neighbouring countries, regardless of region, this would be of considerable assistance in establishing a high standard of diagnostic services.

REFERENCES

1. Brown, P., *in* "Current Diagnosis" 6th Edition (H.F. Conn and R.B. Conn, eds.), p.884. W.B. Saunders, Philadelphia, (1980).
2. Brown, P., *in* "Current Diagnosis" 5th Edition (H.F. Conn and R.B. Conn, eds.), p.126. W.B. Saunders, Philadelphia, (1977).
3. Tjakradinata, D., Oebil, H., and Tjay, J.K., *J. Indon. Paed. Ass. 17,* 11, 385 (1977).
4. Theos, Personal communication (1977, 1981).
5. Thaib, S., Mangun, H., Priatna, A., and Dindin, N., *Bull. Bio Farma IX,* 1, 1 (1972).
6. Thaib, S., and Priatna, A., *Bull. Bio Farma XIV,* 1, 1 (1977).
7. Thaib, S., and Alisyahbana, A., IInd Internat. Symp. on Immunization, Min. of Hlth Rep. of Indon., WHO., Unicef, ICC. and USAID, Jakarta, Nov. 27 - Dec. 1 (1979).

8. Witoelar, S., Thaib, S., and Taryana, A., IInd Nat. Congr. of Indon. Ass. of Neurology, Psychiatry and Neurosurgery, Nov. 17-19, 1980, in Bandung.
9. Thaib, S., In progress.

12

MONOCLONAL ANTIBODIES, RECOMBINANT DNA TECHNOLOGY, AND OTHER NEW APPROACHES

Wolfgang K. Joklik

Department of Microbiology and Immunology
Duke University Medical Center
Durham, North Carolina

The 1970s have witnessed the development of two very powerful methodologies for the study of proteins and nucleic acids. The first of these is hybridoma technology, which provides extremely specific probes for antigenic sites on proteins; the second is recombinant DNA technology which in addition to providing probes for any nucleic acid sequence, permits one to rearrange genetic material in ways undreamt of only a decade ago. Together these two new methodologies permit one to find, isolate and study in exquisite molecular detail any protein and any nucleic acid sequence in any living cell.

Both hybridoma technology and recombinant DNA technology have recently been applied to the detection and identification of minute amounts of viral components and of antibodies against them, and promise to become powerful tools for the diagnosis of viral diseases.

This review will be divided into four parts:

i. Studies on the isolation and characterization of a series of monoclonal antibodies against the proteins of reovirus, which pointed the way to their use in viral diagnosis;

[1]*Supported by grant number AI-08909 from the National Institutes of Health*

VIRAL DISEASES IN SOUTH-EAST ASIA
AND THE WESTERN PACIFIC
ISBN 0 12 484820 6

ii. The identification of unknown orthopoxvirus antisera;
iii. The isolation and characterization of monoclonal antibodies against orthopoxviruses;
iv. The cloning and sequencing of reovirus genes.

A. *The characteristics of a series of monoclonal antibodies against reovirus proteins*

There are three serotypes of virus. As judged by the ability of their genomes to hybridize with each other, serotypes 1 and 3 are related to each other to the extent of about 70%, and serotype 2 is related to both serotype 1 and to serotype 3 to the extent of about 10% (Martinson and Lewandowski, 1975; Gaillard and Joklik, 1982). Not surprisingly, the antigenic determinants on most of the proteins of serotypes 1 and 3 are very similar; but very interestingly, the antigenic determinants on serotype 2 proteins are no more different from those on serotype 1 and 3 proteins than those on the latter differ among themselves. This was shown as follows (Gaillard and Joklik, 1980). Antisera to reovirus serotypes 1, 2 or 3 were added to extracts of cells that had been infected with reovirus serotype 1, 2 or 3, and labelled with [^{35}S] methionine from 10-12 h after infection, when all reovirus-coded

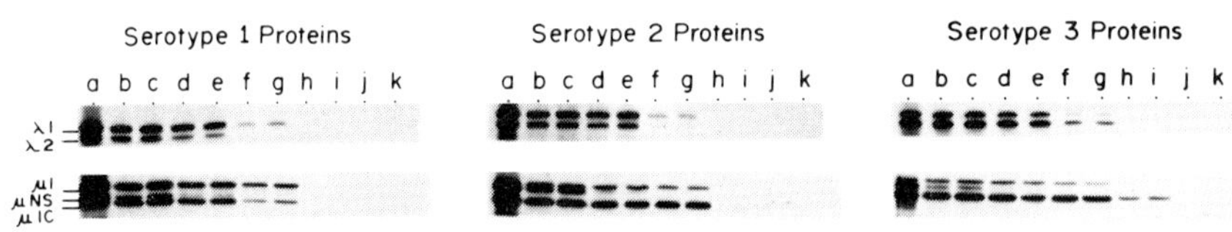

FIGURE 1. RIP analysis demonstrating the efficiency with which proteins encoded by serotypes 1, 2, and 3 are precipitated by antiserum to serotype 2. The panels are regions containing the λ and μ size classes of reovirus proteins that had been excised from SDS-polyacrylamide gels. In all panels lane a is the marker lane (from extracts of [^{35}S] methionine-labelled cells infected with serotypes 1, 2 and 3, respectively); lanes b and c, antiserum dilution 10^{-1}; lanes d and e, antiserum dilution, 10^{-2}; lanes f and g, antiserum dilution, 10^{-3}; lanes h and i, antiserum dilution, 10^{-4}; and lanes j and k, antiserum dilution, 10^{-5}.

proteins were being synthesized at maximum rates. The resulting antigen-antibody complexes were adsorbed to cells of Staph A, and the antigens that had reacted with antibody were identified by polyacrylamide gel electrophoresis followed by autoradiography. It proved possible to quantitate this reaction by adding serial dilutions of antisera to extracts of infected cells and determining that antibody concentration that reacted with one-half of the maximum amount of antigen that could react; the reciprocal of that dilution provides an absolute measure of the affinity of individual antibodies in the antiserum for individual antigens in the cell extract. Fig. 1 illustrates the technique, and Table 1 summarizes the data for all three

TABLE 1

QUANTITATION OF THE SEROLOGIC RELATEDNESS OF REOVIRUS-CODED PROTEINS[a]

Protein	M_r	Approximate number of molecules per virus particle	Location	Coded by serotype	Antiserum against: Strain Abney serotype 1	Strain D/5 Jones serotype 2	Strain Dearing serotype 3
λ1	155,000	100	Core	1	250	180	160
				2	190	200	240
				3	110	140	120
λ2	140,000	100	Core spike/ virion surface	1	230	60	*120*
				2	260	160	*200*
				3	80	240	*1000*
μ1	80,000	24	Core ?	1	660	140	520
				2	400	200	660
				3	200	410	700
μ1C	72,000	550	Virion surface	1	1420	*80*	700
				2	1000	*1100*	1220
				3	700	1780	1100
μNS	85,000	—	Nonstructural	1	40	30	30
				2	40	40	30
				3	60	30	40
σ1	42,000	24	Virion surface	1	*1240*	60	*<10*
				2	*100*	*200*	*<10*
				3	*<10*	*<10*	*2000*
σ2	38,000	200	Core	1	280	*100*	1100
				2	280	*1250*	2300
				3	320	400	820
σ3	34,000	900	Virion surface	1	1000	260	1060
				2	1060	2400	1700
				3	860	1660	680
σNS	36,000	—	Nonstructural	1	40	40	45
				2	30	45	30
				3	50	40	50

[a] *The numbers are the reciprocals of the antiserum dilutions at which 50% of the maximum amount of each protein reacted. Numbers in boxes indicate significant type-specificity.*

reovirus serotypes (Gaillard and Joklik, 1980). It is seen that the antigenic determinants on most of the proteins of all three serotypes, even those of serotype 2, are indistinguishable. In view of the marked dissimilarity between the genomes of serotype 2 on the one hand and those of serotypes 1 and 3 on the other, this indicates that the antigenic determinants on most reovirus proteins have been highly conserved during evolution. There is only one very type-specific protein, σ1, a minor component of the reovirus outer capsid shell, although there are several other proteins that display lesser degrees of type-specificity.

Two immediate applications of this technique are as follows. First, any antiserum against reovirus of unknown serotype can be readily identified by reacting it with extracts of cells infected with either serotype 1, 2 or 3: each antiserum will only precipitate one protein σ1, namely the homologous one, efficiently. Second, if monoclonal antibodies to the three σ1 proteins were available, they would clearly provide highly specific reagents for each of the three reovirus serotypes.

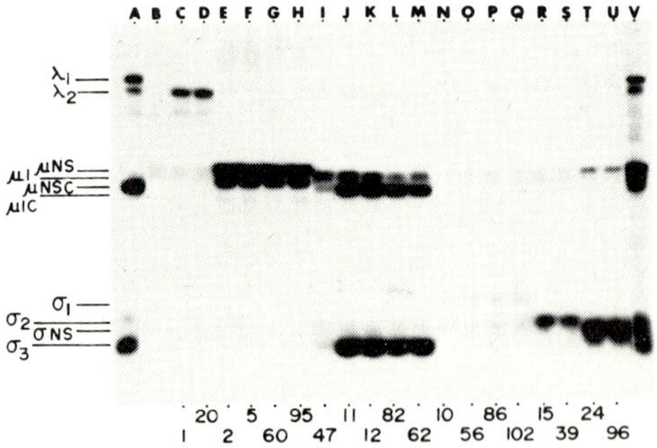

FIGURE 2. Autoradiogram of SDS-urea-7.5% polyacrylamide gel in which the labelled reovirus proteins that reacted with the various hybridoma-secreted IgGs had been electrophoresed. The number of each hybridoma clone is indicated, as is each reovirus-coded protein. Lane A, [^{35}S] methionine-labelled reovirus capsid protein; lane B, cell lysate reacted with the culture supernatant of 45.6.TGl.7 cells (the parental myeloma cell line); lane V, [^{35}S] methionine-labelled infected cell lysate. The direction of electrophoresis was from top to bottom.

With this background information, let us examine the properties of a series of hybridomas that secrete monoclonal antibodies against reovirus-coded proteins. The hybridomas were constructed by infecting mice with reovirus strain Dearing (serotype 3) and fusing cells of their spleens with mouse myeloma cell strain 45.6.TG1.7. Nineteen of the resulting hybridoma cell lines were cloned from single cells and grown up to large amounts in order to isolate sufficient amounts of the antibodies secreted by each. All 19 hybridomas secreted antibodies of the IgG class. The monoclonal antibodies were characterized by causing them to react with reovirus-coded proteins present in extracts of infected cells that had been labelled with $[^{35}S]$-methionine during late stages of the infection cycle; the antigen-antibody complexes were then collected on Staph A and the antigens analyzed in SDS-polyacrylamide gels followed by autoradiography (Lee et al., 1981a). Fig. 2 shows the proteins that reacted with each of the 19 antibodies. Most of the antibodies reacted only with a single protein, but some, like clones 1 and 20; 2, 5, 60 and 95; and 47, 4, 12, 82 and 62, reacted with two, because the proteins against which they are directed (λ 2, μNS and μ1 respectively) exist in infected cells not only in intact form, but also in the form of cleavage products some 5 to 15 kd smaller.

Another reason why some monoclonal antibodies reacted with more than one protein (clones 11, 12, 82 and 62) was the fact that two proteins, namely μ1C and σ3, the major components of the outer capsid shell of reovirus, possess high affinity for each other and exist in infected cells in the form of a complex. When this situation was analyzed in detail (Lee et al., 1981a), it was found that one antibody (clone 47) reacted only with μ1/μ 1C and was unable to precipitate the complex μ1C-σ3, presumably because the antigenic site with which it combined was located in a region that was sterically blocked by σ3. Two other monoclonal antibodies (clones 11 and 12) were capable of reacting with the complex μ1C-σ3, but not with free σ3; their antigenic site must be located on protein μ1C. Another monoclonal antibody (clone 62) was able to react with the complex as well as with free σ3; its antigenic site is therefore on σ3. Finally, one monoclonal antibody (clone 82) was able to react with the complex, but not with free σ3 or free μ1/μ1C, which indicated that its antigenic site involves portions of both μ1/μ1C and σ3 (Fig. 3) (Lee et al., 1981a).

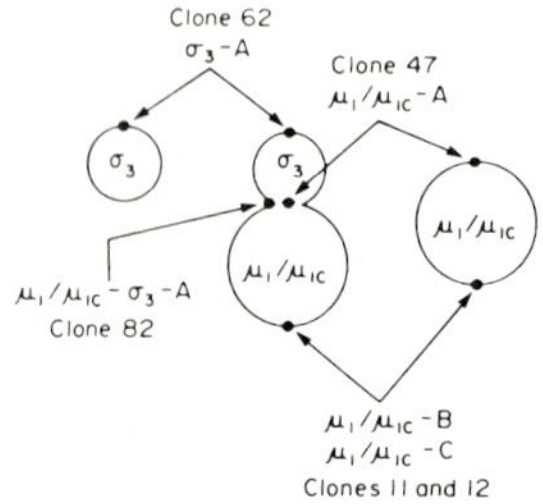

FIGURE 3. Model depicting the putative locations of antigenic sites on polypeptides μ1/μ1C and σ3.

Among the 19 monoclonal antibodies were several that reacted with the same reovirus-coded protein. For example, we isolated four monoclonal antibodies against protein σ1, four against protein μNS, and so on. In order to differentiate between such antibodies, a series of experiments were carried out. The first was to measure the efficiency with which they were able to combine with the proteins of the two heterologous reovirus serotypes, serotypes 1 and 2, relative to that with which they combined with the homologous (serotype 3) protein. The methodology employed here was to react serial dilutions of the monoclonal antibodies with extracts of cells infected with each of the three reovirus serotypes, and to determine the dilution at which 20% of the total amount of protein in the cell extract reacted. The results are shown in Table 2. It is seen that all antibodies against the same protein could be readily differentiated in this manner; in fact, each antibody could be identified by a simple cryptogram of the type 150/39, which signifies the dilutions of a 1 mg/ml solution of antibody that react with 20% of the maximum amount of protein of serotype 1 and 2 proteins respectively, relative to that of the serotype 3 protein, which is taken to be 100. As can be seen, all 19 antibodies are clearly different. Further, it is seen that by far the most type-specific protein is protein σ1, since the four monoclonal antibodies against it are able to react only with the homologous protein, and not with the heterologous ones.

TABLE 2

MEASUREMENT OF THE ABILITY OF THE 19 HYBRIDOMA-SECRETED IgGs TO PRECIPITATE PROTEINS SPECIFIED BY REOVIRUS SEROTYPES 1, 2, AND 3

IgG secreted by hybridoma cell line	Reovirus serotype[a]			Reovirus serotype[b]		
	1	2	3	1	2	3
λ2-A	42	29	75	150	39	100
λ2-B	42	26	64	66	41	100
μl/μlC-A	6060	1307	1600	379	82	100
μl/μlC-B	1960	226	556	352	41	100
μl/μlC-C	606	444	833	73	53	100
μl/μlC-σ3-A	2702	2061	909	267	226	100
μNS-A	2409	185	540	446	34	100
μNS-B	631	669	451	140	148	100
μNS-C	1299	1000	313	415	319	100
μNS-D	13	4.6	12	109	39	100
σ1-A	0[c]	0	69	0	0	100
σ1-B	0	0	222	0	0	100
σ1-C	7	0	952	0.7	0	100
σ1-D	0	0	289	0	0	100
σ2-A	208	566	600	35	94	100
σ2-B	176	139	243	73	57	100
σ3-A	13	0	12	108	0	100
σNS-A	1818	870	3508	52	25	100
σNS-B	2247	2739	4347	52	63	100

[a] *The figures in these three columns are the reciprocals of the dilutions of 1 mg/ml IgG solutions which precipitated 20% of the maximum amount of antigen precipitate. The maximum concentration of each IgG used was 1 mg/ml.*

[b] *The figures in these three columns are those in the first three columns normalized with respect to the serotype 3 (the homologous) value.*

Similar analyses were carried out to determine the efficiency with which these monoclonal antibodies were able to neutralize the infectivity of the three serotypes of reovirus, inhibit hemagglutination by the three serotypes of reovirus, and precipitate virus particles of the homologous serotype. The results are summarized in Table 3 (Hayes et al., 1981). Three proteins gave rise to neutralizing antibody: these were proteins σ1, σ3 and λ2. Neutralization by antibodies against σ1 was essentially type-specific; neutralization by antibody against σ3 was partially group- and partially type-specific; and neutralization by antibodies against λ2 was group-specific. As for the HI activity, this is also an property of antibodies against σ1, σ3 and λ2, and it was almost completely type-specific in all cases. Finally, antibodies against these same three proteins were capable of precipitating reovirus particles.

TABLE 3

NEUTRALIZATION OF HOMOLOGOUS AND HETEROLOGOUS REOVIRUS SEROTYPES BY HYBRIDOMA IgGs[a]

IgG or antiserum	Serotype 1	Serotype 2	Serotype 3
λ2-A	2,100	1,140	1,820
λ2-B	2,220	1,960	2,520
μ1/μ1C-A	–	–	–
μ1/μ1C-B	–	–	–
μ1/μ1C-C	–	–	–
μ1/μ1C-σ3-A	–	–	–
μNS-A	–	–	–
μNS-B	–	–	–
μNS-C	–	–	–
μNS-D	–	–	–
σ1-A	–	–	720
σ1-B	–	–	580
σ1-C	500	–	660
σ1-D	–	–	1,220
σ2-A	–	–	–
σ2-B	–	–	–
σ3-A	40	–	60
σNS-A	–	–	–
σNS-B	–	–	–
45.6.TG 1.7	–	–	–
Rabbit antiserum against serotype 3 σ3	1,275	1,395	1,530
Rabbit antiserum against serotype 3 λ1	–	–	–
Rabbit antiserum against reovirus serotype 1	5,415	735	1,665
Rabbit antiserum against reovirus serotype 2	990	15,310	2,190
Rabbit antiserum against reovirus serotype 3	1,050	320	25,560

HEMAGGLUTINATION INHIBITION OF HOMOLOGOUS AND HETEROLOGOUS REOVIRUS SEROTYPES BY HYBRIDOMA IgGs[a]

IgG or antiserum	Serotype 1	Serotype 2	Serotype 3
λ2-A	120	960	15,360
λ2-B	–	240	1,920
μ1/μ1C-A	–	–	–
μ1/μ1C-B	–	–	–
μ1/μ1C-C	–	–	–
μ1/μ1C-σ3-A	–	–	–
μNS-A	–	–	–
μNS-B	–	–	–
μNS-C	–	–	–
μNS-D	–	–	–
σ1-A	–	–	1,920
σ1-B	–	–	122,880
σ1-C	480	–	245,760
σ1-D	–	–	122,880
σ2-A	–	–	–
σ2-B	–	–	–
σ3-A	–	–	480
σNS-A	–	–	–
σNS-B	–	–	–
45.6.TG 1.7	–	–	–
Rabbit antiserum against reovirus serotype 3 σ3	105	105	13,450
Rabbit antiserum against reovirus serotype 3 λ1	–	–	–
Rabbit antiserum against reovirus serotype 1	294,910	1,150	385
Rabbit antiserum against reovirus serotype 2	1,200	153,600	800
Rabbit antiserum against reovirus serotype 3	2,690	1,345	21,505

RIP OF REOVIRUS SEROTYPE 3 BY HYBRIDOMA IgGs[a]

IgG or antiserum	Percentage precipitation
λ2-A	100
λ2-B	100
μ1/μ1C-A	29
μ1/μ1C-B	7
μ1/μ1C-C	5
μ1/μ1C-σ3-A	65
μNS-A	4
μNS-B	4
μNS-C	4
μNS-D	28
σ1-A	67
σ1-B	52
σ1-C	64
σ1-D	59
σ2-A	2
σ2-B	2
σ3-A	93
σNS-A	1
σNS-B	1
45.6.TG 1.7	1
PBS	1
Rabbit antiserum against reovirus serotype 3 (1:10)	100
Rabbit antiserum against reovirus serotype 3 λ1 (1:10)	2
Rabbit antiserum against reovirus serotype 3 σ3 (1:10)	100
Nonimmune rabbit serum (1:10)	2

[a] *Measurement of the ability of hybridoma IgGs to neutralize reovirus infectivity, inhibit hemagglutination by reovirus, and precipitate reovirus particles. The numbers in the left and center panels are the reciprocals of the dilutions of 10 mg/ml IgG solutions that reduce titers by 50 percent or completely inhibit hemagglutination. The final IgG concentration in the panel on the right was 0.5 mg/ml.*

Two antibodies against μ1/μ1C were also capable of doing this, while the other two antibodies against μ1/μ1C could not.

This analysis showed that the ratios of the efficiencies with which antibodies can combine with antigens, neutralize infectivity, effect HI and precipitate virus particles vary widely. For example, the monoclonal antibody against protein σ3 possessed weak neutralizing and HI activity, but precipitated particles very efficiently; certain antibodies against μ1/μ1C precipitated reovirus particles, but did not neutralize or possess HI activity; and so on. These ratios even vary among the monoclonal antibodies against the same protein. For example, of the four antibodies against σ1, one clearly possesses very weak neutralizing and HI activity but strong binding activity, while others possess relatively stronger HI activity relative to neutralizing activity than others, and so on. Clearly such differences point to the existence of functional domains on the various reovirus proteins, which can be studied using monoclonal antibodies (Hayes et al., 1981).

Finally, using monoclonal antibodies it was also possible to show that protein σ1 is the reovirus cell attachment protein; in fact, protein σ1 can adsorb to cells by itself, and its ability to adsorb is competed for by reovirus particles. Further, protein σ1 is located on the surface of reovirus particles in close proximity with protein λ2 because antibodies against λ2, but not antibodies against μ1/μ1C or σ3, are capable of preventing antibodies against σ1 from combining with protein σ1 (Lee et al., 1981b).

This series of experiments served not only to characterize the monoclonal antibodies against reovirus that we had isolated, but also yielded a large amount of new information. Thus, until then it had not been known that proteins μNS and λ2 existed in cells not only in the form of the uncleaved proteins, but also in the form of cleavage products, which presumably have some function (as yet unknown) during the reovirus multiplication cycle; that protein μ1 is cleaved to its cleavage product μ1C at the time when it forms a complex with protein σ3; that protein λ2, a component of reovirus cores, extends through the outer capsid shell so that it can be "seen" from the outside; that antibodies against the various surface components of reovirus particles differ greatly in their relative ability to interact with and affect various properties of reovirus particles; that protein σ1 is the reovirus cell attachment protein; and that protein σ1 is located on reovirus particles in close proximity to protein λ2. All these new pieces of information were obtained as "fall-out" of the study to characterize the 19 monoclonal antibodies.

For viral diagnostics, the two primary take-home lessons from this series of experiments were that a) when extracts of cells infected with any one of a series of related viruses are mixed with antisera against these viruses or antibodies against their proteins, highly reproducible and specific reaction patterns are obtained that one should be able to use to identify antisera/ antibodies against unknown viruses; and b) it should be possible to identify any virus, given monoclonal antibodies against its group- and type-specific proteins. We are currently trying to exploit these approaches in identifying orthopoxvirus antisera (see below).

B. *The Identification of Unknown Orthopoxvirus Antisera*

We are collaborating with the Smallpox Eradication Program of WHO in attempting to identify the specific viruses responsible for the presence of antibodies to orthopoxviruses in the sera of individuals and animals in East and Central Africa (Zaire, Congo, Gold Coast, Ivory Coast, Sierra Leone, etc.), whereas smallpox was until recently endemic. The most likely candidates are vaccinia virus (from vaccination), monkeypox virus, smallpox virus, or an unknown poxvirus. All these are members of the orthopoxvirus genus which are closely (at least 50%) related as judged by the efficiency with which their genomes hybridize with each other. They are thus related to about the same extent as reovirus serotypes 1 and 3, and it should be possible to differentiate between them and antisera against them by the approaches described above.

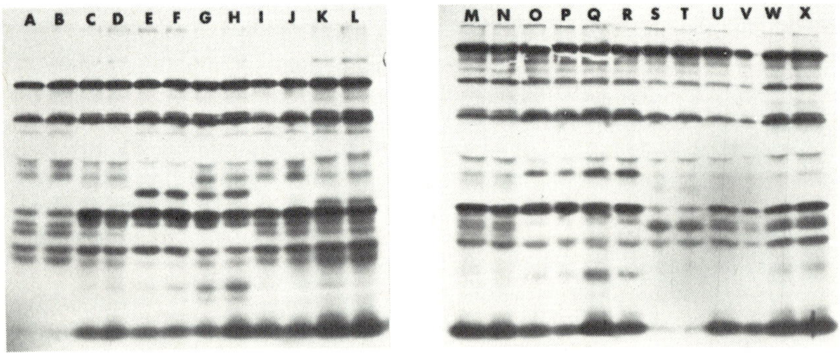

FIGURE 4. Orthopoxvirus proteins specifically precipitated by antisera to various orthopoxviruses. Lanes A to L and M to X, VV and CPV proteins, respectively. Antisera: lanes A and B, CPV; C and D, CPV; E and F, SPV; G and H, MPV; I and J, VV (rabbit antiserum); K and L, VV (mouse antiserum); M and N, CPV; O and P, SPV; Q and R, MPV; S to V, VV (rabbit antisera); W and X, VV (mouse antiserum).

The first of these approaches is illustrated in Fig. 4. Antisera (rabbit or human) to smallpox virus (SPV), monkeypox virus (MPV), cowpox virus (CPV) or vaccinia virus (VV) were added to extracts of cells infected with either CPV or VV and labelled with [^{35}S] methionine from 12-15 h after infection. The antigens in the resulting antigen-antibody complexes were then identified by polyacrylamide gel electrophoresis and autoradiography as described above.

It is seen that the four antisera can be readily differentiated from each other on the basis of their antigen-reaction patterns. It is clear that the ratios of the amounts of antibodies in these antisera to various antigens in the infected cell extracts, and the relative affinities of these antibodies for homologous and heterologous orthopoxvirus proteins are sufficiently different for the various antigen-antibody reaction patterns to be unequivocally differentiable. Further, unknown antisera can be readily identified by reference to these authentic standard antisera. We plan to include extracts of cells infected with MPV in this test in the near future, which should increase the accuracy of the identification of unknown orthopoxvirus antisera still further.

C. *The Isolation and Characterization of Monoclonal Antibodies to Orthopoxviruses*

We have started a program to isolate and characterize monoclonal antibodies against two orthopoxviruses, CPV and VV. The technique is similar to that which yielded the monoclonal antibodies against reovirus: mice are injected

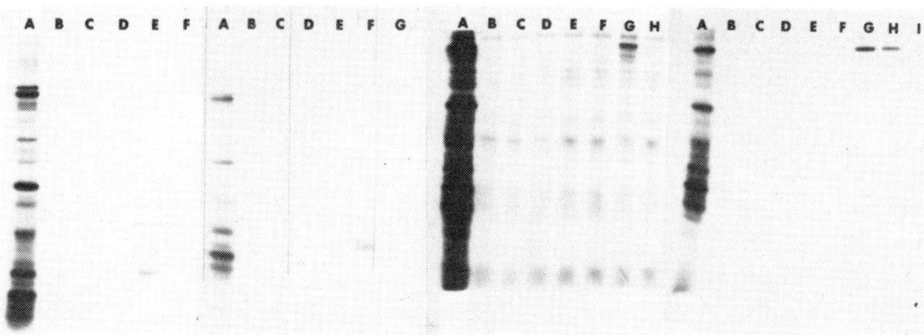

FIGURE 5. Examples of monoclonal antibodies against CPV proteins demonstrated by the RIP technique.

repeatedly with virus, sacrificed, and their spleen cells fused with 45.6.TG1.7 myeloma cells. Among the antibodies secreted by the resulting hybridoma cell lines are the five shown in Fig. 5, which are directed against CPV proteins. Experiments are currently underway to determine the efficiency with which they react with CPV, VV and MPV proteins, that is, to determine the degree of their type-specificity, and whether any of them can be used for specific and unequivocal virus identification.

D. Cloning and Sequencing of Reovirus Genes

Cloning of viral genes, particularly the genes of RNA viruses, can provide very powerful tools for diagnosis. Cloned genes can be highly labelled, thereby providing highly specific and sensitive probes for viral nucleic acids; their restriction endonuclease patterns provide useful information for identifying virus strains; if cloned in vectors in which they can express themselves, they can provide proteins for preparing monospecific antisera which are often much more useful than monoclonal antibodies; and finally, they can be sequenced readily, thereby providing additional information for the unequivocal identification of virus isolates.

We have recently cloned the ten genes of reovirus by polyadenylating both of their strands, transcribing them into cDNA, tailing them with poly(C), annealing them and inserting them into the Pstl site of pBR322. It is easy to clone fragments of reovirus genes; it is much more difficult to clone the entire genes. The only certain way of proving that entire genes have been cloned is to compare the terminal sequences of the cloned inserts with those of the uncloned genes. Fig. 6 shows the sequences at both ends of all ten genes of reovirus serotype 3 (strain Dearing) (Li et al., 1980; Gaillard et al., 1982; Antczak et al., 1982), as well as an example of one of the genes that we have cloned, namely the S2 gene (Esparza et al., 1982). We are currently sequencing the reovirus genes that we have cloned; are engaged in computer analyses to discover which sequence elements cause some reovirus genes to express themselves frequently in infected cells (that is, the protein that they encode is synthesized in large amounts), while others express themselves only very infrequently; are attempting to identify the sequence elements responsible for assembling

THE 5'-TERMINAL SEQUENCES OF THE PLUS STRANDS OF
THE REOVIRUS SEROTYPE 3 GENES

Gene

5'

L1 GCUACACGUUCCACGACAAUGUCAUCCAUGAUACUGACUCAGUUUGGACCGUUCAUUGAGAGCAUUCAG . . . .

L2 GCUAAAUGGCGCGAUGGCGAACGUUUGGGGGUGAGACUUGCAGACUCGUUAUCUUCACCCACUAUUGAGACACGA . . . . . .

L3 GCUAAUCGUCAGGAUGAAGCGGAUUCCAAGGAAGACAAAGGGCAAAUCCAGCGGAAAGGGCAAUGACUCAACAGAGAGA . . . .

M1 GCUAUUCGCGGUCAUGGCUUACAUCGCAGUUCCUGGCGUGAUUCACGUUCGAGUAXCUAUUACUGCUAGAAUCGUU . . . . .

M2 GCUAAUCUGCUGACCGUUACUCUGCAAAGAUGGGGAACGCUUCCUCUAUCGUUCAGACGAUCAACGUCAC . . . .

M3 GCUAAAGUGACCGUGGUCAUGGCUUCAUUCAAGGGAUUCUCCGCUAACACUGAU . . . .

S1 GCUAUUGGUCXGAUGGAUCCUCGCCUACGUGAAGAAGUAGUACGGCUGAUAAUCGCAUUAACGAGUGAUAAUGGAG . . . . . .

S2 GCUAUUCGCUGGUCAGUUAUGGCUCGCGCUGCGUUCCUAUUCAAGACUGUUGGUUUGGUGGUCUGCAAAAUGUGCAU . . . . .

S3 GCUAAAGUCACGCCUGUCGUCGUCACUAUGGCUUCCUCACUCAGAGCUGCGAUCUCCAAGAUCAAGAGGGAUGACGUCGG . . . .

S4 GCUAUUUUUGCCUCUUCCCAGACGUUGUCGCAAUGGAGGUGUGCUUGCCCAACGGUCAUCAGGUCGUGGACUUAAUUAACGCUUU .

Clone S132 (S2 gene)

G_9-GCTATTCGCTGGTCAGTTATGGCTCGCGCTGCGTTCCTA . . . .

THE 3'-TERMINAL SEQUENCES OF THE PLUS STRANDS OF
THE REOVIRUS SEROTYPE 3 GENES

Gene

L1 CGUGUCGUCACUUGGACAGAGAUUCAUGACUUGGAUGCGACAGGAAGGAGGUCAGCGUGAGUCAUCAUGGGUCGUGGUGCGUCAACUCAUC-OH 3'

L2 . . . . . UGAAUCAAUAAUUGUGCACCGGUGAUUAUACCUUGACUCCUCUGUAACUCACUGUCCCUCGUGAGCGCGCCUAAUUCAUC-OH 3'

L3 . . . . CAGGUGCUGGCAUUGG(C)CUCAAUGCUAGUUGGGCCGAUUCAUC-OH 3'

M1 . . . . . . GCGUGAUCGUGACAUGCGUAGUGUGAGUACUAGGUCAAUGGGGUAGGGGGCGGGCUAAGACUACGUACGCGCUUCAUC-OH 3'

M2 . . . . GGUGGUCAACGUGGGUACACACGUUAGGCCGCUCCGCCUGGUGACGCGGGUUAAGGGAUGCAGGCAAAUCAUC-OH 3'

M3 . . . . CUGAUGAGUUGUAAAUAAUCCGUGUAGCAGUGUUGCCCUAAUCCCUUUAAGCCUUCCCGGGCCACAUUCAUC-OH 3'

S1 . . . . GGUGCUGCUAGACCGUUUCGUACCCGCGUAGUUUCACGUGAGGAUXAGACCCACGCGGCACUGGGGCAUUUCAUC-OH 3'

S2 . . . . CGAUUCGAGCCCUUAUCUGAUCAGUCUUGGAGUAGGGUCCCCCCACACCCCUCACGACUGACCACACAUUCAUC-OH 3'

S3 . . . . GUAAUGGGUGAGUGAGCUGAUGUGGUCGCCAAGACAUGUGCCGGUGUCUUGGUGGUGGGUGACGCCUAAUCAUC-OH 3'

S4 . . . . UAACUAAACAACCCAUCUUCACAGCGCCGGGCUUGACCAACCUGGUGUGACGUGGGACAGGCUUCAUUCAUC-OH 3'

Clone S132 (S2 gene)

. . . . CCCCCCACACCCCTCACGACTGACCACACATTCATC-A_{11}-C_{18} 3'

FIGURE 6. The 5'-terminal (Top) and 3'-terminal (Bottom) sequences of the plus strands of the ten genes of reovirus serotype 3 (strain Dearing) (Li _et al._, 1980; Gaillard _et al._, 1982; Antczak _et al._, 1982). The sequences at the two ends of a cloned S2 gene are also shown (Esparza _et al._, 1982).

the ten different species RNA in progeny reovirus particles during the initial stages of morphogenesis; and are introducing the cloned genes both into normal cells and into cells persistently infected with reovirus mutants, in order to identify the functions of the various reovirus-coded proteins.

In summary, both hybridoma and recombinant DNA technology are about to be applied to the problem of virus identification. Owing to the great sensitivity of these new techniques it will be possible to identify viruses much earlier (and much more rapidly) following infection than has been possible so far. Not only will this greatly aid the physician in prescribing appropriate treatment, but it is also an essential prerequisite for the successul introduction of antiviral chemotherapy, which is not useful unless initiated during the early phases of infection.

REFERENCES

Antczak, J., Chmelo, R., and Joklik, W. K. (1982).

Esparza, J., Hudson, R. R., Cashdollar, L. W., Lee, P.W.K., and Joklik, W. K. (1982).

Gaillard, R. K., and Joklik, W. K. (1980). Virology 107, 533.

Gaillard, R. K., and Joklik, W. K. (1982).

Gaillard, R. K., Li, J. K.-K., Keene, J. D., and Joklik, W. K. (1982).

Hayes, E. C., Lee, P. W. K., Miller, S. E., and Joklik, W. K. (1981). Virology 108, 147.

Lee, P. W. K., Hayes, E. C., and Joklik, W. K. (1981a). Virology 108, 134.

Lee, P. W. K., Hayes, E. C., and Joklik, W. K. (1981b). Virology 108, 156.

Li, J. K.-K., Keene, J. D., Scheible, P. P., and Joklik, W. K. (1980). Virology 105, 41.

Martinson, H. G., and Lewandowski, L. J. (1985). Intervirology 4, 91.

Part IV
Control of Viral Diseases

Chairman W. K. Joklik

13

PREVENTION AND CONTROL OF CERTAIN VIRAL DISEASES IN CHILDREN-REVIEW OF THREE PRIORITY PROGRAMMES DEVELOPED BY THE WORLD HEALTH ORGANIZATION

Daniel Tarantola

Communicable Diseases Unit
World Health Organization
Manila, Philippines

I. INTRODUCTION

The World Health Organization carries out a number of programmes aimed at the prevention and control of viral diseases (1). One of them, the Viral Diseases Programme, is oriented towards research and development and is mostly carried out through an extensive network of research institutions and laboratories collaborating with WHO. This programme is quite active in the area of viral hepatitis, influenza, arboviral diseases (including Dengue haemorrhagic fever, yellow fever, other haemorrhagic fevers and Japanese encephalitis). It also serves to a large extent as support to other WHO programmes which have developed as separate entities as they are addressing major public health problems and may benefit from reinforced manpower and financial resources. In particular, the Viral Diseases Programme cuts across three major programme areas which have an important viral component and at the same time have a significant potential for reducing childhood mortality and morbidity:

The Expanded Programme on Immunization (EPI)
The Control of Diarrhoeal Disease Programme (CDD)
The Acute Respiratory Infections Programme (ARI)

Each of these programmes which we shall describe in further detail, is concerned with the prevention and control of viral diseases (Table I), but not exclusively: they may also be concerned with bacterial diseases (Pertussis,

VIRAL DISEASES IN SOUTH-EAST ASIA
AND THE WESTERN PACIFIC
ISBN 0 12 484820 6

TABLE 1. Viruses Concerned in 3 WHO Programmes

EPI[a]	CDD	ARI
Measles	*Rotavirus*	*Influenza A*
Poliomyelitis	*Adenovirus*	*Influenza B*
	Astrovirus	*Influenza C*
	Calicivirus	*Parainfluenza*
	Coronavirus	*Respiratory syncytial*
	Enterovirus	*Adenovirus*
	Other viruses-like objects	*Rhinovirus*
		Enteroviruses

[a]*Although not included in the six target diseases, there is a relationship between this programme and the prevention and control of diseases such as Yellow fever, Hepatitis, Rubella and Mumps.*

Diphtheria in EPI) or parasitic diseases (amoebic dysentery, giardiasis in CDD). The reason for grouping diseases of various aetiology under each of these three programmes is that the control measure applied (for example immunization) is the same or that these diseases share similar symptomatology and mode of transmission (for example viral and bacterial diarrhoeas). These programmes address diseases which are among the major contributing factors to under-5 mortality (Table II), particularly in Africa, Asia and Latin America where the probability of dying before the age of 5 years is more than 3 times higher than in more developed regions in the world.

A review of other successful communicable disease control programmes where *individual* pathogenic agents are involved shows that success followed:

(1) definition of the pathogen and its role in diseases;

(2) an understanding of its ecology, transmission and mode of action;

(3) interruption in the cycle of transmission or disease production at the point of maximal vulnerability with the simplest available technology.

Using these criteria, it becomes apparent that the three programmes under review have reached a different stage of development.

TABLE II. *Major Factors Contributing to Under-5 Mortality*

Age[a]	*Contributing Factors*
Prenatal	*Maternal weight gain less than 6800 grams (15 lbs.)*
Birth	*Birth weight less than 2500 grams (5.5 lbs.)*
1 month	*Neonatal tetanus*
1-12 months	*Whooping cough (pertussis)*
4-36 months	*Diarrhoea and dehydration*
6-48 months	*Malaria*
7-48 months	*Acute respiratory diseases*
8-48 months	*Under nutrition*
9-48 months	*Measles*
10-24 months	*Subsequent pregnancy*

[a]*Although the factors are considered to be most significant in the age groups shown, other age groups may also be significantly affected as, for example, with malaria.*

	EPI	CDD	ARI
Definition of pathogen and of its role	+	+	±
Understanding of ecology and mode of action	+	±	-
Development of a simple technology for control	±	±	-

These programmes have however, a number of similarities. In particular, they address the same target population - mostly children under the age of 5 years - and are implemented by the same category of health personnel: in developing countries they are mostly health centre nurses, health assistants and village health workers.

Also in common they have both a research and a services component, the latter being directed towards the implementation of prevention and control strategies at the level of the community, using the primary health care approach. The research component of these programmes encompasses basic (biomedical) research and operational (field based) research.

As these programmes develop, it becomes increasingly apparent that even when a simple and affordable technology is available, health workers have serious difficulties in applying it; they often lack adequate knowledge of epidemiological, social and behavioural factors which determine the feasibility and effectiveness of any health intervention. Here is an area where operational field based research represents a necessary bridge between basic research and actual implementation of control programmes.

II. THE EXPANDED PROGRAMME ON IMMUNIZATION

The Expanded Programme on Immunization was established as a priority programme by the World Health Organization in 1977. Its long-term objective is to reduce mortality and morbidity from six diseases, namely, diphtheria, pertussis, tetanus, tuberculosis, poliomyelitis and measles, in children of the world, particularly those under the age of 5 years. At the start of the programme, less than 10% of the 80 million children born each year in developing countries received protective immunization services. The six EPI target diseases were estimated to kill approximately 5 million children under 5 years each year and to cripple a similar number. An estimated 20% of the overal mortality in children under 5 years in developing countries was caused by these preventable diseases. Surveys promoted by EPI in the developing world have confirmed the previous estimates of the toll being taken by diseases such as measles, poliomyelitis and neonatal tetanus (2).

In the absence of immunization programmes, some four out of every 1000 school-age children will be disabled by

TABLE III. Poliomyelitis. Survey results on lameness due to poliomyelitis from areas without poliomyelitis immunization programmes.

Country	*Lame children per 1000 schoolage children*[a]	*Source*
Thailand	*2.2*	*W.E.R. No. 26/1979*
Indonesia	*3.1*	*W.E.R. No. 23/1979*
Philippines	*4.0*	*W.E.R. No. 20/1978*
Burma	*4.1*	*S.T.C. Report, 1979*
India (rural)	*4.6*	*J. Hyg. Camb. 1978*
India (urban)	*8.2*	*J. Hyg. Camb. 1978*

[a]*Schoolage is taken as starting at age 5 years. Most surveys have included an upper age limit between 10 and 15 years.*

poliomyelitis (Table III). This estimate does not take into account those who have been afflicted by the disease and have subsequently died, or those who have recovered. Measles, which kills about two per 10,000 cases in the United States of America, kills two hundred per 10,000 cases in the developing world, the figure rising to 1000 or more per 10,000 cases in malnourished populations. Without immunization, almost all children will contract this disease. Neonatal tetanus accounts in many areas for 20-50% of the total infant mortality. Figure 1 shows the reported world incidence rates per 100,000 population for measles, tetanus and poliomyelitis, 1974-1980.

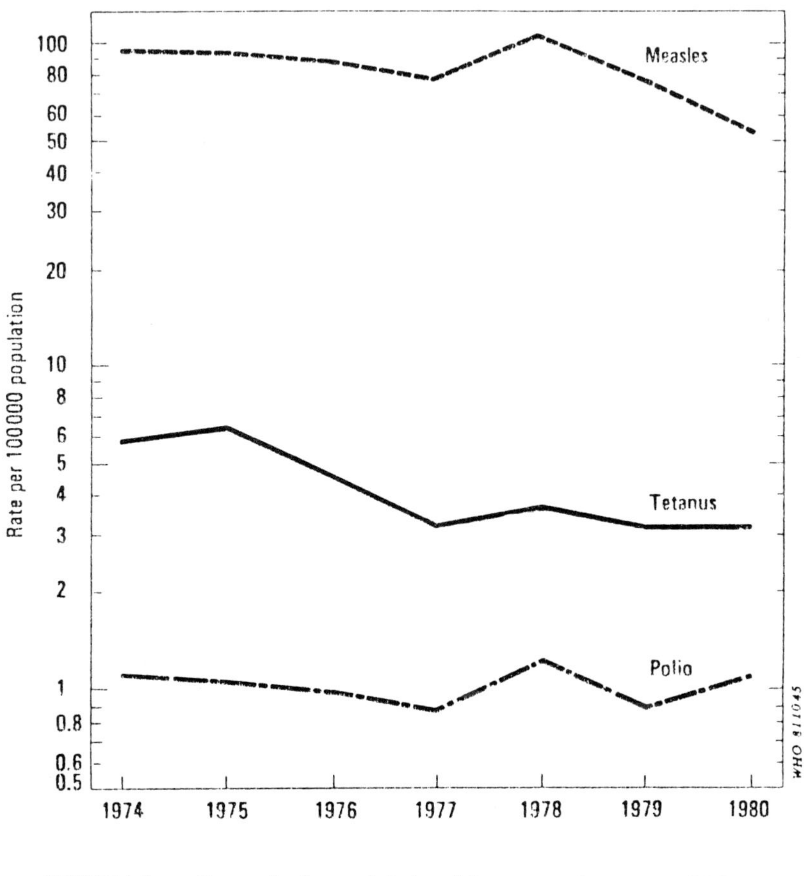

FIGURE 1. Reported world incidence rates per 100,000 population for measles, tetanus and poliomyelitis, 1974-1980.

In expanding the provision of immunization services, attention is first paid to immunizing children and pregnant women who are already utilizing fixed facilities. Next, outreach services are provided to populations which can be reached from the fixed facilities during regularly scheduled weekly or monthly visits. These services should not necessarily be limited to immunization. Once this expansion has been achieved, the far more difficult question of providing services to the population living in more remote areas is addressed.

A significant contribution of WHO to national programmes has been the cooperation provided in formulating national plans. To date, all countries in the world have some sort of immunization programme but there are still some which implement this programme without clear objectives and targets, adequately trained staff and sufficient provision of vaccines and equipment.

To remedy this situation, WHO has given high priority to the training component of the programme. To date, more than 2,000 nationals have participated in courses sponsored by WHO on the planning and management of EPI, on the cold chain or on the quality control of vaccines. While these *ad hoc* training courses were conducted, efforts were made to incorporate newly developed EPI training material in the curricula of national health manpower institutions.

The vaccines used in national programmes should be potent, safe and sufficiently stable to be used in countries where logistics pose a constant problem. The proportion of countries in the South-East Asia and Western Pacific regions using vaccines which conform to WHO requirements is 82% and 78%, respectively.

Most immunization programmes in the developing world, and some in the developed world, lack timely and reliable data concerning immunization activities and impact at national and local levels. To collect, analyze and use these data for reprogramming, WHO has actively collaborated with countries in performing comprehensive programme reviews including immunization coverage surveys and field assessment. Flow of information on activities and epidemiological surveillance still represent weak spots of most programmes in developing or developed countries.

It may be estimated that to date, some 20% of children under the age of 5 years in developing countries are fully immunized. The target of the programme is to make immunization available to all children in the world by 1990.

When EPI was launched, it was felt that the technology already available was sufficiently evolved to provide effective and safe immunization to a significant proportion of children. Research could only receive a limited portion of available resources. Considerable progress however has been achieved at least in two research areas: improvement of vaccines (3) and development of equipment needed for their storage and transport (the cold chain). Measles and poliomyelitis vaccines have become more stable under warm temperatures allowing more than half of the countries in South-East Asia and the Western Pacific regions to use them; this proportion should fast increase so that by 1990 all countries in the world use the vaccine. By the end of 1981, poliomyelitis vaccine was routinely used in 40 of the 42 countries in the two regions.

Meanwhile, new cold chain equipment was developed and alternate sources of energy (kerosene, bio-gas, charcoal, solar energy) were explored.

Indicators which change colour after exposure to certain temperatures over a given period of time have also been developed and are being tested.

More research is urgently required before the programme can further expand its geographic coverage. Special concerns include the development of approaches for delivering services which engage the full support of the community, the improvement of methods and materials relating to sterilization and to the cold chain, the acquisition of additional knowledge concerning the epidemiology of the target diseases, and further improvement in the production and quality control of vaccines.

III. THE CONTROL OF DIARRHOEAL DISEASES

In 1980, WHO reviewed data from available published prospective field studies carried out in the last three decades in which diarrhoeal disease morbidity and mortality had been measured. From these data it was estimated that in 1980 there were some 744 million to 1000 million episodes of acute diarrhoea in children under 5 years of age globally (excluding China), and that about 4.6 million of these resulted in death. The study confirmed that morbidity rates were highest in the first two years of life and particularly in the 6-11 months age group, while mortality rates were equally the greatest (about 20 per 1000) in the under-one and one-year age groups. In the first five years of life the median incidence of diarrhoea was 2.2 episodes per child per year.

From national data it is clear that in most of the developing countries the acute diarrhoeal diseases are among the leading causes of death in infants and young children under the age of five years and one of the first three causes of young childhood morbidity, often accounting for 30% or more of admissions to children's hospitals or wards (4). Moreover, diarrhoeal diseases retard the physical growth and impair the quality of life of young children and, along with malaria, are the major infectious diseases contributing to malnutrition.

At least 25 aetiological agents are responsible for acute diarrhoea, many of which have been discovered only in the last decade (Table IV). Among these, rotavirus is particularly important as a cause of infantile diarrhoea (5).

Significant research findings in the last decade have also made available new knowledge in the areas of diagnosis, treatment and prevention of acute diarrhoeas that can be used as a basis for strengthening control efforts against these diseases.

A resolution adopted by the World Health Assembly in 1978 was the first commitment of Member States to attack the

TABLE IV. Causes of Acute Diarrhoea

BACTERIA	
Vibrio cholerae 01 (Cholera)	*Salmonellae*
Vibrio cholerae Non-01 (Nag)	*Shigellae*
Vibrio parahaemoliticus	*Yersinia enterocolitica*
Enterotoxigenic *Escherichia coli*	*Campylobacter jejuni*
Other *Escherichia coli*	Foodborne Pathogens
Other Gram-Negative Organisms (Klebsiella, Citrobacter, Aeromona)	- *Staphylococcus aureus* - *Clostridium perfringens* - *Bacillus cereus*
VIRUSES	
Rotavirus	Astrovirus
Norwalk and Norwalk-like Agents	Mini-Rotavirus
Others(?) - Adenovirus - Coronavirus - Enterovirus - Calicivirus	SMV
PARASITES	
Entamoeba histolytica	*Giardia lamblia*

problem of *all* acute diarrhoeal diseases on a global scale, within the context of primary health care, and called for a programme that included activities in control, training and research.

The objectives of the Programme are to reduce the mortality caused by acute diarrhoeal diseases; to reduce the morbidity caused by diarrhoeal diseases and their associated ill-effects, particularly malnutrition, especially in infants and young children; and to promote the self-reliance of countries in the delivery of health and social services for the control of diarrhoeal disease.

Although the Programme's activities are mutlidisciplinary and have been directed towards achieving all three objectives, it has been recognized that the greatest immediate impact can be expected in the reduction of mortality.

In order to achieve its objectives, the Programme has been built up on two main components: a health *services* component concerned with the incorporation of existing knowledge on the primary health care programmes; and an action-oriented *research* component, through which support is being given both to applied (or health services) research and to basic (or biomedical) research.

At this stage of development of the global programme, emphasis is given to promoting the formulation and implementation of national CDD programmes applying the following strategies or approaches:

A. *To Reduce Diarrhoea Mortality*

The treatment of acute diarrhoea, as early as possible in the course of illness, with emphasis on *oral rehydration therapy* using a balanced glucose-electrolyte solution, accompanied by the education of mothers to feed children appropriately during diarrhoea and in convalescence (6). The solution recommended by WHO and UNICEF for oral rehydration therapy - ORS - has been proved to be effective for treating almost all cases of dehydration from acute diarrhoea of any aetiology in all age groups, and also to have a beneficial nutritional effect in children (Table V).

*TABLE V. Electrolyte Content of Stool in Acute Watery Diarrhoea and the Electrolyte and Glucose Content in ORS Solution**

		Na^+	K^+	Cl^-	HCO_3^-
Cholera stool					
- adults		140	13	104	44
- children (<5 years)		101	27	92	32
Enteritis stool					
- children (<5 years)		56	25	55	14
	Glucose				
ORS solution	111	90	20	80	30

*Values are expressed in MMOL/L.

B. To Decrease Diarrhoea Morbidity

The encouragement of maternal and child care practices; and the improvement of environmental health practices. These activities are linked with other national and international efforts during the International Drinking Water Supply and Sanitation Decade (1981-1990). During this decade, rural populations, which are largely underserved (Table VI) will receive special attention.

C. To Reduce Diarrhoea Mortality and Morbidity

The detection and control of epidemics, especially of cholera.

*TABLE VI. Estimated Coverage of the Population in Developing Countries with Water and Sanitation Services (1980)**

	Water Supply	Sanitation
Urban population	74%	53%
Rural population	29%	15%

*Based on ECOSOC country reports to the U.N. General Assembly

WHO's collaboration with countries is concentrated in the areas of programme planning, training and evaluation.

It has been clear from the outset that, at the country level, diarrhoeal disease control activities, as an essential component of primary health care, need to be integrated in, or closely linked to activities in related programmes, such as those for maternal and child health, family planning, immunization, nutrition and environmental health. As of January 1982, about 30 countries had formulated plans for national CDD programmes.

Research is the second component of the programme. Project support was initiated in a number of priority areas which included the development of improved and simplified techniques for the laboratory diagnosis of diarrhoea due to rotavirus, enterotoxigenic *E. coli* and *Campylobacter jejuni*. The testing and development of new vaccines and studies on the mode of transmission of specific pathogens (especially rotavirus and *E. coli*) and the evaluation of new products for the treatment of diarrhoea also received WHO support. To manage biomedical research, WHO has created three scientific working groups, one of which is only concerned with viral diarrhoeas (microbiology, epidemiology, immunology and vaccine development).

Support was also provided to operational research and here, priority was given to studies into the aetiology of diarrhoea, investigations of different approaches for delivery of oral rehydration therapy, studies of traditional beliefs and practices regarding diarrhoeal diseases. Although oral rehydration, a proven technology to control diarrhoeal diseases mortality, was available, difficulties were encountered by national programmes in promoting this approach and ensuring the participation of the community members in the programme. Clearly more field-based research is urgently needed in this programme area.

As of January 1982, 75 research projects in 32 countries have received funding from WHO (7).

III. ACUTE RESPIRATORY INFECTIONS

Acute respiratory infections compete with diarrhoeas as the commonest causes of mortality in children under the age of 5 years in developing countries (8).

There are several compelling reasons for WHO to evolve a worldwide control strategy for acute respiratory infections. Among them: the continuing massive morbidity from ARI with its resulting economic losses in all countries; the very high premature mortality from pneumonia-influenza in many of the less developed countries; the existence of vaccines and the need to determine their optimal usage; the emerging antibiotic resistance of many bacterial respiratory pathogens; and the likely prospect of future developments in respiratory syncytial virus vaccines and antiviral substances (9).

With ARI, the problem is quite complex, as many pathogenic agents are involved, each with different ecological needs, methods of identification and modes of action - often acting synergistically and in various combinations.

It has been estimated that infectious agents other than bacteria were responsible for the great majority of cases of acute respiratory diseases. Viruses, the most frequent, belong to several families and the relative frequency of virus association with acute respiratory diseases vary according to age (Figure 2).

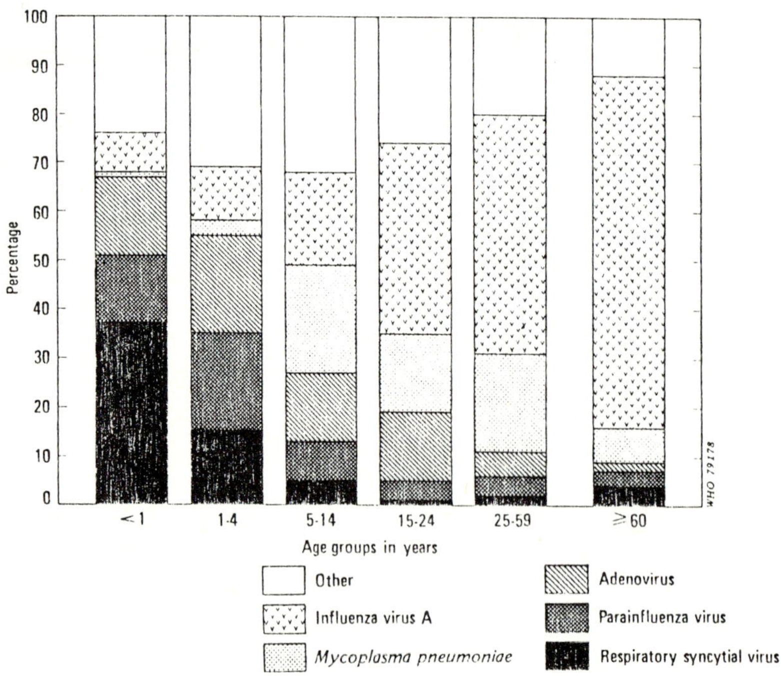

FIGURE 2. Relative frequency of virus association with acute respiratory disease by age.

In view of this complexity, the control programmes that will ultimately evolve are likely to differ from other communicable disease control programmes. One of the functions of such programmes must be the coordination between the many disciplines working on the problem, sometimes with insufficient cross-communication.

WHO created a programme for the prevention and control of Acute Respiratory Infection in 1979. Its objective is to establish a feasible scheme for the detection, treatment and prevention of acute respiratory infections and for the collection of valid information. The first priority set for this programme is the reduction of mortality in infants and children.

The currently available strategies include the upgrading of primary health care in the management of acute respiratory cases, health education programmes, immunization (potent and safe vaccines against measles, whopping cough, diphtheria, pneumococcus and influenza are already available) and the identification of high-risk individuals (10).

As a better knowledge of the problem will have to be acquired before control measures can be recommended for implementation through primary health care nationwide, the immediate approach is to establish ARI units which through active surveillance of a defined population, allow scientific conclusions about aetiology, prevention and control of ARI (11).

The establishment of agreed terminology and criteria for diagnosis will permit comparison between the few studies correlating bacteriological, virological and environmental (including behavioural) factors contributing to ARI. The monitoring of bacterial resistance should indicate the need for adjustment of standardized treatment. The first ARI unit was in Papua New Guinea where a population of about 7,500 is under surveillance implemented through fortnightly visits by project staff. Other units are operating or at their initial stage of development in Malaysia, the Phillipines, the People's Republic of China, India and Thailand.

More biomedical research is needed to obtain the appropriate technology which will determine the success of the ARI programme. There are, however, interventions such as immunization and antibiotherapy which have existed for a rather long time but have not yet been made available to the community in a rational manner as the knowledge of how to develop programmes within a community, and with its active involvement, is still largely lacking.

IV. CONCLUSIONS AND SUMMARY

Three WHO programmes, the Expanded Programme on Immunization, the Control Programme on Diarrhoeal Diseases and the Acute Respiratory Infections Programme are expected to significantly reduce morbidity and mortality in children under the age of 5 years by the direct impact they have on infectious diseases - in particular viral diseases - and the indirect effect they have on other public health problems such as undernutrition.

The technology which is currently available and forms the basis for the development of these programmes represents the successful outcome of intensive biomedical research. The EPI is using vaccines which have proved largely cost-effective and safe; the CDD offers oral rehydration therapy as the most promising approach to the control of mortality due to diarrhoeal diseases while morbidity can be prevented through improvement of feeding practices and environmental sanitation; immunization and improved clinical management are both reliable strategies for the prevention and control of acute respiratory infections.

Although well known to health workers and routinely used in developed countries, the above disease prevention and control measures are not yet available to the larger part of the world population, namely, the peoples of the developing countries. An important factor contributing to this apparent inequity is the lack of knowledge concerning the community structure, its aspirations and its ability to resolve its own problems. As a result, there is a growing gap between biomedical research - which produces the tools and constantly improves them - and actual implementation of programmes for which these tools are intended. To fill this gap, more operational - field-based - research is required. Its aim should be to acquire a better understanding of factors which, within the community, influence the success or failure of different approaches.

ACKNOWLEDGMENTS

In reviewing certain WHO programmes for the control of viral diseases, the writer used documents and publications prepared by several of his colleagues in WHO. Mention must be made of excellent review documents prepared by Dr. R. Henderson (EPI), Dr. M. Merson and Dr. D. Barua (CDD),

Dr. F. Assaad (VIR), Dr. F. Perkins (Biologicals), Dr. I. Riley (ARI).

Gratitude is also expressed to Dr. C.J. Ross-Smith for the advice and guidance he provided in compiling the information.

REFERENCES

1. World Health Organization, Sixth General Programme of Work Covering Specific Period (1978-1983). Communicable Disease Prevention and Control - Global Medium Term Programme, WHO Document (CDS/MTP/80.1).
2. Henderson, R., "Expanded Programme on Immunization, Global Strategies". Address given at the 2nd International Seminar on Vaccination in Africa, Dakar, Senegal, (1981).
3. Perkins, F.T., "Viral Vaccines", *in* Vaccination Des Enfants, Collogue INSERM-CIE-OMS, Paris, (1978).
4. Barua, D., Merson, M., Zahra, A., "Recent Advances in Diarrhoeal Diseases Control". Tenth International Congress on Tropical Medicine and Malaria, Manila, Philippines, In press, (1980).
5. World Health Organization, "Rotavirus and other Viral Diarrhoeas", Report of a sub-group of the Scientific Working Group on Epidemiology and Etiology, Document WHO/DDC/EPE/79.2, Washington (1979).
6. "Oral Rehydration Therapy, An Annotated Bibliography", Pan American Health Organization, WHO, Washington, D.C. (1980).
7. Merson, M., "The Global Problem of Acute Diarrhoeal Diseases and the WHO Diarrhoeal Disease Control Programme". Paper to be presented at the International Symposium on Bacterial Diarrhoeal Diseases, Osaka (1982) Personal communication.
8. Bulla, A., Hitze, K.L., "Acute Respiratory Infections: A Review". *Bull. Wld Hlth Org. 56,* 481 (1978).
9. Viral Respiratory Diseases, Report of a World Health Organization Scientific Group, WHO Technical Reports Series, 642 (1980).
10. Douglas, R.M., "Acute Respiratory Infections". Technical Presentation, 30th Session of the Regional Committee of the WHO, Western Pacific Region, Singapore (1979).

11. Report of the Second Meeting of the Regional Advisory Panel on ARI, WHO Regional Office for the Western Pacific, Manila (1981).

14

VACCINES - NEW DEVELOPMENTS

Robert M. Chanock, M.D

Laboratory of Infectious Diseases
National Institute of Allergy and Infectious Diseases
National Institutes of Health
Bethesda, Maryland 20205

I. VACCINES CURRENTLY OR RECENTLY IN USE

A. Live Attenuated Viral Vaccines

The first vaccine used in man contained live vaccinia virus developed by Jenner almost 200 years ago for the control of smallpox. During the ensuing two centuries, vaccinia virus has had a noble record of success in controlling this disease in many parts of the world. Vaccinia virus also played an essential role in the final eradication of smallpox. These remarkable successes were achieved despite difficulties on occasion with vaccine potency and underattenuation. As the prototype vaccine and the vaccine with the longest history of successful use, vaccinia virus continues to exert a strong influence on the formulation of strategy for the development of new vaccines for the prevention of human virus diseases.

It is ironic that the origin of this most influential of vaccine virus strains remains obscure. Attempts to determine the origin of vaccinia using modern molecular biologic techniques have yielded equivocal results. Vaccinia virus is not identical to either variola virus or cowpox virus, but has features of both, suggesting that it may be a recombinant virus (1).

Subsequent live attenuated viral vaccines have had a clearer lineage than vaccinia virus. Thus, each of the later vaccine viruses was derived from a wild-type human virus that was passaged serially in an unnatural host leading to the emergence of a host range mutant that was partially restricted in its growth in man. In this manner,

VIRAL DISEASES IN SOUTH-EAST ASIA
AND THE WESTERN PACIFIC
ISBN 0 12 484820 6

monkey kidney cell culture was used to derive attenuated mutants of the polioviruses and rubella virus. Attenuated strains of yellow fever virus and measles virus were derived in the same way using chick embryo cell culture. Finally, attenuated mumps virus was selected following serial cultivation in embryonated hens' eggs. In the case of measles virus, satisfactory attenuation required additional mutations that were selected for during growth at suboptimal temperature.

Attenuated host range mutants probably accumulate many mutations making it difficult to define in a precise way the genetic basis of satisfactory attenuation. For example, the type 1 poliovirus vaccine strain is estimated to have undergone 35 base changes during its passage and plaque purification in monkey kidney cell culture (2). Also, recent analysis of an experimental attenuated strain of influenza A virus selected by growth in chick kidney cell culture at suboptimal temperature revealed that each of the 8 viral genes had sustained one or more mutations (3).

In some instances mutant phenotypes (laboratory markers) that correlate with attenuation have been identified, but their actual role in attenuation has not been established. Thus, the genetic basis of attenuation of live vaccine viruses now in use is not known. In a sense, these satisfactorily attenuated mutants are the product of a process of genetic roulette. This is illustrated by the failure of Theiler and associates to produce additional attenuated mutants of yellow fever virus using the protocol that yielded the satisfactorily attenuated 17D strain of virus (4).

B. Inactivated Viral Vaccines

Inactivated whole virus vaccines are now in use for prevention of influenza, poliomyelitis and rabies. In each instance, virus grown in eggs (influenza), monkey kidney cell culture (poliovirus) or human diploid fibroblast cell culture (poliovirus, rabies) is inactivated with formalin. Inactivated poliovirus vaccine is highly effective in preventing disease, while influenza virus vaccine is only partially protective.

In an attempt to increase purity and decrease toxicity, semi-purified influenza virus subunit vaccines were developed. Vaccines of this type containing the hemagglutinin and neuraminidase surface antigens of the virus have proved to be less toxic than inactivated whole virus vaccine, but there has been no increase in protective efficacy.

Finally, the latest inactivated vaccine to be developed is a highly purified subunit preparation that contains the 22 nm surface antigen of hepatitis B virus (HBV) (5). This vaccine, designed to protect against type B hepatitis, is unusual because surface antigen is purified from the blood of chronically infected carriers. Although vaccine prepared in this manner is effective in preventing type B hepatitis, it will not be widely used since it is very expensive as a consequence of the complex purification procedure and lengthy safety test required for its production and certification. This is unfortunate since many of the populations most in need of immunization are in the Pacific and Asia.

C. Relative Advantages and Disadvantages of Vaccines Containing Non-replicating Antigen or Live Attenuated Virus

Non-replicating antigens should be satisfactory for use in prevention of viral diseases in which systemic spread plays an important role in pathogenesis. Thus, inactivated poliovirus vaccine is highly effective in prevention of poliomyelitis. However, it should be noted that the inactivated vaccine is less effective than live attenuated poliovirus vaccine in protecting the gastrointestinal tract from infection. The purified hepatitis B surface antigen vaccine provides significant protection against type B hepatitis, but the duration of this resistance has not been established (5).

My thoughts about immunoprophylaxis against viral infections that affect primarily mucosal surfaces are heavily influenced by the important role played by local immunity in resistance to most respiratory and gastrointestinal pathogens. Infection of the respiratory or gastrointestinal tract induces systemic immunoglobulin and cell mediated immunity as well as local immunity and thus all phases of host defense are brought into play. For these reasons live vaccines offer a potential advantage over non-replicating antigen vaccines for use in prevention of viral diseases limited primarily to mucosal surfaces.

Difficulties associated with inactivated influenza virus vaccine can be cited to support this view. Inactivated influenza virus vaccine provides significant but not complete protection. The vaccine is also less than ideal since it loses it effectiveness when used on an annual basis which is the schedule recommended for individuals in the high risk category (6). The phenomenon of original antigenic sin probably plays a role in the diminished effect of vaccine administered yearly.

Two other factors probably play a role in diminishing the effectiveness of inactivated influenza antigen in prophylaxis. First, in man influenza is primarily a topical infection limited to the respiratory tract. In this situation local immunity within the respiratory tract plays an important role in resistance. It is known that inactivated antigen inoculated parenterally is less effective than infection in stimulating local respiratory tract immunity. Second, cytotoxic T cells play an important role in recovery from influenza virus infection, constituting an integral arm of host defense. Recent studies suggest that inactivated antigen is less effective than infection in inducing this desired cytotoxic T cell response (7). Indeed, inactivated antigen may stimulate a suppressor T cell response that could adversely affect the induction of immunity. These various phenomena may help explain why infection immunity is broader, more effective and more durable than that induced by inactivated influenza virus or subunit antigens derived from the virus.

It should be noted, however, that live viral vaccines are not without their problems. The most serious of these difficulties is genetic instability that is typified by the emergence of virus with altered phenotype during the course of infection with vaccine virus. For example, virus with increased neurovirulence for monkeys is often shed by vaccinees infected with live attenuated poliovirus vaccine (8). Genetic instability was also a problem with the live yellow fever virus vaccine during its early history when some batches of vaccine caused encephalitis (9). It has been particularly difficult to address these problems since the genetic basis of attenuation is not known and hence cannot be studied directly.

III. NEW APPROACHES TO IMMUNOPROPHYLAXIS

A. Non-replicating Antigens

Recent advances in molecular biology and peptide synthesis provide a basis for producing virtually unlimited quantities of purified viral protein for use in immunoprophylaxis. Success of this approach will not be limited by technological constraints. Instead, the issue will be determined separately for each virus by the effectiveness of viral protein in providing protection against disease caused by that virus. As mentioned earlier, it is likely that purified viral proteins will prove more effective in prevention of systemic viral diseases than in those limited primarily to mucosal surfaces. Two separate approaches to the production of purified viral antigens are currently being explored. In both instances the viral genome or viral messenger RNA is cloned in E. coli and its sequence is determined by one of the rapid methods now in widespread use.

Once the nucleic acid sequence is known, the amino acid sequence can be deduced and the stage is set for the production of synthetic peptides for use as immunogens. The feasibility of this approach was first demonstrated by Langbehein, Arnon and Sela who studied a synthetic icosapeptide that represents the immunodominant region of the outer coat protein of MS-2 bacteriophage (10). Initially, a cyanogen bromide fragment of coat protein that reacted with neutralizing antibodies was identified and sequenced. This icosapeptide was then synthesized and conjugated to a synthetic carrier, poly-DL alanine, yielding an immunogen that stimulated the development of neutralizing antibodies in rabbits when administered in Freund's complete adjuvant. Subsequently an adjuvant more suitable for use in man was sought for this prototype synthetic peptide antigen. This led to the observation that the synthetic viral peptide-carrier conjugate was also antigenic when covalently linked to a chemically defined bacterial peptidoglycan, derived from Bacillus megaterium. The antibody response in rabbits, however, was somewhat lower than when Freund's complete adjuvant was used as adjuvant.

Rapid progress in determining the RNA or DNA sequence of various viral genes has simplified the selection of peptides with potential antigenic activity. For example, the base sequences of hepatitis B surface antigen and influenza A virus hemagglutinin have been used by Lerner and associates to identify highly hydrophilic regions that presumably occupy an external location on these viral surface proteins (11,12). Based on this information, short hydrophilic peptides were synthesized and coupled covalently to keyhole limpet hemocyanin (KLH) that served as carrier. When inoculated in combination with Freund's complete adjuvant, many of the hydrophilic HBV peptides stimulated antibodies that reacted with surface antigen of the virion. Similarly, antibodies induced by hydrophilic influenza A virus peptides neutralized virus infectivity in an *in vivo* assay. Apparently these small peptides exist in an equilibrium in which all possible conformations are assumed and the conformation corresponding to that present on the virus surface stimulates antibodies reactive with intact virus. Evaluation of synthetic viral peptides in man awaits the identification or development of an acceptable, effective adjuvant. Perhaps synthetic peptidoglycans such as MDP may serve this function (13).

Cloned viral DNA derived from the viral genome or viral messenger RNA can also be used to transform *E. coli* or yeast to produce the desired viral protein. Successful expression of foot-and-mouth disease virus VP3 capsid protein, HBV surface antigen, and influenza A virus hemagglutinin was recently achieved in *E. coli* (14-15). In each instance cloned viral DNA was inserted in a plasmid downstream from a strong bacterial promoter, such as the lac or tryp promoter, thus assuring efficient expression. Expression from the tryp promoter was enhanced by derepression. Insertion of the viral DNA sequences downstream from the amino terminus of a bacterial gene controlled by the promoter also enhanced expression and facilitated purification of viral antigen in the form of a fused bacterial-viral protein. When the bacterial tryp leader (large L) gene and the last third of the tryp E gene were employed for this purpose, purification was facilitated because the fused viral-bacterial protein was insoluble. Using the tryp operator and tryp leader (L) and a portion of the tryp (E) protein, foot-and-mouth disease virus VP3 was expressed efficiently in *E. coli*, accounting for 17% of protein produced in transformed bacteria (14).

Several factors may limit the effectiveness of viral protein produced by transformed bacteria. First, *E. coli* does not possess a pathway for glycosylation of proteins.

This could limit the usefulness of this method for production of glycoproteins such as influenza A virus hemagglutinin and HBV surface antigen. Transfer of cloned viral DNA into a vector suitable for transformation of yeast might solve this problem because yeast possesses the appropriate glycosylation pathway. Recently a plasmid vector containing a strong yeast promoter was used successfully by Hitzeman and associates to express an interferon gene in yeast (17). Approximately 1% of the protein produced by transformed yeast was interferon that exhibited antiviral activity. Unfortunately, evidence for glycosylation of interferon was not sought.

Second, some proteins such as picornavirus capsid proteins and HBV surface antigen are considerably less antigenic in the dissociated state than when present on the surface of the virus. For example, purified foot-and-mouth disease VP3 capsid protein is 1000 times less antigenic than the same protein present on the surface of intact virus (14).

Decreased antigenicity might be overcome in part by inoculating a large amount of purified antigen combined with a potent immunologic adjuvant. The feasibility of this approach was recently demonstrated by Kleid and associates for foot-and-mouth disease VP3 produced in *E. coli* (14). Administration of this viral capsid protein in Freund's incomplete adjuvant induced serum neutralizing antibodies in cows and these animals were resistant to subsequent challenge with virulent foot-and-mouth disease virus. Success in applying this approach to man requires the development of an acceptable, potent adjuvant that can be used in place of Freund's incomplete adjuvant. Perhaps equally important is the question of duration of immunity, an issue that remains to be investigated.

B. Live Attenuated Virus Vaccines

Viruses bearing specific, identifiable, attenuating mutations represent the live vaccine strains of the future because the genetic basis for attenuation is known and can be monitored directly during all phases of vaccine development, manufacture, and utilization in humans.

C. Negative-strand RNA Viruses

The greatest success in producing and characterizing such attenuating mutations has been achieved with influenza

A virus, whose segmented genome facilitates the segregation and characterization of individual genes. Although current inactivated influenza virus vaccines are effective, they do not provide complete protection nor do they appear to retain their effectiveness when administered annually. For this reason there is renewed interest in the development of a live attenuated virus vaccine that would mimic natural infection in its greater, broader, and more durable immunity.

Several groups have sought to produce mutant influenza genes that would confer a satisfactory level of attenuation upon any virus into which they were transferred by genetic reassortment. In studies performed by Murphy and associates, chemical mutagenesis was used to produce temperature-sensitive (*ts*) mutations on genes that code for nonsurface viral proteins so that the mutant genes could be transferred into reassortant viruses bearing the surface antigens of new epidemic or pandemic strains (18). It is implicit in this approach that chemically induced *ts* mutations are primarily responsible for the attenuation of reassortant viruses bearing *ts* genes. This was shown to be the case for reassortants derived from two different *ts* donor viruses (18).

Although the *ts* genes from one of these donor viruses, *ts*-1A2, conferred a satisfactory level of attenuation upon a series of reassortant viruses, it became clear that genetic instability represented an insoluble problem. During infection of a susceptible child, one of the *ts*-1A2 reassortants underwent a complex set of genetic alterations, including suppression, that led to loss of the *ts* phenotype and restoration of virulence, even though the *ts* reassortant was greatly restricted in its ability to replicate *in vivo*. Genetic instability has also plagued the development of *ts* mutants of RS virus suitable for use in immunoprophylaxis.

Another technique now being actively pursued for rapid attenuation of new influenza A viruses involves the use of a donor virus that grows well at a suboptimal temperature which does not support efficient replication of wild-type virus. The A/Ann Arbor/6/60 (H2N2) donor strain was adapted by Maassab to grow well at 25°C by serial passage at successively lower temperatures (33°C-25°C) in primary chick kidney cell culture (19). This virus was also shown to be *ts* with a shutoff temperature for plaque formation of 38°C (19). Genes from this cold-adapted (*ca*) donor strain were transferred to a succession of new antigenic variants of influenza A virus, and reassortant viruses bearing the ca and ts properties of the attenuated donor virus were isolated. Several reassortants that derived the ca and ts properties from the A/Ann Arbor/6/60 donor virus were shown to be attenuated for ferrets (19). The genes of the A/Ann Arbor/6/60 donor virus responsible for attenuation and for the ca and ts phenotypes have not been fully identified; however, its P3, P2, and NP genes are present in all A/Ann Arbor/6/60 ca reassortants that possess the ca and ts phenotypes (3).

Ideally, reassortant viruses produced by mating the A/Ann Arbor/6/60 ca donor and a new epidemic influenza A virus should receive all their nonsurface viral protein genes from the ca donor and their surface glycoprotein genes from the new variant. Maassab and his associates have produced ca reassortants with this gene constellation by mating the A/Ann Arbor/6/60 ca donor and wild-type virus at 25°C, a temperature restrictive for replication of wild-type virus. Sixty-six percent of ca reassortants produced in this manner have the desired gene constellation (19).

Four separate ca reassortants containing the six transferable genes of the A/Ann Arbor/6/60 donor strain and the surface glycoprotein genes of successive H1N1 or H3N2 wild-type human influenza A viruses were evaluated in susceptible adult volunteers to determine whether genes from the cold-adapted donor regularly confer a satisfactory level of attenuation on new epidemic wild-type viruses. Two of the reassortants induced only a few minor illnesses, whereas the other two reassortants caused a systemic or febrile illness in 3 to 8% of volunteers. In addition, Wright and his colleagues observed that ca reassortants were satisfactorily attenuated in a limited number of doubly seronegative children (20). These results indicate that the six transferable genes present in the A/Ann Arbor/6/60 donor virus can render epidemic influenza A viruses attenuated for fully susceptible individuals.

During replication in susceptible individuals, most of the ca reassortant viruses were stable genetically. Those reassortant viruses that possessed all six transferable A/Ann Arbor/6/60 genes retained the ts and ca phenotypes. However, instability of the ca phenotype was observed with two reassortants that received only five of the six transferable A/Ann Arbor/6/60 genes (18). These findings suggest that the potential for genetic instability exists. What is not clear, however, is the effect of such genetic change on attenuation. Perhaps other silent mutations that have been introduced into genes of the ca donor will provide a safety net that prevents reversion to virulence.

It is clear from this discussion that one of the most urgent needs in immunoprophylaxis is the development of satisfactorily attenuated mutants that are completely stable genetically. Restriction of growth of an attenuated mutant in vivo exerts positive selection for new mutations that allow the virus to grow better and to escape the limitations imposed by its original mutations. We need stable mutants that are unable to escape from their attenuated phenotype by reversion and/or suppression during replication in completely susceptible individuals.

It may be possible to produce stable attenuated reassortant influenza viruses by using an avian influenza A virus that is restricted in primate cells as the donor of attenuating genes (18). In this situation, restriction would be effected by naturally occurring avian influenza virus genes rather than by mutant genes selected by limited passage of human virus in an unnatural host. In studies performed by Murphy in collaboration with Hinshaw, Webster and London, potential avian influenza A donor viruses were evaluated for evidence of restriction of growth in squirrel monkeys. Two of ten influenza A viruses recovered from asymptomatic birds were clearly restricted in their replication in the lower respiratory tract of the squirrel monkey. These two viruses appeared to be of avian origin since they were strongly enterotropic in ducks, a property not exhibited by human influenza A viruses.

Reassortants produced by mating a restricted avian virus with a virulent human influenza A virus are currently under study by Murphy in an attempt to identify the avian influenza gene or genes responsible for restriction of growth in primate cells, as well as possible incompatible human-avian gene constellations that might also restrict growth. Once the restricting avian genes and incompatible human-avian gene constellations are identified,it should be possible to construct an appropriate donor virus by genetic reassortment. Studies in progress indicate the feasibility of this approach. It appears that avian surface antigen genes are not required for restriction of human-avian influenza virus reassortants. On the other hand, the other

6 transferable avian genes can confer the desired level of attenuation on human-avian reassortants. Significantly, infection of monkeys with a restricted reassortant of this sort induces almost complete resistance to challenge with a virulent human H3N2 influenza A virus.

Many of the influenza genes that have evolved over a long period of time in birds differ significantly from the corresponding genes of human influenza viruses when studied by nucleic acid hybridization. Because of these marked differences, it is likely that the avian genes will retain their attenuated characteristics after limited replication in man, and thereby prove to be stable phenotypically.

Another approach to the construction of stable mutants involves deletion mutations that should be stable because they are not subject to reversion, and it is unlikely that they would be easily suppressed by a new mutation at another site on the viral genome. For these reasons we have initiated attempts to produce stable deletion mutations that will render a virus sufficiently defective so that it becomes attenuated, but not so defective that it loses viability. This type of genetic surgery can only be performed on DNA. Hence those viral genomes that are composed of RNA must be transcribed into DNA and then manipulated in this form. This presents us with the difficult problem of transcribing mutant DNA into an RNA form that can be transferred back into an infectious virus.

Before discussing strategy for producing stable mutants for use in immunoprophylaxis, it should be noted that stable, viable deletion mutants of several DNA animal viruses, including the adenoviruses, have been prepared, and some of these mutants exhibit a reduced capacity for viral replication in vitro and in vivo (21-23). This is of interest because reduced replicative capacity is synonymous with attenuation.

The general plan for construction of deletion mutants of negative strand RNA viruses was developed initially by Lai, and Markoff and Sveda for influenza A virus (24,25). In the first phase of this plan, individual virus RNA gene segments were cloned using an Escherichia coli K12 plasmid system. Initially, positive and negative complementary DNA (cDNA) strands were prepared separately by reverse transcription. The positive strands of cDNA were transcribed from genomic RNA segments using a specific dodecamer DNA primer with a sequence complementary to the conserved 3'-terminal nucleotides of virion RNA. The negative strands of cDNA were transcribed from cytoplasmic polyadenylated viral messenger RNA segments using an oligo (dT) primer. The single-stranded DNA molecules from both preparations were annealed to generate double-stranded DNA segments which were then inserted into plasmid pBR322 at the specific Pst I site using the dG/dC tailing technique. The hybrid DNA molecules were then used to transform E. coli, and transformants containing influenza virus gene sequences were identified by hybridization. In this manner, putative full-length influenza virus DNA segments were obtained corresponding to genes coding for the NS proteins (gene 8), the M proteins (gene 7), the neuraminidase (gene 6), the nucleoprotein (gene 5) and the hemagglutinin (gene 4). This approach should be generally applicable to other influenza virus genes as well as to other negative-strand RNA viruses.

Sequence analysis of the terminal nucleotides of most cloned influenza DNA segments indicated that both ends of virion RNA were fully represented. This suggested that these cloned DNAs were complete and contained all the information present in the viral RNA segments from which they were derived. This was verified for the NA, M and NS genes by sequencing the entire cloned DNA. Thus, RNA transcribed from such cloned DNA should have all the control signals for viral gene replication and expression in eukaryotic cells.

In the second phase of the plan, full-length cloned influenza DNA was used to produce influenza RNA in eukaryotic cells (25). A late region deletion mutant of SV40 was used for construction of influenza DNA-SV40 hybrid molecules. The influenza DNA was inserted into the late region of the SV40 genome previously occupied by the deleted sequences that code for SV40 capsid proteins. This type of hybrid DNA molecule was propagated in eukaryotic cells that were coinfected with an early ts mutant of SV40. When cell cultures were incubated at a restrictive temperature, the hybrid influenza DNA-SV40 molecule supplied the function defective in the SV40 early ts mutant and vice versa, thereby permitting both SV40 molecules to replicate. Replication of influenza DNA-SV40 hybrid molecules in eukaryotic cells resulted in transcription of influenza messenger RNA and expression of the appropriate functional influenza protein. Currently Lai, Markoff, Sveda and Lin are investigating the possibility that cloned influenza DNA inserted in the opposite orientation into SV40 may lead to transcription of negative-strand influenza viral RNA. If negative-strand RNA is produced, it may be possible to rescue it from cells by coinfecting with an influenza virus and selecting for reassortant virus particles containing RNA coded for by the cloned DNA. In this manner, stable, site-specific mutations, such as deletions, introduced into the cloned DNA by enzyme surgery, might be transferred back into influenza virus.

D. Positive-strand RNA Viruses

Recently, a complete cloned DNA copy of the positive-strand RNA genome of poliovirus was constructed by joining 3 partial clones of this virus (26). Significantly, the complete cloned DNA was infectious for simian and human cells in culture. This important observation by Racaniello and Baltimore suggests that the cell recognizes the appropriate control signals in the cloned poliovirus DNA and employs those signals to transcribe complete (+) strands of poliovirus RNA that initiate the normal cycle of infection. Construction of deletion mutants of poliovirus and other picornaviruses, as well as other (+) RNA viruses such as togaviruses, should be relatively simple because altered cloned DNA could be transferred directly into infectious virus by transfection of cells in culture. In this manner viable deletion mutants could be identified and evaluated subsequently for attenuation and immunogenicity.

E. Double-stranded RNA Viruses

The control of rotaviral infection in infancy and early childhood represents an important public health challenge since 50% or more of severe pediatric diarrheal disease in most parts of the world is caused by the rotaviruses (27). It should be noted that diarrheal disease is the leading cause of mortality in infants and young children in developing countries. Efforts at immunoprophylaxis have been hampered by the fastidious nature of the human rotaviruses. Until recently, these viruses could not be grown serially to high titer in tissue culture. Fortunately, this obstacle was overcome during the past two years.

The first success in cultivation of human rotavirus was reported by Wyatt and his associates in our laboratory (28). He identified a tissue culture adapted mutant of the Wa strain of type 2 rotavirus that emerged during serial passage of this virus in a permissive animal host, the gnotobiotic piglet. The tissue culture adapted mutant grew to high titer and was shown to be of human origin by polyacrylamide gel analysis of its RNA and by cross-neutralization studies.

Similar efforts to select a culture-adapted mutant of type 1 human rotavirus failed since this virus could not be passaged in piglets. For this reason, Greenberg and his associates developed another strategy which took into account the segmented viral genome of the rotaviruses that belong to the family Reoviridae (29). Since other members of this virus family undergo genetic reassortment with high frequency during mixed infection, he attempted to rescue noncultivatable human rotavirus by coinfection with a cultivatable, temperature-sensitive (<u>ts</u>) mutant of bovine rotavirus.

Noncultivatable type 1 human rotavirus was inoculated into African green monkey kidney cell culture that was coinfected with a <u>ts</u> mutant of a cultivatable bovine rotavirus (29). Selection of the desired viral reassortants was achieved by exposing progeny from the mixed infection to potent, bovine rotavirus antiserum that neutralized bovine rotavirus, but not type 1 human rotavirus. Surviving virus was then plaqued at a restrictive temperature (39°C) to eliminate the <u>ts</u> bovine rotavirus parent and <u>ts</u> reassortants. In this manner, viral reassortants were recovered that (1) grew to high titer in tissue culture, (2) produced plaques with high efficiency, and (3) were specifically neutralized by antiserum to type 1 human rotavirus. Analysis of the RNA segments from these viruses confirmed that reassortment of genes had occurred. Similar reassortants were also produced with noncultivatable type 2 human virus. Recently refinements in tissue culture technique have made it possible to recover strains of each of the three human rotavirus serotypes directly in cell culture.

The scene is now set to evaluate different strains of human rotavirus for attenuation and immunogenicity in man. Manipulation of these strains to produce cold-adapted mutants may yield the desired attenuated viruses. Also, evaluation of a variety of interspecies reassortant viruses in experimental animals and in humans may shed light on the genetic determinants of virulence allowing us to identify certain mixed constellations of animal and human rotavirus genes that render viral reassortants attenuated for man and thus suitable for use in a live attenuated rotavirus vaccine. It should also be noted that antigenic relationships between animal and human rotaviruses may allow us to use the former in prophylaxis of human disease. Several years ago we showed that prior infection of calves with a bovine rotavirus protected these animals against experimental challenge with type 2 human rotavirus (28). Finally, attempts at cloning human rotavirus genes are now underway and success in this area may allow us to construct stable deletion mutants that can be evaluated in man.

F. Double-stranded DNA viruses

Previously, it was shown by our group that oral administration of live type 4 adenovirus in an enteric coated capsule produced a silent infection in the lower intestinal tract that induced effective immunity to type 4 virus (31). This type of silent, selective, enteric adenovirus infection served as the basis for the development of a type 4, type 7 adenovirus vaccine that has effectively controlled epidemic adenovirus disease in military recruits in the U.S.A. during the past 12 years. Concern for the oncogenic potential of adenoviruses has prevented extension of this method of immunization to other adenovirus serotypes, especially those important in pediatric respiratory tract disease. Although intensive efforts to link adenoviruses to human cancer have failed to establish an association, concern for possible oncogenicity lingers on. Perhaps DNA surgery can be combined with enteric vaccination to yield an effective vaccine that will gain acceptance for use in children.

The genes of type 5 adenovirus responsible for cell transformation reside in the left hand 8% of the viral genome. Using a restriction enzyme that cuts at site 4% from the left hand end of the viral genome Jones and Shenk have selected spontaneous deletion mutants lacking this site and often flanking sequences as well (22). Some of these deletion mutants exhibited the following properties desirable for a vaccine virus: (1) viability, (2) restriction of replicative capacity in human cells and (3) inability to transform cells in culture. These observations suggest that it should be possible to derive other mutants with a deletion in the transformation region that renders the affected viruses transformation-defective and restricted in their growth in human cells. The degree of growth restriction represents a critical property because the desired mutants must still be sufficiently competent to infect enough cells *in vivo* to stimulate immunity.

REFERENCES

1. Mackett, M., and Archard, L., *J. gen. Virol. 45*, 683 (1979).
2. Nomoto, A., Kitamura, N., Lee, J., Rothberg, P., Imura, N., Wimmer, E., *Virology 112*, 217 (1981).
3. Cox, N., Konnecke, I., Kendal, A., *in* "Genetic Variation Among Influenza Viruses" (D. Nayak, ed.), p.639. Academic Press, New York, (1981)
4. Theiler, M., *in* "Yellow Fever" (G.K. Strode, ed.), p.39. McGraw-Hill, (1951).
5. Szmuness, W., Stevenes, C., Harley, E., Zang, E., Oleszka, W., William, D., Daovsky, R., Morrison, J., and Kellner, A., *New Engl. J. Med. 303*, 833 (1980).
6. Hoskins, T., Davies, J., Smith, A., Miller, C., and Allchin, A., *Lancet 1*, 33 (1979).
7. Ada, G., Leung, K., Ertl, H., *Immunol. Rev. 58*, 5 (1981).
8. Melnick, J., *in* "Poliomyelitis: Papers and Discussions Presented at the Fifth International Poliomyelitis Conference, Copenhagen, Denmark, July 26-28, 1960" p.384. J.B. Lippincott, Philadelphia (1960).
9. Fox, J., Kossobudzki, S., da Cunha, J., *Am. J. Hyg. 36*, 117 (1942).
10. Langbeheim, H., Arnon, R., and Sela, M., *Immunol. 35*, 573 (1978).
11. Lerner, R., Green, N., Alexander, H., Liu, F., Sutcliffe, J., Shinnick, T., *Proc. Natl. Acad. Sci. USA 78*, 3403 (1981).
12. Lerner, R., Green, N., Olson, A., Shinnick, T., and Sutcliffe, J., *Hosp. Pract. 16*, 55 (1981).
13. Carelli, C., Audebert, F., and Chedid, L., *Inf. Immun. 33*, 312 (1981).
14. Kleid, D., Yansura, D., Small, B., Downbenko, D., Moore, D., Grubman, M., McKercher, P., Morgan, D., Robertson, B., and Bachrach, H., *Science 214*, 1125 (1981).
15. Edman, J., Hallewell, R.A., Valenzuela, P., Goodman, H., Rutter, W., *Nature 291*, 503 (1981).
16. Heiland, I., Gething, M., *Nature 292*, 851 (1981).

17. Hitzeman, R., Hagie, F., Levine, H., Goeddel, D., Ammerer, G., and Hall, B., *Nature 293*, 717 (1981).
18. Murphy, B., and Chanock, R., *in* "Genetic Variations Among Influenza Viruses" (D. Nayak, ed.), p.601. Academic Press, New York (1981).
19. Maassab, H., Spring, S., Kendal, A., and Monto, A., *in* "Negative Strand Viruses and the Host Cell" (B. Mahy and R. Barry, eds.), p.721. Academic Press, New York (1978).
20. Wright, P., Okabe, N., and Karzon, D., *in* "Current Chemotherapy and Infectious Disease" p.1346. ASM Publications, Washington, D.C. (1980).
21. Topp, W., *J. Virol. 33*, 1208 (1980).
22. Jones, N., and Shenk, T., *Cell 17*, 683 (1979).
23. McCance, D., *J. Virol. 39*, 958 (1981).
24. Lai, C., Markoff, L., Zimmerman, S., Cohen, B., Berndt, J., and Chanock, R., *Proc. Natl. Acad. Sci. USA 77*, 210 (1980).
25. Sveda, M., and Lai, C., *Proc. Natl. Acad. Sci. USA 78*, 5488 (1981).
26. Racaniello, V., and Baltimore, D., *Science 214*, 916 (1981).
27. Kapikian, A., Wyatt, R., Greenberg, H., Kalica, A., Kim, H., Brandt, C., Rodriguez, W., Parrott, R., and Chanock, R., *Rev. Infect. Dis. 2*, 459 (1980).
28. Wyatt, R., James, W., Bohl, E., Theil, K., Saif, L., Kalica, A., Greenberg, H., Kapikian, A., and Chanock, R., *Science 207*, 189 (1980).
29. Greenberg, H., Kalica, A., Wyatt, R., Jones, R., Kapikian, A., and Chanock, R., *Proc. Natl. Acad. Sci. USA 78*, 420 (1981).
30. Wyatt, R., Mebus, C., Yolken, R., Kalica, A., James, H., Kapikian, A., and Chanock, R., *Science 203*, 548 (1979).
31. Edmondson, W., Purcell, R., Gundelfinger, B., Love, J., Ludwig, W., and Chanock, R.M., *J.A.M.A. 195*, 453 (1966).

15

STABILITY OF VIRAL VACCINES IN TROPICAL AREAS

C. Huygelen
J. Peetermans
G. Colinet

Biological Division
SmithKline-RIT
Rixensart, Belgium

The objective of the Expanded Programme on Immunization (E.P.I.) of the World Health Organization is to immune all children of the world against six major diseases by 1990. Two of these diseases are of viral origin: polio and measles. E.P.I. is fully operational in most industrialized countries of the world and has recently started in most developing countries. This has led to a substantial increase in the use of these vaccines. Apart from the two virus vaccines mentioned, several others are being used increasingly in many parts of the world, e.g., rubella, mumps, yellow fever, rabies, etc. More than ever before, public health authorities realize that prophylaxis is the cheapest way to combat diseases. It is not only more economical but it also prevents much human suffering which cannot be expressed in money. The cost-benefit ratio is probably more favourable for vaccines than for any other drug or therapy. This may be even more true in less developed countries.

The organization of campaigns, the distribution of the vaccine within the country and its administration to those who need it, are the most expensive parts of immunization campaigns. It is therefore extremely important that the vaccine is still fully potent when it arrives in the field. Use of vaccines which have lost their potency before they are used results in lack of protection of whole populations of children. This affects the confidence of the population and jeopardizes the future of the vaccination programmes,

VIRAL DISEASES IN SOUTH-EAST ASIA AND THE WESTERN PACIFIC
ISBN 0 12 484820 6

especially in developing countries. This may be particularly true for measles, a preventable disease, which still has a mortality rate between 2 and over 20% in various areas of the third world.

TABLE I. Stability of Poliomyelitis Vaccines Exposed at Different Temperatures

Temperatures (°C)	Time	Mean difference with initial titre[a]	
		Sucrose stabilized	Mol. $MgCl_2$ stabilized
+ 45	(days)		
	1	-0.59	-0.47
	2	-1.01	-1.05
	3	-1.69	-1.72
	4	NT	-2.27
	5	NT	-2.92
+ 37	(days)		
	1	-0.20	-0.06
	2	-0.35	-0.32
	3	-0.74	-0.50
	6	NT	-0.70
	8	-1.30	-1.01
	12	NT	-2.00
+ 25	(weeks)		
	1	-0.10	-0.10
	2	-0.30	-0.14
	3	-0.50	-0.32
	6	NT	-0.50
	12	NT	-1.20
+ 2 to + 6	(months)		
	1	0.00	0.00
	6	-0.20	0.00
	8	-0.40	-0.10
	12	-0.55	-0.20
	15	NT	-0.10
	18	NT	-0.30

[a] Log_{10} $TCID_{50}$

Vaccines are usually protected from high environmental temperatures by using a cold chain, and in this respect much progress has been made in various countries with the help of W.H.O. However, it must be realized that cold chains can break down for many different reasons, and therefore, vaccine manufacturers should attach much importance not only to the potency of the product at the time when it leaves the factory, but also to its stability. Accidental exposures to higher temperatures can occur during the transportation from the manufacturer to the country of destination, but in the case of less industrialized countries, they usually occur in the country itself between the time the vaccine leaves the refrigerators in the capital and its arrival in the small villages where a large portion of the target population lives.

Some virus vaccines are freeze-dried, others not. For example, live oral polio vaccine is presented in the liquid form because polio virus is difficult to freeze-dry on an industrial scale without unacceptable loss of titre. Fortunately, this virus is relatively stable in the liquid form and its stability can be improved significantly by the addition of $MgCl_2$ (9). Other vaccines, such as measles, are very labile in the liquid form, but their stability can be improved significantly by lyophilization.

STABILITY OF POLIO VACCINE

To test the stability of the product, samples of trivalent live polio vaccine in $MgCl_2$ or in sucrose solution were exposed in the laboratory to different temperatures for varying periods of time. Preliminary results have been published previously (11). The findings with both preparations are shown in Table I. The figures in the table are the mean differences between the total virus titres obtained at each point studied and the initial potency of the vaccine. At 45°C and at 37°C, the difference between the two preparations is not significant. At 25°C, the difference is more pronounced. At refrigerator temperatures the sucrose containing vaccine showed a loss of 0.4 $\log_{10}$ after 8 months whereas the preparation containing $MgCl_2$ lost only 0.3 $\log_{10}$ after 18 months. The results given in the tables are the total titres of the three types.

Extensive studies have shown that each of the three polio vaccine types is equally stable if the trivalent vaccine is properly prepared and stabilized at the optimal pH.

These results demonstrate that for tropical countries, live oral polio vaccine has to have a high initial titre, and must be stabilized in $MgCl_2$. It must also be handled with much care. The question can be raised here how many vaccination "failures" of live polio vaccines in tropical countries are in fact due to lack or loss of potency of the vaccine used. If and when live oral polio vaccine is used properly, it is able to control the disease, not only in industrialized countries but also in developing countries, e.g., Chile, Costa Rica, Singapore, Hong Kong, Fiji, Western Malaysia and Taiwan (4,5).

STABILITY OF MEASLES VACCINE

In terms of morbidity and mortality, measles is a much more important disease than polio in the third world. Live attenuated measles vaccines have been shown to be safe and immunogenic, producing antibodies in close to 100% of children, provided the children have lost their maternal antibodies at the time of vaccination. Among the measles vaccine strains the Schwarz strain is the most commonly used.

The need for tight control of the stability of measles vaccines can best be illustrated by two trials carried out by W.H.O. during the last years (2,3). These data prove that there were and still are very marked differences in the stability of measles vaccines from different manufacturers.

In our laboratories we made a major effort to improve the Schwarz measles vaccine (Rimevax$^{(R)}$). The results obtained with the stabilized products have been published before (10,11) and therefore, I will summarize them only very briefly here. Table II shows the results obtained at refrigerator temperature, 25°C, 37°C and 41°C respectively. The minimum titre for live measles vaccine is 10^3 TCID 50. As we can see from the tables, the vaccine which has been in use for the last five years can be exposed at 25°C for more than 12 weeks, at 37°C for more than 6 weeks and at 41°C for at least 7 days and still maintain its potency. At refrigerator temperatures, the loss is minimal even after two years or more.

TABLE II. Stability of Rimevax[R] Measles Vaccine Stored/Exposed at Different Temperatures

Temperature (°C)	Time	Mean titre after freeze-drying[a]	Mean titre after storage	Difference
+ 2 to + 6	(months)			
	18	3.69	3.60	-0.09
	18	3.84	3.67	-0.17
	24	3.75	3.56	-0.19
+ 25	(weeks)			
	1	3.79	3.87	+0.08
	2	3.82	3.65	-0.17
	3	3.82	3.73	-0.09
	4	3.80	3.47	-0.33
	6	3.82	3.37	-0.45
	12	3.82	3.10	-0.72
+ 37	(weeks)			
	1	3.89	3.66	-0.24
	2	3.89	3.46	-0.43
	3	4.00	3.51	-0.49
	4	3.89	3.17	-0.72
	6	4.00	3.17	-0.83
+ 41	(days)			
	1	3.84	3.58	-0.26
	2	3.84	3.54	-0.30
	7	3.84	3.13	-0.71

[a] Log_{10} $TCID_{50}$/dose

STABILITY OF RUBELLA VACCINE

Cendevax(R), a live attenuated rubella vaccine, containing Cendehill(R) strain, was developed in our laboratories in the sixties. As shown by results after storage at elevated temperatures for various periods of time, this vaccine is highly stable (10,13).

The potency of several lots of vaccine was studied over a five-year period at refrigerator temperatures. No significant variation in titre was observed over this period. The recommended shelf-life of Cendevax(R) is only 24 months but the results demonstrate that its potency is maintained over a much longer period.

Samples of the vaccine were also exposed to temperatures of 25°C. There was a progressive but slow drop in potency over a period of months, but after six months, the vaccine still had the required potency of 10^3 TCID 50 per dose.

The results obtained at 37°C demonstrate that it takes about 3 months for the titre to drop under 10^3 TCID 50 and more than two weeks at 45°C.

TABLE III. Stability of Cendevax[R] Rubella Vaccine Stored/Exposed at Different Temperatures

Temperature (°C)	Time	Mean titre after freeze-drying[a]	Mean titre after storage	Difference
+ 2	(months)			
to	6	3.60	3.56	-0.04
+ 6	12	3.53	3.53	0.00
	24	3.52	3.44	-0.08
	36	3.73	3.79	+0.06
	60	3.65	3.62	-0.03
+ 25	(weeks)			
	3	3.62	3.57	-0.05
	6	3.62	3.67	+0.05
	10	3.62	3.43	-0.19
	16	3.54	3.23	-0.31
	25	3.64	3.12	-0.52
+ 37	(weeks)			
	1	3.60	3.56	-0.04
	3	3.62	3.45	-0.17
	4	3.62	3.41	-0.21
	6	3.62	3.32	-0.30
	16	3.66	2.98	-0.68
+ 45	(days)			
	2	3.67	3.57	-0.10
	7	3.67	3.36	-0.31
	14	3.67	3.16	-0.51

[a] Log_{10} TCID/dose

Table III shows the results obtained at refrigerator temperature, 25°C, 37°C, and 45°C respectively.

STABILITY OF A COMBINED VACCINE AGAINST MEASLES AND MUMPS

In recent years there has been a growing tendency in most European countries to vaccinate infants simultaneously against measles and mumps.

Rimparix(R) is a combined measles-mumps vaccine developed recently from the Schwarz measles vaccine strain and the Urabe Am 9 mumps vaccine strain. To study the stability of this combined product, samples from vaccine lots were titrated after exposure at 25°C, 37°C, and 45°C. The results are shown in Table IV.

From the results one may conclude that the measles component of the combined vaccine shows the same stability as the measles virus in the monovalent vaccine and that the

TABLE IV. Stability of Rimparix^R Measles-Mumps Vaccine Exposed at Different Temperatures

Temperature (°C)		Mean titre after freeze-drying[a]		Mean titre after storage		Difference	
		Measles	Mumps	Measles	Mumps	Measles	Mumps
+ 25	(weeks)						
	3	3.94	4.79	3.91	4.74	-0.03	-0.05
	6	3.94	4.79	3.84	4.59	-0.10	-0.20
	10	3.94	4.79	3.62	4.41	-0.32	-0.38
+ 37	(weeks)						
	3	3.94	4.79	3.49	4.24	-0.45	-0.55
	4	3.94	4.79	3.33	4.13	-0.61	-0.66
	6	3.94	4.79	3.11	3.93	-0.83	-0.86
+ 45	(days)						
	3	3.94	4.79	3.51	4.23	-0.43	-0.56
	7	3.94	4.79	3.17	3.99	-0.77	-0.80
	14	3.94	4.79	2.70	3.58	-1.24	-1.21

[a] Log_{10} $TCID_{50}$/dose

stability of the mumps component is very similar to that of the measles component.

Accelerated stability tests have been used routinely by our control laboratories for all freeze-dried vaccine batches for more than 15 years. Samples are exposed for 7 days at 37°C and then titrated. These tests give useful information regarding the stability of each vaccine batch. Experience with a great number of different vaccines has demonstrated that the titres found after storage at refrigerator temperatures for two years, were generally higher than the titres observed after the 7 days/37°C test. Apart from the results on human vaccines we also confirm this on a whole range of veterinary vaccines (Table V).

TABLE V. Comparison of the Titres of Different Vaccines After Exposure for 7 Days at 37°C and Those Obtained After Storage for at Least Two Years at 4°C

Vaccine	Titre at release[a]	Titre after two years storage at +4°C[a]	Titre after seven days at +37°C[a]
Avian Bronchitis			
Strain N	4.90	4.35	3.45
Strain H-120	4.97	4.17	3.85
Strain H-52	5.15	4.05	3.65
Newcastle Disease			
Strain Hitcher B1	6.72	6.65	6.54
Strain La Sota	6.71	6.67	6.47
Fowlpox	4.70	4.38	4.13
Infect. Bovine Rhinotracheitis (IBR)	6.19	6.12	5.61
Canine Distemper	4.50	3.67	3.53
Canine Adeno I	5.35	5.33	5.23
Feline Parvovirus	6.37	6.34	6.00
Marek's vaccine	3,075 PFU	2,917 PFU	2,100 PFU

[a] Log_{10} EID_{50}/dose or Log_{10} $TCID_{50}$/dose

In addition to the results reported here in vaccines artificially exposed to high temperatures in the laboratory, we also checked the potency and efficiency of vaccines used under field conditions after accidental or intentional exposure to high temperatures. These results include *in vitro* titration data but also serological results obtained in children with vaccines exposed for variable periods of time to high environmental temperatures. These results were obtained in Belgium (during a heat wave) (12), in Cameroon (8), in Tanzania (7), and more recently in Papua-New Guinea (6). They confirm the laboratory data and allow us to conclude that by carrying out an accelerated stability test in the laboratory on each batch of vaccine, it is possible to predict the stability of the vaccine under adverse conditions.

In September 1981, W.H.O. decided to require an accelerated stability test on each batch of measles vaccine used in E.P.I. Each vaccine batch must be exposed at a temperature of 37°C for 7 days. It is then titrated and the titre compared to that of a vaccine kept in the refrigerator. After 7 days the vaccine should not have lost more than one $\log_{10}$ and must still have a minimum titre of 10^3. The results of a survey published by W.H.O. in 1981 demonstrated that only one manufacturer met these requirements at that time (3). The requirements in our own laboratories are much more stringent than those of W.H.O. After exposure for 7 days at 37°C we accept a maximum loss of only 0.5 $\log_{10}$ instead of 1 $\log_{10}$.

In our hands, the test at 37°C for 7 days has been a reliable tool for predicting the stability of individual batches of vaccine and it is used routinely. However, before a new vaccine is put on the market or whenever production methods are modified, more extensive tests have to be performed at different temperatures in order to be able to calculate the regression lines at different temperatures. Furthermore, attention has to be paid to the fact that some virus preparations have two components: a more labile and a more stable one (1).

In conclusion, it is possible today to produce vaccines with greatly improved heat-stability. Such vaccines offer a higher margin of safety to overcome the problem of unreliable cold chains in tropical countries. However, extensive testing is necessary and all production steps and especially the lyophilization cycles have to be highly standardized in order to avoid batch-to-batch variation.

REFERENCES

1. Allison, L.M.C., Mann, G.F., Perkins, F.T., and Zuckerman, A.J., *J. Biol. Stand. 9,* 185 (1981).
2. Anon., *W.H.O. Wkly Epid. Rec. 54,* 354 (1979).
3. Anon., *W.H.O. Wkly Epid. Rec. 56,* 177 (1981).
4. Borgoño, J.M., and Corey, G., *Develop. Biol. Stand. 41,* 301 (1978).
5. Borgoño, J.M., Vicent, P., and Toro, J., Int. Symp. Potency and Efficacy Vacc., Manila (F.E. André, ed.), Smith Kline-RIT, Rixensart, Belgium, p.73-82 (1980).
6. Climie, A., and André, F., In preparation (1982).
7. De Haes, P., Personal communication (1981).
8. Heymann, D.L., Nakano, J.H., Maben, G.K., and Durand, B., *Brit. Med. J. 2,* 99 (1979).
9. Melnick, J.L., Wallin, C., *Proc. Soc. Exp. Biol. Med. 112,* 894 (1963).
10. Peetermans, J., Colinet, G., Int. Symp. Potency and Efficacy Vacc., Manila (F.E. André, ed.), Smith Kline-RIT, Rixensart, Belgium, p.247-264 (1980).
11. Peetermans, J., Colinet, G., Stephenne, J., Proc. Symp. on Stability and Effectiveness of Measles, Poliomyelitis and Pertussis Vaccines, Zagreb, 61 (1976).
12. Peetermans, J., Colinet, G., and Bouillet, A., *Develop. Biol. Stand. 41,* 259 (1978).
13. Peetermans, J., Colinet, G., Huygelen, C., *J. Biol. Stand. 1,* 179 (1973).

16

VIRAL VACCINATION IN THE MALNOURISHED : A BRIEF REVIEW

John S. Mackenzie

Department of Microbiology
University of Western Australia
Nedlands, Western Australia

It has been estimated that between half and two-thirds of children in developing countries may be suffering from nutritional deprivation (1,2), and are therefore potentially vulnerable to infection. The association between malnutrition, particularly protein-energy malnutrition, and infection has been described as synergistic, with each augmenting the severity of the other in a vicious circle (3-6). On the one hand, infection may precipitate frank malnutrition in those with a marginal dietary intake due to anorexia, vomiting, urinary nitrogen loss, intestinal malabsorption and increased catabolism contributing to significant weight loss, and on the other hand, those with moderate or severe malnutrition have an impaired immunocompetence resulting in an increased susceptibility to and severity of infection. This association is, however, complex and influenced by the interactions of many other diverse factors such as vitamin and mineral deficiencies, parasitic loads and intercurrent infections, genetic predisposition, resistance mediated by non-specific immune mechanisms and virulence of the infectious agent as well as social customs and conditions. Furthermore, it should be stressed that in the clinical situation multiple nutrient deficiencies are usually encountered. The association of malnutrition and infection has been discussed elsewhere in this seminar by L. Mata.

The role of viral infections in precipitating malnutrition and the increased susceptibility of the malnourished to viral diseases have been recently reviewed (7). The purpose of this brief paper is to examine more specifically the importance and efficacy of viral immunization in the malnourished.

VIRAL DISEASES IN SOUTH-EAST ASIA
AND THE WESTERN PACIFIC
ISBN 0 12 484820 6

IMMUNOCOMPETENCE AND MALNUTRITION

Although alterations in immune function are infrequent in the mildly malnourished, those with moderate (60-80% of the Harvard weight-for-age median) or severe (<60% weight-for-age) malnutrition exhibit a significantly impaired immunocompetence which needs to be taken into consideration in assessing the efficacy of viral vaccines. A number of recent reviews and monographs have detailed and discussed immune function in the malnourished (8-15), and only a brief summary will be presented here.

Pathology of lymphoid tissue. A number of pathological changes have been reported in lymphoid tissues, particularly in the severely malnourished, including thymic, splenic and tonsillar atrophy and a depletion of paracortical lymphocytes in lymph nodes.

Cell-mediated immunity. As might be expected from the pathological changes in thymus-dependent areas, cell-mediated immunity is generally depressed and T-cell function profoundly impaired, with absolute or proportionate decreases in T-cell numbers. Cutaneous delayed hypersensitivity reactions are also impaired, and lymphocyte proliferation in response to mitogens and antigens is moderately depressed.

B-lymphocytes and humoral immunity. Although variable results have been reported, B-cell numbers are usually unchanged and serum immunoglobulin levels are normal or elevated in malnourished children. Elevated levels of IgE are often observed as a result of associated parasitic infections. Serum antibody responses to most antigens are generally normal, although depressed responses have been observed in a few studies.

Secretory immunoglobulins. A reduction in secretory IgA has been found in saliva, tears and nasopharyngeal secretions in moderately malnourished children, and impaired secretory antibody responses were demonstrated to attenuated viral vaccines.

Complement. The serum levels of all complement components with the exception of C4 are decreased in malnourished children.

Phagocytosis and opsonization. Polymorphonuclear leucocyte dysfunction has been reported in bacteria-killing capacity, but opsonization and phagocytosis by these cells appears to be normal in the malnourished. Total leucocyte counts are generally normal or elevated.

Interferon. Preliminary studies have indicated that interferon synthesis may be diminished in malnourished individuals.

Other serum proteins and hormones. A number of other serum proteins and hormones have been shown to be deficient in malnutrition, some of which are important in non-specific protective mechanisms. Thus transferrin, lactoferrin, serum albumin and lysozyme levels are significantly reduced, and properdin is presumed to be deficient.

RESPONSES OF THE MALNOURISHED TO VIRAL VACCINES

Numerous undernourished children in developing countries have received viral vaccines during mass vaccination programmes, but although such programmes have been very successful in reducing morbidity and mortality in the vaccinated populations as a whole, it was never possible to ascertain the effects of the vaccines on the malnourished subpopulations. Yet the ability of the malnourished to mount an immune response which is both protective and long-lasting despite their impaired immunocompetence and without post-vaccinal morbidity, is obviously critical in the face of severe, life-threatening infection. Assessment of the effects of vaccination, therefore, has been dependent on small 'research' studies. However, relatively few such studies have been reported, and although a pattern has emerged, some of the findings have been inconsistent. The majority of studies have been concerned with the effects of live measles vaccine (16-21), and to a lesser extent with oral polio (16,17,22), smallpox (20,22-24) and yellow fever (25) vaccines. All, except for one study (23), were conducted with malnourished children.

Antibody Responses to Vaccination

In most reports on humoral immune responses elicited to live measles (16,18-20) and polio (16) vaccines, seroconversion frequencies and humoral antibody levels in children with moderate to severe malnutrition were similar to those in age-matched healthy control children, although the development of specific antibody (to measles) may be delayed (19). In contrast, however, very low antibody levels following administration of both vaccines were observed in a study of Egyptian children suffering from moderate to severe malnutrition compared to healthy controls (17). The reasons for the apparent discrepancy in this latter study are unknown. Secretory IgA antibody responses were significantly impaired in children with moderate to severe malnutrition after immunization with measles and polio vaccines (16). Not only was IgA antibody detected less often in the malnourished children, but its maximum level was significantly lower than in healthy age-matched control children and its appearance was delayed.

Smallpox vaccination in malnourished children has been assessed by the development of a post-vaccinal scar (20,24). In both reports, local reactions to vaccination were comparable to the reactions in healthy children. In a study of smallpox vaccination in chronically starved, undernourished adults, all of whom had received a primary vaccination many years earlier, a normal vaccinial reaction was observed but significantly delayed. Prevaccination neutralizing antibody titres were lower than in healthy control adults, and post-vaccination titres remained persistently lower than in the controls. Furthermore, specific cellular immunity against vaccinia as measured by intradermal tests was considerably impaired.

In a single report, malnourished children were shown to have a marked impairment in humoral antibody production after receiving 17-D yellow fever vaccine (25). However, although the eight malnourished children were all antibody-negative 9-13 days after vaccination, one child was examined 35 days after vaccination and found to be antibody-positive. Thus, development of a humoral response might have been delayed as reported for measles (19), and had they been tested the other children might also have been seropositive at that time.

Post-vaccinal Complications

There have been no reports of major complications following immunization with measles (18,20,21) or smallpox (20,23,24) vaccines, although pyrexia sometimes with coryza was noted in 9 of 14 malnourished children after measles vaccination in one study (19).

It was noted at the beginning of this contribution that infections may precipitate malnutrition in those with marginal dietary intake; the infection resulting in a decrease in the expected weight-for-age. Indeed, even a mild, attenuated virus, 17-D yellow fever vaccine, has been shown to significantly decrease nitrogen retention in older children (26), but few studies have examined the effect of viral immunization on changes in weight-for-age indices. Kielmann (22) found that children below six months of age who were immunized with smallpox or polio vaccines suffered statistically significant reductions in their weight-for-age, and the decrease was considerably greater if they were moderately malnourished. In older children, no significant weight changes were observed after smallpox vaccination (24).

Longevity and Protection

The longevity of the immune response to a viral vaccine in moderately malnourished children has been investigated in a single study. McMurray *et al.* (18) found that high HI antibody titres were maintained for at least 14 months following measles immunization in moderately malnourished Colombian children. Moreover, even a progressive decline in nutritional status failed to adversely affect their antibody levels. The authors suggested that the continued high titres could be related to a booster effect of exposure to wild-type virus in the environment, as well as residual antibody produced in response to vaccination.

However, the most essential consequence of vaccination, the protective capacity of the response, has not been studied. This is particularly important for those diseases in which a cell-mediated response may play a more dominant role in protection than humoral antibody, such as measles. Thus in the malnourished with their significant impairment in cell-mediated immunity, is the induction of a humoral response indicative of protection? This question has been discussed elsewhere (7,21,27), but few studies have addressed the problem. Reduced cell-mediated responses measured by skin test responsiveness and *in vitro* lymphocyte transformation have been reported following measles vaccination in moderately malnourished children, but these circumstances did not exacerbate the infection produced by the vaccine (18). In chronically starved adults, a significantly impaired specific cell-mediated responsiveness was observed after smallpox vaccination, suggesting to the authors that the vaccine might be less effective in protecting against variola infection (23), but neither in this study nor in others describing the results of smallpox vaccination in malnourished children (20,24) was there any report of generalized vaccinia.

The impaired secretory IgA responses in malnourished children after immunization with measles and polio vaccines have also raised some concern that protection may be inadequate when they later encounter wild type virus (16), since earlier observations with inactivated measles vaccine in which a normal humoral response but a poor IgA response were elicited resulted in severe local and systemic reactions. Furthermore, impaired clearance of the subsequently encountered wild-type measles may lead to prolonged replication and shedding of virus, increasing the period of contagiousness and possibly resulting in persistence. In the absence of previous vaccination, viral persistence has been described in wild-type infections of malnourished children leading to further immunosuppression and susceptibility to secondary infections (28). The potential problem of persistency and latency of measles vaccine virus leading to subacute sclerosing panencephalitis in the malnourished has been discussed by Katz (12,29).

Although measles vaccine failure has been reported with previously immunized children falling ill from wild type measles, and in some instances dying (21), a poor immune response associated with malnutrition was not necessarily implicated. It was seen more as a problem of "field conditions" as opposed to "research conditions" in which vaccine viability was suspect because of failure of adequate transport, storage and "cold chain" facilities.

CONCLUSIONS

The studies of viral immunization in the malnourished show a definite pattern in which those with moderate malnutrition respond to vaccination with normal humoral antibody levels and without deleterious post-vaccinal morbidity. Even those with severe malnutrition generally respond adequately, and where impaired humoral responses were reported, serum samples may have been obtained too early to detect a possibly delayed response. Given the high risk of natural exposure to infection in the malnourished, particularly with measles, vaccination is fully warranted; the risk of severe disease or death far outweighing the theoretical dangers of immunization.

Nevertheless, a number of further studies are urgently required to be fully able to assess viral immunization in the malnourished. They include:

(1) the protective efficacy of vaccination, particularly to measles - does vaccination indeed protect and are humoral responses indicative of protection;

(2) the longevity of the immune response - is the response sufficiently longlasting and does subsequent exposure to wild type virus help maintain it, or is revaccination of malnourished children warranted at a later age;

(3) does viral persistence (and possibly latency) in the malnourished occur after vaccination or on subsequent exposure to wild type virus;

(4) adult malnutrition due to famine (23,30) or refugee status - are malnourished adults susceptible to infection, or does immunity attained during childhood persist with adequate protection;

(5) although the most effective age for vaccination to measles is discussed elsewhere in this volume by Dr. Black, in terms of the malnourished child, should immunization be routinely pursued between 6 and 8 months of age (21), and should children at increased risk of exposure due to an epidemic situation or hospitalization be passively immunized if below 6 months of age (19), or vaccinated on the basis that vaccine given even up to three days after contact will produce "vaccine disease" and not wild measles (31).

The above list is by no means exhaustive. To it should also be added the necessity of confirming and extending earlier reports, such as secretory IgA responses in the malnourished, and the need to investigate cell-mediated responses after vaccination, such as T-cell mediated cytotoxicity (32).

REFERENCES

1. Jelliffe, D.B., *Ann. Intern. Med. 79,* 701 (1973).
2. Goldsmith, G.A., *Amer. J. Trop. Med. Hyg. 23,* 756 (1974).

3. Scrimshaw, N.S., Taylor, C.E., and Gordon, J.E., World Health Organization Monograph Series No. 57 (1968).
4. Scrimshaw, N.S., *J. Amer. Med. Assoc. 212,* 1685 (1970).
5. Mata, L.J., *Amer. J. Trop. Med. Hyg. 24,* 564 (1975).
6. Chandra, R.K., *World Rev. Nutr. Diet. 25,* 166 (1976).
7. Mackenzie, J.S., *Papua New Guinea Med. J. 21,* 134 (1978).
8. World Health Organization Memorandum, *Bull. Wld. Hlth. Org. 46,* 537 (1972).
9. Faulk, W.P., Demaeyer, E.M., and Davies, A.J.S., *Amer. J. Clin. Nutr. 27,* 637 (1974).
10. Chandra, R.K., Chakraburty, S., and Chandra, S., *Indian J. Pediat. 43,* 159 (1976).
11. Douglas, S.D., and Schopfer, K., *Clin. Immunol., Immunopath. 5,* 1 (1976).
12. Katz, M., and Stiehm, E.R., *Pediatrics 59,* 490 (1977).
13. Suskind, R.M. (ed.), "Malnutrition and the Immune Response". Raven Press, New York, (1977).
14. Chandra, R.K., and Newberne, P.M., "Nutrition, Immunity and Infection: Mechanisms of Interactions." Plenum, New York, (1977).
15. Glazebrook, P.W., and Davis, G.H.G., *Asian J. Infect. Dis. 3,* 93 (1979).
16. Chandra, R.K., *Brit. Med. J. 2,* 583 (1975).
17. Hafez, M., Aref, G.H., Mehareb, S.W., Kassem, A.S., El-Tahhan, H., Rizk, Z., Mahfouz, R., and Saad, K., *J. Trop. Med. Hyg. 80,* 36 (1977).
18. McMurray, D.N., Loomis, S.A., Casazza, L.J., and Rey, H. *Bull. Pan. Amer. Hlth Org. 13,* 52 (1970).
19. Wesley, A., Coovadia, H.M., and Watson, A.R., *Trans. Royal Soc. Trop. Med. Hyg. 73,* 710 (1979).
20. Ifekwunigwe, A.E., Grasset, N., Glass, R., and Foster, S., *Amer. J. Clin. Nutr. 33,* 621 (1980).
21. Kimati, V.P., Loretu, K., Munube, G.M.R., and Kimboi, F., *J. Trop. Pediat. 27,* 205 (1981).
22. Kielmann, A.A., *Amer. J. Clin. Nutr. 30,* 592 (1977).
23. Saha, K., Mehta, R., Misra, R.C., Chandhury, D.S., and Ray, S.N., *Scand. J. Immunol. 6,* 581 (1977).
24. Brown, R.E., and Katz, M., *Trop. Geograph. Med. 18,* 129 (1966).
25. Brown, R.E., and Katz, M., *Trop. Geograph. Med. 18,* 125 (1966).
26. Gandra, Y.R., and Scrimshaw, N.S., *Amer. J. Clin. Nutr. 9,* 159 (1961).
27. Edelman, R., *in* "Malnutrition and the Immune Response" (R.M. Suskind, ed.), pp.47-75. Raven Press, New York, (1977).

28. Dossetor, J., Whittle, H.C., and Greenwood, B.M., *Brit. Med. J. 1,* 1633 (1977).
29. Katz, M., *in* "Malnutrition and the Immune Response", (R.M. Suskind, ed.), pp.421-427. Raven Press, New York, (1977).
30. Chizea, D.O., *J. Amer. Med. Wom. Assoc. 29,* 499 (1974).
31. Morley, D.C., *in* "Potency and Efficacy of Vaccines", (F.E. André, ed.), p.176. Smith-Kline-RIT, Rixensart, Belgium, (1980).
32. Whittle, H.C., and Werblinska, J., *J. Clin. Exp. Immunol. 42,* 136 (1980).

17

ANTIVIRAL AGENTS

John Beale

Wellcome Research Laboratories
Beckenham, Kent

In the last few years the prospects for antiviral chemotherapy have been transformed. For years the outlook had seemed very dim and only a few investigators were active in the field. The reasons are not far to seek. In most virus diseases, by the time the disease is clinically manifest, most of the viral replication has occurred, so that antiviral agents have little time to act. Moreover, until relatively recently, the possibility of finding targets for selective antiviral action seemed remote and most antiviral agents had emerged from other research mainly looking for anti-tumour agents. It is now apparent that there are many phases of the virus replicative cycle that are open to selective inhibition. A listing of licensed antiviral agents 10 years ago is very small and other agents available in the research phase were also limited. The situation now is more hopeful, although the delay between discovery of an antiviral drug and its use in medicine is long. Another key reason for the relative lack of interest in antiviral drugs has been the immense successes of viral vaccines. For example, since World War 2, we have had introduced successively poliomyelitis, measles, rubella, mumps and hepatitis vaccines. Vaccines against herpes viruses based on the successful living modified or attenuated virus concept have proved more difficult. This is mainly because of latency but also because of the association of some of them with malignant disease. They have become prime targets for antiviral chemotherapy.

The agents that are now licensed for use in man are given in Table I.

Methisazone was the first antiviral drug to be used in man on any scale (1). It has been shown to have two uses,

VIRAL DISEASES IN SOUTH-EAST ASIA
AND THE WESTERN PACIFIC
ISBN 0 12 484820 6

TABLE I. *Antiviral Agents Licensed for Sale in a Major Country 1981*

1.	Methisazone	Prophylaxis smallpox
2.	Idoxyuridine	Herpes keratitis
3.	Trifluorothymidine	Herpes keratitis
4.	Vidarabine	Herpes keratitis Herpes encephalitis
5.	Amantadine Rimantadine	Prophylaxis influenza A
6.	Acyclovir	Herpes keratitis Herpes in immunocompromised patients

the prevention of smallpox in contacts and the treatment of complications of smallpox vaccination. It is not effective in the treatment of smallpox. It is a toxic drug, its use being limited by the nausea and vomiting it produces. Fortunately, it is no longer needed since smallpox has been eradicated as a result of the WHO campaign using smallpox vaccination.

The major successful antiviral agents have been the nucleoside analogues. The first of these to be discovered was idoxuridine by Herrman in 1961 (2), and subsequently was shown by Kaufmann (3) to be effective in the treatment of herpetic keratitis in rabbits and man. Idoxuridine has proved very valuable over the years for the treatment of herpetic keratitis. It has some problems: first, it is not always effective; approximately 85% of dendritic ulcers heal in two weeks on treatment with drops or ointment. The drug is toxic to corneal epithelial cells and this is a problem for patients needing long term or repeated treatment. It is also less effective in deep seated disease, and generally is not effective for the treatment of local herpes simplex or zoster on the skin unless given in dimethyl sulphoxide; also, resistant strains occur. Other nucleoside analogues, cytarabine, vidarabine and its monophosphate, have also been tried locally and are not as effective as idoxuridine. The best of this group of compounds for local use so far used has been trifluorothymidine; it is superior in solubility and can be used as a 1% solution. Although it is licensed for use on herpes simplex keratitis only, it seems likely from animal studies that it should be active locally against other DNA viruses, especially adenovirus infections of the eye and herpes zoster, but no controlled clinical trials have been conducted. Carefully controlled trials of efficacy are of vital importance in antiviral chemotherapy. These must involve a double-blind randomized design with a comparison either with placebo or a standard form of therapy. Objective measurements of the course of disease and virus isolation are important.

The history of antivirals is of uncontrolled studies of an agent, leading to equally uncontrolled enthusiasm, followed by controlled studies showing much less striking results. Interferon is now going through this period of proper evaluation but two other examples will suffice. First, cytarabine was introduced for the treatment of herpes zoster infection, mainly in leukaemic children, but a later controlled trial (4) showed that the drug was without any beneficial effect and at high doses was clearly toxic. A second example is the use of acyclovir amongst immunocompromised patients with herpes simplex. Uncontrolled use of the drug in the U.K. on a named patient basis led to much enthusiasm about the efficacy of the drug, but no data could be analysed to show unequivocally that the drug was effective. This was readily forthcoming when a properly controlled trial was carried out.

The analogues of pyrimidine and purine nucleosides discussed so far appear to work on a common pattern, although it has only been firmly established for idoxuridine. It is converted to the triphosphate and incorporated into DNA. It is not a selective agent; its differential effect on viruses, as opposed to cells, depends on a favourable therapeutic index resulting from pharmacokinetic properties and greater turnover of viral DNA during replication compared with cellular DNA.

The first compound in this series to prove effective when given systemically is vidarabine. It is less active than cytarabine and idoxuridine in cell cultures but can be administered intravenously up to 15 mg/kg daily by slow infusion over a 12 hour period. Drug used in this way has been shown to be effective in the treatment of herpes zoster in the immunocompromised, in herpes simplex in the newborn and for herpes simplex encephalitis (5). Studies of its use, either as the parent drug or its monophosphate in chicken pox in leukaemic children, in patients with hepatitis B and cytomegalovirus, are underway and there must be reasonable optimism for their success.

A new generation of more selective agents has recently been discovered. The first of these to reach clinical use is acyclovir. It was first discovered by Schaeffer at the Wellcome Research Laboratories in the U.S.A. He made a series of acyclic nucleosides in order to determine the

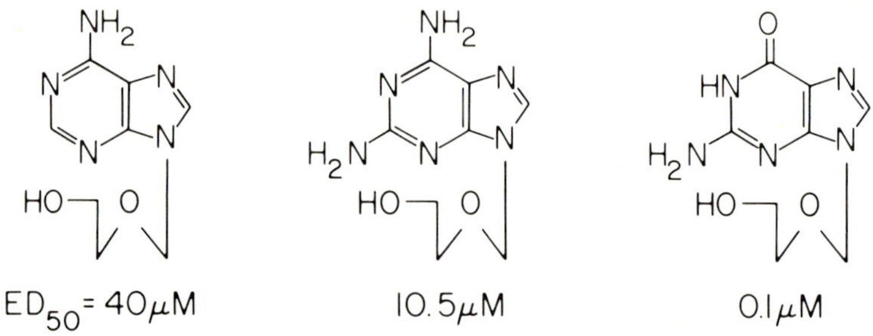

3 U **134 U** **248 U Acyclovir**

FIGURE 1. Increasing activity of antiviral compound.

minimum structure that would bind to the enzyme adenosine deaminase. Compounds of this general sort were investigated by Schaeffer, Bauer and their colleagues at the Wellcome Research Laboratories for antiviral activity (6). They were examined semiquantitatively in diffusion assays against herpes simplex, amongst other viruses. This technique is a simple, rapid means for primary screening. However, in order to guide the chemical work, a more accurate method is required and Bauer introduced an ED50 method using plaque reduction and expressing the comparative activity of compounds in molar terms. The results of such estimates (Figure 1) show that compounds of greater activity can be selected. Acyclovir was the most active antiviral compound when it was found, although others more active on a molar basis have been found since. Elion and her colleagues (7) showed that acyclovir is selectively phosphorylated to the monophosphate by virally encoded thymidine kinase and then to the triphosphate, which acts on the viral DNA polymerase. The evidence for this mode of action came first from studies of the amounts of monophosphorylated and triphosphorylated compound present in virus infected, as opposed to control, cells. Resistant mutants have also revealed that the main mode of action is the conversion to monophosphate by viral enzyme since thymidine kinase deficient mutants are resistant to the drug. They are also non, or poorly, pathogenic for mice and relatively poor at producing latent virus. However, resistant mutants also occur at the level of the polymerase and these remain pathogenic for mice on intracerebral injection. So far, resistant mutants do not appear to be an important problem clinically, but it is early days to assess their eventual role. Controlled studies have shown the drug to be effective in the treatment of herpetic keratitis, herpes simplex in the immunocompromised, genital herpes and herpes zoster in normal and immunocompromised hosts.

The drug appears to have some effect *in vitro* on the replication of Raji strain of EB virus, but it is not yet known whether it will show any clinical benefit in patients with infectious mononucleosis or EB virus tumours, for example, nasopharyngeal carcinoma.

There are some other drugs that have been described that may join acyclovir as more selective herpes virus chemotherapeutic agents. The most promising of these is bromovinyl deoxyridine, described by De Clercq *et al.* (8).

One of the major targets for antiviral agents is the viral respiratory disease complex. This seems to be an unpromising field for vaccines because of the number of aetiological agents involved. Of course, the relative mildness of respiratory diseases means that special care needs to be taken about the safety of any antiviral drugs. The most important agent is influenza and an antiviral effect in the prevention of the disease in contacts was described nearly 20 years ago. It was not really taken seriously as a prophylactic agent because of the promise of influenza vaccines. There was so much known about the antigens and genetics of influenza virus that the solution to the problem of making an effective influenza vaccine seemed a matter of time. The recent reappraisal resulting from the problems with the swine flu vaccine in the U.S.A. in 1976 and the results of the trials in an English boarding school, Christ's Hospital, described by Hoskins and his colleagues (9) has led to renewed interest in amantadine and rimantadine, especially in the U.S.A. (10). There is no doubt that these drugs are effective in preventing the disease and will probably be given a more prominent place in public health programmes for the control of the disease in future. They are an encouragement to those seeking antiviral agents against influenza. An attractive idea that is reported by Purnell Choppin and his colleagues, is that oligopeptides homologous with the constant hydrophobic regions of the haemagglutin molecule of influenza inhibit growth of the virus. Attempts at Wellcome to repeat this observation have been unsuccessful, although the similar approach to an inhibitor of measles was readily confirmed.

Amantadine is active in cell culture against a range of other viruses besides influenza A, parainfluenza 1, 2, 3, respiratory syncytial virus and rubella. These *in vitro* observations have not been followed up by well-controlled studies in man.

Like acyclovir, mutants of influenza A viruses resistant to amantadine have been readily isolated *in vitro*, but so far they do not seem to be clinically important.

Recently, drugs active against rhinoviruses have been described. One of these, enviroxime, has been shown to be marginally effective in the prevention of rhinovirus infection in man (11). It will not be satisfactory for use because 15 out of 26 subjects had nausea and 6 vomited. Four of 22 subjects who had placebo were also nauseated. This is an unacceptable level of toxicity for a common cold cure.

Flavones, for example, have been described which inhibit most rhinoviruses and Bauer and his colleagues at Wellcome have reported on the antirhinovirus activity of flavans (12). One of these compounds, 4',6-Dichloroflavan is the most active synthetic antiviral compound, being active at 0.07 M. This is a similar degree of activity to interferon. Studies with 4',6-Dichloroflavan are being carried out at present at the Common Cold Unit. The fact that it will act in the vapour phase suggests that local treatment may be a possible mode of effective application of the drug, but this can only be discovered by a properly controlled challenge study of the sort possible at the Common Cold Unit at Salisbury.

Interferon is the ideal antiviral drug, a natural, relatively non-toxic substance active against all viruses. It is the ideal complement to a drug like acyclovir, which is very selective depending on a viral encoded enzyme so that its action is very limited to a few viruses. Unfortunately, until recently, interferon has been so impure and in such short supply that studies of its antiviral effects have been limited. However, a number of controlled studies have been carried out which show that very low doses are effective against a range of viruses (13). Thus, it has been found to depress yellow fever in monkeys, though an experiment to repeat this observation in man failed because we could not regularly detect viraemia when the 17D yellow fever vaccine strain was given to volunteers. It was shown to prevent the take of vaccinia virus in the skin. It is active against herpes simplex in the eye and after trigeminal surgery; it has also been shown to be active against varicella zoster in the immunocompromised. In challenge studies in man it has activity against rhinoviruses and rubella virus, but not against influenza, although Soloviev has reported a reduction of influenza A in contacts given a small dose of interferon intranasally. Interferon also reduces the DNA polymerase level of chronic hepatitis B carriers. Merigan has now embarked on a proper trial of the effect of interferon on

TABLE II. Classification of Interferons - IFN 1980

Name	Alternatives	No. of Species	Inducer	Acid Stability
	Type 1			
Alpha (α)	Leucocyte	8 peptides 15-26 K MWt.	Viruses and DS RNA	Stable
	Lymphoblastoid			
	Type 1			
Beta (β)	Fibroblast	1 peptide 15 K MWt.		
	Type 2			
Gamma (γ)	Immune	Unknown	Mitogens Antigens	Unstable

hepatitis B, although there are indications that vidarabine monophosphate is also effective.

There is sufficient promise from these studies with crude interferon to carry out studies with the pure material now available. Interferons are complicated mixtures; the current classification is shown in Table II. It seems that β and γ interferons are single polypeptides and both have been cloned in bacteria. Work with these agents produced in this way is awaited with interest. α interferon is available from leucocytes mainly prepared by Cantell in Finland, and from lymphoblastoid cells. Studies of lymphoblastoid material has shown that at least 9 polypeptides are produced, one of which is a glycoprotein. All these polypeptides have interferon activity and the material produced by the techniques of Finter, Fantes and Johnston (14) are better than 80% pure (15). One disappointment in the use of pure interferon, either from leucocytes, lymphoblastoid cells or α 2 interferon from genetic manipulation has clearly shown that there are undesirable side effects from the use of interferon. The different α interferons have different biological activities, for example, the interferons that are not taken up by a monoclonal antibody to interferon described by Secher and Burke (16) are more active in mouse cells than α 2 interferon. There is merit, therefore, in clinical work in using mixtures of interferon as the standard preparation to compare the activities of single component interferon.

The achievements of antiviral chemotherapy are slight until now, but the prospects for the future, both short term and long term, are bright.

REFERENCES

1. Bauer, D.J., *in* "The Specific Treatment of Virus Diseases". MTP Press Ltd., Lancaster, (1977).
2. Herrman, E.C., *Proc. Soc. Exp. Biol. Med. 107,* 142 (1961).
3. Kaufman, H.E., *Proc. Soc. Exp. Biol. Med. 109,* 251 (1962).
4. Stevens, D.A., Jordan, G.W., Waddell, T.F., and Merigan, T.C., *New Eng. J. Med. 17,* 289 (1973).
5. Whitley, R.J., and Alford, C.A., *in* "The Human Herpesviruses. An Interdisciplinary Perspective" (A.J. Nahmias, W.R. Dowdle, R.F. Schinazi, eds.), p.475. Elsevier North Holland Inc., Amsterdam, (1981).
6. Schaeffer, H.J., Beauchamp, L., de Miranda, P., Elion, G.B., Bauer, D.J., and Collins, P., *Nature 272,* 583 (1978).
7. Elion, G.B., Furman, P.A., Fyfe, J.A., de Miranda, P., Beaucham, P.L., and Schaeffer, H., *Proc. Natl. Acad. Sci. USA 74,* 12 (1977).
8. De Clercq, E., Descamps, J., Maudgal, P.C., Missotten, L., Leyten, R., Verhelst, G., Jones, A.S., Walker, R.T., Busson, R., Vanderhaeghe, H., and De Somer, P., *in* "Developments in Antiviral Therapy" (L.H. Collier and J. Oxford, eds.), p.21. Academic Press, London (1980).
9. Hoskins, T.W., Davies, J.R., Smith, A.J., Allchin, A., Miller, C.L., and Pollock, T.M., *Lancet I,* 105 (1976).
10. Monto, A.S., Gunn, R.A., Bandyk, M.G., and King, C.L., *J.A.M.A. 241*, 1003 (1979).
11. Phillpotts, R.J., Jones, R.W., Delong, D.C., Reed, S.E., Wallace, J., and Tyrrell, D.A.J., *Lancet I*, 1342 (1981).
12. Bauer, D.J., Selway, J.W.T., Batchelor, J.F., Tisdale, M., Caldwell, I.C., and Young, D.A.B., *Nature 292,* 369 (1981)
13. Scott, G.M., and Tyrrell, D.A.J., *Br. Med. J. 1*, 1558 (1980).
14. Finter, N.B., Fantes, K.H., and Johnston, M.D., *Dev. Biol. Standardization 38,* 343 (1978).
15. Fantes, K.H., and Allen, G., *J. Interferon Res. 1*, 465 (1981).
16. Secher, D.S., and Burke, D.C., *Nature 285*, 446 (1980).

18

THERAPEUTIC POTENTIAL OF MONOCLONAL ANTIBODIES

P.C. Doherty
A.D. Lopes
N. Greenspan
W. Gerhard

The Wistar Institute
36 and Spruce Street
Philadelphia PA 19104

The capacity to reproducibly generate monospecific immunoglobulin (Ig) molecules is currently revolutionizing the analysis of a great variety of questions in experimental biology (1,2). This hybridoma technology also offers immense possibilities for developing new approaches (or for improving on old ones) to many persistent problems in human disease (3). The diagnostic potential of these reagents is obvious, and is currently being energetically developed by a great number of small, new commercial enterprises. Preparation of diagnostic kits for use *in vitro* (eg for venereal disease), and specific probes for imaging tumors *in vivo*, is well advanced.

The hybridoma approach also offers the potential for producing enormous amounts of highly purified, well defined Ig populations. Have we at last been provided with the 'magic bullet' for use *in vivo* against tumors and viruses?

However, before such therapeutic possibilities are explored in man, it is obviously necessary to first analyse their efficacy in animal models. The present paper summarizes some early studies on the administration of large amounts of virus-specific monoclonal antibodies to mice infected with influenza and rabies viruses. The results of these, as yet incomplete, experiments are both encouraging, and show pointers to potential problems.

VIRAL DISEASES IN SOUTH-EAST ASIA
AND THE WESTERN PACIFIC
ISBN 0 12 484820 6

THERAPEUTIC INTERVENTION IN INFLUENZA AND RABIES MODELS

The success achieved so far with the therapeutic use of monoclonal antibodies is in two experimental models of virus-induced neurological disease. In the first, and less practically relevant, system adult mice were injected intracerebrally (i.c.) with $10^{2 \cdot 5}$ mouse LD_{50} of A/WSN influenza virus. This produces an invariably fatal disease, with death occurring on day 5 or 6. Such mice can be saved by intravenous (i.v.) administration of a large dose (0.5 mg) of influenza hemagglutinin (HA)-specific monoclonal antibody (4) as late as 2 to 3 days after i.c. challenge.

The mechanism of protection seems to be that the process of virus growth itself causes the blood-cerebrospinal fluid (CSF) barrier to break down. This occurs at about the same time (day 3) in mice injected variously with different γ3-class Ig (complement fixing) populations which either bind to the virus, or have no affinity at all for A/WSN. There is thus no evidence that the exogenously-administered antibody interacts with mouse complement to destroy virus-infected cells in the blood-CSF barrier. High concentrations of the monoclonal Ig are found in CSF within a few hours, the titre being greater for an antibody that does not bind to A/WSN. This presumably reflects that it is not adsorbed by viral antigen present in the brain.

Mice injected with the virus-specific antibody survive, while those given the irrelevant Ig die. The mechanism of protection may be that the virus in brain is directly neutralized by the antibody: the influx of Ig is not accompanied by any obvious change in the level of inflammatory response. Mice injected with A/WSN and treated in this way have remained clinically normal for as long as one year. A more complete account of the experiments is given in reference 5.

Comparable results were achieved when mice injected i.c. with ERA rabies virus were dosed i.v. with a large amount of virus-specific monoclonal antibody, as late as 2 days after challenge. Such mice remain clinically normal in the long term though, in 2 of 15 animals tested, virus was isolated from the brain on day 14. Even so, these experiments raised the possibility that virus-specific monoclonal antibodies might be used for post-exposure treatment in rabies.

VARIANT VIRUSES AND THE NEED FOR AN Ig 'COCKTAIL'

Less success was achieved when comparable studies were done with the fast-growing Hep isolate of rabies virus (Dr T.J. Wiktor, personal communication). The reason for this is that, with a virus that grows to high titre, the monoclonal antibody simply selects for antigenic variants. Such variants are considered to be generated at frequencies as high as $10^{-4.0}$ for rabies stocks, $10^{-5.0}$ to $10^{-6.0}$ for standard influenza strains (6,7). Again, virus titres remain low following i.c. challenge with A/WSN (5), so that the chance that variants will emerge is relatively slight. Little success has been achieved with post-exposure treatment of mice infected intranasally with influenza viruses, as the virus grows to a high titre in the lung (8).

The way to circumvent the problem of emergence of variants is to use at least two, different monoclonal antibodies which bind to distinct sites on the virus. The probability that variants will emerge under these conditions is then greatly diminished, as the frequency of variants which bind neither should be approximately 10^{-10} (6). Any therapeutic protocol would thus need to incorporate at least two monoclonal Ig populations.

Two antibodies might not, in the practical sense, be sufficient. It is now known that many rabies virus isolates that were thought to be antigenically homogeneous do not bind a variety of rabies-specific monoclonal Ig populations (7). The need is thus to identify antigenic determinants on the rabies virus glycoprotein that are present on most, if not all, rabies viruses. The aim would then be to make a cocktail of, say, 3 or 4 monoclonal antibodies that bind to different, highly-conserved antigenic determinants (associated with neutralization) on the rabies virus glycoprotein.

MONOCLONAL ANTIBODIES AND HOST RESPONSE

A further problem that needs to be considered when proposing the therapeutic use of monoclonal antibodies concerns the potential effects of such treatments on other aspects of the immune response. Most of our effort to date in this regard has been concerned with the virus-immune T cell, the operator in cell-mediated immunity. A fairly comprehensive series of experiments (9) has shown quite clearly that post-exposure treatment with influenza HA-specific monoclonal antibody will, at the most, only partially inhibit the subsequent T cell response. This is in accord with other findings that T cell effector function, measured *in vitro*, is generally blocked to a fairly limited extent by the concurrent presence of virus-specific monoclonal antibody (10,11). The reason for this is that the virus-immune T cell response is very polyclonal, and only a few of the virus-specific T cell clones seem to focus onto regions of the viral HA molecule that bind the monoclonal antibody (12).

Other potential problems exist if it is considered necessary to dose people repeatedly with mouse-derived monoclonal antibodies over a protracted period. This is one reason why so much effort is being put into making monoclonal antibodies of human cell origin (13). Even when this is routinely possible it is obvious that people given the same monoclonal antibody repeatedly may themselves develop an antibody response to the binding site (anti-idiotype) or to more conserved regions (anti-allotype) of the exogenously-administered Ig populations.

Present experiments have also raised the possibility that mixtures of viruses and monoclonal antibodies may be useful for immunization. Mice injected with influenza virus neutralized in the presence of a vast excess of monoclonal Ig are primed for a secondary T cell response. We do not yet know whether this reflects that the virus-Ig complexes can stimulate T cell memory, or if the priming is due to variant viruses which are not bound by the monoclonal antibody in question. These experiments are currently being repeated with two different monoclonal antibodies, used separately or together.

SUMMARY

Treatment with large amounts of virus-specific monoclonal antibody may serve to protect mice injected intracerebrally 2 to 3 days previously with relatively slow-growing strains of influenza and rabies viruses. However, much less success is achieved in mice injected with viruses that grow rapidly to a high titre, as the monoclonal antibody may simply select for the emergence of variants which are not neutralized by the Ig molecule in question. The solution to this difficulty is to use a 'cocktail' of different monoclonal antibodies, which bind to distinct regions on the viral glycoprotein. People may be expected to develop anti-idiotype and anti-allotype responses if injected repeatedly with the same monoclonal antibody over a protracted period. Even so, the fact that the Ig molecules in question constitute a well-defined, and reproducible, reagent should allow the use of different antibody populations for subsequent exposures. Another intriguing possibility is that virus-monoclonal antibody mixtures may ultimately be of value for vaccination protocols.

REFERENCES

1. Köhler, G., and Milstein, C., *Eur. J. Immunol. 6*, 511 (1976).
2. Koprowski, H., Gerhard, W., and Croce, C.M., *Proc. Natl. Acad. Sci. USA 74*, 2985 (1976).
3. Scharff, M.D., Roberts, S., and Hammona, P.T., *Hosp. Prac. 16*, 61 (1981).
4. Gerhard, W.U., Yewdell, J., Frankel, M.E., Lopes, A.D., and Staudt, L., *in* "Monoclonal Antibodies" (R.H. Kennet, T.J. McKearn and K.B. Bechtol, eds.), p. 217. Plenum Press, New York, (1980).
5. Doherty, P.C., and Gerhard, W., *J. Neuroimmunol. 1*, 227 (1981).
6. Yewdell, J.W., Webster, R.G., and Gerhard, W.U., *Nature (Lond.) 279*, 246 (1979).
7. Wiktor, T.J., and Koprowski, H., *J. exp. Med. 152*, 99, (1980).
8. Lopes, A.D., PhD thesis, University of Pennsylvania (1982).
9. Greenspan, N., and Doherty, P.C., *Hybridoma, in press* (1982).
10. Effros, R.B., Frankel, M.E., Gerhard, W., and Doherty, P.C., *J. Immunol. 123*, 1343 (1979).
11. Frankel, M.E., Effros, R.B., Doherty, P.C. and Gerhard, W., *J. Immunol. 123*, 2438 (1979).
12. Doherty, P.C., *in* "Proceedings of the 4th International Congress of Immunology" (J. Dausset and M. Fougereau, eds.), p. 563. Academic Press, New York (1980).
13. Croce, C.M., Linnenbach, A., Hall, W., Steplewski, Z., and Koprowski, H., *Nature (Lond.) 288*, 488 (1980).

Part V
National Overviews

Chairman F. L. Black

Co-Chairman R. L. Doherty

19

VIRAL DISEASES IN INDIA - A NATIONAL OVERVIEW

Khorshed Pavri and Jeanette Rodrigues

National Institute of Virology
Pune, India

INTRODUCTION

Nearly 15% of the world's population exists in India which has only 2.4% of the world's total land area. Demographic data collected during the 1981 census re-emphasize the glaring variations between the different States. For example, the population density ranges from 7/sq.km. in Arunachal Pradesh to 654/sq.km. in Kerala. The overall average urban population is around 22-25%; it varies from 6-7% in Arunachal Pradesh, 30% in Maharashtra, to more than 90% in the Union Territories like Delhi and Chandigarh. Literacy (reading and writing with understanding in any language) is yet another parameter with marked variation. Among the States, Kerala with around 65% literacy among females almost towers over the others ranging from around 11 to 35%.

The health statistics in India cover some viral diseases like chickenpox, measles, poliomyelitis, influenza and rabies from hospital based data. However, the absence of evidence (records) does not necessarily mean evidence of absence of a certain disease. On the other hand, over-diagnosis and misdiagnosis are common, particularly during epidemic situations. In such circumstances, "all-India" health statistics cannot reflect the actual extent of viral diseases. Keeping all these limitations in view, we have attempted to review the major problems according to the disease syndromes, using the available information which is rather scanty.

VIRAL DISEASES IN SOUTH-EAST ASIA
AND THE WESTERN PACIFIC
ISBN 0 12 484820 6

ACUTE GASTROENTERITIS

Diarrhoeal diseases, excluding cholera, account for nearly 1.4 million deaths in children annually. The lack of simple and sensitive diagnostic facilities has hampered studies to determine the role of viruses. Studies in South India indicate that 22-66% of hospitalised cases were associated with human rotaviruses (1).

At present, no specific control measures for viral diarrhoeas are envisaged in the absence of general improvement of various environmental factors, including availability of safe drinking water. Oral rehydration therapy and health education are the most effective tools.

POLIOMYELITIS

The incidence of poliomyelitis in Greater Bombay is about 1 paralytic case per 1000 children in the age group 0-9 years (2). Poliomyelitis is increasingly being recognised in different parts of the country including rural areas. Oral poliovirus vaccine was introduced in 1961 and a marked reduction in paralytic polio has been observed among the small minority of the privileged urban well-to-do class who have access to potent vaccine. In most parts of the country, polio vaccine is not available due to problems of transport and storage. Hence, the impact of vaccination on the incidence of paralytic polio cannot be ascertained. There is, however, evidence of occurrence of paralytic polio in the triple vaccinated children. The Government of India has now initiated surveys by cluster sampling to estimate the prevalence of residual polio paralysis among 5 to 9 years old children, with the objective of determining the areas of high, moderate and low incidence. Immunization will be taken up first in the "high" prevalence area to cover at least 70-80% of eligible children. Without entering into the controversy of the "live" versus "killed" vaccine, we feel that if periodic well-organised community campaigns are held for mass immunization of all children under 5 years, it will produce a noticeable impact.

VIRAL HEPATITIS

Viral hepatitis is widely prevalent in the country. Hepatitis A virus (HAV) is endemic and by the age of 5 years, 90% of children acquire antibodies (3). Our studies on paediatric patients reveal a distinct age specific distribution, the mean age being 6.5 years and the mode 5 years for HAV, and the mean of 11.8 years and the mode 15 years for hepatitis B virus (HBV). Thus HBV also occurs in older children and adults and is responsible for about 20-30% of the sporadic cases of hepatitis. Mixed HAV-HBV infections were not recorded.

The rate of chronic carriers of HBsAg by DCIEP varies and is lower (0.6-5.85%) than the prevalent rates in south-east Asia, China and tropical Africa. The higher carrier rate of 5.85% was found in the tribal population of Arunachal Pradesh (4). Data on serious consequences of chronic persistent HBV infection are meagre but the incidence of hepatoma is lower than that reported in the countries of high endemicity. Only a few blood banks and the large private hospitals utilize the 3rd generation methods for detection of HBsAg. In the absence of planned follow-up investigations, there is no information on the role of non-A/non-B virus(es) or even HBV in post-transfusion hepatitis.

Most of the extensive epidemics of water-borne hepatitis as well as a proportion of the sporadic cases among the adults are attributed to neither HAV nor HBV. This is being discussed separately.

ACUTE RESPIRATORY INFECTIONS (ARI)

ARI constitute a major cause of morbidity and mortality in all age groups. Aetiological information is inadequate but malnutrition is an important determinant of mortality (5).

A systematic year-round study of viral ARI had been made at Calcutta amongst 38 members of 6 families living in a crowded slum area. Viruses were isolated from 13% of the 1716 throat swab specimens collected. Recovery of viruses was the highest during the post-monsoon season (September-October) and myxoviruses formed the largest group (6). Studies on respiratory viruses were made in rural areas near Calcutta where a high level of respiratory virus activity was recorded among the village communities living in poor hygienic conditions (7).

Continuous monitoring at Pune for influenza, carried out by our Institute (as one of the WHO National Monitoring Centres), indicates that the influenza viruses play a very important role in the aetiology of ARI, particularly among children. All the currently circulating influenza A and B virus strains have been isolated and there is serological evidence of the occurrence of these influenza viruses also in rural areas around Pune (4).

EXANTHEMATOUS DISEASES

After the eradication of smallpox, the common childhood exanthematous diseases are chickenpox and measles. Measles is not considered as severe a public health problem as in Africa. It is, however, a masked problem which needs investigation, particularly in children with malnutrition or tuberculosis. The estimated incidence rate for measles is 19 cases per 1000 population. Seroepidemiological surveys show that the median age of infection is between 2-4 years (8). The all-India seasonal distribution shows a high level of incidence in the first 4 or 5 months of the year, with a peak in March-April. The case fatality rate ranges between 1-3%. This percentage represents only deaths directly attributed to measles and would be much higher if indirect mortality due to belated complications were to be included. The availability of a live effective vaccine, administered in a single dose, is an attractive attribute for its inclusion in the expanded programme on immunization.

ENCEPHALITIS AND ENCEPHALOPATHIES

Viral encephalitis in sporadic or epidemic form and encephalopathies of uncertain origin cause heavy mortality in India. Although sporadic cases far outnumber those due to acute epidemic encephalitis, the latter receives much greater publicity. For example, when in 1978, epidemic Japanese encephalitis (JE) was recognised in the most populous State of India, viz. Uttar Pradesh for the first time, there was tremendous panic. In that year, 23,446 cases of encephalitis were recorded in the entire country. Surpirsingly in 1977, even though 31,995 cases of encephalitis were recorded, this did not cause as much concern because of the absence of large outbreaks.

JE, a mosquito-borne virus infection, usually affects the lowest socio-economic group living around the rice growing rural and suburban areas. Children below 15 years of age have been mainly affected in South India, whereas in North India all age groups were affected. The male-female ratio is approximately between 1.5:1 and 2:1. Prior to 1970, cases of JE were recorded only from South India. However, from 1973 onwards, outbreaks have also occurred in North and North-east India. The epidemic situation is often manifested in years of heavy rainfall following a period of drought. Sporadic cases occur but are generally missed. The pattern of distribution is diffuse, there being on an average 1-1.5 cases per village. The case fatality ranges from 25% to 45% (9).

Insecticide spraying is a useful control measure against adult mosquitoes but is rather impractical, because of the need to spray large, widely scattered areas. Vaccination using killed JE virus vaccine manufactured in India is being considered.

Rabies encephalitis occurs throughout the year in all parts of the country. Over 1,500 human deaths due to rabies are reported annually. The National Committee on Zoonoses has given top priority to the control of canine rabies. A comprehensive programme has been planned but its effective implementation will depend on the people's cooperation.

VIRAL HAEMORRHAGIC FEVERS

Kyasanur Forest disease, a tick-borne flavivirus disease, was first recognized in 1957; it is restricted to a small area in Karnataka State and affects all age groups. It has a seasonal incidence (January-June) coinciding with the peak activity of the nymphal stage of the vector and with the period of the greatest human activity in the forest. A killed formalinised vaccine has been developed which appears to be reasonably effective. Control measures against the ticks and tick bites have been recommended (10).

Haemorrhagic fever due to mosquito-borne viruses, i.e. dengue and chikungunya, was reported in Calcutta in 1963. Usually, however, epidemics of dengue have manifested as "classical" dengue fever and have affected approximately 25-50% of the population. All the four serotypes of dengue virus are present in India, mainly in urban areas with known prevalence of *Aedes aegypti*. Recent studies in Maharashtra have shown that the rapid development of road transport plays an important part in the dispersal of *A. aegypti* resulting in outbreaks of dengue fever in newer areas (11).

During epidemics, control measures, i.e. spraying of malathion in ultra low volume and pyrethrum indoors, against adult *A. aegypti* and source reduction against larvae is recommended. In the inter-epidemic period, use of larvicides like "Abate" in domestic water storage containers and other breeding sites, like tyre depots, should be undertaken.

ACUTE HAEMORRHAGIC CONJUCTIVITIS

Among the "new" diseases afflicting humans in the last decade, acute haemorrhagic conjunctivitis has caused very extensive epidemics. Coxsackie virus A 24 and enterovirus 70 have been incriminated. Enterovirus 70 infection has more serious consequences being associated with neurological complications - a polio-like disease and isolated cranial nerve palsies, mainly in adults (12).

CONCLUSIONS

This overview reflects an iceberg phenomenon. In the absence of public health laboratories for microbiologic diagnosis, this function devolves on the larger city hospitals and/or the National or State research laboratories.

As a WHO Collaborating Centre for Reference and Research for Arboviruses, the NIV carries out a combined programme of training and supplies of serological reagents for arboviruses. For polio and other enteroviruses there are, at present, 5-6 laboratories in larger cities including the WHO-designated National Laboratories at Bombay and Vellore. All these facilities need augmentation. There is an urgent need for development of a good reagent programme whereby standard quality serological reagents would be available at the field laboratories for diagnostic investigations.

An important factor in the control of communicable diseases is the degree of literacy of the population which influences the effectiveness of health education. Control of disease is also interlinked with environmental factors.

In a poor environment, nutritional deficiencies are compounded by worm infestations and diseases like malaria, tuberculosis and leprosy. A large number of cases of gastroenteritis, ARI and encephalopathies are probably due to multiple aetiology. For a vast majority of our people, sufficiency of drinking water, fuel and food remains a seasonal luxury. Therefore, community-based epidemiological studies are necessary to determine the exact role of viruses and the seasonal pattern of interaction with other factors.

REFERENCES

1. Steinhoff, M.C. and John, T.J., *Indian J. Paediat. 47*, 317 (1980).
2. Chodankar, V.P., *J. Indian Association Communicable Diseases 4*, 52 (1981).
3. Gandi, B.M., Joshi, Y.K. and Tandon, B.N., *Lancet 2*, 374 (1981).
4. National Institute of Virology - Unpublished data.
5. Verma, I.C. and Menon, P.S.N., *Indian J. Paediat. 48*, 37 (1981).
6. Ota, K.W. and Bang, F.B., *Am. J. Epidemiol. 95*, 371 (1972).
7. Kloene, W., Bang, F.B., Chakraborty, S.M., Cooper, M.R., Kulemann, H., Ota, M. and Shah, K.V., *Am. J. Epidemiol. 92*, 307 (1970).
8. Rey, M., *Expanded Programme on Immunization Bulletin 4*, 12 (1981).
9. Japanese encephalitis in India - Information Document, Pune, National Institute of Virology (1980).
10. Pavri, K.M., *Proceedings Workshop Zoonoses Public Health Importance*, National Institute Communicable Diseases/WHO, New Delhi (1981). (In Press).
11. Mahadev, P.V.M., Dhanda, V. and Shetty, P.S., *Indian J. Med. Res. 67*, 562 (1978).
12. Wadia, N.H., Wadia, P.N., Katrak, S.M. and Misra, V.P., *Lancet 2*, 528 (1981).

20

VIRAL DISEASES IN SRI LANKA: A NATIONAL OVERVIEW

Tissa Vitarana

Medical Research Institute (M.R.I.)
Colombo, Sri Lanka

I. INTRODUCTION

Sri Lanka is an island 22 miles South of India having a land area of about 25,000 square miles and a population of approximately 15 million. Colombo the capital has a population of over 600,000. About 85% of the population live in the rural areas.

Information on the incidence of different virus diseases in Sri Lanka is obtained by the Epidemiology Unit, Colombo from (1) notifications (rabies, chicken pox, polio, viral hepatitis and encephalitis are notifiable), (2) a study of hospital records and (3) mortality data from the Registrar General's Office. Most data presented here is probably an under estimate of the real situation.

II. VIRAL DISEASES OF THE NERVOUS SYSTEM

From the point of view of mortality this is the most important group of viral diseases and the annual figures for the 10 years since 1971 have been summarised in Table I.

VIRAL DISEASES IN SOUTH-EAST ASIA
AND THE WESTERN PACIFIC
ISBN 0 12 484820 6

TABLE I. Incidence of Viral Diseases of the Nervous System

	Rabies		Encephalitis		Poliomyelitis	
	No.	Deaths	No.	Deaths	No.	Deaths
1971	270	270	833	341	330	9
1972	295	295	872	357	297	9
1973	377	377	1313	513	360	48
1974	347	347	912	417	603	88
1975	288	288	983	400	190	16
1976	257	257	1166	387	258	28
1977	312	312	967	350	127	11
1978	242	242	1217	360	153	12
1979	214	214	1484	425	141	4
1980	153	153	1293	362	264	31
Annual Average	276	276	1030	391	272	26
				(38%)		(9.6%)

Rabies

Due to its importance the rabies figures have been separated from encephalitis due to other causes. There was an average of about 300 cases of human rabies per year up to 1978 but, with the introduction of the eradication programme in 1979, there has been a drop in cases and the average for the 10 years was 276. The main source of infection is the stray dog, but cats and sylvatic sources like the jackal and mongoose also play a minor role. The eradication programme is based on immunizing domestic dogs and eliminating strays.

Viral Encephalitis

Acute encephalitis due to other causes accounts for an average of 1030 hospital admissions each year, with an average case fatality rate of 38% (a range of 25% to 45%). Cases occur sporadically and there have been no major epidemics - though a few outbreaks have occurred.

Table II gives the results of a limited virus study by Vitarana *et al.* (9). It is seen that Japanese Encephalitis (JE), mumps and measles are the main causes. Enteroviruses (polio, coxsackie and echo) and herpes simplex have also

TABLE II. Viral Aetiology of Encephalitis - Serology Specimens Received at MRI (1972-1981)

	JE	*Measles*	*Mumps*	*Adeno*	*H.simplex*	*Vaccinia*
1972	*4*	*2*	*2*	*0*	*0*	*0*
1973	*0*	-	-	-	-	-
1974	*0*	*0*	*1*	*0*	*0*	*0*
1975	*0*	*3*	*0*	*2*	*0*	*0*
1976	*3*	*0*	*1*	*0*	*1*	*0*
1977	*2*	*2*	*2*	*0*	*0*	*0*
1978	*2*	*0*	*0*	*0*	*0*	*0*
1979	*0*	*1*	*0*	*0*	*0*	*0*
1980	*1*	*0*	*0*	*0*	*0*	*0*
1981	*1*	*0*	*0*	*0*	*0*	*0*
Total	*13*	*8*	*6*	*2*	*1*	*0*
%	*43.3*	*26.7*	*20.0*	*6.7*	*3.3*	*0*

been implicated by isolation. There have been 3 cases with high Group B arbovirus HI antibodies that were negative for JE by NT, but positive for Dengue. The aetiology of many cases is unknown.

The results of serological surveys done by Vitarana *et al.* suggest that JE occurs mainly in the West, where domestic pig rearing is common, and in Kurunegala, Anuradhapura, Batticaloa and Tissamaharama where large rice fields and wild pigs occur. Among twelve domestic pigs tested, ten had quite high levels of HI and NT antibodies against JE. As yet the prevalence of JE is not considered to be high enough to warrant an immunization programme. JE vector field studies are going on at the moment.

In the last ten years there have been 26 cases of Subacute Sclerosing Panencephalitis (SSPE) diagnosed at the MRI.

Poliomyelitis

Poliomyelitis is endemic in Sri Lanka and occurs in nearly all the towns, being maximal in Colombo. There have been an average of 272 cases each year in Sri Lanka with a case fatality rate of 9.6% in the last ten years. Epidemics seem to occur once in five to six years (e.g., 603 cases in 1974) and are usually due to Polio type 1, which is also the predominent type at other times. But in 1980 type III was predominent. This was unusual.

Polio occurs mainly in young children (e.g., in 1978 - 91.8% were under 5 years of age with 45.7% in the 1+ year group). The immunization status of 76 polio cases studied in 1978 showed that 59.2% had no doses, 10.5% one dose, 19.7% two doses and 10.5% three doses. The latter could be considered vaccine failures, and are seen more in areas distant from Colombo. Another problem is that many children fail to take the third dose.

Coxsackie and Echo viruses have been sporadically associated with paralytic illness (e.g., Coxsackie B_1, B_2, B_3, B_4 and B_5, Echo 9, 12, 13, 14, 17, 19 and 23).

III. DENGUE

Dengue infections are endemic in Sri Lanka and, on the basis of isolations, types 1, 2 and 3 (and possibly 4) have been active in the last two years. Serological evidence of Dengue activity was first tested for and found in 1962 but it was the Chikungunya epidemic of 1965 followed by the Dengue epidemic of 1966 that focused attention on the condition. During the epidemic, Dengue types 1 and 2 were isolated (2). A feature was the low incidence of DHF/DSS (the maximum recorded for any year was 26 cases with 6 deaths in 1966). Since 1970 there have been only one to four cases of DHF per year.

Serological surveys done in 1966 (3) and 1976 (4) have confirmed the occurrence of Dengue in most major towns, but not in Nuwara Eliya (elevation 6000 feet), or in smaller towns in the hill country and Dry Zone. The highest prevalence is in the capital, Colombo, where over 50% of children are infected by the age of six years. In the congested northern parts of Colombo this figure exceeds 70%. Though infection rates as high as 32% have been recorded in these areas, recent studies give a value of about 15%.

Samarawickrema and Mendis have shown that in Colombo *Aedes aegypti* predominates though *Aedes albopictus* increases towards the south and the periphery. In the other towns both are present but in variable proportions. In 1977 the average Breteaux Index for the 47 wards of the city was 30.1 (range 0 to 122), but values of over 200 and 300 have been obtained in some wards since then.

The enigma is why the occurrence of DHF is so low in Sri Lanka despite a high endemicity of dengue.

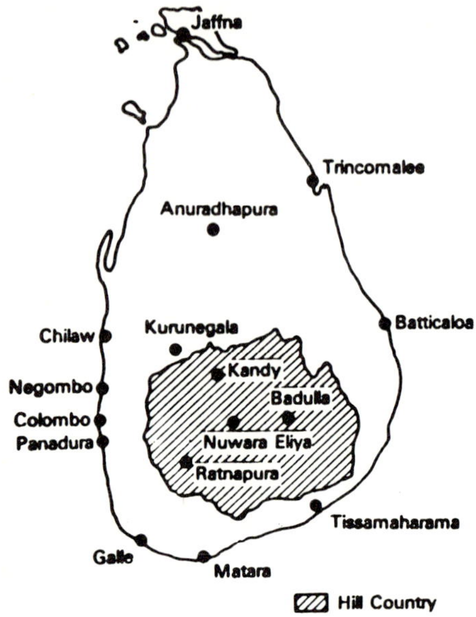

FIGURE. Map of Sri Lanka.

IV. VIRAL HEPATITIS

Viral hepatitis is a serious clinical problem and in 1976 there were 14,816 hospital admissions (a morbidity rate of 107/100,000 population). From 4,995 routine specimens received at the MRI in the five years up to 1981 approximately 25% were positive for HBsAg (immunodiffusion followed by RIA). In the absence of routine testing for anti-HAV IgM no information is available on the incidence of HAV and non-A, non-B hepatitis. However, an age-stratified serological study of the 16 main towns in the island done in 1976 (5) showed an anti-HAV prevalence (by solid-phase RIA) of 76.4%, and that the majority of the population are infected early in life (see Table III). A study in Colombo (6) showed an anti-HAV prevalence of 76.9% and as much as 91% being affected under 9 years of age.

TABLE III. Detection of Anti-HAV by RIA in a Survey of 16 Major Towns (1976)

Age (years)	1	1-4	5-9	10-19	20-39	40-59	60+	Total
No. tested	10	64	68	151	142	142	68	645
Anti-HAV+Ve	0	17	38	134	128	118	58	493
% Anti-HAV+Ve	0	26.6	55.9	88.7	90.1	83.1	85.1	76.4

V. INFLUENZA

Type A and B influenza are endemic in Sri Lanka and often 2 strains of type A have been isolated in the same year, e.g., A/USSR/90/77 and A/Texas/1/77 in 1979, A/Victoria/3/75 and A/England/864/75 in 1977, and A/Portchalmers/1/73 and A/England/864/75 in 1976 (7).

VI. ROTAVIRUS

In a one year study (8) at the Childrens Hospital 98 (30%) of the stools from 326 diarrhoea cases were positive for rotavirus by enzyme immunoassay. It occurred throughout the year, but more in the rainy season. The incidence was lowest in infants below three months (13.3%) and highest in those up to 2 years of age (34.6%).

VII. RUBELLA

In the five years (1976-1980) specimens were received at the MRI from 311 babies and on testing by HI, 7 were positive and 22 others were possible positives for the rubella syndrome. There were nine pregnant mothers who had contracted rubella in the first trimester. Regrettably maternal rubella is not grounds for legal termination of pregnancy and immunization is not available in Sri Lanka.

VIII. CONJUNCTIVITIS

Outbreaks and epidemics of conjunctivitis, sometimes haemorrhagic, have occurred once in about two to three years. Coxsackie A24 and adenovirus type 7 have been isolated repeatedly, but not enterovirus 70 (10).

ACKNOWLEDGMENTS

My thanks to Dr. Y. Hermon, the staff of the Virology Department, MRI and the Epidemiology Unit, Colombo for their assistance.

REFERENCES

1. Hermon, Y.E., and Anandarajah, M., *Cey. Med. J. 19,* 93 (1974).
2. Hermon, Y.E., and Anandarajah, M., *Indian J. Med. Res. 60,* 221 (1972).
3. Vesenjak-Hirijan, J., Hermon, Y.E., and Vitarana, T., *Bull. Wld. Hlth. Org. 41,* 243 (1969).
4. Vitarana, T. *et al., Proc. Sri Lanka Assoc. Adv. Sci., 7* (1976).
5. Vitarana, T. *et al., Asian J. Infect. Dis. 2,* 247 (1978).
6. Moritsugu, Y. *et al., Asian J. Infect. Dis. 3,* 33 (1979).
7. Fernando, N.I., Personal communication.
8. Mendis, L.N. *et al., Proc. Sri Lanka Assoc. Adv. Sci. 2* (1981).
9. Fernando, N.I., Personal communication.
10. Vitarana, T. *et al.,* Unpublished observations.

21

VIRAL DISEASES IN BANGLADESH

M.N. Islam

Department of Virology
Institute of Postgraduate Medicine and Research
Dacca

A.Q. Khan
A.M. Khan

Institute of Epidemiology and Disease Control[1]
Dacca

During the period of 1960 to 1966 Dengue virus was isolated from many countries of South-East Asia (1-8). Although laboratory facilities for investigating Dengue virus infection were not available in Bangladesh, the outbreak of so called "Dacca fever" in 1964 was shown to be Dengue virus infection by serological investigation conducted in Thailand (9). However no study was undertaken until the late seventies to explore the incidence of Dengue and Japanese B encephalitis virus (JE) in Bangladesh. In 1979, a serological survey was started among the school children in different parts of the country to delineate the prevalence of antibody against Dengue and JE viruses. In addition, in view of the fact that a high proportion of patients in big hospitals suffer from liver diseases, an effort was made to explore the incidence of hepatitis type-B virus infection among these patients and to determine the prevalence of HBsAg among the apparently healthy persons.

[1] *The Institute of Epidemiology and Disease Control, Dacca, is now amalgamated with the National Institute of Preventive and Social Medicine.*

VIRAL DISEASES IN SOUTH-EAST ASIA
AND THE WESTERN PACIFIC
ISBN 0 12 484820 6

MATERIALS AND METHODS

Specimens of blood were collected from children and patients and sera were stored at $-20^{\circ}C$ if not tested immediately. Sera were tested for antibody against Dengue and JE viruses by Haemagglutination Inhibition (HAI) and HBsAg by Counter Current Immunoelectrosmophoresis (CIEOP). Sera for detecting Dengue and JE virus antibody were collected from Dacca, the capital city situated in the central part of Bangladesh, Chittagong city in the south-eastern part of the country, Kushtia and Khulna towns situated in the south-western part, Thakurgaon villages in the northern part and Sylhet in the north-eastern part of the country.

RESULTS

Table I shows a wide variation in the Dengue virus antibody among the school children. Sex distribution of Dengue antibody (Table II) does not show marked variation except in the city of Dacca where the prevalence was significantly higher ($p<0.01$) in females than in males. Age distribution of Dengue virus antibody (Table III) does not show any significant variation, although perhaps the eleven to fifteen year age groups constituted the group with peak prevalence. Antibody against JE virus (Table IV) was detected in all the areas so far studied. A particularly high prevalence was obtained in north-eastern (Sylhet) and south-western (Kushtia) parts of the country. Prevalence of JE antibody does not show any significant variation between males and females nor is there any variation in the prevalence in different age groups.

Table V shows the detection rate of HBsAg in apparently healthy persons and patients. A high proportion (19.3%) of

TABLE I. Prevalence of Dengue Antibody in Different Parts of Bangladesh

Place studied	*No. tested*	*Positive*	*%*
Dacca city	*1,314*	*79*	*6.0*
Chittagong city	*639*	*26*	*4.6*
Kushtia and Khulna town	*1,375*	*176*	*12.8*
Thakurgaon village	*768*	*3*	*0.4*

TABLE II. Sex Distribution of Dengue Antibody

Place Studied	Males			Females		
	No. tested	Positive	%	No. tested	Positive	%
Dacca city	300	8	2.6	1,014	71	7.0
Chittagong city	393	19	4.9	246	7	2.8
Kushtia and Khulna	462	60	12.9	913	116	12.7
Thakurgaon	544	1	0.2	224	2	0.8

commercial blood donors who are almost the exclusive source of blood in Bangladesh are HBsAg carriers. The impact of such a high carrier rate among the blood donors has been reflected in a high incidence (53.6%) of hepatitis type-B virus infection among the patients with post-transfusion hepatitis. Among the patients with hepatitis without any history of blood transfusion a high proportion (29.4%) suffer from hepatitis type-B virus infection. However the incidence is significantly lower ($p<0.01$) than that obtained in the patients with post-transfusion hepatitis. In a group of 204 apparently healthy adult male villagers, 15 (7.4%) were found to be positive for HBsAg.

DISCUSSION

Although the feeling among the medical practitioners about the presence of Dengue and JE virus infections in Bangladesh has prevailed for a long time, laboratory

TABLE III. Age Distribution of Dengue Virus Antibody

Age groups	Percentage of sera with dengue antibody		
	Dacca city	Chittagong city	Kushtia and Khulna
3 - 5 years	5.6%	-	-
6-10 years	5.4%	4.5%	9.1%
11-15 years	6.6%	5.5%	14.3%
16-18 years	4.2%	-	11.3%

TABLE IV. Prevalence of JE Virus Antibody

Place Studied	No. tested	Positive	%
Chittagong	712	17	2.4
Sylhet	137	31	22.6
Kushtia	629	93	14.8

facilities were not available to confirm this. From the above data, however, it has become obvious that these viruses are widely distributed in this country. A wider availability of laboratory facilities could diagnose a proportion of patients who have perhaps been treated for some other conditions. Although around 10-15% (10) of patients in medical units in big hospitals suffer from liver diseases and a high proportion of them suffer from hepatitis type-B virus infection, the magnitude of the problem in the population at large is not yet known. Extensive studies should be conducted employing more sensitive techniques to explore the hepatitis situation in Bangladesh, and a routine screening of blood donors should be introduced to prevent post-transfusion type-B hepatitis virus infection.

TABLE V. HBsAg in Apparently Healthy Persons and Patients

Groups tested	No. tested	Positive	%
Commercial blood donors	419	81	19.3
Apparently healthy villagers	204	15	7.4
Patients with post-transfusion hepatitis	56	30	53.6
Patients with hepatitis without a history of blood transfusion	509	149	29.4

SUMMARY

A serological survey was conducted among the school children of different parts of Bangladesh for Dengue and JE virus antibody by employing the HAI technique. Prevalence of Dengue virus antibody ranged from 0.4 to 12.8% and antibody against JE virus was detected in 2.4 to 22.6% of children in different parts of the country. HBsAg was detected in apparently healthy persons and patients with hepatitis by employing CIEOP. Whereas the prevalence of HBsAg was 7.4% among the apparently healthy villagers, it was as high as 19.3% among the commercial blood donors. HBsAg was detected in a significantly higher proportion of patients (53.6%) with post-transfusion hepatitis than the patients (29.4%) with hepatitis without any history of blood transfusion.

REFERENCES

1. Hammon, W.McD., Rudnick, A., and Sathe, G.E., *Science 131*, 1102 (1960).
2. Dasaneyavaja, A., Robin, Y., and Yenbutra, D., *J. Trop. Med. Hyg. 66*, 35 (1963).
3. Halstead, S.B., and Yamarat, C., *J. Public Health 55*, 1386 (1965).
4. Lim, K.A., Rudnick, A., and Chan, Y.C., *Singapore Med. J. 2*, 158 (1961).
5. Chan, Y.C., *Bull. Wld. Hlth. Org. 35*, 61 (1966).
6. Lim, K.A., Chan, Y.C., Phoon, W.O., and Hanam, E., *Bull. Wld. Hlth. Org. 30*, 227 (1964).
7. Rudnick, A., *Bull. Wld. Hlth. Org. 35*, 62 (1966).
8. Sarker, J.K., Pavri, K.M., Chatterjee, S.N., Chakravarty, S.K., and Anderson, C.R., *Indian J. Med. Res. 52*, 684 (1964).
9. Aziz, M.A., Graham, R.R., and Gregg, M.B., *Pak. J. Med. Res. 6*, 83 (1967).
10. Meeting of the National Collaborators on "Studies on Chronic Liver Diseases Including Liver Cell Carcinoma in Bangladesh", 28th-30th November, 1978, Dacca, Bangladesh.

22

VIRAL DISEASES IN BURMA

Mi Mi Khin

Virology Research Division
Department of Medical Research
Rangoon, Burma

Seroepidemiological studies in urban and semiurban populations have revealed that measles and rubella occur from 6 months after birth, and 50% have antibodies by the end of the first year of life. Anti-HAV was positive in 80% by the 4th year of age, and 100% positive at 30 years. The overall rate positive for HBsAg was found to be 10.1%, and no differences were observed between the urban and rural populations. Natural infections with poliovirus are common in early childhood, and by the 5th year of life a high percentage (75%) have acquired immunity to all 3 types. Among the arboviral infections chikungunya and Japanese encephalitis appeared mainly in sporadic forms, and occasional mild epidemics. However dengue epidemics occur annually with a peak season during June to September. Serological findings of other viral infections were mumps (60%), Epstein Barr virus (22%), influenza A (54%) and influenza B (17%). Virus isolation studies have confirmed that the excretion rate of enteroviruses (polio and nonpolio) was 40%. In 1968 the community in Rangoon experienced the influenza/A2/Hong Kong/68 variant epidemic, and the isolation rate was 47%. All 4 serotypes of dengue viruses were recovered in the annual epidemics of dengue haemorrhagic fever, with a case fatality rate of 2-4% a year. Dengue type 2 appeared to be the predominant serotype, causing both severe and mild infections. Case studies of acute diarrhoea in children under 2 years by electron microscopy revealed that rotavirus was responsible in 31.5% of the cases. Although other common viral infections are clinically observed, their incidence/prevalence has not yet been studied due to low national priorities.

VIRAL DISEASES IN SOUTH-EAST ASIA
AND THE WESTERN PACIFIC
ISBN 0 12 484820 6

GEOGRAPHY AND CLIMATE

The Socialist Republic of the Union of Burma lies between latitude 10° and 28°N, and longitude 92° and 101°E in South-East Asia covering 676,552 square miles, with a greater portion within the tropics and a lesser subtropical region. Basing on the geography Burma can be divided into 3 parts, namely delta area, dry zone and the hilly regions. There are three seasons, the wet monsoon (late May to October), cool (November to February), and the dry hot (March to May) climatic conditions.

The population of the country in 1973 was 28.8 million (approx.) and the urban population consitutes 23.25% of the total population. The annual rate of population growth is 2.2%.

According to the national health profile infections due to viruses (rabies, poliomyelitis, diarrhoea, dengue haemorrhagic fever, and Japanese encephalitis) are among the 2nd ten priority health problems. Hepatitis, influenza and measles rank among the 4th and 5th ten priority health problems respectively.

RUBELLA AND MEASLES

Seroepidemiological studies in the semiurban and urban population of children and young adults in 1970 in 3 different towns of Burma indicated that rubella infections start from 6 months and measles infections occur by the 9th month after birth, and 50% of infants studied showed the presence of haemagglutination-inhibiting antibodies by the end of the 1st year of life.

VIRAL HEPATITIS

Serological studies in the general population showed anti-HAV antibodies by radioimmuno assay (RIA) method to be present in 80% at age 4, 96.2% at 20 and 100% at age 30 years.

The hepatitis B antigen (HBsAg) percent positive rate by RIA in the general population was 5.5% at pre-school age, 9.2% in 5-9 years, 17.4% in 15-19 years and 4.2% after 50 years of age. The overall rate is 10.1% with 11.5% in males and 9% in females. There was no difference in the positive rate between rural (10.4%) and urban population (9.5%).

Post transfusion hepatitis studies by reverse passive haemagglutination (RPHA) have revealed that out of 160 patients transfused with unscreened blood, 13.12% developed antigenaemia, 3.7% had antigenaemia and hepatitis, and 6.25% developed hepatitis without antigenaemia.

POLIOMYELITIS

In Burma the actual incidence of both paralytic and nonparalytic forms of poliomyelitis is not known. Various serologic surveys have been conducted at different periods in various parts of Burma. These results have revealed that natural infections with the 3 types of polioviruses at one time or the other is common in Burma. Neutralizing antibodies were detected in infants below 1 year of age and by the 5th year of life virtually 75% had acquired antibodies to all 3 types of polioviruses (1-3). These results have provided useful data for determining the susceptible age group for mass control with the oral vaccine.

ENTEROVIRUS (polio and non-polio)

A study on the excretion of enteroviruses was carried out in Mandalay in 1968 and in Taunggyi and Moulmein in 1970. The positive isolation rate was 42.1% in Mandalay, 57.4% in Taunggyi and 59.1% in Moulmein. The results clearly indicated that infection was predominantly occurring during the nursery period (1-3 years), when the children of low socio-economic groups are generally left exposed to unsanitary environmental surroundings. The various types of enteroviruses identified were adeno, poliotype 3, coxsackie A and B, and echo viruses (2). High excretion of non-polio enteroviruses among the young children, who will be the chief candidates for vaccination, brings up the possibility that such natural infections may seriously hamper the efficacy of the oral vaccination, as interference may occur between the polio vaccine strain and the non-polio enteroviruses. High isolation rates probably suggest the existence of some conditions favourable for the invasion of enteroviruses. However since there were no epidemics of aseptic meningitis and other symptoms caused by enteroviruses, it seems that these viruses may be of low pathogenecity.

ARBOVIRAL INFECTIONS

Dengue/dengue haemorrhagic fever (DHF) is endemic in Burma, and since 1970 epidemics have regularly occurred in the delta region, and by 1974 cases of dengue haemorrhagic fever were reported from other areas of Burma. Although clinical cases confirmed by laboratory diagnosis occur throughout the year, a definite epidemic season is noted yearly during the wet monsoon months which corresponds with the increase in the vector *Aedes aegypti*. Virological studies conducted at the Pacific Biomedical Research Centre in Hawaii in 1976 have shown that all 4 serotypes of dengue viruses were prevalent. Isolation of the dengue viruses was conducted by the intrathoracic inoculation of mosquitoes (4) and the isolation rate in 1976 was found to be 52.5%. However in the subsequent years (1977-1980) the isolation rate varied from 20-30%. It was interesting to note that dengue type 2 and 3 serotypes were commonly recovered from both the nonshock and shock cases of DHF (Table 1).

Dengue 2 was the predominant serotype isolated from the shock patients irrelevant of whether it was a primary or secondary infection. On the other hand, among the nonshock patients dengue 2 and 3 serotypes were isolated with almost equal frequency during primary and secondary infections (Table 2).

Of the total number of DHF patients confirmed serologically by haemagglutination inhibition (HI) tests the rate of primary infection was found to be between 12-15% from 1976 to 1980. Among the incidence of acute communicable diseases in Burma in 1977, there were 5,364 cases of DHF and the case fatality rate was 4.4%.

TABLE 1. Dengue Virus Isolation According to Disease Severity (1976)

Disease severity	*Dn 1*	*Dn 2*	*Dn 3*	*Dn 4*
Shock	*1*	*38*	*11*	*1*
Non shock	*21*	*30*	*39*	*4*

TABLE 2. Ratio of Frequency of Occurrence of Dengue Serotype According to Antibody Response

Disease severity	*Dn 1*	*Dn 2*	*Dn 3*	*Dn 4*
Primary infection shock	*0.07*	*0.69*	*0.23*	*0*
Secondary infection shock	*0.02*	*0.68*	*0.26*	*0.03*
Primary infection non shock	*0.26*	*0.35*	*0.38*	*0*
Secondary non shock	*0.13*	*0.35*	*0.45*	*0.06*

A country wide survey on the prevalence of dengue and chikungunya in 1973-1974 have shown that these infections were widely distributed in Burma (5).

A small outbreak of presumed Japanese encephalitis was first reported in 1974, and similar outbreaks in the neighbouring towns were reported in the following year (6). A country wide survey of the prevalence of JE antibody was carried out in 1976. Since the HI antibodies were broadly reacting to a member of group B (dengue), only a monotypic response to JE virus was considered and a low incidence found in some areas. An outbreak of equine encephalitis occurred among the horses in the breeding center in 1977, and JE virus was isolated from an autopsy brain specimen (7). In 1978, 2 human cases were confirmed as JE by neutralization tests (8). A small study was conducted in a semiurban area in Rangoon in 1979 to provide some epidemiological information on JE infections among human and porcine populations. JE neutralizing antibodies were found in 90% of the porcine and only 10% of the human population, predominantly from those over 11 years of age (9).

MUMPS

This is a common childhood disease and by 7 years of age 60% of the children have had the infection.

EPSTEIN BARR VIRUS (EBV)

Using the indirect fluorescent antibody technique, the presence of EB virus antibodies was studied in 1971. The results showed that 22.2% of the population exhibited the presence of EB virus antibodies (10).

INFLUENZA TYPE A and B

Yearly outbreaks of the mild form of influenza are reported based on clinical evidence. However an epidemic of a severe form occurred in September and October of 1968, and influenza type A2/HK/68 was isolated from throat washings (11). The isolation rate was found to be 47%. A few months after the outbreak, the prevalence rate of this variant was found to be 32.8% in the population of Rangoon.

A study of pyrexia of unknown origin (PUO) occurring during the monsoon months in 1971, 1972 and 1973 revealed that 54.3%, 28.6% and 21.1% of the patients demonstrated a four fold or greater sero-conversion to influenza A2/HK/68. Likewise a study of the PUO during June to September in 1969 revealed that 40% of the cases were due to influenza B. A further study in 1972 also revealed that 17% of the infections were due to influenza type B (12).

VIRAL DIARRHOEA

A study of acute diarrhoea in children below 2 years with vomitting as a predominant symptom was carried out in 1977. Rotavirus was detected by the electronmicroscope in 6 of the 19 specimens (31%) (13).

HAEMORRHAGIC CONJUNCTIVITIS (HC)

Epidemics of acute haemorrhagic conjunctivitis have been known since 1971. Since then epidemics of varying intensity have occurred at intervals of 3-5 years, with the last epidemic in 1980 involving about 50% of the population in Rangoon. Antibodies against HC virus were found in some sera collected in Mandalay and Moulmein between 1968 and 1970 which indicates that this virus had already been in Burma since 1968 (14).

ACKNOWLEDGMENTS

I would like to acknowledge thanks to Dr. Khin Maung Tin and Soe Thein from the Department of Medical Research and Dr. Than Swe from the National Health Laboratory for providing some data on viral infections in Burma.

REFERENCES

1. Tokuda, M., Ann. Rep. Inst. Virus Res. 13, 38, Kyoto University, Kyoto (1970).
2. Tokuda, M., Virus Research in Burma, p.59, Kyoto University, Kyoto (1972).
3. Than Swe and Mi Khin Khin Soe, Unpublished data (1980).
4. Rosen, L. and Gubler, D., *Am. J. Trop. Med. Hyg. 23,* 1153 (1974).
5. Thaung, U., C. Khai Ming, Than Swe and Soe Thein, *South East Asian J. Trop. Med. Pub. Hlth. 6,* 276 (1975).
6. Thaung, U., Noi, J., Than Swe and C. Khai Ming, *Burma Med. J. 21,* 151 (1975).
7. Than Swe, Khin Khin Soe and Than Aung, Unpublished data (1977).
8. Soe Thein, Than Swe and Than Aung, *Burma Med. J.*, in press.
9. Mi Mi Khin and Khin Aye Than, Unpublished data (1979).
10. C. Chai Ming, Soe Thein, Thaung, U., Tin U., Khin Nwe and Diwan, A.R., *J. Trop. Med. Hyg. 77,* 260 (1974).
11. Tokuda, M., Imai, J. and Mi Mi Khin, Ann. Rept. Inst. Virus Res. 12, 107, Kyoto University, Kyoto (1969).
12. Mi Mi Khin, Unpublished data (1969).
13. Thane Toe and Thein Than, Unpublished data (1977).
14. Tokuda, M., Personal communication (1979).

23

VIRAL DISEASES IN THAILAND - A NATIONAL OVERVIEW

Nadhirat Sangkawibha

Department of Medical Sciences
Ministry of Public Health, Bangkok, Thailand

Thailand is a Southeast Asian country comprising 72 provinces. It is divided into four geographical regions, Central, Northern, North-Eastern and Southern. The Central Region is a flat terrain, the North is mountainous, the North-East is a plateau and the South is a peninsula.

In 1980, the estimated population of Thailand was about 47 million of which 85% lived in rural areas. The major health problems are infectious diseases, including many viral diseases.

The annual notifications of viral diseases in Thailand have increased remarkably during the past decade. The reasons for this include the improvement of the reporting system, expansion of health services to the rural areas, a greater public interest in using the government hospital services and a natural increase of the diseases.

The epidemiological and virological features of viral diseases which are major health problems in Thailand are described herein.

JAPANESE ENCEPHALITIS (JE)

From 1964 to 1966, a few cases of Japanese encephalitis with virological confirmation were recorded in Sukhothai, Phitsanulok, and Korat Provinces (1). In 1969, a large outbreak of Japanese encephalitis occurred in Chiang Mai valley,

VIRAL DISEASES IN SOUTH-EAST ASIA
AND THE WESTERN PACIFIC
ISBN 0 12 484820 6

Northern Region of Thailand. The causal agent of this epidemic was confirmed to be Japanese encephalitis virus (JEV) which had characteristics similar to the JaGar#01 JEV strain (2). In the following years, outbreaks have occurred in the same area and have spread to surrounding areas.

The number of officially reported viral encephalitis cases has increased condiderably during the past ten years, with the peak of 2,387 cases and 439 deaths in 1980.

The epidemics of viral encephalitis in Thailand are found to have been clearly associated with season. Each year epidemics of viral encephalitis occur consistently between June and August, with a peak in July. This period is the beginning of the rainy season. The outbreaks occur in rural areas where there are plenty of rice plantations and pig farms. The disease is distributed all over the country, but the Northern Region is the area of highest incidence.

Blood specimens collected on filter papers have been submitted from hospitals in most provinces for laboratory confirmation. Each year, specimens from about 20-30% of the total reported cases were serologically examined by the HI test. JE infection was confirmed in 33.9%, 36.0%, 43.1% and 57.7% of the total cases for which paired blood specimens were submitted in 1977-1980, respectively. The serodiagnosis of JE in Thailand in 1977-1980 by region is summarized in Table 1.

The majority of JE cases were in the age group 5-9 years (34%), with the next most common age group being 10-14 years

TABLE 1. Serodiagnosis of JE in Thailand, 1977-1980

Regions	No. reported (M.R./100,000)	Patients tested No.	Patients tested % examined	% JE confirmed
Central	1,154 (2.0)	405	35.1	32.8
Northern	3,669 (9.5)	1,162	31.7	55.0
North-Eastern	2,438 (3.8)	488	20.1	42.4
Southern	451 (2.0)	96	21.3	29.2
Total	7,712 (4.2)	2,151	27.9	46.8

(24%). The ratio of JE cases in males to cases in females was 1.34:1. The age distribution of JE confirmed cases was very similar to that of the reported cases, except that the percentage of JE confirmed cases was lower in children aged under 5 years. This may be because most viral encephalitis in young children is caused by other viruses.

For JE control, the insecticide spraying has been undertaken occasionally in places where frequent outbreaks have occurred. At present, there is no definite programme for JE control in Thailand.

DENGUE HAEMORRHAGIC FEVER (DHF)

Since the first outbreak of DHF in Bangkok in 1958 (3), the disease has occurred continuously. During the past decade, DHF has spread throughout the country from large urban areas to small towns. Cases have been reported from every province and also from rural areas. Even with mosquito control, in 1980 there were 42,487 reported cases, which was the highest number ever recorded. The North-Eastern Region, which had 40% of population of Thailand, was the area of the highest morbidity (117 cases/100,000 population), followed by the Central, Northern and Southern Regions respectively.

The epidemics occur in the rainy season, usually starting in mid-April with the peak in July or August and declining in November. During December to March, the disease occurs sporadically. Large epidemics have been recorded every one or two years. The morbidity rate from this disease has increased but the case fatality rate has declined from 3.4% in the past to 0.8% in 1980 (4).

Of 14,117 serologically confirmed dengue cases, about 50% were in the 5-9 year age group, with the next most commonly affected age groups being 10-14 and 1-4 years old, respectively. About 2% of the total DHF patients reported were under 1 year of age, and 5.2% was ages 15 and over. The ratio of disease in females to males was 1.15:1.

In 1977-1980, blood samples from clinical cases were submitted from hospitals in most provinces for serological testing. The results were shown in Table 2. More than 90% of the confirmed dengue cases were secondary antibody response. Each year during the past decade all four types of dengue

TABLE 2. Serodiagnosis of DHF in Thailand, 1977-1980

Regions	*No. reported (M.R./100,000)*	*Patients tested No.*	*Patients tested % examined*	*% Dengue confirmed*
Central	*38,205 (67.0)*	*8,675*	*22.7*	*65.0*
Northern	*20,065 (52.5)*	*4,312*	*21.5*	*61.8*
North-Eastern	*43,326 (67.2)*	*6,898*	*15.9*	*71.1*
Southern	*4,604 (20.4)*	*1,661*	*36.1*	*65.2*
Total	*106,200 (58.3)*	*21,546*	*20.3*	*66.3*

virus were isolated from patients in Bangkok, but dengue type 2 was found to be the most common, occurring in 71% of all isolated (5).

During 1976 to 1980, space spraying with ULV 96% malathion was undertaken in the municipal areas of 52 provinces with high incidences of DHF. This was carried out twice during the dry season (December to April) and 3 times during the epidemic seasons (May to November). Beginning in 1981, a long term programme which based on health education and community participation for the control of *Ae. aegypti*'s breeding place is being implemented. The treatment of water containers with 1% ternephos sand granules is emphasized in the programme.

POLIOMYELITIS

The first outbreak of poliomyelitis occurred in Bangkok in 1952, during which 349 cases of paralytic disease were admitted to hospitals. This disease has occurred continuously ever since. There are reported cases all year round with the peak during October to January. Virological and epidemiological studies in Bangkok showed that children in the age group of 4 months to 4 years were of greatest risk of developing paralytic poliomyelitis (6). There was a high rate of enterovirus infections (30%) among children under 5 years old (7). The mass administration of OPV immunization was carried out in Bangkok in 1969 and has been followed by routine immunization of children under 1 year of age.

During the past ten years, while the incidence of poliomyelitis in Bangkok was decreasing, there was an increasing incidence in provincial areas.

In 1978, a survey to determine the prevalence of residual paralysis from poliomyelitis was undertaken in children aged 5 to 10 years in selected areas of two provinces of each region of Thailand and Bangkok (8). The prevalence rates of paralysis analysed by type of community indicated that the Bangkok rate was low (0.62/1,000) and the rural rate (2.34/1,000) was slightly higher than the urban rate (2.06/1,000).

There were 1,082 reported poliomyelitis cases in 1979, which was the highest number ever recorded. It appears that poliomyelitis in Thailand is a disease affecting urban and rural communities. The provinces of the lower part of the North and those of the upper part of the Central Region are the areas with highest incidence in the country.

Of 1,240 laboratory confirmed poliomyelitis cases during 1974-1980, 31.5% were under one year of age and 77% were under 5 years. The incidence of poliomyelitis was higher in males than females by a ratio of 1.47:1.

About 60% of cases tested had a positive isolate, and by serological testing of paired sera, about 80-90% of cases were confirmed as poliomyelitis. All three types of poliovirus were found, but type 1 virus was the predominant virus responsible for outbreaks.

Serological surveys to detect levels of antibodies to poliovirus in children in Bangkok Metropolis undertaken in 1976 and 1979, Korat Municipality, 1976, and rural areas of Chainat Province, 1979, confirmed that children under three years of age in Korat Municipality and Chainat rural areas had a much lower immunity to the three types of poliovirus than did children of the same age in Bangkok (9,10).

Since 1970, besides the routine administration of polio vaccine in Bangkok, polio vaccination has been given in the municipal areas of provinces of higher incidence. The nation-wide expansion of the polio vaccination programme was started in 1977 in 102 municipal areas of 13 provinces. In 1980, 647 communities of all 72 provinces were covered, including rural areas of 28 provinces. More than 400,000 children aged under 1 year were immunized.

It should be noted that the incidence of poliomyelitis in 1980 and 1981 was remarkably lower than in previous years (4). This may be due to the effectiveness of the OPV vaccination programme or to the immunity induced by the large epidemics of 1979.

VIRAL HEPATITIS

Viral hepatitis is endemic in Thailand. In 1980, 2,413 cases (M.R. 26.9/100,000) were reported with a case fatality rate 0.6% (4). The disease occurs all year round and has a peak between May and October. The notifications of viral hepatitis from each region are not markedly different. All ages are affected, with predominance in the age group 15-24 years. Males are affected more than females in a ratio of 1.62:1.

The prevalence of HBsAg among blood donors and the general population, as determined by CIE, is 7-10% (11-13). The rates of HBsAg carriage in rural and urban areas are not different.

Over 20% of children aged 1-4 years have anti-HBs and the prevalence rises with age, reaching 60-70% after age 15 (14). Family contact is an important source of HBV infection. Among HBsAg carriers, 55.88% have e-antigen and 5.88% have anti-e (15).

HAV is also common. Studies by Burke et al., 1981 showed that 97% of Thai adults 16 years of age and older were anti HAV positive (16).

In children less than 15 years old, the cause of viral hepatitis was HAV in 69%, HBV in 11%,simultaneous HAV and HBV in 7%,and HNANB 12%. Among patients 15 years of age or older the proportion was HAV 18%, HBV 51%, simultaneous HAV and HBV 3%, and HNANB 28% (17).

VIRAL DIARRHOEA

Diarrhoeal disease is the most common cause of morbidity in Thailand. The occurrence of acute diarrhoea is endemic, with peaks occurring in June and in January. About 40% of reported cases of acute diarrhoea occur in children under 5 years old.

Virological studies using electron microscopy showed that out of 179 stool samples from children under 3 years with acute diarrhoea, 30.7% contained rotavirus, 2.8% adenovirus and 2.2% were enteric-like virus (18). Rotavirus particles were found rather more frequently in females than males and were most common in the age group between 6-11 months. The incidence was highest during the period September to February.

REFERENCES

1. Bunnag, T., et al., *Am. J. Epidemiol. 50,* 590 (1976).
2. Yamada, T., et al., *Biken J. 14,* 167 (1971).
3. Hammon, W.McD., Rudnick, A. and Sather, G.E., *Sciences. 131,* 1102 (1960).
4. Ann. Reports, Division of Epidemiology, Ministry of Public Health, Thailand (1975-1981).
5. Nisalak, A. and Burke, D.S., *Dengue Newsletter. 7,* 34 (1981).
6. Trisnanonda, M., et al., *Ann. Trop. Med. Parasitol. 64,* 433 (1970).
7. Sangkawibha, N., et al., *Southeast Asian J. Trop. Med. Pub. Hlth. 6,* 3 (1975).
8. Ward, N.A., WHO Assignment Report, Nov.-Dec. (1978).
9. Ann. Report, Virus Res. Inst., Department of Medical Sciences. Ministry of Public Health, Thailand (1976).
10. Jayavasu, C., et al., *Southeast Asian J. Trop. Med. Pub. Hlth,* in press (1981).
11. Kun-Anake, C., Sangkawibha, N. and Pojanagaroon B., *Bull. Dept. Med. Sci. 19,* 85 (1977).
12. Thongcharoen, P., et al., *J. Med. Ass. Thailand. 59,* 546 (1976).
13. Ann. Reports, Thai Red Cross Blood Centre (1979-1980).
14. Grossman, R.A., et al., *Am J. Epidemiol. 101,* 144 (1975).
15. Pongpipat, D., Suvatte, V. and Assateerawatts A., *J. Med. Ass. Thailand. 69,* 26 (1979).
16. Burke, D.S., et al., *Am. J. Epidemiol. 113,* 245 (1981).
17. Burke, D.S., and Snitbhan. R., Proceeding of the Third Asia Congress Pediatrics, Bangkok, Thailand, Nov. 19-29 p. 213 (1979).
18. Sanguanwongse, S., Jayavasu. C. and Sangkawibha, N., *Bull. Dept. Med. Sci. 23,* 1 (1981).

24

NATIONAL OVERVIEW ON THE INCIDENCE OF MAJOR VIRAL DISEASES IN MALAYSIA

S. K. Lam

Department of Medical Microbiology
University of Malaya
Kuala Lumpur, Malaysia

In common with most countries in South East Asia and the Western Pacific, there is a wide spectrum of viral infections in Malaysia. In this overview, viruses of major importance will be presented and some factors that affect viral disease patterns will be discussed.

ACUTE RESPIRATORY INFECTIONS (ARI)

It has been established in many countries, both temperate and tropical, that viruses are responsible for 20-50% of cases of mild and severe respiratory disease in adults and children. In the University Hospital in Kuala Lumpur, respiratory diseases account for 14% of all admissions in the Paediatric Unit alone.

Our interest in ARI goes back some 10 years, when we began a study to determine the role of viruses in hospitalized children with lower respiratory tract infections, admitted to the University Hospital. Our initial study involved the examination of paired sera by complement fixation tests from 101 patients aged up to 10 years. Of these children 32.6% showed serological evidence of infection to one or more viral agents (1). Below 6 months the frequency of respiratory syncytial virus infection was only 9.5% and increased to 33% in the 2-3 year old age group. Parainfluenza viruses, adenoviruses and influenza A virus were of moderate importance as causes of ARI.

VIRAL DISEASES IN SOUTH-EAST ASIA
AND THE WESTERN PACIFIC
ISBN 0 12 484820 6

Follow-up studies, firstly by virus isolations and then by immunofluorescence on clinical specimens, have been carried out over the last five years and these studies again emphasized the importance of viruses in ARI. Rhinovirus and influenza A viruses were more commonly associated with upper respiratory tract infection. Respiratory syncytial virus and parainfluenza viruses were particularly important in bronchiolitis in children under 2 years of age. There were several instances where mixed virus infections were seen. In bronchopheumonia and pneumonia, the important viruses involved were the parainfluenza viruses and measles virus. Rhinoviruses appeared to play a significant role in lower respiratory tract infection, either by themselves or as mixed infections.

ACUTE GASTROENTERITIS

This has long been recognized as a major public health problem in developing countries; in tropical countries it may account for approximately 30% of hospital admissions. Recent evidence has indicated that viruses are responsible for the majority of diarrhoeal episodes in infants and young children and may account for malnutrition due to associated malabsorption. The most important virus involved in viral diarrhoea is the rotavirus.

A study was started in July 1975 to determine the importance of rotavirus in viral diarrhoea in children admitted to the University Hospital. Up to December of that year, stools from 130 patients were examined by electron microscopy and 28% of the specimens were positive for rotavirus; 8% of the specimens contained adenoviruses. Since then, all cases of diarrhoea were examined by electron microscopy. The data collected for 1978-1980 showed that rotavirus diarrhoea was present throughout the year and the highest incidence was in May and June. The positive percentage ranged from 10.7 to 34.3, with an average of 21.1%.

The age incidence of cases in 1980 showed that rotavirus was an important cause of viral diarrhoea in children under 2 years of age, particularly in those aged 0-6 months. These data also included an explosive outbreak of rotavirus diarrhoea in two small towns north of Kuala Lumpur. The significant finding here was that the cases were dotted around a particular water supply system and at that period the *E. coli* count in the pipe water was found to be high, indicating a possible water-borne spread. There were seven deaths among the approximate 600 cases reported.

Adenoviruses were occasionally encountered in stool specimens examined by electron microscopy and only one specimen examined so far contained calicivirus.

MEASLES

In developing countries where malnutrition is common, measles is a serious communicable disease and ranks among the ten leading causes of death in childhood. In Malaysia the number of notified cases ranged from 7,189 in 1976 to 8,727 in 1980. However, this is only the tip of the iceberg as many cases are not reported. The disease is endemic and cases are seen throughout the year with a peak incidence between April and July. In one hospital-based study (2), 25% of children developed complications. The Malays had a significant higher rate of complication compared with the Chinese and the Indians. The most frequent complications were respiratory tract infections (73%) e.g. bronchopneumonia and bronchitis, followed by acute gastroenteritis (14%) and encephalitis and meningitis (7%). The nutritional status of 42% of measles cases was adversely affected for 10-21 months following an attack. There was a case fatality rate of 3% in this study.

The age at which measles occurred was similar to other developing countries, with a peak from 6 months to 4 years. However, a high percentage of children developed measles before their first birthday. This implies that Malaysian children need to be immunized at an earlier age than those in developed countries. A pilot immunization programme against measles has already started in Malaysia.

RUBELLA

Rubella outbreaks occur in Malaysia every three to four years and the last major outbreak was in 1979-1980. A sero-epidemiological study conducted in West Malaysia (3), revealed that only 48% of females had antibody to rubella by the age of 15, compared with about 80% in temperate countries. Among the three major ethnic groups, the Chinese had the highest percentage of positives (65.2%).

These findings have not changed significantly over the past ten years and a recent survey carried out in Sarawak, East Malaysia, also showed that only 50% of the female population had antibody to rubella at child-bearing age. In spite of the high susceptibility to rubella, the incidence of congenital infections is not excessive. This may be due to innate resistance in the local population, to virulence difference in the local rubella strain and also to the fact that rubella virus spreads less efficiently in the tropics.

Rubella immunization has not received priority in the national expanded programme of immunization. Hopefully, this may change over the years once the measles immunization campaign comes to a successful conclusion.

ARBOVIRUS INFECTIONS

The main arboviruses causing human infections are the four dengue types. Analysis of data over the past five years shows that dengue is endemic in Malaysia and that the incidence begins to increase around April and May of each year and reaches a peak around June and July. The pattern seen in 1980 is fairly typical of dengue disease in Malaysia.

The age distribution showed that young adults were more prone to dengue infection and that there was no significant difference in incidence between the sexes. The highest incidence was seen among the Chinese (47.6%) followed by the Malays (39%). The incidence among the Indians was only 7.3%. The high incidence in the Chinese was due mainly to the fact that this ethnic group live in crowded, urban areas. The distribution of cases analysed on socio-economic factors showed that the incidence was highest in the lower income group in each of the ethnic classes.

HEPATITIS B INFECTION

It has been estimated that about 200 million people in the world are carriers of hepatitis B virus and are therefore at risk to chronic liver diseases, including liver cancer. Of these, 170 million live in Asia. One out of every ten patients admitted to hospital in the South East Asian region suffer from chronic liver disease.

In Malaysia, a study conducted in 1972, using counter immunoelectrophoresis, showed that the carrier rate among healthy blood donors in Kuala Lumpur was seventeen times higher that that reported in developed countries (4). Subsequently, using the more sensitive reverse passive haemagglutination test, we found that the carrier rate was about 7%. Studies are currently going on to determine the association between the carrier rate and the occurrence of liver diseases in Malaysia.

REFERENCES

1. Ong, S.B., Lam, K.L. and Lam, S.K., *Bull. Wld. Hlth. Org. 52,* 376 (1975).
2. Chen, S.T., *Med. J. Malay. 34,* 18 (1979).
3. Lam, S.K., *Bull. Wld. Hlth. Org. 47,* 127 (1972).
4. Kamath, S. *et al*, *S.E. Asian J. Trop. Med. Publ. Hlth. 4,* 159 (1973).

25

VIRAL DISEASES IN SINGAPORE - A NATIONAL OVERVIEW

S. Doraisingham

Department of Pathology
Ministry of Health
Singapore

Major viral infections in Singapore are caused by the respiratory viruses, dengue, Japanese encephalitis and hepatitis viruses.

1. RESPIRATORY VIRUSES

Respiratory viruses are the major cause of morbidity. A surveillance programme for influenza has been in existence since 1973. Twenty specimens are sent weekly from out-patients with influenza-like illness for virus isolation and the results from these specimens together with those from inpatients with respiratory illness are used to monitor influenzal activity throughout the year.

The influenza viruses exhibit a seasonal variation in incidence, an increase occurring from April to June or July when major epidemics usually occur, and again towards the end of the year (Fig. 1). These peaks appear to be associated with periods when the day to day fluctuation in temperature is maximal (J.E. Pakiam, personal communication). In contrast to H3N2 strains, H1N1 strains of influenza A were usually isolated in greater numbers towards the end of the year. Outbreaks due to influenza B virus occurred during the alternate, odd-numbered years 1975, 1977 and 1979, either following or immediately preceding those due to the A virus.

VIRAL DISEASES IN SOUTH-EAST ASIA AND THE WESTERN PACIFIC
ISBN 0 12 484820 6

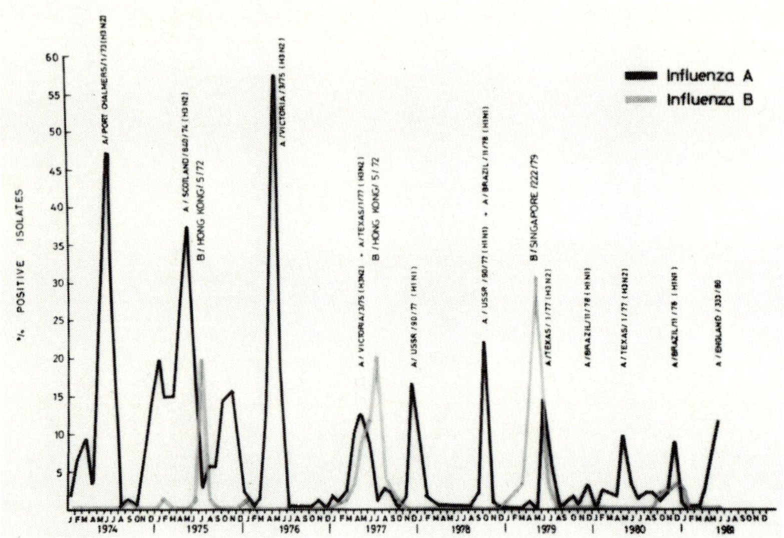

FIGURE 1. Influenza virus isolations in Singapore, January 1974 - June 1981.

Of the other respiratory viruses, respiratory syncytial virus (RSV) is the most important cause of infection in young children, annual outbreaks occurring in the middle or second half of the year (Fig. 2). Parainfluenza virus types 1 and 3 are most active during the first four months. From 1977-81 it was observed that type 1 infections peaked in the alternate years 1977, 1979 and 1981, while type 3 peaked in 1978, 1980 and 1981 as well. Type 3 is the most frequently encountered type, and type 2, the least. Adenoviruses and rhinoviruses are isolated irregularly throughout the year, adenovirus types 1,2,3,5 and 6 being serotypes commonly isolated from respiratory specimens.

The majority of RSV, parainfluenza type 3 and rhinovirus isolates from hospitalised children come from infants under 1 year of age, peak isolations for RSV and rhinoviruses occurring in those under 6 months. These viruses are usually isolated from children with bronchiolitis, bronchitis or bronchopneumonia, while parainfluenza types 1 and 2 usually come from patients with laryngitis or croup (1).

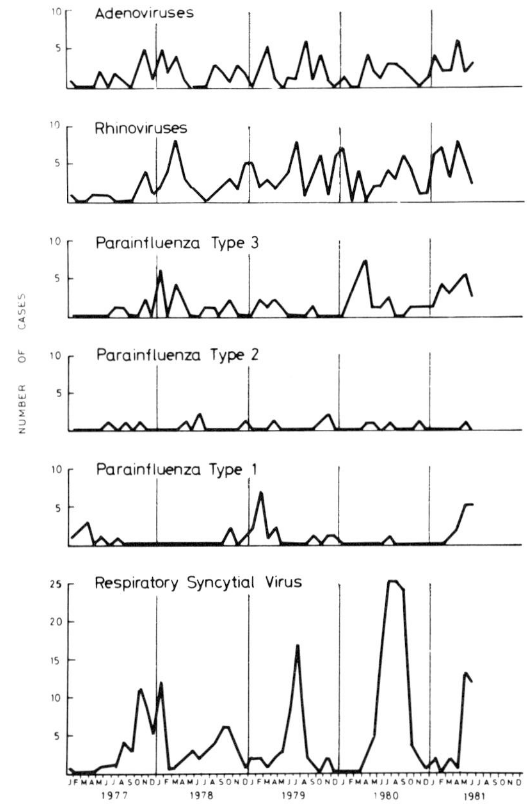

FIGURE 2. Distribution of respiratory viruses by month in Singapore, January 1977 - June 1981.

2. DENGUE HAEMORRHAGIC FEVER

Dengue haemorrhagic fever (DHF) first appeared in Singapore in 1960 when 70 hospitalised cases were reported (2). Thereafter, outbreaks were reported almost annually until 1968 (Fig. 3). In 1969, a national Aedes control programme was started and since then outbreaks have occurred at 5 year intervals (3).

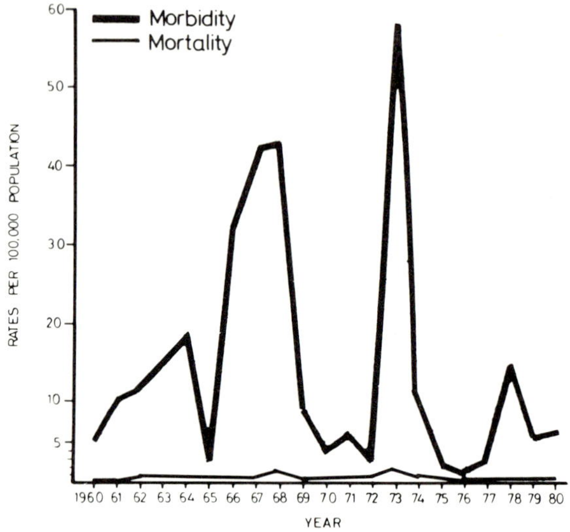

FIGURE 3. Reported morbidity and mortality rates of DHF in Singapore, 1960 - 1980. (Courtesy Dr. K.T. Goh, Ministry of the Environment)

The first outbreak in 1960 was a relatively mild one in which older children and adults were mainly affected. In 1962 the picture changed: younger children were being affected, and the more severe manifestations of shock and haemorrhage were seen (4). The largest recorded epidemic occurred in 1973 when 1187 cases were notified (5).

In the 1973 epidemic, peak morbidity and mortality rates occurred in the 1-4 year age group, but in subsequent years, the peak morbidity rate shifted to the 15-24 year age group. Among the three major ethnic groups in Singapore, Chinese, Malays and Indians, the morbidity rate is highest among the Chinese.

All 4 types of the virus have been responsible for infection, but type 4 is the least common type. Types 1 and 2 have been isolated from the two vectors, *Aedes aegypti* and *Aedes albopictus* (6,7). The former is considered to be the primary vector because the distribution of human cases corresponds more closely to its breeding sites: in the city centre and in urban satellite towns.

3. JAPANESE ENCEPHALITIS

Japanese encephalitis is endemic in Singapore and cases occur throughout the year with a biannual increase in incidence around April and October. Infection is widespread, for a study in 1955 revealed that about 70% of the population above the age of 12 years in Singapore, Malaya and Borneo had neutralising antibody to the virus (8). Antibody has also been found to be widely distributed among horses (9) and pigs (A.C. Lim, personal communication), and pigs are considered to be an important reservoir of infection.

In contrast to dengue, Japanese encephalitis cases occur mainly in the rural areas of Singapore in association with Culex breeding sites. The virus has been isolated from *Culex tritaeniorhynchus*, one of the vectors (10).

Human infection has always been sporadic, with the morbidity rate being highest in the 5-14 year age group and among Indians. A study extending from 1956 to 1962 showed that 52% of children surviving the acute phase and followed up for periods varying from a few months to 6 years, had either physical or mental sequelae, behavior disorders or a combination of two or three of these (11).

4. VIRAL HEPATITIS

The reported annual incidence of viral hepatitis in Singapore varied from 13-41.9 per 100,000 population from 1977-1980. Hepatitis B cases are notified throughout the year, whereas non-B hepatitis is associated with a sharp increase in notifications periodically (12). A study in 1975 on 67 patients hospitalised for acute viral hepatitis showed that infection was due to hepatitis A virus (HAV) in 30%, to hepatitis B virus (HBV) in 46%, and to hepatitis non-A non-B virus (HNANBV) in 24% (13).

The age-specific morbidity rate for all forms of hepatitis is highest in the 15-34 year age group (12,14), but the mean age of patients with HNANBV infection was found to be significantly higher than that of patients with either HAV or HBV infection (13). Among the three major ethnic groups, the carrier rate of HBsAg is highest among the Chinese (13.6% by rPHA) and lowest among the Indians (6%), but the morbidity rate for all forms of hepatitis is highest among the Indians (12,14,15).

Cases of HBV infection have been traced to various parenteral procedures including the use of contaminated tattoo needles. Large outbreaks of non-B hepatitis predominantly affecting adult Chinese have been traced to the consumption of inadequately-cooked molluscs (14).

About two-thirds of Chinese patients with chronic hepatitis were HBsAg positive by RIA (16). Further, over 70% of patients with hepatocellular carcinoma (HCC) were found to be HBsAg positive, a rate 6-10 times higher than that of the general population. The incidence of HCC is highest among the Chinese and lowest among the Indians, corresponding to the HBsAg carrier in the three major ethnic groups (15,17,18).

5. IMMUNISATION AGAINST VIRAL DISEASES

Three viral vaccines are included in the national immunisation programme: polio, measles and rubella. Oral polio vaccine was first used in Singapore in 1958 when type 2 vaccine was successfully used to abort an epidemic due to the type 1 virus (19). In 1962, oral polio vaccine was included in the national programme, and coverage now exceeds 90% of the live births (20). The effect on the incidence of polio has been dramatic (Fig. 4).

Measles immunisation of infants at 13 months and rubella vaccination of female primary school-leavers at 11+ years were started in 1976. Around 50% of women in the reproductive age group are non-immune to rubella (21).

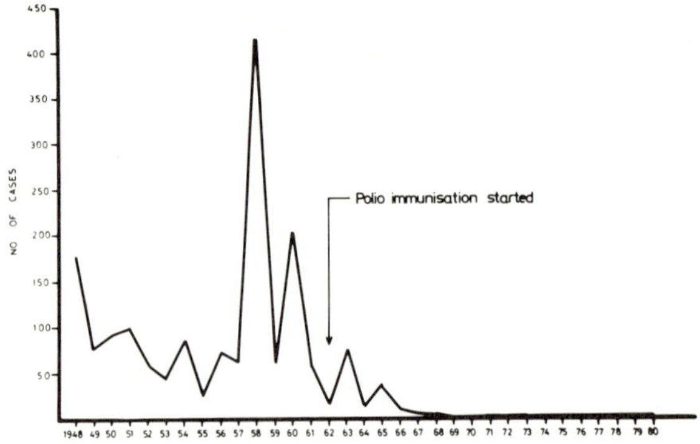

FIGURE 4. Notification of Poliomyelitis Cases, 1948-80. Courtesy Dr. K.T. Goh, Ministry of the Environment.

ACKNOWLEDGMENTS

I wish to express my sincere gratitude to Dr. K.T. Goh, Professors L.H. Lee, Y.C. Chan and S.H. Chan for vital information, and the staff of the Quarantine and Epidemiology Department for the preparation of figures and tables.

REFERENCES

1. Doraisingham, S., and Ling, A.E. *Ann. Acad. Med. Singapore, 10,* 69 (1981).
2. Chew, A., Ho, Y., Lee, Y.K., Gwee, A.L., Khoo, O.T., Lim, C.H., and Wells, R. *Lancet 1,* 307 (1961).
3. Goh, K.T. *Asian J. Inf. Dis. 2,* 25 (1978).
4. Wong, H.B. *Ann. Acad. Med. Singapore 10,* 91 (1981).
5. Chan, K.L., Ng, S.K., and Chew, L.M. *Sing. Med. J. 18,* 81 (1977).
6. Chan, Y.C., Ho, B.C., and Chan, K.L. *Bull. WHO 44,* 65 (1971).
7. Rudnick, A., and Chan, Y.C. *Science 149,* 638 (1965).
8. Hale, J.H., and Lee, L.H. *Ann. Trop. Med. and Parasit. 49,* 293 (1955).
9. Hale, J.H., and Witherington, D.H. *Ann. Trop. Med. and Parasit. 48,* 15 (1954).
10. Hale, J.H., Colles, D.H., and Lim, K.A. *Ann. Trop. Med. and Parasit. 51,* 17 (1957).
11. Phoon, W.O., and Lim, K.A. *Sing. Med. J. 4,* 11 (1963).
12. Goh, K.T. *Ann. Acad. Med. Singapore 9,* 136 (1980).
13. Chan, S.H., Oon, C.J., and Seah, C.S. *Lancet 2,* 469 (1981).
14. Goh, K.T. *Ann. Acad. Med. Singapore 10,* 25 (1981).
15. Chan, S.H. Epidemiological News Bulletin Vol.3, 15 (1977).
16. Chan, S.H. *Ann. Acad. Med. Singapore 9,* 179 (1980).
17. Chan, S.H., Simons, M.J. and Oon, C.J. *JNCI, 65,* 21 (1980).
18. Shanmugaratnam, K. *Sing. Med. J. 14,* 69 (1973).
19. Hale, J.H., Lee, L.H., Doraisingham, M., Kanagaratnam,K., Leong, K.W., and Monteiro, E.S. *Brit. Med. J. 1,* 1541 (1959).
20. Lee, L.H., and Lim, K.A. *Sing. Med. J. 18,* 34 (1977).
21. Doraisingham, S., and Goh, K.T. *Ann. Acad. Med. Singapore 10,* 238 (1981).

26

VIRAL DISEASES IN INDONESIA

Soeprapti Thaib

Virus Department
Perum. Bio Farma
Bandung, Indonesia

PICORNAVIRIDAE

A. *Poliomyelitis*

Successive serological studies have shown a significant increase in the number of triple-negative children, from 11% to more than 50% in 1978, in all sections of the population (1-6).

In polio outbreaks during 1976-77 in various regencies, attack rates in the 0-4 year age group of up to 90% were observed, with estimated paralytic polio incidence rates between 3.5-8.0/100,000, and also prevalence paralytic rates between 4-7/10,000 in the 0-14 year age group. Polio cases were also detected in adults, clinically diagnosed as polyneuritis and encephalitis (1,2). The largest outbreak of poliomyelitis was in Bali in 1976.

Since then, polio has become a public health problem, and vaccination has been included in the EPI starting with basic immunization in infants.

B. *Echo and Coxsackie Viruses*

These viruses have been involved in infantile diarrhoea and aseptic meningitis cases (7,8) similar to polio virus. They were also isolated from various water systems and reservoirs in Bandung, and a continuous circulation of enteroviruses seems to occur throughout the year (4,9).

VIRAL DISEASES IN SOUTH-EAST ASIA
AND THE WESTERN PACIFIC
ISBN 0 12 484820 6

Coxsackie B_3 virus was found to be responsible in cases diagnosed as encephalitis.

TOGAVIRIDAE

A. Dengue

Dengue was first discovered in Indonesia in 1779. During the 1920s various names were given to the disease. The diagnosis at that time, however, was based on clinical symptoms alone, without laboratory confirmation.

During the late 1960s serological studies on B Group arbovirus antibodies in the healthy population in Bandung, have indicated that dengue is endemic (10,11).

The first positive DHF/DSS cases from Jakarta in 1968 were serologically diagnosed by Bio Farma (12). Since the early 1970s dengue has become a serious problem, occurring in epidemics with a peak incidence of more than 10,000 cases in 1973. All 4 types of dengue virus were isolated from patients in various cities/regions in Indonesia, not only from pediatric but also from adult cases (13-16). At present 20 out of 27 provinces are affected, the vectors being *Ae. aegypti* in urban areas and *Ae. albopictus* in rural areas (17).

A study of the sex distribution has revealed a preponderance of females over males with hemorrhagic symptoms, shock and death (18,19). The highest proportional attack rate has been in the 5-10 year age group (18,19). The differences among races present in Indonesia is not clear, but during the epidemics in Central and East Java, there was the impression that more children of Chinese origin were affected than pure Indonesians (20). It was generally observed that a peak incidence is frequently seen at the end of the rainy season, March or April, with a few occasional exceptions (18,19,21).

Eradication and health education programs have kept the number of cases to less than 1,000 a year and CFR of less than 2%.

B. Japanese B. Encephalitis (JBE)

This virus is also present in Indonesia, as shown by serological studies in the healthy population and in pigs slaughtered in Bandung; also by virus isolation from mosquito vectors in Jakarta. Viral encephalitis will become a health problem in Indonesia, a CFR of around 25% is noted in Bandung. JBE has also been incriminated in a special study of encephalitis still in progress. The diagnosis has been based mainly on the presence of a significant increase of CF antibodies in sera, and also the presence or increase of HI antibody in paired CSF specimens, since brain biopsies can not be done due to various reasons (22-24).

C. Rubella

Serological studies in 1970-71 in Bandung revealed that 80% of all ages were positive for rubella haemagglutination-inhibiting (HI) antibodies, but this incidence of seropositives had dropped dramatically in a recent study in 1979-80 to between 8% and 49%, particularly in the one month to 14 year age group. This latter study has indicated that there is a considerable risk for women of childbearing age (3,25,26).

In Bandung, the virus has been isolated from throat swabs and urine of babies with congenital anomalies, accompanied by successive HI titre rises over more than 6 months in the babies compared to a constant titre in their corresponding mothers. Rubella cases in children clinically diagnosed as suspect DHF were serologically rubella positive, also by virus isolation from throat swabs (26). At present many cases are recognised in children as well as in adults. A survey of congenital cataracts in an ophthalmic hospital in Bandung has revealed an average incidence of at least 2 cases/month during 1979-81.

Whether rubella has become a health problem and vaccination should be included in the EPI, needs further studies in other areas similar to those done in Bandung (26).

ORTHOMYXOVIRIDAE

A. Influenza

Severe outbreaks of influenza in Indonesia occurred during the Asian and Hongkong influenza pandemics in 1957 and 1968, respectively. The virus laboratories in Bandung and Jakarta have isolated influenza A type viruses in 1962, 1966, 1968 and 1979, including the Russian and Swine type A viruses.

PARAMYXOVIRIDAE

A. *Mumps*

Mumps is endemic in Indonesia, as shown by a serological study on mumps HI antibodies in the healthy population and various animal species in 1971 in Bandung (27).

It occurs sporadically, occasionally in small outbreaks, and complications have so far never been reported, although mumps virus has been found to be responsible for aseptic meningitis and encephalitis cases (8,23,24).

B. *Measles*

Measles has become a public health problem in Indonesia since 1977, when outbreaks were reported from various regions in the country with CFRs ranging from 2.9-25%. It started in the island of Lombok with 12,508 cases and a CFR of 2.9%, followed by smaller outbreaks in several regencies (28). The 1-4 year age group has been the most affected, and nutritional status has had an important influence on the response and outcome of the disease, as proved by the fact that most of the victims and deaths occurred under bad nutritional conditions. No differences were found between urban and rural areas. Serological studies were done and vaccination trials are in progress. The Government will most probably include measles vaccination in the EPI.

RHABDOVIRIDAE

Rabies

Since the second world war, the prevalence of rabies has increased, not only in the number of species acting as reservoir hosts, and in animal bites and human cases annually, but in the number of affected provinces (22 out of 27 provinces), despite the introduction of the Rabies Ordinance in 1926 (29). The endemicity in the provinces varies considerably, depending on local habits, social structure and culture, population density and local dog numbers.

Studies have revealed that 95% of cases occur in dogs, less than 3% in cats, about 1% in monkeys, and less than 0.2% in cattle, horses, water buffaloes and other species

(30). Human rabies is very rare, but in highly endemic areas, 4-21 fatal human cases have been reported annually, such as in the province of North Sumatra (population about 7 million), with 4000 animal bites each year. The dog population has increased enormously (North Sumatra - 500,000), but generally less than 50% are vaccinated. The number of cases in urban areas is higher than in rural areas, due to the denser human and dog populations and, in particular, the increase in urbanization over the last decade. Sylvatic rabies does not appear to constitute a health problem, with only 2 positive cases so far detected in civet cats.

OTHER VIRUSES

A. Smallpox

Thanks to the WHO world-wide smallpox eradication programme in 1967, the incidence decreased dramatically, from over 100,000 cases yearly during the early 1960s to zero by February 1972. Since February 1974, Indonesia has been free from smallpox (31).

B. Varicella

Chickenpox is endemic, occurring sporadically or in small outbreaks among children. Complications (i.e. encephalitis) have so far never been reported, or otherwise not recognized.

During November-December 1981, severe adult cases clinically indistinguishable from smallpox were seen in Bandung. However, they were shown not to be a pox virus by cultivation on the chorioallantoic membrane of embryonated chicken eggs.

C. Herpes Simplex

Herpes febrilis/labialis is frequently seen at the outpatient clinic of the Dermatology Department in Bandung, occasionally also in the form of aphthous stomatitis in young children of the low socio-economic level.

However, herpes virus hominis has been found to be responsible also for aseptic meningitis and encephalitis cases (24).

D. Hepatitis Virus

Hepatitis type A virus seems to be endemic in Indonesia, whereas the incidence of serum hepatitis is lower than that caused by type A virus.

Studies on the presence of HBs antigen by Elisa, CIEP and RPHA in various cities among certain population groups (blood donors, infants, umbilical cord blood, etc.) have revealed positives ranging between 0.5-25% (in press).

E. Trachoma

This disease is the second most important cause of blindness in Indonesia after xerophthalmia among children, particularly those in lower socio-economic groups, and is due in part to malnutrition (32). As is well-established, the prevalence of trachoma is closely associated with overcrowding (urbanization), personal hygiene, poverty and fly density (being the mechanical vectors).

REFERENCES

1. Soewarso, T.I., Epid. Bull. Rep. Indon., 2nd quarter, 26 (1978).
2. Thaib, S. and Alisyahbana, A., IInd Internat. Symp. on Immunization, Min. of Hlth. Rep. Indon. WHO., Unicef, ICC. and USAID., Jakarta, 27 Nov. - 1 Dec. (1979).
3. Thaib, S., Madhar, E., Mangun, H. and Priatna, A., *Bull. Bio Farma VII:* 2, 35 (1970).
4. Thaib, S., Dindin, N. and Mangun, H., *Bull. Bio Farma VIII:* 1, 25 (1971).
5. Thaib, S. and Madhar, E., *Bull. Bio Farma XI:* 2, 11 (1974).
6. Thaib, S. and Priatna, A., *Bull. Bio Farma XIV:* 1, 29 (1977).
7. Thaib, S., Nafsiah and Rumini, M., *Bull. Bio Farma IV:* I, 29 (1967).
8. Thaib, S., Mangun, H., Priatna, A. and Dindin, N., *Bull. Bio Farma IX:* 1, 1 (1972).
9. Thaib, S. and Soengkono, *Bull. Bio Farma V:* I, 1 (1968).
10. Goen, L.S., Madhar, E. and Odah, *Bull. Bio Farma I and II*, 1 (1964, 1965).
11. Thaib, S. and Madhar, E., *Bull. Bio Farma V:* 2, 10 (1968).

12. Sulindro, Wulur, H., Karsono, A. and Thaib, S., *J. Indon. Med. Ass. 19*, 417 (1969).
13. Thaib, S. and Madhar, E., *Bull. Bio Farma XI:* 2, 30 (1972).
14. Thaib, S. and Madhar, E., *Bull. Bio Farma XI:* 2, 19 (1974).
15. Trastotenoyo, M., Anggoro, S., Sumantri, A.G. and Thaib, S., *J. Indon. Paed. Soc. 15*, 5-6, 169 (1975).
16. Kusumobroto, H., Notopuro, H. and Thaib, S., 2nd Nat. Congr. Indon. Assoc. Pathol., Jogyakarta, September (1973).
17. Thaib, S., SEAMEO BIOTROP III Training Course in Ectoparasite Biology, Bandung, Jan. 17 - Feb. 26 (1977).
18. Thaib, S., *Bull. Bio Farma IX:* 1, 22 (1972).
19. Thaib, S., IVth Intern. Congr. for Virol., The Hague, The Netherlands, Aug. 30 - Sept. 6 (1978).
20. Trastotenoyo, M., Personal communication (1973).
21. Thaib, S., *Bull. Bio Farma XIV:* 2, 15 (1977).
22. Thaib, S. and Priatna, A., *Bull. Bio Farma VIII:* 2, 32 (1971).
23. Thaib, S. and Priatna, A., *Bull. Bio Farma XIV:* 1, 1 (1977).
24. Thaib, S., Thesis in press.
25. Thaib, S. and Madhar, E., *Bull. Bio Farma VIII:* 1, 1 (1971).
26. Thaib, S., *Bull. Bio Farma XVII:* 1, 1 (1980).
27. Thaib, S. and Dindin, N., *Bull. Bio Farma VIII:* 2, 1 (1971).
28. Thaib, S., IInd Intern. Symp. on Immunization, Min. of Hlth. Rep. of Indon., WHO, Unicef, ICC and USAID, Jakarta, Nov. 27 - Dec. 1 (1979).
29. Thaib, S., *Bull. Bio Farma XV:* 1, 1 (1978).
30. Hardjosworo, S. and Partoatmodjo, S., A sectoral and regional study, Min. of Education, School of Veter. Medic., Min. of Hlth. and Agriculture (1977).
31. Thaib, S., *Bull. Bio Farma XI:* 2, 39 (1974).
32. Sugana Tjakrasudjatma, Inaugural Speech, April 9 (1980).

27

VIRUS DISEASES IN CHINA

Chi Ming Chu

Institute of Virology
Chinese Academy of Medical Sciences
Beijing, China

There are many virus diseases of importance in a vast country like China. In this summary report, only a few will be described in some detail, others will be briefly mentioned.

I. VIRAL HEPATITIS

Viral hepatitis is probably the most important virus disease in China. Recent historical records revealed three peaks in the years 1958-1960, 1965-1967 and 1969-1972 respectively. The incidence in Beijing varied from 64.2 to 384.8/100,000 for the years 1959-1972. In the high prevalence year 1972, a survey of different population groups in Shanghai revealed incidences varying from 200 to 1,500/100,000. A study in Beijing in 1980 showed that out of 145 hospitalized cases of acute hepatitis with jaundice in adults, 45 (31%) were diagnosed as hepatitis A, 44 (30.3%) as hepatitis B, 2 (1.4%) as mixed hepatitis A and B infection, 44 (30.3%) as non-A and non-B and 10 (6.9%) as hepatitis due to other causes. Since the tests for HBV used were not the most sensitive ones, there may be an overestimation of the proportion of non-A non-B at the expense of B. In another study of 88 cases of chronic hepatitis, 78 (89.8%) were found to possess one or more HBV markers by RIA and only 9 (10.2%) could be diagnosed as non-B.

Hepatitis A in China is predominantly a disease of childhood with highest incidence in the preschool age group. The

VIRAL DISEASES IN SOUTH-EAST ASIA
AND THE WESTERN PACIFIC
ISBN 0 12 484820 6

disease is most prevalent in the autumn and winter in North China, but a seasonal peak is not so distinctive in South China. Spread is mainly by close contact in families, nurseries and kindergartens, but water-borne outbreaks have been described. A recent national survey of 2,685 sera from representative urban and rural population groups in 29 provinces for HAV antibody by IAHA test showed an average positive rate of 71.4%, being lowest in Shanghai (41.1%) and highest in Shanxi (92%). The positive rate by age was 25% for infants under 1 year, 58% for the age group 6-7 and attained a peak of 83.4-91.4% at 15-30.

Hepatitis B is more frequent in adults with a tendency to become chronic in a proportion of cases. Studies on hepatoma suggest that HBV may be one etiological factor in this cancer, but the peculiarly high incidence in certain areas of prevalence suggests that other factors may also be involved. The national survey mentioned above covering 277,186 persons yielded an overall HBsAg positive rate by RPHA test of 8.75%, being higher in rural (10.1%) and lower in urban (7.89%) populations. The positive rate was already high (8.86%) in children under 5, reached a peak (12.5%) at 5 years and then declined gradually, with a secondary elevation at 30-40 years. The distribution of HBsAg subtypes showed interesting features: adr was predominant (78%) in populations to the North of the Yangtze River; adw was predominant (76%) to the South and ayw was the predominant subtype in Xicang and to some extent in Xinjiang.

There is a strong tendency for family clustering of HBV infection. Vertical transmission from mother to newborn infants plays a major role. Thus, out of 22 newborn infants of HBsAg positive mothers, 12 became positive within 6 months (2 at 1-2 months, 7 at 3-4 months, 3 at 4-6 months) and only one above 6 months. All 6 babies of HBsAg positive mothers were infected. These data emphasized the importance of transmission from mothers to infants during or immediately after childbirth. Many of the infected babies become asymptomatic chronic carriers. Horizontal transmission in the family also plays a role in other age groups.

Prophylaxis of hepatitis A includes epidemiological control and the use of γ-globulin for contacts. Control of hepatitis B includes screening of blood donors and strict sterilization requirements for injection instruments. An HBV vaccine prepared from the plasma of HBsAg positive donors is under clinical trial. In view of the vast importance of mother to infant transmission, interruption by vaccination of newborns of HBsAg positive mothers is being studied.

II. INFLUENZA

Fifteen large or medium-size epidemics of influenza occurred between the years 1953-1981, all being due to influenza A virus. Four of these were parts of the two pandemics, namely, those in 1957 and 1957-1958 represented respectively the first and second waves of the H2N2 pandemic and those in 1968 and 1970-1971 were waves of the H3N2 pandemic. The 1977 epidemic was due to both H3N2 and H1N1, while the smaller epidemic in the winter of 1979-1980 in North China was due to H3N2 variants, and the smaller epidemic in the summer of 1981 in South China was again due to H1N1. The course of antigenic shift and drift coincided with what happened in the rest of the world. By chronological order, the Hong Kong/107/71-like variant of H3N2 was first detected in China in September 1971 and the Bangkok/1/79-like variant of H3N2 was first detected (retrospectively) in China in March 1979, both being earlier than similar variants reported abroad. The other H3N2 variants were detected later. As these were usually first found in Guangdong province, they were probably imported. Influenza B virus did cause localized epidemics in 1964-1965 and in 1973, but more frequently they were isolated from sporadic outbreaks. There is no statistical data concerning excess mortality due to influenza and pneumonia in China, but since influenza is a reportable disease, deaths were often reported during epidemics, especially in remote rural areas. As an example, the total numbers of cases and deaths reported in 1980 were 2,937,931 and 556 respectively, but there must be considerable under-reporting. Except for the first wave of pandemics, influenza epidemics invariably occurred during the winter in North China, whereas in South China, there were often two epidemic peaks, one in the winter-spring season and the other in the summer season. The summer peak was often the predominant one and may be the only one in some years.

A cold-adapted live vaccine prepared from the current strain of influenza A virus has been produced since 1968 and used mainly for prophylaxis in healthy adults. Several clinical trials demonstrated an average protective efficacy of about 70%.

III. EPIDEMIC HEMORRHAGIC FEVER

Epidemic hemorrhagic fever with renal syndrome has been known to exist in Heilongjiang province in Northeast China since 1935. The disease apparently spread from mountainous areas to agricultural regions after 1955. Presently, cases have been reported from 18 provinces and 2 municipalities, although the distribution is characteristically spotty. The number of cases reported in 1980 was 30,464 with 1960 deaths. The main reservoir host is *Apodemus agrarius*, although in forestry areas, bank voles and red-backed voles, and in marshy grassland, certain *Microtus* species are also suspected. Contamination of broken skin or mucosa with infected rodent excreta is a recognized route of infection. Transmission by aerosol or by mites are also considered possible by some epidemiologists. Recently, virus strains have been isolated from naturally infected *Apodemus agrarius* by inoculation of Apodemus caught in disease-free areas and of A549 cells. Antigens prepared from these sources reacted positively in an immunofluorescent test with sera from patients convalescent from epidemic hemorrhagic fever as well as from Korean hemorrhagic fever, but not with sera from normal persons or patients with various other diseases in non-endemic areas. Significant antibody rise was demonstrated in paired sera of most clinical cases. Similarly, 97% of paired sera from 193 cases of epidemic hemorrhagic fever also reacted positively with Korean hemorrhagic fever antigen in one or both samples. These results indicate that the two diseases are immunologically closely related, if not identical.

Effective control of epidemic hemorrhagic fever had been achieved in localized endemic areas by reduction of wild rodent population to less than 1%. Early diagnosis, early rest and early treatment on the spot had reduced the case mortality rate in most places from over 10% to about 5%. Prophylactic treatment of shock, uremia, pulmonary oedema and heart failure is emphasized. In recent years, peritoneal or blood dialysis has improved the success of therapy.

IV. ARBOVIRAL DISEASES

There are three arboviral diseases of clinical and epidemiological importance in China, namely, Japanese B encephalitis, Russian spring-summer encephalitis and dengue fever. Only Japanese B encephalitis has a wide distribution and is of general importance.

Japanese B encephalitis was first recognized by serology and virus isolation in the 1940s. At present, with the exception of Xicang, Xinjiang, Qinghai in the high altitude western part, there have been case reports from all other provinces, but the disease is most prevalent in the central and eastern parts of China, where surface water is abundant and the average temperature in July exceeds 20°C. The years of high incidence were 1957, 1966 and 1971. Since 1971, there has been a steady decline in incidence, largely attributed to the wide use of an inactivated vaccine for children under 10 years of age. For the year 1980 in Beijing, the morbidity has been reduced to 2.5/100,000 and case mortality to about 5%. In recent years, however, the disease has shown a tendency to extend northward and to involve higher age groups. The main vector is *Culex tritaeniorhynchus* and pigs serve as the main amplifying host. Preventive measures consist of mosquito control and the use of vaccine. Large scale control of *Culex tritaeniorrhynchus* which breeds in the rice field, however, has proved to be difficult. An inactivated vaccine prepared in hamster kidney cell culture has given over 80% protection in controlled trials and is now widely used. Several live vaccine strains (strain 5-3, 2-8, 14-2) have been developed and tested in small scale trials in man, but they did not seem to induce lasting antibody. However, live vaccine has been effective in the protection of ponies against encephalitis and of swines against abortion.

Russian spring-summer encephalitis was first recognized in 1952 and is restricted to the forest areas of the Northeast. Virus has been isolated from *Ixodes persulcatus*, *Haemaphysalis concinna* and *Dermacentor silvarum* and transovarian transmission demonstrated. The first species is probably the most important vector. An inactivated hamster kidney vaccine is used for prophylaxis. The incidence has been very low in recent years.

Dengue fever had been introduced into the coastal provinces of China during the Second World War by Japanese troops, but apparently failed to persist. Recently, the disease was reintroduced three times during 1978-1980 : type 4 in 1978, type 1 in 1979 and type 3 in 1980. The former two types were transmitted by *Aedes albopictus* and the affected areas were restricted to certain coastal counties near Hong Kong. The last type, however, spread to a wider area, involving the Hainan Island and the coastal regions of Guangdong and Guangxi provinces and was mainly transmitted by *Aedes aegypti*. Cases with hemorrhagic tendency were frequently encountered, but no genuine dengue hemorrhagic fever or shock syndrome has been identified.

V. OTHER VIRAL DISEASES

The mass application of live vaccines has considerably reduced the incidence of poliomyelitis and measles in China. The polio situation is described in another report. The use of live measles vaccine since 1966 has levelled epidemic peaks and altered the bi-yearly epidemic periodicity characteristic of measles before the vaccine era. However, there were still 570,037 reported cases and 3,862 deaths in 1980, mainly in remote areas. The locally developed measles vaccine strains, Zhangchun 47 and Shanghai 191, have been found to be comparable in reactogenicity and immunogenicity to the Schwarz and L16 strains in parallel trials. However, in at least three long term studies in isolated island or hyperimmunized populations, there was always a proportion turning sero-negative after 5 years. Epidemiologically, cases with antibody falling below a critical level may either contract typical or atypical measles or undergo inapparent infection with rise in antibody. There is also a shift of incidence to higher age groups. These observations have led to the adoption of revaccination practice in certain provinces.

Rabies had been very rare in the 1950s, but the incidence has increased in recent years in rural areas where dogs are raised for economic purposes. An inactivated hamster kidney vaccine is now prepared for human use. Vaccination of dogs has been found effective in the control of rabies.

Pneumonia in young infants due to adenovirus type 3 and type 7 had been prevalent in the late 1950s and early 1960s causing high mortality, but in recent years, milder pneumonia due to respiratory syncytial virus has become predominant. However, even lately, about one third of hospitalized cases of pneumonia complicating measles have been found to be caused by these two types of adenovirus. The etiology of "autumn diarrhoea" in infants has recently been attributed mainly to rotavirus.

China was also involved in the pandemic of epidemic hemorrhagic conjunctivitis in 1970-1971. Virus was isolated in Shanghai and was later identified as enterovirus 70. Occasional outbreaks have been reported in recent years.

28

A REVIEW OF VIRAL DISEASES IN HONG KONG

W.K. Chang

Virus Unit
Medical & Health Department
Hong Kong

Hong Kong is one of the most densely populated places in the world. The overall density per square kilometre at the end of 1980 was 4,850, but in urban areas the density was over 25,000 people per square kilometre. The total estimated population was 5.15 million with 25.3 per cent under the age of 15. The high population density with a large number of young people facilitates rapid dissemination of viruses especially those infections which are transmitted by the respiratory route or through close personal contacts.

Diagnostic virology facilities have been gradually established since 1960. Data collected from laboratory diagnostic activities and surveillance reveal the occurrence and distribution of various groups of viruses. Table I shows the laboratory evidence of viral and associated infections in the past five years from 1976 to 1980 in Hong Kong.

Adenoviruses

Adenoviruses were most commonly encountered in acute respiratory disease and pharyngoconjunctival fever. Adenovirus 3 was prevalent from 1976 to 1979, while type 7 was more common in 1979-80. Adenovirus types 1, 2, 5 and 14 were associated with a small proportion of all adenovirus infections.

VIRAL DISEASES IN SOUTH-EAST ASIA
AND THE WESTERN PACIFIC
ISBN 0 12 484820 6

TABLE I. *Laboratory Evidence of Viral and Associated Infections in Hong Kong, 1976-1980*

Virus type	1976	1977	1978	1979	1980
Adenovirus	36	44	33	69	39
Influenza A(H3N2)	136	115	1	82	20
Influenza A(H1N1)	-	36	107	-	27
Influenza B	3	62	4	78	7
Parainfluenza	38	44	43	14	31
RS virus	-	1	1	4	9
Mumps virus	21	8	14	14	3
Measles virus	5	11	3	2	12
Rhinovirus	-	1	1	0	8
Coxsackie A	2	18	0	4	4
Coxsackie B	36	23	18	69	60
Echovirus	9	48	25	34	21
Poliovirus	-	-	-	-	2
Herpes simplex	14	32	21	29	61
Varicella-zoster	5	1	-	5	4
CMV	59	43	66	55	65
EB virus	-	-	-	-	1
Rubella virus	13	128	8	11	39
Congenital rubella	-	15	2	2	4
Japanese encephalitis	2	4	-	4	-
Hepatitis B	564	868	1273	1631	1532
Rabies	-	1*	-	-	2
Rotavirus	9	-	-	1	3
M. pneumoniae	2	-	34	22	7
Chlamydiae psittaci	-	1	1	4	5

*Imported case

Myxo- and Paramyxoviruses

The influenza A virus was the dominant myxovirus. In 1976, scattered outbreaks and sporadic cases due to A/Victoria/3/75 (H3N2) were observed throughout the year. This variant caused a medium-size epidemic in April-June 1977. The H1N1 subtype was first encountered in November 1977, and prevailed continually up to August 1978. H3N2 subtype - mainly A/Texas/1/77 - was the most common influenza A virus in 1979, while in 1980, both A/USSR/77 (H1N1) and A/Bangkok/1/79 (H3N2) were in circulation at the same time.

Increased activity of influenza B virus was observed in 1977 and 1979. The peak incidence of influenza B in 1977 followed the outbreak of influenza virus A (H3N2) in July. In 1979, the type B virus was in concurrence with A virus (H3N2).

The incidence of parainfluenza viruses constituted about 18% of all myxo- and paramyxoviruses infections in 1976-80. Type 1 and type 3 were the common and important causative agents of lower respiratory illnesses in young children.

Respiratory syncytial virus infection was confirmed in a few cases in routine diagnosis in 1976-80. The incidence might be much higher. In a previous planned serological study, RS was found to be the most important cause of pneumonia and bronchiolitis in infants under 12 months.

Mumps is endemic and occurs sporadically. Data in this report was obtained mainly from hospitalized patients of which 29% had CNS involvement and 9% with complication of orchitis.

Prior to 1968, measles was a common childhood disease which showed a distinct biennial pattern with exacerbation every alternate winter and spring. The introduction of measles vaccine since December 1967 significantly reduced the disease incidence and its mortality, and children under 3 years of age are now less frequently affected. An analysis of 497 measles cases in 1976 showed 431 (87%) had not been vaccinated. The vaccination failure rate at Maternal and Child Health Centres was estimated to be 0.1%.

Enteroviruses

Enteroviruses are widely distributed in the community. An average of 15% of children under 5 years of age were asymptomatic excretors of an enterovirus at any one time. Activity of different types of enteroviruses varied from time to time; e.g. coxsackie B3 prevailed in 1976, A9 and echovirus 11 in 1977, coxsackie B2 and echovirus 14 in 1978, coxsackie B3 and echovirus 1 in 1979 and coxsackie B1 in 1980. In an epidemic of a specific type, for instance, coxsackie B3 in 1976, the virus was usually found in association with various clinical entities, such as febrile illness, respiratory disease, pleurodynia, meningitis and myocarditis.

Poliomyelitis has markedly decreased since 1963 when oral poliovaccine was combined in the expanded immunization programme. The incidence of poliomyelitis fell from an annual average of 208.6 cases in 1958-62 to 53.6 in 1963-67 and 11.8 in 1968-72. Four cases were recorded in 1973. The disease was absent in the following 6 years. Then two cases of poliomyelitis reappeared in 1980, and three cases in 1981.

Two outbreaks of acute haemorrhagic conjunctivitis due to enteroviruses occurred in Hong Kong. In 1971, both enterovirus type 70 and coxsackie A24 were incriminated, and in 1975 coxsackie A24 variant was the causative agent.

Herpesviruses

Herpesviruses, including herpes simplex, varicella-zoster, cytomegalovirus and Epstein-Barr viruses, are endemic in Hong Kong. In general, most children are exposed to these viruses in early life.

Herpes simplex virus infections are common in Hong Kong. The relative prevalence of the two serotypes HSV-1 and HSV-2 at different ages has not been determined. Varicella-zoster virus was mainly associated with skin diseases, and rarely with CNS involvement.

Cytomegalovirus was associated with a wide variety of clinical symptoms in infants and young children. CMV antibody was demonstrated in 94% of blood donors between 20 and 40 years of age. It postulates that the potential risk of a woman becoming infected for the first time during pregnancy would well be under 6%. Tests on newborns showed a prenatal infection rate of 1 in 500 births (0.2%). CMV infection was quite common in postnatal period and early infancy. A surveillance based on virus isolation and serological tests (Table II) revealed that excretor-rate in infants rose rapidly after birth to 24% at 3 months of age. Fifty per cent of children in the second year of life showed serological evidence of exposure to the virus. In cultural examination of high cervical swabs from women after second trimester, CMV was isolated in 6% of the specimen. The presence of CMV in the birth canal, breast milk and probably in maternal saliva and urine as well as CMV excretors in siblings constitute the sources of infection.

Only one case of infectious mononucleosis due to Epstein-Barr virus was diagnosed in 1980. Antibody to EBV VCA is commonly detected indicating that most people have been infected in early childhood.

TABLE II. Incidence of CMV Antibody and Excretors in Children

Age (Months)	CMV antibody (CFT)		CMV excretor	
	Number tested	Number positive (%)	Number tested	Number positive (%)
Newborn	100	96 (96%)	500	1 (0.2%)
½ - 1	N.T.*	-	51	4 (7.9%)
1 - 2	N.T.	-	50	6 (12.0%)
2 - 3	N.T.	-	50	12 (24.0%)
3 - 4	N.T.	-	50	12 (24.0%)
4 - 6	50	21 (42%)	100	21 (21.0%)
7 - 12	50	24 (48%)	308	85 (27.6%)
13 - 24	50	25 (50%)	42	9 (21.4%)
25 - 36	50	27 (54%)	49	5 (10.2%)
37 - 48	50	31 (62%)	N.T.	-

*N.T. - Not tested

Rubella virus

An epidemic of rubella occurred in the spring of 1977 after a lapse of 14 years. The outbreak was imminent in the population as low immunity was revealed in a serological study in 1976 that 53.3% of persons at 21-30 years of age did not have rubella haemagglutination-inhibition antibody. Morbidity rate of the epidemic could not be ascertained because rubella is not notifiable. However, of 105 laboratory confirmed cases, 59 (56.2%) belonged to the age-group of 21-30 years. There were 15 cases of congenital rubella detected at the end of the year.

Sporadic cases continued to occur in the following years with a moderate increase in 1980. Follow-up studies showed that about 30% women of child-bearing age remained seronegative in 1978-80. Rubella vaccination was added to the immunization programme in September 1978. The vaccine is given to girls aged 11 to 14 years and women of child-bearing age for the prevention of congenital rubella.

Japanese encephalitis virus

Japanese encephalitis virus is the only arbovirus detected in Hong Kong. The disease in human is sporadic, while the antibody to this virus is commonly detected in pigs.

Hepatitis viruses

Viral hepatitis is a major health problem in Hong Kong. Both hepatitis A and B viruses occur endemically with periodic outbreak of hepatitis A once every three years.

In 1981, 256 cases of acute hepatitis were tested for anti-HAV IgM and hepatitis B surface antigen. The results showed 22.3% had serological evidence of hepatitis A infection and 41% were positive for HBsAg.

A serological survey was carried out in 1979 to study the prevalence of anti-HAV and HBsAg/anti-HBs in different age-groups (Table III). Anti-HAV positivity rate increased with advancing age, reaching 90% at 50 years of age. A sharp rise was observed at the age between 11 and 30 years. The distribution of HBsAg and anti-HBs indicated that many children acquired hepatitis B infection at early age and a significant proportion at adolescence. The HBsAg carrier rate is high in the population reaching 11.4% in the age-group of 21-30 years. Although HBsAg is less prevalent in females, about 6% of women at child-bearing age are carriers. Maternal transmission and early postnatal infection play an important role in the epidemiology of hepatitis B in Hong Kong.

TABLE III. Percentage Distribution of Hepatitis A and B Markers

Age-group	*Anti-HAV*	*Hepatitis B markers*		
		HBsAg	*Anti-HBs*	*HBsAg+Anti-HB*
1 - 10	*12.7%*	*3.3%*	*10.3%*	*13.6%*
11 - 20	*44.7%*	*8.7%*	*27.9%*	*36.6%*
21 - 30	*75.0%*	*11.4%*	*34.4%*	*45.8%*
31 - 40	*82.9%*	*9.7%*	*44.8%*	*54.5%*
41 - 50	*90.2%*	*9.6%*	*55.8%*	*65.4%*
51 & over	*90.0%*	*8.6%*	*68.8%*	*77.4%*

Rabies virus

There was one case of rabies in 1977, but it was an imported case with no public health risk. An outbreak occurred in October 1980 after a lapse of 25 years. A total of 3 human cases, 15 rabid dogs and one cat was detected. The outbreak was finally contained and subsided in 6 months.

Rotavirus

Rotavirus was scarcely detected in the past years due to the lack of laboratory facilities. Its existence in Hong Kong was first confirmed in a WHO collaborative study in 1976 that 9 (34.6%) of 26 diarrhoeal cases were associated with this virus. The introduction of Elisa test in 1981 has corroborated its prevalence in Hong Kong.

Mycoplasma Pneumoniae and Chlamydia Psittaci

Mycoplasma pneumoniae infection was rarely encountered before 1977. There was a marked increase of pneumonia cases in association with this agent in 1978. The disease affected persons of all age, ranging from 3 months to 58 years.

Pneumonia in association with chlamydia psittaci was rare, but since 1979, the incidence has increased slightly. Most laboratory-confirmed cases (60%) were over 50 years of age.

Summary

Many viral diseases are endemic in Hong Kong and infections occur early in life. The immunization programmes against poliomyelitis and measles have dramatically changed the epidemiological pattern of these two important diseases. Poliomyelitis has almost completely disappeared. The introduction of rubella vaccine will hopefully reduce the incidence of congenital rubella. Hong Kong is vulnerable to the spread of viruses from other parts of the world, such as acute haemorrhagic conjunctivitis in 1971 and rabies in 1980. Effective control of these viral diseases has to depend on early detection of the causative agents.

29

VIRAL DISEASES IN THE PHILIPPINES: AN OVERVIEW

Veronica F. Chan

Department of Medical Microbiology
Institute of Public Health
University of the Philippines
Manila, Philippines

For health statistics, the Philippines is divided into 13 regions consisting of 73 provinces and 60 cities, the 13th region being the national capital region composed of 4 cities and 13 municipalities.

TABLE 1. Ten Leading Causes of Morbidity and Mortality Rate/100,00 Population, Philippines, 1977

Morbidity		*Mortality*	
Cause	*Rate*	*Cause*	*Rate*
Influenza	*614.1*	*Pneumonia*	*105.1*
Gastroenteritis & colitis	*464.5*	*Tuberculosis, all forms*	*70.7*
Bronchitis, emphysema & asthma	*400.5*	*Diseases of the heart*	*62.2*
Tuberculosis, all forms	*238.0*	*Gastroenteritis & colitis*	*40.1*
Pneumonias	*231.2*	*Diseases of the vascular system*	*35.0*
Malaria	*66.6*	*Malignant neoplasms*	*31.1*
Measles	*61.5*	*Accidents*	*25.2*
Whooping cough	*47.6*	*Avitaminosis & other nutritional deficiencies*	*22.3*
Malignant neoplasms	*46.1*	*Bronchitis, emphysema & asthma*	*14.1*
Dysentery, all forms	*45.7*	*Measles*	*11.8*

VIRAL DISEASES IN SOUTH-EAST ASIA
AND THE WESTERN PACIFIC
ISBN 0 12 484820 6

In the past decade, morbidity and mortality statistics indicate that 2 viral diseases, influenza and measles, were among the ten leading causes of morbidity, but only measles was among the ten leading causes of mortality. Malnutrition has also consistently been one of the ten leading causes of mortality. The respective ranking of these diseases are shown in Table 1 for the year 1977 (1).

Incidence of some of the viral diseases is widespread nationwide, while others show significant difference between urban and rural areas (Table 2). Influenza is maintained as the first cause of morbidity in 8 out of 13 regions. Measles, whether it be in the provinces or in the national capital region ranks on the average as the 7th cause of morbidity. Other viral diseases of the same pattern of occurrence are infectious hepatitis and viral encephalitis. In contrast, rabies is the only viral disease that occurs more commonly in the rural than in urban areas. The opposite pattern of occurrence of rabies is noted in dengue H-fever, varicella and poliomyelitis.

While the reported morbidity patterns vary in urban and rural areas, and in different regions, it is very difficult to infer that such variations are real. A 1962 survey showed that underregistration of deaths was found as high as 27.3% in 32 provinces and 18 cities for the years 1959 to 1962. How much of these variations are due to differential completeness of reporting in the different parts of the country, and how much is due to real geographic differences cannot be determined. Be that as it may, one thing is certain; the reported figures are subject to this differential completeness of reporting cases and deaths. The findings of a recent lameness survey favors the suspicion that geographical variation is largely due to differences in reporting in the different areas. In a recent lameness survey among 12,055 children Ward *et al* (2) reported that poliomyelitis is just as prevalent in rural as in urban areas.

TABLE 2. Frequency of Occurrence of Some Viral Diseases by Place, Philippines

Urban > Rural	*Urban = Rural*	*Urban < Rural*
Dengue H-fever	*Influenza*	*Rabies*
Poliomyelitis	*Measles*	
Varicella	*Infectious hepatitis*	
	Viral encephalitis	

Notifiable viral diseases include acute poliomyelitis, dengue H-fever, infectious hepatitis, influenza, measles, varicella, viral encephalitis, rabies, smallpox and yellow fever. The case and death rates of ages below 10 years old as compared for all ages are shown in Table 3. Attention is called to the high mortality rate among infants due to measles.

For the decade 1967 to 1976, it was noted that deaths from notifiable diseases showed a continued declining trend except for viral encephalitis and influenza which increased in 1976. Measles and influenza presented irregular trends on account of outbreaks at almost yearly intervals.

In 1980, we reported the results of an incidence study conducted among infants and children below 10 years of age residing in the national capital region (3). Viruses that caused viral infections with the highest incidence rates were cytomegalo and adeno viruses. Second only in order of frequency of occurrence were viral infections due to respiratory syncytial, rubella, mumps and herpes simplex viruses. Among the low frequency occurring viral infections were those due to influenza types A and B, parainfluenza types 1, 2 and 3, and varicella-zoster viruses. Lymphocytic choriomeningitis virus was a very rare cause of infection.

Seasonal variation was observed in the incidence of these viral infections. Many of these viral infections had the tendency to occur during the dry months from January to June, as opposed to only two (respiratory syncytial and influenza type B) which occurred more commonly during the rainy months from July to December, and only influenza due to type A viruses occurred throughout the year.

Vaccination against poliomyelitis is the only one included in the Extended Program of Immunization which was launched in January, 1980 throughout the country. Prior to 1980, oral polio vaccine was first introduced in August 1967 on a large scale in the national capital region, and from 1968 to 1970, regions #4, 6, 9 and 11 were included. Since then, pediatricians were the source of immunizations but mainly in the urban areas among children of middle to high-income groups. Such a history of immunization program partly explains the occurrence of poliomyelitis outbreaks in recent years.

TABLE 3. *Notifiable Viral Diseases: Reported Cases and Deaths by Age-Group Rate/100,000 Population, Philippines, 1977*

Viral Diseases	All Ages		Under 1 Year		1 - 4 Years		5 - 9 Years	
	Cases	Deaths	Cases	Deaths	Cases	Deaths	Cases	Deaths
Influenza	614.1	6.4	1,453.2	22.1	634.9	8.0	570.4	2.7
Measles	61.5	11.8	283.6	93.3	210.4	53.5	129.1	7.7
Infectious hepatitis	16.4	1.7	15.0	6.2	15.5	0.9	16.4	0.9
Acute poliomyelitis	3.2	0.8	16.6	4.4	11.6	3.3	3.5	0.6
Varicella	2.6	0.1	4.7	0.6	6.2	0.2	5.9	0.2
Dengue H-fever	1.6	0.5	2.3	0.7	3.2	1.0	3.6	1.1
Viral encephalitis	0.8	0.4	3.5	2.0	1.5	1.0	1.0	0.4
Rabies	0.6	0.6	0	0	0.4	0.4	0.8	0.8

ACKNOWLEDGMENT

We are grateful to Dr. A. Savinov, Medical Officer, Virus Diseases, World Health Organization, Geneva, Switzerland for providing us with the various CF viral antigens used in the incidence study.

REFERENCES

1. Valera, J.P., Faraon, A.O., Ludovice, Z.O. and Bonoan, T.M., *in* "Philippine Health Statistics, 1977", Ministry of Health, Manila, Philippines (1977).
2. Ward, N.A., Dizon, J.J., Casabal, G.T., Sale, G.J. and Zaraspe, R., *WHO Wkly. Epidem. Rec. 56*, 377 (1981).
3. Chan, V.F., Soriano, L., Limson, B.M., Madraso, E.D., Rosete, S., Bagoyo, R., Almagro, E., Reyes, Z., Salenda, S., Rayo, L. and Gazmen, J., *Phil. J. Microbiol. Infect. Dis.* (in press).

30

VIRAL DISEASES IN PAPUA NEW GUINEA - A NATIONAL OVERVIEW

Michael P. Alpers

Papua New Guinea Institute of Medical Research
Goroka, Papua New Guinea

Papua New Guinea (PNG) is an independent country of 462,840km^2 consisting of the eastern part of the island of New Guinea and hundreds of adjacent islands. Its topography contains much variety, including a central cordillera 80-250 km wide, with the highest point 4519m. The population in 1980 was 3,007,000, and the average annual growth rate since 1966 2.3%. The percentage living in rural areas is 87%, ranging by province from 76% to 99%. The average population density is 6km^{-2} with a range between provinces of 0.6 to 21. There is extreme linguistic diversity, with over 700 languages spoken. Rural life is based on subsistence horticulture, though cash cropping is becoming increasingly important. Rural society is usually grouped into hamlets loosely combined into villages. The expectation of life was 59 years in urban areas and 51 years in rural areas in 1976. The infant mortality rate is high but is declining; on the basis of the 1971 census, urban infant mortality rate was estimated to be 63 and rural 123 (1). The age structure of the population is typical of a developing tropical country - the percentage under 15 years of age was 43 in 1971 and 45 in 1976.

Health services are based on a hierarchical system, with aid posts in rural areas serving a few thousand people, health sub-centres, health centres, provincial hospitals and regional base hospitals. Rural health services throughout the country in 1979 included 169 health centres, 209 health sub-centres and 1916 aid posts; the average population per rural health facility was 1180. Rural health services, in particular immunizations and nutritional care of mothers and infants, are also carried out by the community health nursing service.

VIRAL DISEASES IN SOUTH-EAST ASIA
AND THE WESTERN PACIFIC
ISBN 0 12 484820 6

Routine immunizations are given to children for diphtheria, pertussis, tetanus, tuberculosis, poliomyelitis and, in the highlands, pigbel. The decision has recently been taken to add measles vaccination. A monthly bulletin of selected morbidity statistics in PNG (EPINT) is issued by the Department of Health. In the last 12 months EPINT has reported outbreaks of influenza-like disease from many provinces. A typical report is that of an outbreak in June 1981 in the West Sepik in which 3370 cases were seen; of these 86 had pneumonia and there were 8 deaths (CFR 0.2%). Measles outbreaks were also reported in 1981. At the Kapuna Health Centre from March to June, 70 cases of measles were seen with the following complications: mild enteritis (53%), severe enteritis (10%), pneumonia (34%), thrush (26%), and bacterial conjunctivitis (11%); lung abscess and encephalitis occurred in a few cases; three cases died (CFR 4%). Another useful general reference for disease problems is Bell's book on the Diseases and Health Services of Papua New Guinea (2).

Influenza Influenza is an important endemic and epidemic disease of PNG; some epidemics have been associated with high case fatality rates, particularly in remote rural areas at high altitude. Influenza was reported in 1892, 1899 and 1907; though the pandemic which appeared in Australia in 1919 did not reach PNG, a less serious form of the disease was epidemic in the Western Province at that time (3). There were epidemics of influenza in 1931, 1964 and 1969 (4). Of the 1969 epidemic one view was that it "was less serious than reports at the time suggested" and "was not widespread" (3). However, between July and October 1969 more than 3000 deaths were recorded from influenza and its complications; the case fatality rate in some areas of the Southern Highlands was 2%; and many of the deaths were only reported when the study of mortality was undertaken (4). This particular epidemic was investigated also by Gajdusek (5). Bell suggests that "reduction of mortality in future epidemics will rely on fast reporting, better-equipped peripheral health centres, district action plans and "fire teams" that can be assembled and dispatched within 24 hours to an area reporting an outbreak" (4). This has not yet been achieved and similar problems can be expected with the next epidemic of influenza. Penicillin is recommended to combat complications and influenza vaccine is not used; it has been suggested also that more widespread use of pneumococcal vaccine may help prevent mortality from epidemic influenza.

Measles Measles is responsible for much morbidity in PNG. However, it does not have the mortality that has been reported from some parts of Africa. The hospital CFR was 0.4% in over 11,000 cases of measles between 1962 and 1969 (6). Although at that time it was considered that measles was not sufficiently severe to warrant routine immunization, this view was challenged and with the advent of heat-stable vaccines the policy has been changed.

Andrew Hall (unpublished manuscript 1980) studied an epidemic of measles in rural Gulf Province and pointed out that since the peak of infection occurred in an older age group than that observed in urban areas, the optimum age for immunization in rural PNG should be 9 months. Hazlett, Blake and Nurse found age stratification in measles antibodies in nearby populations, indicating recurrent epidemics and susceptibility of a large number of individuals into adolescence (7).

Chicken pox is a relatively common disease and is usually mild. However, serious cases do occur and of 2,925 patients admitted with the disease to hospitals in 1968-1972 39 died, giving a hospital CFR of 1.3% (8). *Mumps* is endemic and mild. Hazlett, Blake and Nurse have shown a pattern of acquisition of antibodies in rural Pawaian populations similar to that found in other parts of the world where the disease is endemic, with 100% of adults being serologically positive (7). *Rubella* is not seen as a problem and rubella vaccine is not used.

Poliomyelitis Bell records known epidemics of paralytic poliomyelitis in PNG in 1936, 1948, 1952, 1962, 1963, 1965 and 1970 (9). In 1970 in Madang 26 cases were seen, of which 10 were from rural communities. In the same year in a rural outbreak in Tari 23 cases were recorded. The proportion of susceptible individuals is high in rural communities, despite the absence of hygiene. Vaccination programs are bedevilled by the problems of delivery and maintaining the potency of the vaccine. Benfante and Gajdusek reported a serological survey for 18 enterovirus antigens in populations in the Eastern Highlands (10). Though prevalence studies over time between 1957 and 1964 indicated increasing acquisition of antibodies and the overall antibody prevalence rate for polio 3 was 60%, rates for polio 1 and polio 2 were much lower; thus many individuals were susceptible to poliomyelitis - and to other enterovirus infections. Coxsackie B viruses appear to have been introduced earlier than type A and prevalence rates were much higher; rates for echoviruses were also high. Outbreaks of Bornholm disease have been reported in the past from various parts of PNG.

Arbovirus Disease Sabin isolated strains of dengue types 1 and 2 from soldiers in PNG during World War II (11). French et al. isolated Murray Valley encephalitis virus from a patient in Port Moresby in 1956 (12). Anderson et al. found antibody to MVE virus widespread in the lowlands (13). Anderson, Doherty and Carley found serological evidence of alphavirus infection in the same lowland populations (14). Wisseman et al. showed that antibodies to both alphaviruses and flaviviruses were prevalent among the inhabitants of lowland regions but that in the highlands there was a striking dissociation between the two groups; flavivirus antibodies disappeared above about 1500m, whereas alphavirus antibodies were still found at higher altitudes (15). Work and Jozan found in two areas of the Purari River drainage antibodies to both alphaviruses (20% positive) and flaviviruses (40% positive) (16). There was an increasing trend with age indicating persistent or cyclic virus transmission. The viruses were apparently maintained in a local vertebrate reservoir. Neutralization testing against MVE and Kunjin of sera positive to flavivirus by HI indicated that most responses were to other flaviviruses. A similar situation probably obtains for alphaviruses. Andrew Hall (unpublished manuscript 1980) studied arbovirus antibodies in urban and rural communities in the Gulf Province and found that alphavirus antibodies were more prevalent, and acquired earlier in life, in rural than in urban areas; of the flaviviruses dengue was more prevalent in urban areas (63% in adults) than rural (5% in adults), whereas MVE was more prevalent in rural areas (91% against 27% in adults). Three clinical syndromes are important in this context: tropical polyarthritis, encephalitis and dengue. Tropical polyarthritis is common in both highland and lowland regions and may in many cases be viral in origin, though evidence for Ross River virus has so far been usually absent. Localized epidemics of encephalitis are frequently reported in PNG, but no investigations rigorous enough to incriminate a particular virus have yet been carried out. Dengue has been documented in urban outbreaks (17) but the disease is diagnosed much more often clinically than it is virologically. Dengue haemorrhagic fever or shock syndrome has not yet been reported.

Diarrhoeal Disease Diarrhoeal disease is the second most common cause of death in hospital in children under 4 years old (18). In no disease is malnutrition so important, especially at weaning. Weanling diarrhoea was the commonest cause of hospital admission in the age group 6-18 months; 48% of these children were considered malnourished (19). Though exact definitions have yet to be worked out it is clear that malnutrition is an important problem in PNG at the time of weaning, when a vicious cycle between infection and malnutrition is readily set up. Viruses are probably profoundly important in the aetiology of diarrhoeal disease in PNG. Shann et al. found rotavirus infection in 54 of 66 children (82%) under 2 years old with diarrhoea of less than 4 days duration requiring admission to hospital; no rotavirus particles were detected in stools of 11 children treated as outpatients (20). Rotavirus infection is thus likely to be the major cause of serious diarrhoea in young children and a suitable vaccine would be of great value.

Pneumonia and Acute Respiratory Infections Although the immediate causes of pneumonia are bacterial, a large number of respiratory viruses are known to be circulating in rural and urban communities. Since pneumonia is the most serious disease in Papua New Guinea and the most important cause of admission to hospital, the importance of respiratory viruses in initiating pneumonia must be given serious consideration. Influenza and measles have been discussed separately. In studies carried out at the Institute of Medical Research (which has the only medical virus laboratory in PNG) a wide range of respiratory viruses have been isolated from children with pneumonia and acute respiratory infection; no one virus or group of viruses stands out as being the most important endemic initiating pathogen. Under these circumstances one looks to the pneumococcus and haemophilus for providing a preventive vaccine.

Skin Infection Skin infections are an important cause of morbidity, but are uncommonly viral. Warts occur in all age groups. Molluscum contagiosum is highly prevalent in young children; investigation of the antigenic strains which cause the disease in PNG has yet to be carried out.

Hepatitis In PNG carriage rates to hepatitis B virus are high, with HB antigen rates between 5 and 25% and antibody rates between 15 and 30%, as measured in surveys, though the actual rate is probably much higher (21).Woodfield described 65 cases of hepatitis amongst Papua New Guineans and concluded that most Papua New Guineans with viral hepatitis have hepatitis A, although a small proportion do have hepatitis B (21). Of expatriates, medical personnel are likely to get hepatitis B and others hepatitis A. Hepatitis B virus is probably involved in the aetiology of primary liver cancer, which is the fourth most common cancer in PNG and the most common in highland males. Woodfield, Endo and Matsuhashi found that 82% of 72 patients with hepatocellular carcinoma were positive for hepatitis B antigen (22).

Herpes Simplex Infection Herpes simplex virus has been isolated from a number of cases of acute respiratory infection but no particular clinical importance has been attached to these infections. The possible role of HSV in the aetiology of cancer has not been looked at in PNG; however, it is important to note that cancer of the cervix is the most common reported cancer in women.

Epstein-Barr Virus Lang, Garruto and Gajdusek showed early acquisition of antibody to EBV in populations in the highlands, with 100% of adults aged 15-29 being positive (23). Infectious mononucleosis is restricted to expatriates. Burkitt lymphoma is an important tumour in PNG, which has the only focus of the disease outside of Africa. The incidence varies markedly: the highlands with 37% of the population has only 9% of reported cases; Madang Province with 7% of the population has 24% of reported cases; and West Sepik Province with less than 4% of the population has 14% of reported cases. It has been generally assumed that Burkitt lymphoma in PNG is EBV-associated, though this has not yet been rigorously demonstrated.

Cytomegalovirus Infection As with EBV, CMV antibodies are acquired early (23). The prevalence and titre of CMV antibody decreased with age among highlanders but was still 74% in individuals over 30 years of age. Persistence of infectious virus in adults leads to the spread in infants; antibody protects against maternal and congenital infections.

Kuru Kuru is the main slow viral subacute spongiform encephalopathy found in PNG though there has been a confirmed case of Creutzfeldt-Jakob disease. Kuru occurs in a restricted area largely confined to the Okapa District of the Eastern Highlands Province. Over 2560 cases have been documented since investigations of the disease began in 1957. Though the annual kuru mortality has fallen from over 200 in 1957 to just under 20 in 1981, the disease is still the most important health problem to the people of the South Fore, where it is anticipated that the disease will continue for another decade before finally disappearing.

REFERENCES

1. McDevitt, T.M., *Asian and Pacific Census Forum* 8, 5 (1981).
2. Bell, C. Ed. "The Diseases and Health Services of Papua New Guinea". Dept Publ. Hlth, Port Moresby (1973).
3. Warburton, M.F., *Med. J. Aust.* Spec. Suppl. 1, 14 (1973)
4. Bell, C.O. *in* C. Bell, ed. *loc.cit.*, p. 200.
5. Gajdusek, D.C., *in* "Journal June 1st 1969 - March 3rd 1970" p. 247-308. National Institute of Neurological Diseases and Stroke, National Institutes of Health, Maryland (1971).

6. Bell, C.O. *in* C. Bell, ed. *loc. cit.*, p. 204.
7. Hazlett, D.T.G., Blake, N.M., and Nurse, G.T., *in* "Purari River (Wabo) Hydroelectric Scheme Environmental Studies", Volume 8 (M. Alpers, ed.), p. 55. Office Environment & Conservation and Dept. Minerals & Energy, Port Moresby (1980).
8. Bell, C.O., *in* C. Bell, ed. *loc. cit.* p. 357.
9. Bell, C.O., *in* C. Bell, ed. *loc. cit.* p. 218.
10. Benfante, R.J., and Gajdusek, D.C., *Papua New Guinea Med. J. 21,* 124 (1978).
11. Sabin, A.B., *Am. J. Trop. Med. Hyg. 1,* 30 (1952).
12. French, E.L., Anderson, S.G., Price, A.V.G., and Rhodes, F.A., *Am. J. Trop. Med. Hyg. 6,* 827 (1957).
13. Anderson, S.G., Price, A.V.G., Nanadia-Koia, and Slater, K., *Med. J. Aust. 2,* 410 (1960).
14. Anderson, S.G., Doherty, R.L., and Carley, J.G., *Med. J. Aust. 1,* 273 (1951).
15. Wisseman, C.L.Jr., Gajdusek, D.C., Schofield, F.D., and Rosenzweig, E.C., *Bull. W.H.O. 30,* 211 (1964).
16. Work, T.H., and Jozan, M., *in* "Purari River (Wabo) Hydroelectric Scheme Environmental Studies", Volume 8 (M. Alpers, ed.), p. 29. Office Environment & Conserv-ation & Dept Minerals & Energy, Port Moresby (1980).
17. Zigas, V., and Doherty, R.L., *Papua New Guinea Med. J. 16,* 42 (1973).
18. Biddulph, J., *in* C. Bell, ed. *loc. cit.*, p. 191.
19. Biddulph, J., and Pangkatana, P., *Papua New Guinea Med. J. 14,* 7 (1971).
20. Shann, F.A., Germer, S., Lansdown, S., Bugg, H.C., Bishop, R.F., and Barnes, G.L., *Med. J. Aust. 2,* 153 (1980).
21. Woodfield, D.G., *Trop. Geogr. Med. 27,* 399 (1975).
22. Woodfield, D.G., Endo, Y., and Matsuhashi, T., *Aust. New Zeal. J. Med. 4,* 3 (1974).
23. Lang, D.J., Garruto, R.M., and Gajdusek, D.C., *Am. J. Epidem. 105,* 480 (1977).

31

VIRUS DISEASES IN THE PACIFIC ISLANDS

J.A.R. Miles[1]

Wellcome Virus Laboratory
Tamavua Hospital
Suva, Fiji

The relative importance of various virus diseases differs very little between tropical countries and not very much between the tropics and the temperate zone. Respiratory viruses are the main infectious cause of morbidity throughout the world but their importance in mortality is far more variable. In the Pacific Islands they are usually among the four most frequent causes of death.

In developing countries diarrhoeal diseases are second to respiratory in importance and, where they have been studied in infants, rotaviruses are the most important causative agent.

Both hepatitis A and B are endemic and mosquito-borne viruses are more important than in the temperate zone. The latter are considered in other papers in this seminar.

I want first to look at what is happening about infantile diarrhoea, to consider the peculiarities of the epidemiology of the "flu" syndrome in the islands and then to look at the endemicity and epidemicity of certain other viruses under island conditions.

INFANTILE DIARRHOEA

Infantile diarrhoea is an important cause of morbidity

[1]*Present address: Cappell Avenue, Lake Hawea, New Zealand*

VIRAL DISEASES IN SOUTH-EAST ASIA
AND THE WESTERN PACIFIC
ISBN 0 12 484820 6

and a significant cause of mortality throughout the islands of the Pacific and in many parts the incidence is increasing. The number of notifications of infantile diarrhoea in Fiji has risen from 1960 to 1980. The number in 1960 was 3,295 and that in 1980 was 12,830 (Table 1). Except for two slight dips there has been a steady rise throughout the period which is approximately fourfold over all while the population has increased by about 50%. It is clear that there has been a large increase in incidence. In our current survey potentially pathogenic bacteria have been found in 18.5% of cases, rotavirus in 69%, in some cases associated with bacteria. No potential pathogen has been identified in about 17%. The highest incidence of rotavirus infection in Fiji appears to be in wettest months February to April. Whether the increase in cases relates mainly to an increase in virus diarrhoea is not known, but there is some evidence that it does relate to bottle feeding which has increased to a great extent especially among the urbanised islanders.

In Papua New Guinea, the government has been so convinced of this that early in 1967 they banned the free sale of infant feeding bottles and allowed them only to be sold by chemists on prescription. In Port Moresby General Hospital in 1975 and 1976, 10% of admissions for gastroenteritis and 26% of deaths were in children under 6 months of age. Since then this group has provided only 6% of admissions and one death out of 22. The proportion of infants bottle fed in Port Moresby has fallen from 35 to 12%. The drop in mortality may relate to the introduction of oral rehydration as well as the fall in the number of cases.

Island authorities are convinced that bottle feeding is a major cause of the increase in infantile gastroenteritis and certainly, under conditions in which many island households live, bottles are not sterilised and are prepared with contaminated water. Further the cost of powdered milk and still more of infant formulas is too high for people on low

TABLE 1. Fiji - Notifications of Infantile Diarrhoea

Year	*No. of notifications*
1960	*3,295*
1965	*5,669*
1970	*6,988*
1975	*9,352*
1980	*12,830*

incomes, so feeds are often inadequate and malnutrition is an additional problem.

THE "INFLUENZA" SYNDROME

Influenza is a notifiable disease in the Pacific Islands and the notifications are reported to the South Pacific Commission and appear in the SPC monthly epidemiology bulletins. These notifications are usually based on a clinical syndrome and the limits of what is notified vary from group to group. The most conservative is New Caledonia where more than 150 notifications in a month clearly indicates an epidemic, while the most liberal is Fiji where there have been less than 2000 notifications in only three months in the last six years and nothing less than 4000 notifications in a month can be regarded as possibly epidemic. The highest number of notifications in any one month was 26,751 in the influenza A (HINI) epidemic in February, 1981, in Fiji.

For notification purposes "influenza" is a febrile illness with respiratory symptoms and malaise and probably often includes febrile colds. Apart from orthomyxovirus epidemics none of the agents causing epidemics of "flu" have been identified.

In the temperate zone, respiratory virus disease is maximal in the late winter and spring. This is not true in the Pacific Islands. In Fiji, over eight years for which detailed data are available, the highest incidence is in March and there is a secondary peak in October.

In 1969, there were epidemics in all the island groups with data available from SPC except Vanuatu (New Hebrides). The peak incidence was February for American Samoa, March for Fiji, French Polynesia and Western Samoa, April for Cook Islands, New Caledonia and Papua New Guinea, June for Tokelau, July for TTPI which is in the nothern hemisphere, August for Wallis, September for Kiribati (Gilbert Islands) which straddles the equator and October for Tonga. Thus among 12 groups reporting epidemics, nine were in autumn and two in the spring and one indefinite. Table 2 shows the timing of epidemics in Fiji over 9 years for which adequate data are available. There were seven autumn and five spring epidemics and in only one year was there a small spring epidemic without the autumn one.

I have examined the data available from SPC and attempted to define the "flu" epidemics for different groups for each year in which that group has sent in reports for every

TABLE 2. Fiji - Months of Peak "Influenza" Notification: 9 Years

Year	Autumn	Spring
1966	May	None
1967	No epidemic incidence	
1968	April	August
1969	March	November
1973	None	September
1975	March	October
1976	March	None
1977	February	October
1978	April	None

month. From 1975 to 1980 twenty-nine epidemics occurred in the autumn and thirty in the spring. The variability of the timing of epidemics is not confined to any one group, nor does it appear, as I had originally thought, to be the direct result of introduction of viruses circulating in both Northern and Southern Hemispheres to countries with a large tourist industry.

It now appears to me that the autumn epidemics are essentially wet season epidemics. The secondary smaller outbreaks in spring I cannot explain although it is possible that they are an overflow from temperate zone outbreaks. In 1981, we have endeavoured to find what agents are circulating in the spring but have had no success. We have not been attempting to isolate rhinoviruses.

MEASLES

It is well known that when measles was first introduced to the Pacific Islands it was a highly fatal disease. By now it is no more serious than in Australia and New Zealand and in the 1973-74 annual report of the Fiji Ministry of Health, following the 1974 epidemic, there was the statement "The disease was relatively mild and no death was reported. Because of these factors and the high cost of measles vaccine no attempt was made to immunise the public against the disease".

In 1966 Black published a paper on the conditions required for endemicity of measles and concluded that a population of about 500,000 with an annual intake of new susceptibles of 15,000 was required for measles endemicity (1).

Table 3 shows monthly notifications of measles from SPC epidemiology reports for 1975 to 1980 together with the figures given for the population of each group for 1976 in the 13th edition of the Pacific Island Year Book (2). Reporting from many island groups was very incomplete, but the overall picture is very much in line with Black's findings and Fiji and Papua New Guinea are the only countries where it appears probable that measles is endemic.

CHICKENPOX, HEPATITIS AND RUBELLA

Table 4 shows that chickenpox and viral hepatitis are endemic in Fiji. Recent evidence suggests that this is true of virus A as well as virus B. The percentage of HB_s antigen carriers varies greatly between different Fiji communities (3). It is likely that notification of rubella is very poor, but I think the figures strongly indicate that

TABLE 3. Notification of Measles - Number of Months with and without Reported Cases 1975-1980

Country	*Months +ve*	*Months -ve*	*Population in 1976*
Tokelau	*0*	*20*	*1,575*
Nauru	*8*	*22*	*7,500*
Wallis & Fatuna	*15*	*27*	*9,192*
Cook Is.	*13*	*19*	*18,128*
American Samoa	*28*	*21*	*30,600*
Kiribati	*15*	*36*	*54,500*
Tonga	*23*	*24*	*90,072*
Vanuatu	*26*	*12*	*100,425*
TTPI	*15*	*35*	*109,975*
New Caledonia	*46*	*6*	*133,233*
French Polynesia	*40*	*10*	*137,382*
Western Samoa	*42*	*6*	*151,515*
Fiji Is.	*68*	*2**	*588,068*
P.N.G.	*29*	*0*	*2,828,600*

**January and June, 1976*

TABLE 4. Fiji: Chickenpox, Hepatitis and Rubella No. of Months with and without Notifications

	Chickenpox	Hepatitis	Rubella
+ve	84	84	37
-ve	0	0	47
Total	84	84	84

the virus is not endemic. I did not obtain a breakdown of the figures for 1971-76 but there was a rubella epidemic in Fiji in 1971. In 1973 and 1976, there were no notifications of rubella and in 1975 only three. We found that in some of the more isolated small islands in the Fiji group rubella has been absent for 20 or more years (4). Because of this finding, the Ministry of Health has introduced rubella vaccination.

Analysis of our data from that study indicated that on the average, 50% of susceptibles were infected by rubella virus at each introduction. Apparently this is not a virus which can remain latent except in congenitally infected infants and it is not able to sustain itself in a population sufficient to maintain endemic measles.

PARAMYXOVIRUSES

We have published data on a survey for antibodies including those for paramyxoviruses in some of the more isolated populations in the Fiji group (5).

There was a quite low proportion of the population with complement fixing antibodies against each of the viruses tested, but no age group completely lacked antibody. Our recent work on the 18 man over-wintering party at South Pole Station has indicated that para-influenza viruses can survive for at least an 8 month period in so small an isolated group (6). It does appear likely that in the lower degree of isolation of small and remote Pacific Islands these viruses can remain endemic. Certainly there is no evidence of the sort of low resistance to infection shown by the natives of Tristan da Cunha when transferred to England, or in migrants from small remote Pacific Islands arriving in New Zealand, although epidemics of colds are reported following the arrival of ships at, for instance, the Tokelaus.

CONCLUSION

The virus problems of Pacific Islands are very similar to those of larger developing countries, but most of them lack the size of population necessary to keep viruses encemic except for those which are able to maintain a latent state in their hosts. Because of this, some special problems exist as in those small islands where young women, at their time of maximum fertility, are completely lacking in antibodies to rubella virus.

ACKNOWLEDGMENTS

This study was supported by the Medical Research Council of New Zealand and the Wellcome Trust.

REFERENCES

1. Black, F.L., *J. Theor. Biol. 11*, 207 (1966).
2. Inder, S. (ed.), *Pacific Islands Year Book* (13th ed.), Pacific Publications, Sydney (1978).
3. Austin, F.J., Maguire, T. and Miles, J.A.R., *Amer. J. Trop. Med. Hyg. 23*, 489 (1974).
4. Macnamara, F.N., Mitchell, R. and Miles, J.A.R., *J. Hyg. (Camb.) 71*, 825 (1973).
5. Miles, J.A.R., Macnamara, F.N. and Mitchell, R., *Human Biol. in Oceania 2*, 79 (1973).
6. Muchmore, H.G., Parkinson, A.J., Humphries, J.E., Scott, E.N., MacIntosh, D.A., Scott, L.V., Cooney, M.K. and Miles, J.A.R., *Nature 289*, 187 (1981).

32

VIRUS DISEASES IN NORTHERN AUSTRALIA

N.F. Stanley

Department of Microbiology
University of Western Australia
Perth, Western Australia

The history of virus diseases in Northern Australia above the 19th parallel of latitude represents a rapidly changing pattern since Caucasian intrusion. Attempts to understand it require recognition of the following environmental factors:

(1) A low population density compared with southern latitudes.
(2) A distinct wet and dry season in a tropical environment geographically part of South-East Asia.
(3) A mixed population of Aboriginal people and Caucasians with different life-styles.
(4) An increasing population of white people developing the north for irrigated agriculture, mining, tourism, etc.
(5) The introduction of animals of economic and domestic significance and consequently increasing numbers of feral animals that can act as amplifier hosts.
(6) The establishment of major extensive permanent tropical wetlands in the north by creation of lakes and irrigated agriculture (1, 2).
(7) Increased movement of people (including refugees) from South-East Asia.

It is proposed to consider these environmental factors under the following headings:

A. Population and environment.
B. Human infection.
C. Conclusions and recommendations.

VIRAL DISEASES IN SOUTH-EAST ASIA
AND THE WESTERN PACIFIC
ISBN 0 12 484820 6

A. POPULATION AND ENVIRONMENT

Table I shows the 1979 figures for three Australian States whose territories extend north of the 19th parallel of latitude, which is the geographic area I propose to consider.

The table is misleading as only a small portion of Western Australians and Queenslanders live in the north and during the dry season there is a great influx of "visitors" across the entire area. In addition, although many Aboriginal people live in the north, it is difficult now to define Aboriginal numbers. Ecologically and virologically, the way of life (especially hygiene) is the important factor. The major environmental factors as far as virus infections are concerned have been: the intrusion of Caucasians into the Australian continent and attempts to develop Australia's north by mining, irrigated agriculture, breeding cattle, tourism and associated activities. These have resulted in (a) the introduction of animals that can act as amplifier hosts for arboviruses (e.g. cattle, buffalo, horses, pigs, donkeys, goats and cats); (b) the introduction of viruses such as measles to "virgin soil" Aboriginal populations; (c) the creation of townships in proximity to water, and (d) the creation of man-made lakes. To these ecological changes we must add the increased movement of humans by air and the legal and illegal movement of refugees. This sparsely populated area is about to undergo rapid development which requires increased population densities in tropical Australia - so far free from such infections as rabies, Japanese B encephalitis and Chikungunya virus. I believe the surveillance required for the detection of viruses has not kept pace with environmental modifications and in some areas we have little idea what may be present or what agents could be introduced (3).

TABLE I. Caucasian and Aboriginal Population Estimates for States with Territory above the 19th Parallel of Latitude

	Caucasian	*Aboriginal*
Northern Territory	*115,900*	*23,751*
Queensland	*2,197,400*	*41,345*
Western Australia	*1,242,800*	*20,126*

B. HUMAN INFECTION

For many years respiratory and enteric infections have represented significant morbidity and mortality in our Aboriginal people, especially children, and greatly in excess of Caucasian illness. To present a glimpse of the changing scene, I propose to examine briefly selected aspects of infections with some viruses listed in Table II.

Poliomyelitis

Paralytic poliomyelitis is exceedingly rare in Aboriginal people. Prior to the introduction of vaccination, the Caucasian population of Australia was subject to the usual epidemics. It was clear, from Miles *et al.* studies in the early 1950s (4, 5) that Aboriginal children acquired antibody to all three types of poliovirus at a very early age; and although I have studied the disease since the 1950s, I have not seen one case of paralytic poliomyelitis.

Hepatitis A

This is a picornavirus with faecal-oral transmission similar to poliovirus. The ecological situation may well be similar to poliomyelitis with the early acquisition of antibody in children and little clinical acute viral hepatitis due to hepatitis A virus in Aborigines. With Caucasians in the north, the situation is different, and our recent experience has been that Caucasians may be severely affected by hepatitis A, due to very few possessing antibody and by moving into northern areas where the virus is active.

Rotavirus

Hospitalization of Aboriginal people is frequently associated with respiratory and gastro-intestinal-genital infections. Although bacteria and chlamydia play important roles here, several careful studies have not revealed that rotavirus is significantly more important in Aboriginal than white children.

TABLE II. Viruses Referred to in the Text

Poliovirus	*Influenza A*
Hepatitis A	*Arboviruses*
Rotavirus	*Dengue*
Hepatitis B	*Ross River virus*
Measles	*Murray Valley encephalitis*

Hepatitis B

As far as the carriage of HBsAg is concerned, this is significantly higher (3% to 24%) in our Aboriginal people than in the Caucasian population (<0.1%). Following Barrett's observations (6, 7) on an unusual distribution of hepatitis B surface antigen serotypes in some Aboriginal communities in North Queensland, it would be interesting to extend the examination over a wider geographic range as well as ascertaining if other types are found in low frequency.

Measles

The early studies of Adels and Gajdusek (8) on measles antibody in Australasian and Micronesian populations pointed out that some Aboriginal communities in Queensland, Northern Territory and Western Australia represented "virgin soil" situations. "Virgin soil" outbreaks did occur in Cape York communities in 1944 and in 1953. In the latter epidemic the Edward River community escaped.

As far as I can ascertain measles vaccine is now widely employed, in addition to triple antigen and polio vaccine, so, as predicted by Gajdusek in 1963, this has been a good opportunity to test the efficacy of measles vaccination in remote and isolated communities.

Influenza A

It appears that influenza in the north has offered no distinctive pattern that needs elaboration. Between epidemics it does not appear to be a significant contributor to respiratory tract infections.

As a general comment, viral infections of Aboriginal children very early in life compared with Caucasians are not confined to enteroviruses but also extend to herpesviruses such as Epstein-Barr virus (EBV) and cytomegalovirus (CMV).

I draw attention to John Pope's (9) observation of an interesting antibody pattern in Aboriginal people in West Cape York Peninsula. High prevalence of antibody in the 1-5 year age group (not associated with clinical disease) was similar to that of sera from Papua New Guinea and endemic Burkitt's lymphoma regions of Uganda. Lang *et al.* (10) reported similar findings with both EBV and CMV in Papua New Guinea.

Arboviruses

A large number of alpha-, flavi, orbi- and rhabdoviruses have been isolated from arthropods, but there are only three human diseases that are endemic and of public health significance: Australian encephalitis, dengue and epidemic polyarthritis. Although important, the animal arbovirus infections, bovine ephemeral fever, bluetongue virus and Akabane disease will not be considered here.

1. Dengue. The history of dengue in Australia is as fascinating and challenging as in any other country. The elimination of *Aedes aegypti* in most of Australia except Queensland has led to its control. In the past dengue viruses have caused extensive outbreaks in Australia, primarily in the coastal north-east regions of Queensland.

It was early this century that Australian studies by Bancroft in 1905 and Cleland *et al.* in 1916 (11) showed that *Aedes aegypti* was the major vector. In spite of that most significant contribution and almost 80 years later we still have the vector in Queensland even in an airport passenger lounge. The importation of cases of dengue thus represents a potential threat for local spread in the areas where *Aedes aegypti* breeds and also *Aedes scutellaris scutellaris*; and this indeed has just occurred in 1981. At the time of writing there have been 17 confirmed clinical cases (type 1) in coastal Queensland towns and Thursday Island (12). The clinical cases and distribution are currently being evaluated but may have involved so far about 150 cases on Thursday Island. Although 1898 saw severe cases with haemorrhage, shock and death, the DHF/DSS does not appear to be a problem in Australia now.

2. Epidemic Polyarthritis and Ross River Virus (RRV). Until 1979, outbreaks appear to have been confined to Australasia. RRV has been isolated from five genera of mosquitoes and antibody to the virus has been found in a variety of Australian vertebrates, including marsupials.

Virus activity and the clinical disease occur throughout the country and foci of persistence are not confined to tropical areas. In Australia, *Aedes vigilax* and *Culex annulirostris* are important vectors. Following the spread of RRV to the Pacific Islands by viraemic air travellers in the last 3 years, *Aedes polynesiensis* appears to be an important vector in at least three areas.

3. Australian Encephalitis and MVE. Table III records the known outbreaks of Australian encephalitis.

It is only since the 1950s that serological studies, effective mosquito captures and sentinel animals have been used to examine MVE and Kunjin ecology. Fig. 1 shows the clinical cases that have occurred during the 1974 outbreak and since that time. The endemic/epidemic pattern is represented pictorially in Fig. 2.

TABLE III. Numbers of Cases of Australian Encephalitis in all States of Australia since 1917[a]

Year	*WA*	*NT*	*Qld*	*NSW*	*Vic.*	*SA*	*Totals*
1917			*44*	*70*	*13*		*114*
1918			*5*	*49*			*67*
1922			*75*				*75*
1925			*11*	*10*			*21*
1951				*10*	*34*	*1*	*45*
1956					*3*		*3*
1971			*1*	*1*			*2*
1974	*1*	*5*	*10*	*5*	*27*	*10*	*58*
1978	*8*						*8*
1979	*2*						*2*
1981	*8*	*1*	*2*				*11*
Totals	*19*	*6*	*148*	*145*	*77*	*11*	*406*

[a]*The numbers refer to clinically recognizable cases, usually confirmed by serology after 1951.*

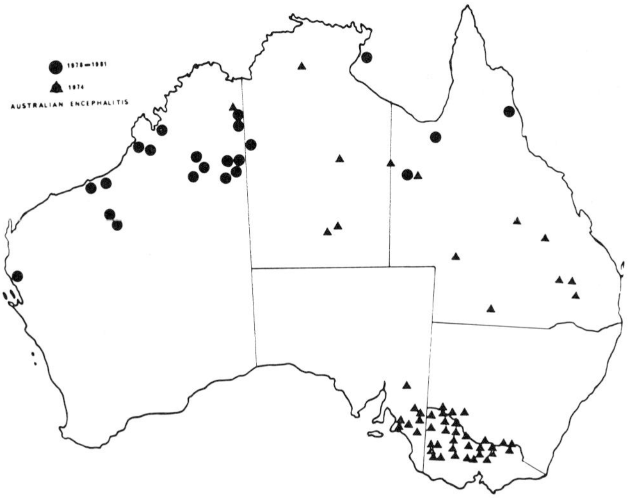

FIGURE 1. Australian encephalitis: location of clinical cases during the 1974 outbreak and cases occurring since that outbreak.

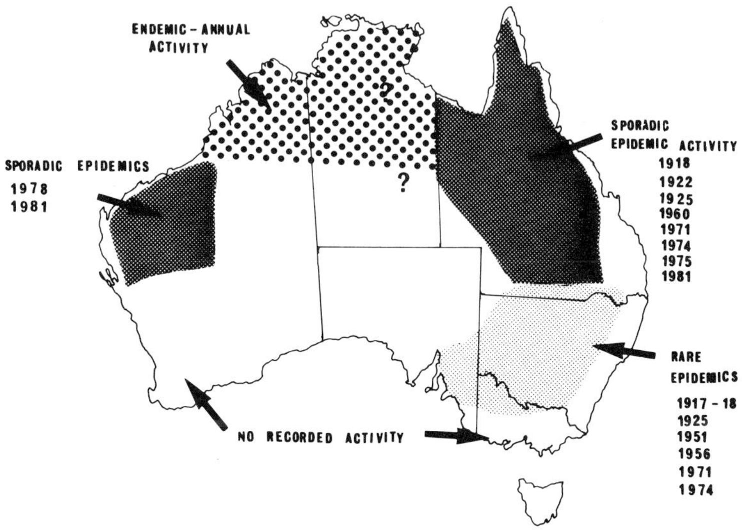

FIGURE 2. Endemic/epidemic pattern of Australian encephalitis.

C. CONCLUSIONS AND RECOMMENDATIONS

Due to the changing scene and the proposals for development of Australia's north, I suggest that more extensive surveillance should be attempted for this area of Australia. Not only should this include arboviruses known to exist on the continent but also those known to be endemic immediately to the north, as well as for antibodies to arenaviruses, RVF and some others. As part of this surveillance, I would also like to see far better communication between virologists of South-East Asia and the Western Pacific through an integrated information service. This meeting should consider that suggestion.

REFERENCES

1. Stanley, N. F., *Search 3*, 7 (1972).
2. Stanley, N.F., *in* "Man-made Lakes and Human Health" (N.F. Stanley and M.P. Alpers, eds.), p. 103. Academic Press, London, (1975).
3. Stanley, N. F., *in* "Changing Disease Patterns and Human Behaviour" (N.F. Stanley and R.A. Joske, eds.), p. 151. Academic Press, London, (1980).
4. Miles, J.A.R., *Med. J. Aust. 2*, 773 (1953).
5. Miles, J.A.R., Stokes, L.J., and Ames, P.G., *Med. J. Aust. 2*, 482 (1955).
6. Barrett, E.J., *in* "Hepatitis B" (G.E. Logan, ed.), p. 207. Abbott Labs., Sydney, (1975).
7. Barrett, E.J., *Aust. N.Z. J. Med. 6*, 106 (1976).
8. Adels, B.R., and Gajdusek, D.C., *Am. J. Hyg. 77*, 317 (1963).
9. Pope, J.H., Walters, M.K., Scott, W., and Gunz, F.W., *Int. J. Cancer 12*, 689 (1973).
10. Lang, D.J., Garruto, R.M., and Gajdusek, D.C., *Am. J. Epid. 105*, 480 (1977).
11. Cleland, J.B., Bradley, B., and McDonald, W., *Med. J. Aust. 2*, 179 (1916).
12. Comm. Dis. Int. Bulletin No. 81/23, Nov. 20, (1981).

Part VI
Specific Viral Diseases

A.
Respiratory Viruses

Chairman J. S. Mackenzie
Co-Chairman W. G. Laver

33

RESPIRATORY VIRUSES -- AN OVERVIEW

Robert M. Chanock

Laboratory of Infectious Diseases
National Institute of Allergy and Infectious Diseases
National Institutes of Health
Bethesda, Maryland 20205

I. MORBIDITY AND MORTALITY OF ACUTE RESPIRATORY TRACT DISEASE

In health surveys, acute respiratory tract disease is usually found to be the leading cause of morbidity and this pattern appears to be the same in all parts of the world. For example, in the Cleveland family study, 60 percent of all acute conditions were ascribed to acute respiratory tract disease (1). In another large prospective study carried out in Tecumseh, Michigan, the overall incidence was observed to be 3 acute respiratory illnesses per person per year. Incidence was highest in infants, 6 illnesses per year, and decreased progressively with age to 1.5 illnesses per year for individuals 50 years and older (2). Acute respiratory tract illness is no longer a leading cause of death in developed countries. However, in developing countries it continues to be a leading contributor to mortality, especially during the first few years of life when it vies with acute gastrointestinal tract disease for first position. It has been estimated by WHO that 4 to 5 million deaths in Asia, Africa and Latin America can be attributed to acute respiratory tract disease each year (3).

II. ROLE OF VIRUSES IN ACUTE RESPIRATORY TRACT DISEASE

Thirty-five years ago, only two respiratory viral pathogens were known. Except for type A and type B influenza, acute viral respiratory disease was largely an uncharted area. During the 1950s and 1960s the situation changed dramatically with the discovery of many new

VIRAL DISEASES IN SOUTH-EAST ASIA
AND THE WESTERN PACIFIC
ISBN 0 12 484820 6

respiratory viruses (4-7). Concurrent epidemiologic and clinical studies defined the natural history of infection and clinical presentation of these newer respiratory viruses. During the 1970s, discovery of new viruses abated and investigative efforts were directed primarily at achieving a better understanding of basic properties of the newer respiratory viruses, as well as pathogenesis of disease and mechanisms of immunity.

The efforts of the past 35 years have yielded a rather detailed picture of viral etiology and epidemiology of acute respiratory tract disease. At present, 144 or more different viruses belonging to 8 separate genera are known to be involved in acute disease of the respiratory tract (Table). In addition, it is clear that viruses are responsible for the major share of acute respiratory tract illnesses that affect individuals of all ages in every locality.

III. CLINICAL-EPIDEMIOLOGICAL CORRELATES

Different viruses belonging to the same genus or different genera can cause the same disease syndrome. Conversely, many of the respiratory viruses can produce a spectrum of effects ranging from mild illness to serious, often life-threatening disease. This means that the virus responsible for an individual illness cannot be identified with certainty from the clinical history and physical findings. Etiologic diagnosis can only be established through the study of appropriate specimens in the laboratory.

Although laboratory studies are required for final etiologic diagnosis, there are a number of clinical and epidemiological correlates that are extremely helpful in suggesting the identity of the virus responsible for an individual illness. For example, in infants and young children, RS virus is the most important cause of bronchiolitis or pneumonia during the late fall, winter, or early spring (8). In this setting, RS virus represents the presumptive etiologic agent until proven otherwise. Presumptive diagnosis can be made with more confidence if laboratory studies indicate that RS virus is prevalent in the community. However, this information is not absolutely necessary since yearly epidemics of RS virus infection are associated with a dramatic increase in hospitalization of infants with bronchiolitis, an event that signals prevalence of the virus in the community (8).

VIRUSES THAT CAUSE RESPIRATORY DISEASE IN MAN

Genus	Serotypes No.	Serotypes No. that cause resp. disease	Most important manifestations of infection
Mastadenovirus	38	8	Pharyngitis, lower respiratory tract disease--infants, children, adults
Coronavirus	3	3	Upper respiratory tract disease--all ages
Herpesvirus			
Simplex	2	1	Stomatitis and pharyngitis--children, young adults
CMV	1	1	Pneumonia--young infants
Influenzavirus*	3	3	Influenza, pneumonia--adults; croup--children (Types A and B). Mild upper respiratory tract disease (Type C)
Paramyxovirus	5	5	Croup, bronchitis, pneumonia--infants, children
Pneumovirus (RS)	1	1	Bronchiolitis, pneumonia--infants, children
Enterovirus	67	12	Pharyngitis--children, adults
Rhinovirus	110+	110+	Upper respiratory tract disease--all ages

*Segmented genome. Influenza A undergoes antigenic shift followed by progressive drift, influenza B undergoes only drift.

In a similar manner, parainfluenza viruses are strongly linked to the croup syndrome (acute laryngotracheobronchitis) (9). An increase in incidence of croup usually signals increased activity of one or more of these viruses in the community. Temporal pattern is also important since the parainfluenza viruses are most active during the fall or spring. Influenza A virus is the next most important cause of croup in children and during influenza epidemics, this virus can become the major etiologic agent. During epidemic intervals, the influenza viruses also play an important role in pediatric pneumonia. Finally, adenovirus types 1, 2, 3, 5, 6, and 7 play a significant role in pediatric pharyngitis and lower respiratory disease (10). Presumptive diagnosis of adenovirus disease in infants and children is difficult because these viruses do not produce a characteristic illness nor do they usually exhibit an epidemic pattern. The situation differs for young adults in military training where the presumptive diagnosis of adenovirus infection can be made with reasonable confidence because most epidemics of febrile respiratory disease in military recruits are caused by type 4, 7, 14 or 21 adenovirus.

Each of the above viruses also cause mild disease that falls within the common cold syndrome. However, the rhinoviruses are the most important cause of common colds that afflict individuals of all ages, particularly during the fall and spring (6). The coronaviruses also play a significant role in the etiology of colds, especially during the winter (11).

The patterns just described are rather well fixed and do not vary significantly from year to year except for the influenza A and B viruses that exhibit an unpredictable variation in epidemic pattern. When epidemics do occur, the influenza viruses can become the major cause of febrile respiratory disease in individuals of all ages.

IV. ETIOLOGIC PERSPECTIVE

How much respiratory tract disease can now be explained by the known viral pathogens? The answer appears to be approximately 50 percent overall, although it is higher in some syndromes and lower in others. For example, about two-thirds of pediatric bronchiolitis is associated with RS virus (8). The same estimate can be made for the parainfluenza and influenza viruses in the croup syndrome. Fifty percent or more of pediatric pneumonia can now be explained by RS virus, the parainfluenza viruses, the influenza viruses, and the adenoviruses (12,13). In addition, cytomegalovirus (CMV) may account for up to 20 percent of pneumonia in very young infants admitted to the hospital (14).

Two-thirds or more of febrile respiratory illness in adults can be linked to influenza A virus when this virus is epidemic. However, during non-epidemic intervals, febrile respiratory disease still occurs with high frequency so that the total amount of this syndrome caused by influenza virus is less than 20 to 30 percent. Clearly, other viruses capable of causing febrile respiratory disease in adults await discovery.

When standard tissue culture techniques are used for virus isolation, approximately 30 to 40 percent of adults with a cold yield a cultivatable virus . Rhinoviruses can be recovered from one-fourth of patients with a cold, while other viruses such as influenza A and B viruses, parainfluenza viruses, RS virus, and adenoviruses account for the remaining isolates. As shown by Larson and associates, these isolation rates represent an underestimate because the frequency of virus recovery can be increased significantly when nasal wash specimens are studied exhaustively by a variety of techniques in addition to standard tissue culture methods (15). These investigators initially studied nasal secretions from 38 colds using standard tissue culture techniques. Negative specimens were subsequently studied in tracheal and nasal organ cultures and in volunteers. Later, fluids from organ cultures and nasal washings from ill volunteers were examined in standard tissue cultures and by electron microscopy. In the first phase of the study, 14 viruses were recovered using standard tissue culture techniques (11 rhinoviruses, 2 parainfluenza viruses, and 1 influenza A virus). Another 11 secretions yielded a virus when the additional studies were performed (4 rhinoviruses and 7 coronaviruses). Also, virus-negative specimens from 5 colds induced illness in volunteers. The overall proportion of the 38 secretions that yielded a virus was 65 percent, while an additional 13 percent contained a presumed viral agent that was transmissible in volunteers. These observations underscore the fastidious nature of many of the viruses responsible for the common cold, especially the coronaviruses, which could not be detected by standard methods. The importance of coronaviruses in this study is consistent with the observation that 15 percent of patients with a cold develop a serologic response to one or more of the human coronaviruses (11).

Pneumonia in civilian adults is the one form of acute respiratory disease in which viruses do not appear to play a major role. Virus infection can be detected in only 16 to 25% of this type of pneumonia (16-18). Influenza A virus is clearly the most important of the respiratory viruses in adult pneumonia and, when this virus is epidemic in the community, the rate for pneumonia in adults doubles or triples (19).

V. GEOGRAPHIC VARIATION

Respiratory viruses do not exhibit significant geographic variation with respect to prevalence, pattern of infection, or pattern of disease. For example, in every large population in which appropriate studies have been performed, RS virus has been observed to cause an extensive epidemic every year. In each instance, high attack rates for infection and febrile respiratory disease in infants and young children have been recorded during the epidemic interval. Furthermore, the major manifestations of serious RS virus disease in this age-group, i.e., bronchiolitis and pneumonia, have remained constant throughout the world. Finally, the relative importance of RS virus in these respiratory syndromes has not varied. Each of the other respiratory virus groups exhibit this same constancy in their epidemiology and clinical presentation. This is not surprising since the respiratory viruses do not have an intermediate host or an insect vector. Instead, with the possible exception of influenza A virus, they depend upon man for their spread and survival.

What does vary significantly with location is severity and outcome of disease. In developed countries the mortality rate for severe pediatric lower respiratory tract disease has been reduced to a relatively low level. In contrast, the rate remains 5 to 25 times higher in the developing countries and this accounts for a significant proportion of the many deaths that occur during the first few years of life.

VI. SEVERITY OF DISEASE

Although the basis for the observed differences in severity of respiratory disease in different countries is not known with certainty, several factors can be suggested. First, overcrowding and large family size may be important since they are now known to play a role in severity of RS virus disease in infancy. Studies in the United Kingdom indicate that the risk of serious RS virus disease requiring hospitalization is directly related to the number of siblings and density of room occupancy (20). There is also a suggestion from these studies that exposure to environmental pollutants also increases the risk of more severe RS virus disease. Based upon observations made in Latin America, malnutrition also appears to play an important contributory role in increasing the severity of acute respiratory disease (21). Finally, the availability and quality of medical care probably also plays a role in the outcome of acute respiratory disease.

VII. OTHER MANIFESTATIONS OF INFECTION

One of the more serious consequences of repeated infections with respiratory viruses is recurrent otitis media. This commonly produces a loss of hearing that leads to learning difficulties and problems in social adjustment. If hearing loss is not detected and corrected in early childhood, the affected individual may suffer irreversible auditory damage and never realize his/her true potential. In the past few years it has become clear that acute respiratory viruses constitute primary etiologic determinants of otitis media with effusion. During a prospective study of infants and young children, Henderson and his colleagues observed that the incidence of otitis media increased fivefold following infection with RS virus (22). A significant increase in otitis media was also observed for adenoviruses (4.3-fold), influenza viruses (4.2-fold) and parainfluenza and mumps viruses (2.3-fold). In contrast, colonization with pneumococci or *Hemophilus influenzae* had a smaller but significant effect on occurrence of otitis media -- 1.4 to 1.8-fold increase over intervals when these bacteria were not present. It was estimated that prevention of infection by the respiratory viruses identified as etiologically significant in this study would effect a greater reduction in otitis than prevention of colonization by pneumococci or *Hemophilus influenzae*.

VIII. SPREAD OF INFECTION

For many years it was assumed that the primary mode of spread of respiratory viruses was by aerosol. Recent studies involving rhinovirus and RS virus suggest that another method of spread may be more important for some viruses. Efficient transmission of rhinovirus requires close contact that allows exposure to virus-containing secretions at short range. Gwaltney and colleagues, observed that rhinovirus infection was not transmitted efficiently among volunteers by small or large particle aerosol (23). In contrast, infection was easily transmitted to volunteers by contaminating their hands with infectious secretions and then allowing them to autoinoculate their nasal or conjunctival mucosa. Gwaltney also demonstrated that the hands of individuals with naturally occurring colds are commonly contaminated with virus that could serve as a source for transmission to others by hand-to-hand contact. Finger-to-eye and finger-to-nose contact are normal and frequent aspects of human behavior that provide a means for self-inoculation and infection.

RS virus also appears to require close contact for efficient transmission. Recently, Hall and her associates observed that adult volunteers did not become infected when exposed at a distance to infants with RS virus disease (24). In contrast, volunteers who touched infectious secretions and then touched their nasal or conjunctival mucosa did become infected. Volunteers also readily acquired infection when they cuddled infants with RS virus disease. If direct contamination with infected secretions does play a major role in the transmission of rhinovirus and RS virus infection, intervention may be possible by application of simple principles of hygiene.

IX. RECOVERY AND IMMUNITY

Until recently, little was known of the immune mechanisms that bring about resolution of respiratory viral infection. Most of the new information on this important issue comes from studies of experimental influenza A virus infection in mice. Initially, antibody was thought to play the major role in the resolution process. Thus, Virelizier observed that thymus-deprived mice were protected against an otherwise lethal disease by administration of physiologic amounts of antibody just prior to infection (25). In contrast, transfer of spleen cells from immune mice did not confer protection.

More recent studies by Ada and his colleagues indicate that H2 restricted, cytotoxic T cells (Tc) do play a role in recovery (26). Mice were protected from fatal influenza virus disease by transfer of syngeneic Tc derived from mice infected 4 to 6 days earlier with influenza virus. Ada and his colleagues also showed that passive transfer of influenza specific Tc suppressed replication of virus in the lungs of recipient mice.

The Tc response is quite rapid and coincides with resolution of infection, while antibody develops somewhat later. This suggests that cell-mediated immunity may play a more important role than antibody in resolution. Unlike antibody, which tends to persist, the Tc response is evanescent and diminishes rapidly during convalescence. Earlier, Virelizier failed to demonstrate a role for Tc in resolution of infection because he used spleen cells harvested late after infection. In contrast, Ada and colleagues used spleen cells collected at the height of the Tc response.

It is likely that future studies will show that Tc also play an important role in resolution of infection by other respiratory viruses that mature at the cell membrane. Clearly, cytotoxic T cell response and memory must be taken into consideration when various immunoprophylactic modalities are being evaluated for effectiveness. The genetics of this response may also help explain variation in severity of human influenza, as well as divergent patterns of immunity. It should be noted that recent studies by Shaw and Biddison indicate an influence of HLA genes on cytotoxic activity of T cells against influenza virus infected target cells (27).

The relative importance of systemic and local antibodies in defense against respiratory virus infection is still being debated 30 years after the issue was first raised. It is known from studies in volunteers that local antibodies are associated with resistance to mild upper respiratory disease caused by RS virus, type 1 parainfluenza virus or rhinovirus (28). Serum antibodies do not show this correlation. Also, there is compelling epidemiologic evidence that moderate-to-high levels of serum neutralizing antibodies to RS virus are not highly protective against serious RS virus disease during infancy (8).

In contrast, little is known about the effectiveness of cell-mediated immunity in resistance. One of the few bits of information available concerns infants who received an inactivated RS virus vaccine and developed a strong RS-specific cell-mediated immune response (as measured by lymphocyte transformation in vitro) (29). They were not protected against subsequent naturally occurring RS virus infection and disease.

Conflicting views of the importance of local and systemic immunity may have their origin in differences in effectiveness of these forms of immunity in different portions of the respiratory tract. As mentioned earlier, local antibody appears to correlate well with resistance in the upper respiratory tract. With viruses other than RS virus, systemic immunity may be more important in the lower tract. Experimental evidence to support this hypothesis was recently provided by Rhampal and associates (30). They observed that administration of antibody protected mice from pulmonary consolidation and death during influenza A virus infection. In contrast, the trachea was not protected and underwent extensive desquamation following unrestricted virus replication in this area.

Finally, it should be noted that prior infection stimulates a broader, more effective and more durable immunity to influenza than does inactivated vaccine. Since infection stimulates all aspects of the immune response, it may well be that this type of comprehensive immunity is required for effective resistance to serious respiratory tract disease involving the lower tract.

X. PREVENTION

Prevention of most or all acute viral respiratory tract disease through immunoprophylaxis will be difficult to achieve because of the large multiplicity of viruses involved. However, a small number of viruses -- influenza A and B viruses, RS virus, types 1, 2 and 3 parainfluenza virus and certain of the adenoviruses (types 1, 2, 3, 4, 5, 7, 14 and 21) -- cause a major share of serious disease. Thus, effective vaccines for these viruses could dramatically alter the pattern of severe lower respiratory disease.

REFERENCES

1. Dingle, J., Badler, G., Jordon, W. (1964). In "Illness in the Home," Press of Western Reserve University, Cleveland.
2. Monto, A., Napier, J., Metzner, H. (1971). Am. J. Epid. 94:269.
3. Walsh, J.A., and Warren, K.S. (1979). N. Engl. J. Med. 301:967-974.
4. Huebner, R., Rowe, W., and Chanock, R. (1958). In "Ann. Rev. Microbiol.," 12 (C. Clifton, S. Raffel, and M. Starr ed.), p. 49-76.
5. Chanock, R., Bell, J., and Parrott, R. (1961) In "Perspectives in Virology," 2, (M. Pollard, ed.), p. 126-138.
6. Tyrrell, D. (1965). In "Common Colds and Related Diseases," Edward Arnold, London, p. 45-57.
7. McIntosh, K. (1974). "Current Topics in Microbiology and Immunology," 63, 85-129.
8. Chanock, R., Kim, H.W., Brandt, C., and Parrott, R. (1982) In "Viral Infections of Humans" 2nd ed., (A.S. Evans, ed.) (In press).
9. Chanock, R., Parrott, R., Johnson, K., Kapikian, A., and Bell, J. (1963). Amer. Rev. Resp. Dis. 88:152-166.
10. Brandt, C., Kim, H., Vargosko, A., Jeffries, B., Arrobio, J., Rindge, B., Parrott, R., and Chanock, R. (1969). Am. J. Epid. 90:484-500.
11. McIntosh, K., Kapikian, A., Turner, H., Hartley, J., Parrott, R., and Chanock, R. (1970). Am. J. Epidem. 91:585-592.
12. Chanock, R., and Parrott, R. (1965). Pediat. 36:22-39.
13. Tyrrell, D. (1965). Br. Med. J. 2:1166-1167.
14. Stagno, S., Brasfield, D., Brown, M., Cassell, G., Pifer, L., Whitley, R., and Tiller, R. (1981). Pediat. 68:322-329.
15. Larson, H., Reed, S., and Tyrrell, D. (1980). J. Med. Virol. 5:221-299.
16. Mufson, M., Chang, V., Gill, V., Wood, S., Romansky, M., and Chanock, R. (1967). Am. J. Epid. 86:526-544.
17. Sullivan, R., Dowdle, W., Marine, W., Hierholzer, J. (1972). Arch. Intern. Med. 129:935-1942.
18. Foy, F., Cooney, M., McMahan, R. Grayston, J. (1973). Am. J. Epid. 97:93-102.
19. Foy, H., Cooney, M., McMahan, R., Grayston, J. (1975). JAMA 241:253-258.

20. Gardner, P. (1978). Br. Med. J. 2:796-798.
21. Puffer, R., and Serrano, C. (1973). "Patterns of Mortality in Childhood," PAHO Sci. Publ. 262, Washington, D.C.
22. Henderson, F., Collier, A., Clyde, W., and Denny, F. (1976). In "Program and Abstracts 16th Interscience Conference on Antimicrobial Agents and Chemotherapy," 188, October 27-29, 1976.
23. Gwaltney, J., Moskalski, P., Hendley, J. (1978). Ann. Int. Med. 88:463-467.
24. Hall, C. and Douglas, R. (1981). J. Ped. 99:100-103.
25. Virelizier, J. (1975). J. Immunol. 115:434-439.
26. Ada, G., Leung, K., Ertl, H. (1981). Immunol. Rev. 58:5-24.
27. Shaw, S. and Biddison, (1979). J. Exp. Med. 149:565-575.
28. Chanock, R., (1971). In "The Secretory Immunologic System," (D.H. Dayton, P. Small, R. Chanock, eds.) p. 167-182, U.S. Government Printing Office, Washington, D.C.
29. Kim, H., Leikin, S., Arrobio, J., Brandt, C., Chanock, R., and Parrott, R. (1976). Ped. Res. 10:75-78.
30. Ramphal, R., Cogliano, R., Shands, J., Small, P. (1979). Inf. Immun. 25:992-997.

34

PROBLEMS ENCOUNTERED IN MEASLES IMMUNIZATION IN DEVELOPING COUNTRIES

Francis L. Black

Department of Epidemiology and Public Health
Yale University, New Haven, CT

Measles can be controlled. I think that the records of Singapore, Hong Kong and the United States last year prove that. The annual incidence of the disease in the U.S. has probably been reduced more than 1000 fold. Of the 3000 cases which were still reported in 1981, many were contracted outside the country or directly derived from an introduced case and others were not actually measles.

One of the largest outbreaks last year consisted of 106 reported cases in Westchester County, N.Y. (1). This outbreak was associated with six introductions, from Venezuela, Portugal, France and England. We were able to get serum specimens from 23 cases (Table 1). In seven of these cases (30%), there was no change in measles antibody level and we believe that they were not, in fact, measles. The vaccine has done nothing to reduce the incidence of measles-like diseases and they now loom much larger relative to the small number of continuing cases of measles. Five cases were in persons who had not been vaccinated, but nearly half the group had been vaccinated. Five of these were only vaccinated when less than 15 months old. Six (26%) had been immunized according to currently recommended protocols, three when less than 15 months and again later, and three only when more than 15 months old. All those who had been first vaccinated at less than 15 months developed high IgG titers without IgM, as if they had been sensitized to measles antigen prior to the current infection. The twice vaccinated individuals are of special concern and I will return to them later. Two of the three who had been first vaccinated at the recommended time behaved as if they had never been vaccinated and I suspect errors must have

VIRAL DISEASES IN SOUTH-EAST ASIA
AND THE WESTERN PACIFIC
ISBN 0 12 484820 6

TABLE 1. Reactions to Measles Infection During an Outbreak in Westchester County, N.Y. 1981

No.[a]	Age	Age at Vaccine	Titer at Days After Rash Onset 0-4	5-10	11-14	15-62	*
Fully Susceptible, Unvaccinated							
1	11mo	--	40[b]				+++
2	16mo	--	80[b]			640	+++
3	16yr	--	10			380[b]	+++
4	19	--		135[b]		380[b]	++
5	21	--			640[b]		+++
Secondary Responses in Prematurely Vaccinated							
6	14	?		2560		1510	++
7	14	9mo	160			1510	++
8	16	10mo	1800			1280	+
9	10	12mo	1070			535	+++
10	12	13mo	190			2560	+++
11	13	9mo,7yr	230			1280	+
12	17	11mo,8yr		67		1280	++
13	10	12mo,8yr	230			3020	++
Secondary Responses in Appropriately Vaccinated							
14	14	34mo	160			2560	+
Primary Responses Where Vaccination Failed							
15	14	7yr	5120[b]			5120[b]	+++
16	14	11yr	40[b]			450[b]	+++

*Severity of clinical diseases.
[a]Seven other children diagnosed as having measles showed no serological response.
[b]Measles specific IgM present.

occurred in maintenance, administration or recording their vaccinations.

Although measles vaccination has been highly successful in the developed countries of the world, it has been much less successful in developing areas where, for many decades, it has taken a much heavier toll of life. The initial problem is that measles occurs earlier in life in these areas.

This may be exemplified by comparing the measles age incidence collected by Iman in Egypt (2) with the prevaccine era age distribution in New Haven, Conn. (3) (Fig. 1). In Egypt 68% of all cases occurred in the first 3 years of life,

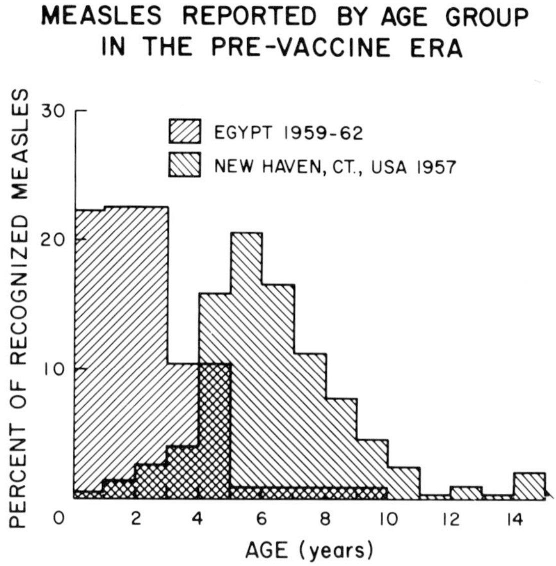

FIGURE 1. Measles reported by age group in the pre-vaccine era.

whereas in New Haven only 5% of the reported cases were in this age bracket. The early cases are more likely to be fatal and hence, their prevention is of primary importance. In Brazil 43% of all measles deaths occur before the first birthday and at least 50% before 15 months of age when vaccination is recommended in the U.S. (4). Obviously, vaccinating as recommended on the U.S. schedule would not be satisfactory in these circumstances.

There have been two proposals for adapting a measles vaccination program to areas where measles occurs early; the WHO has recommended, on the basis of a study done in Kenya, that vaccine be given at 7 1/2 months of age (5); the Centers for Disease Control in the U.S. has recommended that measles vaccine be given twice, once as early as 6 months of age and again at about 15 months (6). I will examine the problems inherent in both approaches in turn.

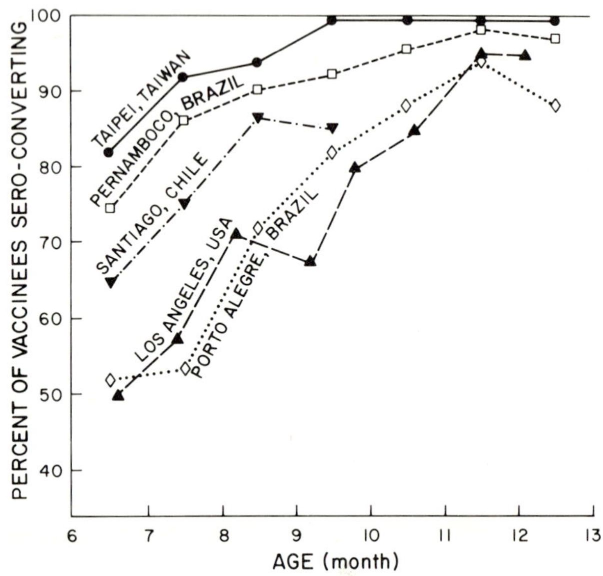

FIGURE 2. Seroconversion rates after vaccination at various ages.
References for data: Taiwan (7), Pernambuco, Santiago and Porto Alegre (8) and Los Angeles (9).

Figure 2 shows the seroconversion rates of children in selected populations who were vaccinated between six and thirteen months of age. The highest seroconversion rates are seen in Taipei and Pernambuco and lowest in Porto Alegre or Los Angeles. To test these differences we used a mathematical model: when the log of the number of children converting over the number of immunologically refractory children is taken as the Y axis, a straight line plot against age accounts for 98% of the variance in the South American studies. Using this plot we can estimate the age at which any particular proportion of seroconversion can be expected. The age for 80% seroconversion is given in Table 2.

With data of this type, one can, with reasonable measles mortality or morbidity incidence data, calculate the age at which a single dose of measles vaccine will have the greatest direct effect. If vaccine is given too early it fails to immunize many children, too late, and many get measles and die before they are vaccinated. A plot of the proportion of deaths expected to continue after vaccination at different ages in two areas of Brasil is given in Figure 3.

The vaccine would be most effective given in Recife at 8.5 months of age, but best at 11 months in Porto Alegre. It is disappointing, however, that the maximal direct effect which could be achieved is 65% protection in Recife and 52% in Porto Alegre.

Furthermore, conducting a full age-specific vaccine response trial, such as these, is a major undertaking. Even when 500 children in appropriate age groups are tested before and after vaccination we are left with 95% confidence limits for the optimal age plus or minus a month or more.

TABLE 2. Age at which 80% Vaccinees Seroconvert

Locale	Number Tested	Age in Months[a]		1976 Per Capita Income in $US	Ref.
Taiwan-Taipei	112	5.8		809	7
Kenya-Nairobi	164	7.0		221	5
Ecuador	236	7.7		652	8
Chile-Santiago	235	8.1		681	8
Costa Rica	62	8.5		1093	8
Brasil-Recife	516	7.0	)		
Sao Paulo	212	8.0	8.3)	1252	8
Rural Para	456	9.0	)		
Porto Alegre	438	9.3	)		
USA-Naugatuck, CT	147	8.8	)		10
Los Angeles	681	10.1	9.3)	6969	9
Cincinati, Ohio	182	10.1	)		11

[a] Calculated by $Y=\beta_0 + \beta_1 X$ where $Y=\ln \frac{\text{Number converting}}{\text{Number refractory}}$

and X = age in months

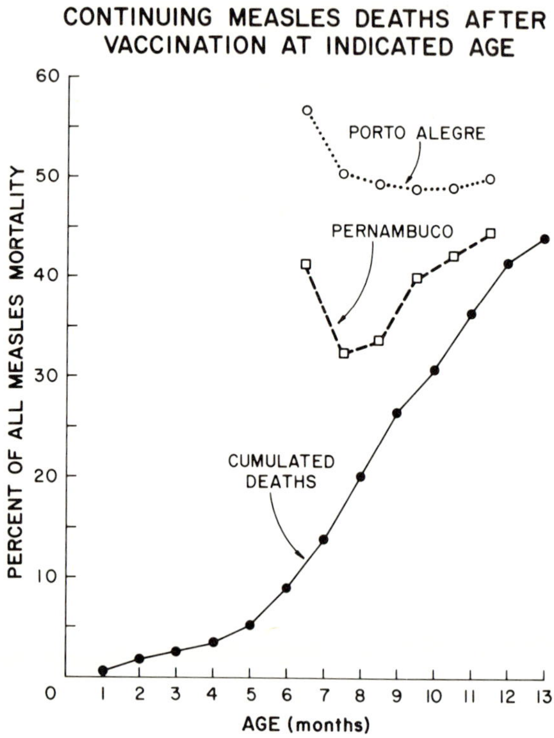

FIGURE 3. Cumulated age-specific reported measles deaths in Brasil 1977-1979 as percent of all reported measles mortality and continuing mortality to be expected in Porto Alegre or Pernambuco if children were vaccinated at the indicated ages and if the nationwide mortality data held for the individual regions.

We need to find out what determines these differences in response rate, so that they can be predicted without testing every locality. Our first assumption was that the age when seroconversion becomes possible, is dependent on stage of economic development. Per capita income for each country is given in Table 2. This does correlate with seroconversion age, but not closely enough to permit accurate predictions of optimal age from income data. No data was available from the different areas of Brasil and Taipei is out of line.

Estimation of seroconversion rates could be calculated quite easily if differences in efficiency of transfer, and in rate of metabolism of passively acquired antibody, are insignificant, and the duration of passive protection is dependent on the mother's measles antibody titer. Measles titers in Connecticut women of child bearing age are substantially higher than those of the mothers of our Chinese vaccinees and this difference is sufficient to account for at least a large part of the difference in response rates in children from the two areas (Table 3).

You will note that titers are lower in younger Connecticut women, about half of whom probably derive their immunity from vaccination. In the future measles susceptibility and vaccine response rates in Connecticut will approach those seen now in Taiwan.

With regard to the CDC proposal for giving two doses, the problem is that a first dose of vaccine, given too soon to elicit protective levels of immunity, may nevertheless, modify the response to a second dose so that antibody levels elicited by a second dose are not maintained, but fall back to very low levels. We studied this phenomenon in Brasilian children who failed to develop protective levels of antibody after the first vaccination. All of 29 who were revaccinated and tested three weeks later had significant titers at that time (Table 4). However, at best, these titers were lower than those in children not previously sensitized, and 3 to 18 months later the titers in 19 of 41 children had fallen back below 5, the minimal level we usually find protective. One might hope that these children would have been able to mount an accelerated immune response when infected with wild virus. However, the previously vaccinated Westchester, New York children, referred to earlier, nevertheless developed a disease which was clinically recognizable as measles. Mild and moderate cases were

TABLE 3. Measles Antibody in Taiwanese and Connecticut Women

	Age of Women	No.	Geom Mean Titer	80% Titers Less Than:	80% Response Age Expc.	Obs.
Taiwan	25-38yrs	75	47.5	160	7.6mos	6.5
	19-24	42	50.4	160	7.6	
CT,USA	24-29	50	226	640	10.2	10.6
	13-19	50	143	320	9.2	

TABLE 4. Measles HI Antibody after Revaccination of Children First Vaccinated at Less than 12 Months of Age Without Seroconversion

	No.	*% >5*	*GMT*
3 weeks after revaccination	*21*	*100*	*29*
3 to 18 months after revaccination	*38*	*67*	*10.5*

more frequent in this group than in the unvaccinated group. It is particularly disturbing that revaccination of children who had first been prematurely vaccinated did not give protection. If we follow the CDC recommendation for an early dose of vaccine followed later by another dose, we can expect to encounter this problem. We do not yet know how frequently it will occur because we have no denominators in the Westchester study.

Whether one uses a single dose of vaccine at the optimal age for prevention of measles, or two doses at appropriately spaced intervals, there is another problem which will only exert its effect in the next generation. The earlier the vaccine is given, the lower the titers that are elicited. The titers elicited in South American children at 12 months of age are barely one tenth of the titers which are elicited by wild measles in older persons (Table 5), and the titers elicited at six months of age are only one third of those observed after vaccination at twelve months. Titers in children revaccinated after initial vaccine failure are not higher than, but only equivalent to those, in infants of seven months who responded on the first occasion. If these titers retain their relative levels into adulthood, the children of mothers who had been vaccinated when they were twelve months old will be susceptible to measles four months sooner than children of women who were naturally immunized after infancy, and the children of women who had been vaccinated when six months old or revaccinated after initial failure to respond will be susceptible two months sooner still. Unless we can control measles in these countries within twenty years we may be faced with increasing incidence rates in infants soon after birth when the mortality is highest.

As you see, there are still serious technical problems in the presently available methods for measles vaccination in developing countries. It is not simply a matter of

TABLE 5. Measles Hemagglutination Inhibition Antibody Titer 3 to 6 Weeks After Infection with Wild or Attenuated Virus and Estimated Duration of Protection in Offspring

	No.	Geom Mean Titer	Mean Protection in Months[a]
Natural Measles in Adults	19	845	10.0
Further Atten. Vaccine in Adults	433	305	8.0
Further Atten. Vaccine at 12 mos.	202	86	5.6
Further Atten. Vaccine at 6 mos.	350	26	3.5
Revaccinated at 2 yrs after Initial Vaccine Failure	59	39	4.0

[a]Assuming that titers will decline 3-fold before stabilizing, a 39 day half life for passive antibody in the child, and a minimal protective titer of 2.5.

transposing the methods which have been so successful in more prosperous areas. I am, nevertheless not pessimistic. The success of a measles control campaign could be assured, I believe, if it were carried out intensively. Even 50%, successful coverage would reduce the amount of circulating virus by 50%, and double the average time interval between loss of maternally derived protection and infection with virus. If we can raise the average age of infection in this way, we can, at a later date, delay the age at which vaccine is given, until those ages at which better titers are elicited. The essential goal is to mount intense, comprehensive vaccination programs to reduce measles virus circulation before the vaccinated generation reaches adulthood.

REFERENCES

1. Smith, F.R., III., R.M. Raciti, and Black F.L. Reported measles in persons immunologically primed by prior vaccination. Westchester County, N.Y. 1981, in preparation.
2. Imman, I.Z.E., Hosny, A., Alfy, L.B., and ElRai, F. *Arch.ges.Virusforsch. 16*, 48 (1965).

3. Black, F.L. *Conn. J. Immunol. 83*, 74 (1959).
4. Fundacao Servicos de Saude Publica, Ministerio de Saude; Sistema de informacoes sobre mortalidade. Obitos por Sarampo X idade. Internal communication 23/09/80.
5. Ministry of Health of Kenya and World Health Organization. *Bull. W.H.O. 55*, 21 (1977).
6. Immunization Practices, Advisory Committee Measles Prevention. *Morb. Mort. Wkly. Rpts. 27*, 427 (1978).
7. Lee, Y-L, Black, F.L., Chen, C-L, Wu, C-L and Berman, L.L. *J. Pediat.*, in press.
8. Pan American Health Organization and Ministries of Health of Brasil, Chile, Costa Rica and Ecuador. *Bull. Pan Amer. Hlth. Org.*, in press.
9. Wilkins, J., Wehrle, P.F. and Portnoy, B. *Am. J. Dis. Child. 123*, 190 (1972).
10. Schlederberg, A.E., Pamm, S.H., Landrigan, P.J. and Black, F.L. *Am. J. Epidemiol. 97*, 402 (1973).
11. Linneman, C.C., Dine, M.S., Bloom, J.E. and Schiff, G.M. *Am. J. Dis. Child. 124*, 53 (1972).

COMMENTS DURING DISCUSSION

ON THE GLOBAL ERADICATION OF MEASLES

K.M. JOHNSON (U.S.A.) In view of both emerging scientific knowledge and estimated costs, would Dr. Black comment on his current thoughts concerning the feasibility of global eradication of measles virus?

F.L. BLACK (U.S.A.) I expect that U.S. authorities will be logically able to claim measles eradication from that country by their self-appointed deadline of October, 1982. This can be based on interruption of measles transmission in that country. It will, however, have more symbolic than practical significance, because, as already mentioned, introductions of measles from outside the U.S.A. are frequent. It is not likely that quarantine of unvaccinated persons arriving at the U.S. border would be acceptable because it would entail long delays for the travellers. Until measles is brought under control in the rest of the world this situation will persist. In controlling measles elsewhere, the cost of about 30 cents per dose is easily justifiable in almost all economic settings and does not present an insuperable obstacle. We do, however, need to know more about the questions I have raised concerning vaccine administration before efficient programmes can be developed in many countries. When that is done, we should be able to reduce the measles incidence to approximately the level of smallpox at the initiation of that eradication campaign. Then, and only then, can we contemplate world-wide eradication. I do believe, however, that eradication will then be technically possible.

ON MEASLES IMMUNIZATION AND HERD IMMUNITY

T. JACOB JOHN (INDIA) Both WHO and CDC recommendations focus on an optimum age for measles immunization. This assumes that mothers will be motivated and will bring their children to fixed immunization clinics at these recommended points of age. This is unrealistic in many communities in developing countries.

In India we are developing and testing a new concept. Measles is a seasonable disease in India and other countries in the region. Therefore vaccine could be given just prior to the measles season to susceptible children above one year by mobile teams. This is done once each year as annual "pulses" of immunization. In such immunized communities, measles does not seem to affect infants below one year because of "herd immunity". Thus we are able to confine measles immunization to children at an age when the immune response is very good, and yet perpetually postpone outbreaks of measles - it is during outbreaks that infants of 6 to 11 months catch their measles.

35

INFLUENZA — EPIDEMIOLOGY AND ANTIGENIC VARIATION

Chi Ming Chu

Institute of Virology
Chinese Academy of Medical Sciences
Beijing, China

In recent years, influenza research has made tremendous progress. Yet, this disease is as much beyond human control as ever before. This paradox can be attributed mainly to the extraordinary antigenic variability of the influenza virus, which in fact has served as the principal impetus for further investigations. This review does not pretend to cover all aspects of recent developments. Rather it will deal with certain aspects most relevant to the epidemiology of this disease.

I. SOME NOTABLE EVENTS OF INFLUENZA EPIDEMIOLOGY IN THE H3N2 ERA

In contrast to the relatively plain and straightforward evolutionary course of H2N2 influenza, the H3N2 era since 1968 has been marked by many episodes and surprises, some of which are undoubtedly due to more intensive surveillance, while others are due to improved methodology for the study of influenza virus.

A. *A High Frequency of Epidemic Mutants*

The H2N2 virus drifted slowly after 1957 and an antigenically distinct epidemic strain did not appear until 1964. The H3N2 virus however has been remarkable in giving rise to a series of antigenically distinct mutants causing repeated

VIRAL DISEASES IN SOUTH-EAST ASIA
AND THE WESTERN PACIFIC
ISBN 0 12 484820 6

epidemics. Early variations occurred in both hemagglutinin and neuraminidase. This trend was first reported by Schild *et al* (1) in 1974 with the successive appearance of A/Hong Kong/107/71, A/England/42/72, A/Port Chalmers/1/73 and has continued since then with A/Victoria/3/75, A/Texas/1/77 and A/Bangkok/1/79. However, in our analysis with chicken antisera, drift after 1977 has been of lesser magnitude and more multi-directional, resulting in the co-circulation of several mutants.

B. *Natural Infection of Many Species*

H3N2 viruses have been found to cause natural infection of pigs, calves, chickens, gibbons, etc. Since its first isolation in pigs by Kundin (2) in 1968, serological evidence and virus isolation have conclusively demonstrated that pigs are frequently infected by successive mutants of H3N2 virus causing epidemics in man, with no apparent symptoms (3,4). Infection of pigs occurred after human epidemics so that H3N2 infections are passed from man to pigs and no instance of transmission from pigs to man has been reported. There is no evidence for the persistence of H3N2 virus in pigs, though two strains of Hong Kong/68-like virus were isolated in Hong Kong in 1976, at a time when Hong Kong/68 virus was believed to be already extinct in man (5). Recently, A.P. Kendal (personal communication) has found the oligonucleotide map of these pig viruses to be similar to that of A/Aichi/2/68, a prototype Hong Kong/68 strain.

C. *The Swine Influenza Episode*

The localized swine influenza outbreak at Fort Dix, New Jersey, in 1976 is familiar to everyone. The origin of this outbreak remains obscure. Genetic analysis of the New Jersey strains failed to distinguish them from genuine swine virus and no evidence for recombination was found in spite of the co-circulation of swine and Victoria/75-like H3N2 virus during the same outbreak (6). Subsequent investigation in the U.S.A. revealed that swine influenza did occasionally pass from pig to man, but with no subsequent spread. Recently, W. Bean (personal communication) has obtained evidence that the first swine virus isolated from man, Mayo Clinic/103/74, is indeed a recombinant with genes 1, 2, 3 and 5 derived from Hong Kong/68.

D. *Recurrence of H1N1 Virus with Subsequent Co-circulation and Recombination of H3N2 and H1N1*

Both these events constitute unique situations in the modern history of influenza (7,8). However, considering the relatively short period of virological study, they may not be so unique in the long run and may simply reflect the limitation of our present day knowledge. Several authors have reported that the 1977 H1N1 virus is closely similar to the "Scandinavian" H1N1 variant prevalent around 1950, both antigenically and genetically (9,10). Both H3N2 and H1N1 have evolved in antigenic drift since 1977. A delicate balance appears to have developed with none able to replace the other. As a result of co-circulation, at least two recombination events seemed to have occurred between these two subtypes, one resulting in a virus with A/Brazil/11/78-like surface antigens (H1N1) and 4 internal genes (P1,P2,P3, NP) from H3N2 and the other, with A/USSR/90/77-like surface antigens (H1N1) and 5 genes (P1,P2,P3,NP,M) from H3N2 (11, 12). The former had caused epidemics in 1978-1979 in the U.S.A. and Japan, but was eventually replaced by non-recombinant H1N1 viruses (12).

E. *Naturally Occurring Temperature-sensitive (ts) Strains*

The first naturally occurring *ts* strain of H3N2 virus was discovered in 1973, but it was not until 1977 when a large number of *ts* strains were found among fresh isolates of the newly recurrent H1N1 virus that attention was drawn to the general nature of the phenomenon (7,13,14). A systematic study revealed the existence of *ts* strains among all human subtypes of influenza A virus, but the proportions varied from 8% to 82% at different times. Some strains consisted of a mixture of *ts* and ts^+ particles. A clinical trial of natural *ts* strains of H1N1 virus in antibody-free volunteers revealed that human virulence closely paralleled their shut-off temperature (15). By complementation recombination test, the *ts* lesion of two H3N2 strains was located on the NP gene and that of two H1N1 strains, on the M gene (16). The prevalence of *ts* strains in 1977 H1N1 virus has been correlated with a high proportion of inapparent infection among antibody-free schoolchildren. The finding of a large number of temperature-sensitive and presumably attenuated strains of influenza virus in nature has obvious clinical and epidemiological implications and deserves further investigation.

II. MECHANISMS OF ANTIGENIC DRIFT

The differentiation between antigenic drift and antigenic shift of influenza virus, at first defined empirically to denote respectively the frequent minor antigenic changes within a subtype and the less frequent major changes characterizing subtype transition, has gained a sound scientific basis in that they correspond respectively to minor or major changes in the amino-acid sequence of the HA or NA molecules. These advances are made possible by the application of molecular genetic techniques such as peptide mapping, polyacrylamide gel electrophoresis of viral RNA, nucleic acid hybridization, oligonucleotide mapping, monoclonal antibody and sequencing of cDNA copies of viral RNA.

The genome of influenza virus consists of 8 segments, each encoding one or two proteins (17). Thus, in the order of size, the first three segments encode the three polymerases, P1,P2 and P3; the fourth segment encodes hemagglutinin (HA); the fifth and sixth segments encode either nucleoprotein (NP) or neuraminidase (NA) depending on the strain; the seventh segment may encode two matrix proteins (M1,M2); and the eighth segment encodes two non-structural proteins (NS1,NS2). Antigenic variation involves changes in HA and NA genes, but other genes (or combination of genes) are involved in other biological properties.

There is unanimous opinion that antigenic drift arises as a result of point mutation (change of single nucleotides and single amino acids) on the HA or NA genes, and selection by the immune pressure of the population. As the hemagglutinin molecule is the principal antigen involved in protective immunity, much work has been concentrated on the structure of HA and delineation of antigenic sites on the molecule.

Utilizing the recently developed recombinant DNA and rapid nucleotide sequencing techniques and in some cases the more difficult amino-acid sequencing method, the complete sequences of at least 8 influenza A virus HA have been worked out, including one H7 (fowl plague virus), one H1 (WSN), one H2 (Japan/305/57) and five H3 (NT/60/68/29c, Aichi/2/68, Memphis/102/72, Victoria/3/75 and Duck/Ukraine/63) (18,19).

The gross structure of HA has been described (20). The HA and NA appear as glycoprotein spikes attached to the viral membrane. Each HA spike is composed of 3 HA molecules. Starting from the N-terminus, each HA molecule consists of a hydrophobic signal peptide of 16-18 residues and two disulfide-bonded polypeptide chains; an HA1 chain of about 330 residues and an HA2 chain of about 220 residues, connected by an arginine residue. During maturation of HA, the signal peptide is processed away and the arginine linkage between HA1 and HA2 is proteolytically cleaved. Cleavage is essential for infectivity of the virus, since it generates the hydrophobic N-terminus of HA2 which probably functions in fusion with cell membrane during infection. The C-terminus of HA2 is also hydrophobic and is responsible for anchoring to the lipid bilayer.

The antigenic character of the virus resides largely in the HA1 chain which is also the principal site of mutation during antigenic drift, whereas the HA2 chain is relatively conserved. Comparing the Aichi/68 and Victoria/75 strains of H3N2 isolated 7 years apart, there are 67 nucleotide differences (3.8%) and 29 amino-acid changes (5.1%) of which 22 (6.7%) occur in HA1 and only 4 (1.8%) occur in HA2 (18). Thus, there is 95% amino-acid homology between these two H3 strains, in marked contrast to the low percentage of homology between H1 and H2 (69%), H1 and H3 (37%), H2 and H3 (40%). This has served as the main argument for the fundamental difference between drift and shift.

Evidently, not all amino-acid changes are of equal importance in causing antigenic changes of the virus. Laver *et al* (21) have analysed laboratory mutants of H3N2 selected by monoclonal antibody in comparison with changes detected in field strains. The monoclonal mutants usually showed only single amino-acid changes and only mutants changed at residue 144 and 145 of HA1 could be distinguished from the wild type by heterogeneous sera. Changes at residues 142-146 have been found in field strains suggesting amino-acid replacement at these positions may be of epidemiological importance. By similar analysis, one critical site for drift in H1N1 has been located at an epitope recognized by monoclonal antibody 264 (22). Webster and Laver (23) delineated at least 3 non-overlapping antigenic areas on the HA of an H3N2 strain (A/Mem/1/71). This corresponds well with the finding of 4 distinct epitopes on the HA of PR8 (24). Thus, amino-acid changes at a small number of critical sites are responsible for antigenic drift.

Recently, the three dimensional structure of the HA of A/Hong Kong/1968 was resolved and the antibody-binding sites determined (25,26). The two structurally distinct regions consist of a triple-strand coil of α-helices extending 76 Å from the membrane and a globular region of anti-parallel β-sheet containing the receptor-binding site and the variable antigenic determinants, located on top. Thus, each molecule forms a loop, starting at the membrane by the N-terminus of HA1, extending 135 Å distally and folding back to enter the membrane by the C-terminus of HA2. In combination with monoclonal antibody studies, 4 antigenic sites each involving a limited number of amino-acids in close proximity were delineated. An amino-acid substitution, by virtue of its difference in size or charge, may cause antigenic changes by steric hindrance, charge repulsion or conformational changes at the locus. However, conformational changes at a distant locus distinct from the site of amino-acid substitution cannot be excluded.

Preliminary studies with monoclonal mutants and field strains also suggest that once an amino-acid has changed, it does not change again on further drift, thus imposing an apparent restriction to the limit of antigenic drift (27).

It must be emphasized that mutation is not limited to the HA gene. In fact, mutation appears to occur with equal frequency on all genes of influenza virus (28). The N1 or N2 neuraminidase gene appears to drift even more extensively than HA (up to 30% of amino-acids) (29). Cloning and sequencing of other genes have been reported and many studies are in progress. In view of the finding of recombinants of H1N1 and H3N2 in co-circulation, it is probable that recombination between two co-circulating variants of the same subtype may also occur, thus contributing to changes in antigenicity and other biological properties.

Techniques simpler than sequencing, such as peptide or oligonucleotide mapping and RNA hybridization may be employed in strain studies and surveillance. Examples of characterization of the New Jersey strains of swine influenza virus, of the 1977 H1N1 virus and of the recombinants of H1N1 with H3N2 have already been described. In addition, Young and Palese (30) have traced the geneology of sequential H1N1 mutants isolated at the beginning of its recurrence in 1977. Nakajima *et al* (12,31) have applied these techniques to the surveillance of H1N1 mutants between 1978 and 1980. It seems certain that these simpler techniques for genotyping together with monoclonal antibody will soon become indispensable tools for epidemiological surveillance.

III. ORIGIN OF PANDEMIC STRAINS

The mechanism of antigenic shift giving rise to a different subtype which usually causes a pandemic is still unresolved. Laver and Webster (32,33) first suggested that H3N2 may have arisen from the recombination of H2N2 with an unknown animal virus antigenically related to A/Duck/Ukraine/1/63 (H3N8) or A/Equine/1/Miami/63 (H3N8). Since then, this hypothesis has been advanced along several lines.

Firstly, extensive ecological studies in animals have revealed a large number of subtypes of influenza, particularly among avian species. All known human HA and NA, either in the same combination as found in man or in other combinations have been identified in animals such as ducks or pigs (34). These could serve as a rich source for recombination with human virus or even for direct transmission to man.

Secondly, recombination has been demonstrated to occur in nature and even in man. Evidence has been presented to indicate that recombination in the intestinal tract of ducks may explain the concurrent existence of multiple combinations of HA and NA in this species (35). As mentioned above, H1N1 and H3N2 have been found to recombine in man.

Thirdly, interspecies transmission certainly occurs in nature, such as transmission of H3N2 from man to pig and of swine virus from pig to man. Recently, a fowl plague-like virus (H7N7) genetically like avian but replicating like a mammalian virus was found to cause lethal infection in seals, suggesting another instance of inter-species transmission (36).

Fourthly, sequencing of A/Duck/Ukraine/1/63 HA revealed that the HA of this virus is at least as close to Aichi/2/68 as Aichi/2/68 is to Victoria/3/75 - a fact which virtually proves that human H3N2 arose by recombination of H2N2 with a Duck/Ukraine-like virus (19).

Thus, there is considerable evidence for the recombinational origin of H3N2. There is also some evidence that H2N2 may have originated from the recombination of H1N1 with an unknown virus from which the H2 and N2 genes were derived (37). However, it is possible that H2 may have originated from H1, since there is 69% homology of amino-acid sequence between the two, and the first H2N2 strain, A/Guiyang/1/57, has a large degree of cross-reaction by several serological tests with late H1N1 of the Dutch/56 group (38). Further studies are needed to clarify this point.

The biggest difficulty with the recombinational theory is related to the recurrence of H1N1 in 1977 which was found to be antigenically and genetically closely similar to H1N1 prevalent around 1950. The only plausible explanation is that the old H1N1 virus has persisted in a non-replicative latent state in either man or animals. There were reports in the literature concerning the persistence of the influenza genome, perhaps in the form of a DNA copy of viral RNA in host cells (39,40), but they have been received with great skepticism. There were also reports of well documented but unexplained sporadic recurrence of old virus believed to be extinct at the time. One such case is an H1N1 virus isolated in England in 1960 (41). Other cases were the isolation of Hong Kong/68-like virus from pigs in Hong Kong in 1976 and from an Australian child in Adelaide in 1979 (42). In the latter two cases, the viruses were found to be antigenically and genetically closely similar to A/Aichi/2/68. In view of these facts, it seems worthwhile to re-investigate the possibility of latent infection in influenza virus. If it turns out that the influenza virus genome (or some of its genes) is indeed capable of persisting in certain hosts, it is not difficult to imagine that the persistent genome may be reactivated as H1N1 did in 1977, or it may recombine with a current virus to generate H2N2 in 1957 or H3N2 in 1968. A unitarian view on the origin of pandemic virus would then be possible.

Any postulate on the origin of pandemic influenza virus has to take recognition of the apparent localized region of its origin. Thus, H2N2 virus first appeared in February 1957 in the western part of Guizhou province in Southwest China (43). H3N2 was first reported in July 1968 in Hong Kong (44). H1N1 in 1977 was first isolated in May in the southeast part of Liaoning province in Northeast China (7). Why should all these pandemic viruses originate in or around China? Several possibilities might be mentioned, such as the abundance of certain animal reservoir hosts, intimate contact between man and such hosts, peculiarity of viral flora, or conditions favoring the persistence of the virus genome. The recent isolation from pigs in Beijing of several strains of influenza C virus (45) not found elsewhere argues strongly for more extensive and intensive surveillance of influenza ecology in China.

IV. OPTIMAL GENE CONSTELLATION AND ANTICIPATION OF PANDEMIC OR EPIDEMIC STRAINS

It is evident that not all antigenically distinct strains can cause epidemics. The virus must have the right antigenic structure as well as high virulence and transmissibility. These criteria require an optimal gene constellation dependent on the characteristics of the constituent genes and perhaps also on the proper cooperation between different genes. This concept was first introduced by Rott and Scholtissek (17,46) when they discovered that substitution of one or two genes of fowl plague virus by that of human influenza strains through recombination may result either in partial or complete loss of virulence, or retention of virulence, depending on the specific gene replaced as well as on the origin of derivation from the donor. The genetic requirements for transmissibility are unknown, but may be even more complicated. It is probable that many more mutants and recombinants arise in nature than those actually detected. Some just appear and disappear. Others only cause sporadic infections or localized outbreaks. Only those fittest in gene constellation can ever get the chance of becoming epidemic. The important problem from the viewpoint of prophylaxis is, how can we recognize and anticipate such strains. We are just beginning to approach this problem. From the tremendous progress made in recent years, the prospect of anticipating the trend of antigenic drift seems to be bright. The possibility of anticipating future pandemic viruses is still remote and will depend on the progress in our knowledge concerning their origin.

REFERENCES

1. Schild, G.C., Oxford, J.S., Dowdle, W.R., Coleman, M.T., Pereira, M.S. and Chakraverty, P., *Bull. Wld. Hlth. Org. 51*, 1 (1974).
2. Kundin, W.D., *Nature 228*, 857 (1980).
3. Stuart-Harris, C.H. and Schild, G.C., *in* "Influenza, the Virus and the Disease", p. 4. Edward Arnold, London (1976).
4. Guo, Y.J., Fan, R.L., Qu, F.Z., Wang, M. and Zhu, J.M. (Chu, C.M.), *Acta Microbiol. Sin. 21*, 379 (1981). (In Chinese).
5. Shortridge, K.F., *Science 196*, 1454 (1976).
6. Palese, P. and Schulman, J.L., *Nature 263*, 528 (1976).
7. Kung, H.C., Jen, K.F., Yuan, W.C., Tian, S.F. and Chu, C.M., *Bull. Wld. Hlth. Org. 56*, 913 (1978).
8. *W.H.O. Weekly Epidemiological Record 56*, 33 (1981).
9. Kendal, A.P., Noble, G.R., Skehel, J.J. and Dowdle, W.R., *Virology 89*, 632 (1978).
10. Nakajima, K., Desselberger, U. and Palese, P., *Nature 274*, 334 (1978).
11. Young, J.F. and Palese, P., *Proc. Natl. Acad. Sci. USA 76*, 6547 (1979).

12. Nakajima, S., Cox, N.J. and Kendal, A.P., *Infect. Immun. 32*, 287 (1981).
13. Chu, C.M., Tian, S.F., Ren, G.F., Zhang, Y.M., Zhang, L.X. and Liu, G.Q., *J. Virol.* in press.
14. Oxford, J.S., Corcoran, T. and Schild, G.C., *J. Gen. Virol. 48*, 383 (1980).
15. Ren, G.F., Zhu, J.M. (Chu, C.M.), Tian, S.F., Zhang, L.X., Qu, F.Z., Chen, C.R. and Wang, S.Q., *Chinese Med. J. 60*, 526 (1980). (In Chinese).
16. Tian, S.F., Zhang, Y.M., Liu, G.Q. and Zhu, J.M. (Chu, C.M.), *Chinese J. Microbiol. Immunol. 1*, 308 (1981).
17. Scholtissek, C., *Curr. Top. Microbiol. Immunol. 80*, 139 (1978).
18. Min Jou, W., Verhoeyen, M., Fang, R.X., Devos, R., Huylebroeck, D. and Fiers, W., *in* "Molecular and Cellular Aspects of Microbial Evolution" (M.J.Carlile, J.F. Collins and B.E.B. Moseley, eds.), p. 235. Cambridge University Press, (1981).
19. Fang, R.X., Min Jou, W., Huylebroeck, D., Devos, R. and Fiers, W., *Cell 25*, 315 (1981).
20. Waterfield, M.D., Espelie, K., Elder, K. and Skehel, J.J., *Brit. Med. Bull. 35*, 57 (1979).
21. Laver, W.G., Air, G.M. and Webster, R.G., *J. Mol. Biol. 145*, 339 (1981).
22. Nakajima, S. and Kendal, A.P., *Virology 113*, 656 (1981).
23. Webster, R.G. and Laver, W.G., *Virology 104*, 139 (1980).
24. Gerhard, W., Yewdell, J., Frankel, M.E. and Webster, R., *Nature 290*, 713 (1981).
25. Wilson, I.A., Skehel, J.J. and Wiley, D.C., *Nature 289*, 336 (1981).
26. Wiley, D.C., Wilson, I.A. and Skehel, J.J., *Nature 289*, 373 (1981).
27. Laver, W.G., Air, G.M., Dopheide, T.A. and Ward, C.W., *Nature 283*, 454 (1980).
28. Air, G.M., Bok, J. and Hall, R.M., *J. Supramol. Struct. Cell. Biochem., Supplement 5*, 354 (1981).
29. Bok, J., *J. Supramol. Struct. Cell. Biochem., Supplement 5*, 370 (1981).
30. Young, J.F., Desselberger, U. and Palese, P., *Cell. 18*, 73 (1979).
31. Nakajima, S., Nakajima, K., Takeuchi, Y. and Sugiura, A., *J. Infect. Dis. 142*, 492 (1980).
32. Laver, W.G. and Webster, R.G., *Virology 48*, 444 (1972).
33. Laver, W.G. and Webster, R.G., *Virology 51*, 383 (1973).
34. Hinshaw, V.S., Webster, R.G. and Rodriguez, R.J., *Arch. Virol. 67*, 191 (1981).

35. Hinshaw, V.S., Bean, W.J., Webster, R.G. and Sriram, G. *Virology 102*, 412 (1980).
36. Hinshaw, V.S., Bean, W.J. and Webster, R.G., *J. Supramol. Struct. Cell. Biochem., Supplement 5*, 371 (1981).
37. Scholtissek, C., Rohde, W., von Hoyningen, V. and Rott, R., *Virology 87*, 13 (1978).
38. Liu, G.Q., Gong, X.C., Zhu, J.M. (Chu, C.M.), Ren, G.F., Fan, R.L. and Yuan, W.Q., *Scientia Sinica 8*, 1061 (1980).
39. Simpson, R.W. and Iinuma, M., *Proc. Natl. Acad. Sci. USA 72*, 3230 (1975).
40. Zdanov, V.M., *Nature 256*, 471 (1975).
41. Isaacs, A., Hart, R.J.C. and Law, V.G., *Bull. Wld. Hlth. Org. 26*, 253 (1962).
42. Moore, B.W., *Virology 109*, 219 (1981).
43. Chu, C.M., *J. Hyg. Epid. Microbiol. Immunol. 2*, 1 (1958).
44. Chang, W.K., *Bull. Wld. Hlth. Org. 41*, 349 (1969).
45. Guo, Y.J., unpublished data.
46. Rott, R., Orlich, M. and Scholtissek, C., *Virology 19*, 54 (1976).

36

INFLUENZA IN SOUTH-EAST ASIA

Yukio Yamazi

Department of Microbiology and Immunology
Nippon Medical School
Tokyo, Japan

Yasue Takeuchi

National Institute of Health
Tokyo, Japan

Kiyoaki Satsuta
Hideo Noriki

Department of Hygiene and Public Health
Nippon Medical School
Tokyo, Japan

Kanai Chatiyanonda

Virus Research Institute
Bangkok, Thailand

Concerning the epidemiology of influenza, there is a hypothesis of the temperate epidemic zone and the tropical virus-reservoir zone. Japan corresponds to the former, and South-East (SE) Asia to the latter zone. This is supported by the following facts: (1) influenza occurs alternately in the two areas (December-March in Japan, and May-November of the rainy season in SE Asia), and it occurs sporadically in SE Asia even in the other months; (2) new variants of the

VIRAL DISEASES IN SOUTH-EAST ASIA
AND THE WESTERN PACIFIC
ISBN 0 12 484820 6

virus were isolated in SE Asia several months prior to the isolation in Japan, according to past records.

One hundred and thirty-six strains of influenza isolated from patients in Thailand and the Philippines during the period of August 1979 - August 1981 were studied by HI tests.

Results with 40 strains of AH1 viruses showed that the subtype was isolated even in August 1979, and the antigenic drift of A/USSR/92/77, A/Brazil/11/78 and A/England/403/80 occurred one or two years behind Japan. Survival of particular drift variants will make SE Asia the virus-reservoir (Table I).

Results with 84 strains of AH3 viruses showed that A/Tokyo/1/77 (A/Texas/1/77)- and A/Bangkok/1/79-like variants cocirculated during the period of August 1979 - January 1981, and the A/Bangkok/1/79 variant was isolated four months prior to its isolation in Japan; whereas a new variant, A/Bangkok/137/80 and 138/80 appeared in May 1980 and it was isolated also in January and August 1981 (A/Bangkok/211/81 and 212/81). A similar variant was isolated in Japan in February (A/Kyoto/C-1/81) and in March (A/Niigata/102/81), and all of the six AH3 Japanese isolates in December 1981 belonged to this variant (Table II). Analysis of the new drifted strains with monoclonal antibodies, produced by hybridoma cultures obtained after fusion of sensitized mouse spleen and NSI cells, is under study.

All of the 12 strains of type B viruses isolated after May 1980 were similar to B/Singapore/222/79 or B/Yokohama/1/80 as in Japan.

These findings confirm the hypothesis of the circulation of influenza virus in the areas of SE Asia and Japan and they should provide a substantial clue to the elaboration of influenza vaccines.

TABLE I. Number of AHI Virus Strains Isolated in Thailand During the Period of August 1979 - August 1981

Time and Areas		Variants					
		USSR[c]	USSR-Brazil	Brazil[d]	Brazil-England	England[e]	?
August 1979	CM[a]	6	0	0	0	0	0
May 1980	Thai	0	2	3	0	0	1
October 1980-January 1981	BKK[b]	0	0	0	2	0	0
June-August 1981	BKK	0	0	3	8	0	0
August 1981	CM	0	0	9	5	1	0

[a] Chiang Mai
[b] Bangkok
[c] A/USSR/92/77
[d] A/Brazil/11/78
[e] A/England/403/80

TABLE II. *Haemagglutination Inhibition Reactions of AH3 Viruses*

	Ferret antisera						
	A/Tok/ 1/77	A/Tex/ 1/77	A/BKK/ 1/79	A/Aic/ 1/80	A/BKK/ 211/81	A/Kyo/ C-1/81	A/Nii/ 102/81
A/Tokyo/1/77	512	512	128	128	128	1024	128
A/Bangkok/1/79	1024	1024	1024	1024	512	2048	128
A/Aichi/1/80	2048	1024	512	1024	512	2048	128
A/Bangkok/211/81	32	32	32	64	512	256	256
A/Kyoto/C-1/81	128	64	64	64	256	1024	128
A/Niigata/102/81	64	64	32	128	512	512	256
A/Satsuporo/C-1/81	64	32	32	32	128	512	64
A/Satsuporo/C-2/81	64	64	32	32	128	512	64
A/Satsuporo/C-3/81	64	64	32	32	128	512	64
A/Hokkaido/11/81	128	128	64	64	128	1024	128
A/Hokkaido/2/82	128	128	32	64	128	1024	64
A/Sendai/C-559/81	128	64	32	64	512	512	512

37

ANALYSIS OF VARIATION AMONG HAEMAGGLUTININ GENES OF INFLUENZA A VIRUSES

Adrian Gibbs
Gillian Air[1]
Graeme Laver

Virus Ecology Research Group
Research School of Biological Sciences
Australian National University
Canberra, A.C.T.
Australia

The haemagglutinin genes of about 55 isolates of influenza A viruses from all serological subtypes have been sequenced; ten fully, the others partly and these include a set of 39 isolates whose 3' (N-terminal) 300-350 nucleotides have been sequenced using a synthetic primer, reverse transcriptase and the dideoxy method; the latter are called here the 'short' sequences. All the sequences are clearly related, and were aligned unequivocally using the predicted amino acid sequence they encode, with particular emphasis placed on cystein residues and hydrophobic residues; up to 16 gaps (1%) had to be inserted to allow alignment of the most dissimilar sequences.

The percentage differences between all pairwise comparisons of the aligned sequences was assessed both for the nucleotides and the predicted amino acids.

Classifications computed from both the nucleotide and amino acid differences of the 'short' sequences produced dendrograms in which the isolates unequivocally fell into the

[1]*Present address: Department of Microbiology, University of Alabama, Birmingham, Alabama, U.S.A.*

VIRAL DISEASES IN SOUTH-EAST ASIA AND THE WESTERN PACIFIC
ISBN 0 12 484820 6

13 known serological subtype groupings. The most dissimilar sequences (e.g. those of H1 or H2 and H3) differed by around 70% in both amino acids and nucleotides.

A 'minimum spanning network' was computed from the data for the full sequences of the HA1 portion of ten H3 subtype isolates. The nucleotide and amino acid data produced the same relative networks, and their shape correlated with the year in which each isolate was obtained (Fig. 1).

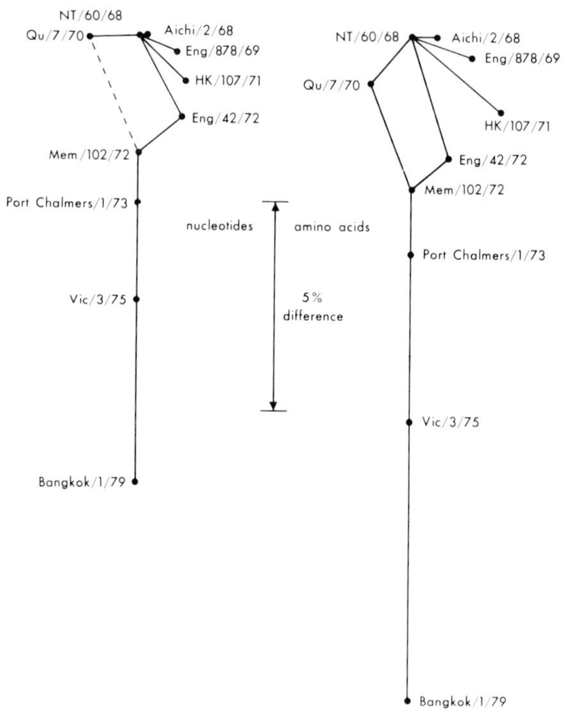

FIGURE 1. MINSPAN analyses of sequence differences of the HA1 genes of ten H3 isolates; scale indicates difference between any directly linked pair.

The most dissimilar sequences in the H3 'networks' (i.e. Aichi/2/68 and Bangkok/1/79) differed by 7% and 10% in their nucleotide and amino acid sequences, respectively. These results, if extrapolated to the differences expressed in the dendrogram, where the overall difference was 70% (i.e. 35%

since H1 or H2 diverged from H3) would suggest that the HA gene arose sometime between 1926 and 1942.5. This is of course nonsense.

The possible reason why rates of change during antigenic 'drift' in human epidemics may not be safely extrapolated to deduce times of origins of subtypes (i.e. 'shift' differences) can be seen when the amino acid and nucleotide differences between all pairs of 'short' sequences are plotted against one another (Fig. 2). Differences between isolates of different subtypes range from around 20% to 75%,

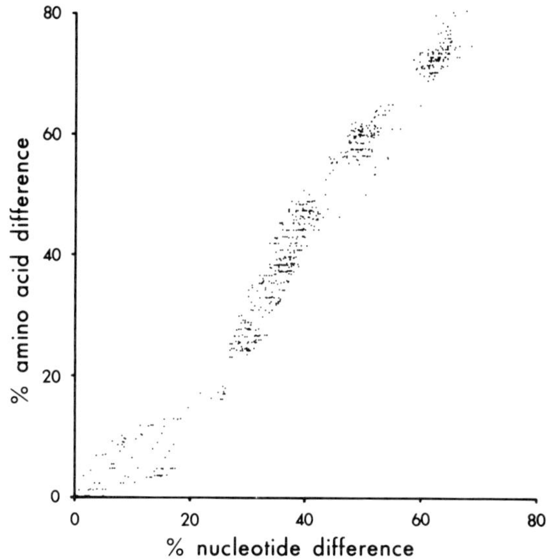

FIGURE 2. Graph showing the relationship between nucleotide and amino acid sequence differences for all pairwise comparisons of 39 'short' HA sequences.

closely grouped around a line with a slope of about 1.4 amino acid differences/nucleotide difference. By contrast, the differences between sequences of the same subtype were scattered (Fig. 3), and were of two types; those comparing human isolates fell near a line with a slope of about 1.1 amino acid difference/nucleotide difference (as in the H3 series) but the bird isolate differences fell near a line with an initial slope of about 0.2 amino acid differences/nucleotide difference but which increased sharply to join the main line of the between subtype comparisons. Counts of the numbers of nucleotides differing in the 1st, 2nd and 3rd positions of each codon showed that most within-subtype differences (drift), especially in bird isolates, are in the 3rd position and result in no amino acid change.

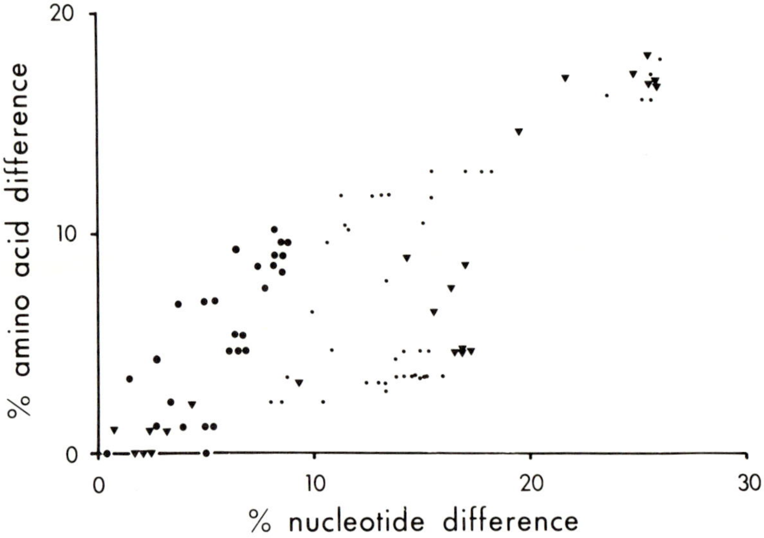

FIGURE 3. Enlarged portion of Fig. 2 indicating particularly the comparisons between pairs of bird isolates (▼), and between pairs of human isolates (●), of the same subtype.

These results may be interpreted most simply as indicating that in human infections, in contrast to bird infections, a much greater proportion of mutational change of the HA1 gene results in amino acid changes; base changes in the 1st and 2nd position of each codon are accepted as well as 3rd position changes. The trend of the bird comparisons in Fig. 3 leading to that of the between-subtype ('shift') comparisons in Fig. 2 would be predicted from the structure of the genetic code if one assumes that mutations are random but that there is selection against amino acid changes. This trend most likely represents mainstream HA evolution, and its rate clearly cannot be deduced from the rate of change observed during human epidemics, when a different set of constraints seems to operate.

The structure of the HA subunit and the position of the antigenic sites on it have been reported (1,2). These sites constitute about 20% of the sequence. Examination of the 'minimum' spanning network' calculated from the H3 'drift' data supports this estimate. The sum of the amino acid sequence differences between isolates on the main pathway of the network was 16.4%, yet a direct comparison of the sequences of the first and last isolates was only 10.1%. The simplest explanation for this discrepancy is that mutational changes are mostly occurring in only about 20% of the sequence (i.e. in the antigenic sites) and some are reverting; inspection of the sequence differences confirm this. If all the sequence was mutable, an observed overall change of 10% would have most probably resulted from a sequence of changes of 11%; calculated from Poissonian principles (3) and indicating 1% reversion. If however only 20% of the sequence was mutable then 50% of that mutable part must change to given a 10% overall change. A 50% change would have probably involved a series of sequential changes of 83% in the mutable 20% portion, and if all those changes had been recorded, 16.6% would have been found to change overall; a 16.4% change was observed.

REFERENCES

1. Wilson, I.A., Skehel, J.J., and Wiley, D.C., *Nature 289*, 266 (1981).
2. Wiley, D.C., Wilson, I.A., and Skehel, J.J., *Nature 289*, 373 (1981).
3. Dayhoff, M.O., "Atlas of Protein Sequence and Structure', Vol. 5, p. 95 (1972).

38

DO VIRAL MATURATION SITES INFLUENCE DISEASE PROCESSES?[1]

Richard W. Compans
Michael G. Roth
Firelli V. Alonso
R.V. Srinivas
Georg Herrler
L.R. Melsen

Department of Microbiology
University of Alabama in Birmingham
Birmingham, Alabama

Herbert Meier-Ewert

Virologische Abteilung
Institut fur Med. Mikrobiologie
Techn. Univ. Munchen, W. Germany

Our laboratories have been investigating aspects of the maturation of enveloped viruses at distinct plasma membrane domains in the MDCK line of canine kidney cells. These cells form tight junctions which divide the plasma membrane into two domains, apical and basolateral, and it has been observed (1) that the budding process of certain enveloped viruses occurs exclusively at one or the other of these membrane domains. Influenza and parainfluenza viruses are assembled by budding at the free apical surface, whereas the maturation of VSV in this cell line occurs at basolateral membranes beneath tight junctions. Results obtained in our previous studies on virus infected MDCK cells (2-5) include the

[1] *Supported by U.S.P.H.S. grant AI12680, NSF grant PCM80-06498, and the Deutsche Forschungsgemeinschaft.*

VIRAL DISEASES IN SOUTH-EAST ASIA
AND THE WESTERN PACIFIC
ISBN 0 12 484820 6

following: (1) Although the viral maturation site is apparently determined by the site of membrane insertion of viral glycoproteins, the information for directional transport of glycoproteins resides in the polypeptide portion, and not in the carbohydrate portion, since polarized maturation continues to occur under conditions where glycosylation is completely blocked by tunicamycin. (2) The sorting mechanisms responsible for directing the glycoproteins of VSV and influenza virus to separate surface domains continue to operate in doubly infected cells, since polarized maturation of viruses at opposite membranes continues in such cells. (3) The sodium ionophore monensin selectively blocks the transport of the VSV glycoprotein to MDCK cell surfaces, whereas transport of the influenza viral glycoproteins is unaffected. (4) No correlation can be made between the maturation site and the presence or absence of sialic acid in viral glycoproteins, since influenza C virions, which contain sialic acid, bud at apical membrane domains like influenza A virus, which lacks this sugar component.

In this paper, we have focused on the possible biological consequences of virus maturation at restricted membrane domains. For example, the maturation site of an envelope virus may be correlated with the pattern of its spread in an infected vertebrate organism. Virus maturation at restricted membrane domains may also limit the access of components of the immune system to virus particles or virus-coded cell surface antigens. The maturation site may also influence the type of cytopathology resulting from virus cell interaction.

Parainfluenza viruses, which are restricted to the respiratory tract, were previously shown (1) to be assembled by budding at apical surfaces of MDCK cells, like influenza virus. To investigate whether any correlation may be made between the site of virus maturation and the pattern of virus spread in an infected organism,we compared the maturation site of parainfluenza viruses with that of measles virus, a virus with similar structural properties that produces a generalized infection. As shown in Figure 1, the formation of measles virions and the alignment of viral components was observed to occur exclusively on apical surfaces of MDCK cells, as was found for parainfluenza viruses. The inset shows a virus particle with surface projections in discrete clusters, corresponding to the positioning of the underlying measles nucleocapsids. These results indicate that viruses which have very different patterns of spread in a natural infection may exhibit similar maturation sites. However, it should be noted that the MDCK cell system may not accurately reflect the natural infection process, and it will

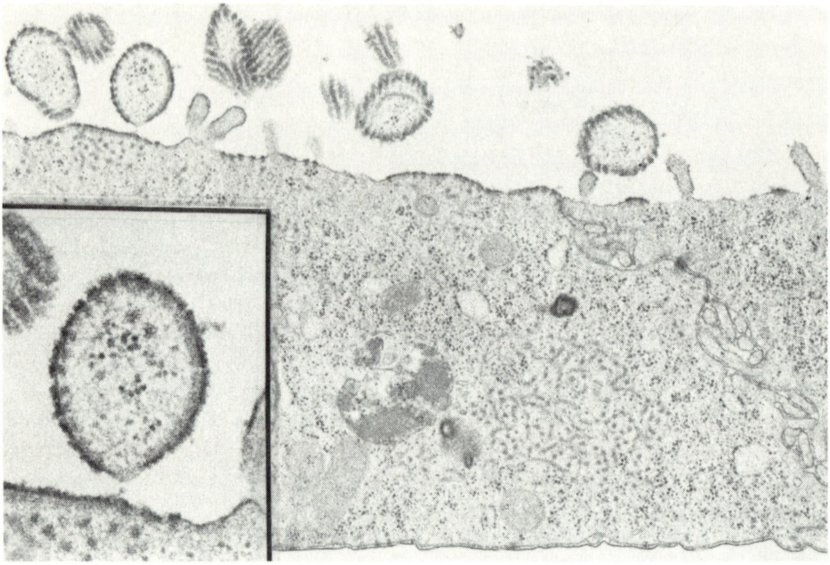

FIGURE 1. Maturation of mealses virus at apical surfaces of MDCK cells. The inset shows a single particle at higher magnification. Magnification = 18,000; inset = 45,000.

be of interest to examine other viruses and cell types to further investigate the biological consequences of virus maturation at restricted membrane domains.

In a previous report (6), we described the effects of antibody on plaque formation by VSV and influenza virus in MDCK cells. Whereas VSV plaques in BHK21 cells were completely prevented when antibody was included in the overlay medium, VSV plaque formation in MDCK cells occurred with equal efficiency in the presence or absence of antiviral antibody. In these cells, viral maturation occurs beneath tight junctions, and the junctional complexes prevent the passage of large molecules such as antibodies; therefore, virus is able to spread from cell to cell and form a plaque. With influenza virus, which forms at apical membranes, plaque formation is completely prevented in the presence of antibody. These results indicate that restriction of viral glycoproteins to specific cell membrane domains may limit the accessibility of viral antigens to components of the immune system.

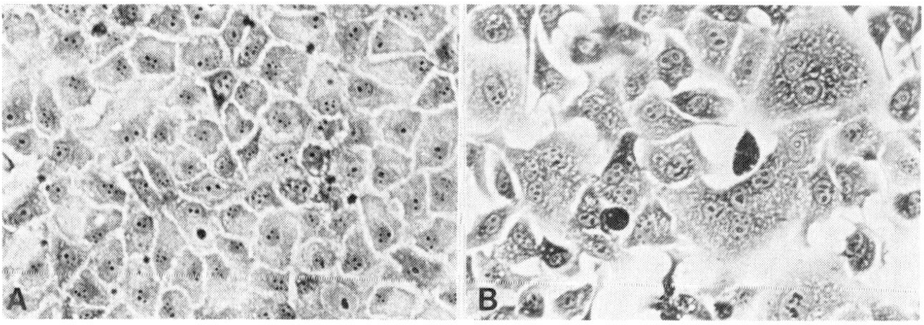

FIGURE 2. Effect of EGTA on Sendai virus-induced fusion of MDCK cells. After virus adsorption (20,000 HAU in 50 μl, 1 hr, 0°C), cells were maintained 2 hr at 37°C prior to fixation in May-Grunwald's stain. (A) Cells untreated prior to virus adsorption. (B) Cells pretreated 10-20 min at 37°C with 2mM EGTA in calcium free medium.

Striking differences were observed previously (7,8) following infection of two different cell types with the paramyxovirus SV5. After infection with SV5 virus, monkey kidney cells continue to appear morphologically normal. In contrast, infected BHK21 cells rapidly fuse into giant syncytia. It was suggested that these differences reflected properties of the two cell membranes. However, primary monkey kidney cells, like MDCK cells, are epithelial and maturation of SV5 occurs at the free apical surface. If the initiation of cell fusion required an intermediate involving viral glycoproteins in a bridging structure between adjacent cells, a virus budding exclusively at the apical surface might be unable to cause fusion. Further, when concentrated virus preparations are applied to cell monolayers, the junctional complexes would prevent virions from forming simultaneous contact with two adjacent cells. To test the idea that resistance to fusion may be correlated with cellular architecture, we compared the susceptibility of MDCK cells to fusion by Sendai virus with or without pretreatment with EGTA, which causes disruption of the junctional complexes. As shown in Figure 2, following exposure of intact MDCK monolayers to concentrated Sendai virus, the cells appear morphologically normal. However, when the virus is applied following brief treatment with EGTA, significant fusion is observed. These results indicate that susceptibility or resistance of cells to virus-induced fusion may depend on the viral maturation site and cellular architecture, and that epithelial cells are resistant to fusion by viruses which form by budding at apical cell surfaces.

SUMMARY

We have demonstrated that maturation of VSV at basolateral membranes of MDCK cells confers upon the virus the ability to spread and form plaques in the presence of antibody. The resistance of cells to parainfluenza virus-induced cell fusion is also dependent on intact junctional complexes in epithelial cells. We have not, thus far, demonstrated a relationship between virus maturation sites and the pattern of virus spread in infected vertebrate hosts.

REFERENCES

1. Rodriguez Boulan, E., and Sabatini, D.D., *Proc. Natl. Acad. Sci. USA 75,* 5071 (1978).
2. Roth, M.G., Fitzpatrick, J.P., and Compans, R.W., *Proc. Natl. Acad. Sci. USA 76,* 6430 (1979).
3. Roth, M.G., and Compans, R.W., *J. Virol. 40,* 848 (1981).
4. Alonso, F.V., and Compans, R.W., *J. Cell Biol. 89,* 700 (1981).
5. Herrler, G., Nagele, A., Meier-Ewert, H., Bhown, A.S., and Compans, R.W., *Virology 113,* 439 (1981).
6. Roth, M.G., and Compans, R.W., *J. Virol. 35,* 547 (1980).
7. Holmes, K.V., and Choppin, P.W., *J. Exptl. Med. 124,* 284 (1962).
8. Compans, R.W., Holmes, K.V., Dales, S., and Choppin, P.W., *Virology 30,* 411 (1966).

39

SEROEPIDEMIOLOGICAL STUDIES ON HUMAN ANTIBODY TO INFLUENZA C VIRUS[1]

Herbert Meier-Ewert
Cornelia Pfeil-Putzien
John P.M. Clerx

Virologische Abteilung
Institut für Med. Mikrobiologie
Technische Universität München
Munich, W. Germany

INTRODUCTION

Since influenza C virus was first isolated in 1947, it has been recognized as a human pathogen (1). Because it was long difficult to propagate the virus in tissue culture, influenza C virus is the least studied member of the orthomyxovirus group. Only recently, a number of results concerning the structural components and replication process of influenza C virus have been obtained and have stimulated new interest in this human pathogen (2,3). The three immunological types of influenza viruses (type A, B and C) share most of the major biochemical characteristics including a multisegmented genome, viral polypeptides with similar functions, as well as the mode of intracellular replication (4,5,6,7). However, a significant difference exists between influenza C virus and other orthomyxoviruses in the nature and function of the viral glycoproteins. In contrast to influenza A and B viruses, the receptor destroying enzyme (RDE) activity shown by influenza C viruses is not a α-neuraminidase (2,8). In addition, although serological and

[1]*This research was supported by the Deutsche Forschungsgemeinschaft.*

VIRAL DISEASES IN SOUTH-EAST ASIA
AND THE WESTERN PACIFIC
ISBN 0 12 484820 6

epidemiological studies indicate a world wide distribution of influenza C virus (9,10), the extent of antigenic variation among different isolates of influenza C virus, collected over a period of some thirty years in different continents, seems to be much less pronounced compared to type A and B influenza viruses, as revealed by haemagglutination inhibition (HI) tests (11,12), as well as by RNA genome oligonucleotide fingerprinting analyses (13).

In this report we have investigated the prevalence of serum antibody to influenza C virus in human sera collected in Europe, Africa, Asia and Australia, using the standard HI procedure. In addition, we used HI positive and HI negative sera for immune-precipitation as an alternative method for demonstration of specific antibody.

MATERIALS AND METHODS

Human sera samples were collected from patients admitted to a general hospital for reasons other than respiratory illness, from blood donors, or from volunteers. Although most of the sera were collected recently, some of the Australian sera were obtained from Australian Aborigines in Northern Australia in 1959. Allantoic fluid containing four HA units of influenza C virus strain Johannesburg (JHB) 1/66 was used as antigen in a standard microtitre HI technique (14). Prior to HI tests, all human sera were treated with trypsin-periodate, to attempt removal of non-specific inhibitors. ^{35}S methionin pulse-labelled chicken kidney cells infected with influenza C/JHB/1/66 virus were used as antigen in an assay in which antigen-antibody complexes are removed from the reaction mixture by adsorption to protein A bearing *Staphylococcus aureus* cells (15).

RESULTS

Sera of donors from Australia, West Germany, Kenya and Malaysia were analysed for HI activity against influenza C virus using routine HI titrations (Table I). Prevalence of HI activity was found to high levels varying from 59% to 93% seropositivity. The highest incidence of HI-positive sera (93%) was demonstrated in Kenya. When the sera were divided according to the age groups of <10 years and >10 years it could be shown that the percentage of seropositivity was

TABLE I. HI Activity of Human Sera for Influenza C Virus

	Australia	W. Germany	Kenya	Malaysia
No. of sera tested	238	96	106	47
% Seropositive[a]	88	59	93	59
Mean geometric titre	19	12	14	22

[a] Defined as titres ≥8

similar, apart from Germany where the group <10 years of age exhibited significantly lower positivity.

To determine that the HI activity was attributable to antiviral antibody rather than nonspecific inhibitors, we used eight HI-positive sera (HI titre of 32) and four HI-negative controls to precipitate viral antigens. None of the sera bound significant amounts of the haemagglutinin. No difference was observed between HI positive and HI negative sera in binding of any of the viral antigens.

DISCUSSION AND CONCLUSIONS

These results confirm other reports which showed high antibody levels against influenza C virus in human sera as measured by HI activity (9-11). The serological data obtained by HI titration suggests that influenza C virus circulates to an even higher extent in the populations of countries with subtropical or tropical climates, as compared to the more temperate middle European zones. However, the failure of HI-positive sera to react with viral antigens in the immune precipitation assay casts some doubts on the specificity of HI tests in measuring antibody against influenza C virus. The immune precipitations that have been done with 12 human sera suggest that inhibitors other than specific antibody are involved in the reported high prevalence of HI titres against influenza C virus (10,11, this report). A careful re-evaluation may therefore be needed.

TABLE II. HI Activity of Human Sera for Influenza C Virus in Different Age Groups

Age of serum donor (years)		Australia	W. Germany	Kenya	Malaysia
<10	No. of sera tested	-	51	49	10
	% positive sera[a]	-	43	96	60
	Mean geometric titre	-	11	14	20
>10	No. of sera tested	238	45	57	37
	% positive sera[a]	88	78	91	57
	Mean geometric titre	19	12	13	22

[a] Defined as titres ≥8

ACKNOWLEDGMENT

We thank Drs. W. Dechant, Kenya, J.S. Mackenzie, Australia, G. Tannock, Australia, and S.K. Lam, Malaysia for providing us with the sera for this study.

The expert technical assistance of Doris Wimmer is gratefully appreciated.

REFERENCES

1. Taylor, R.H., *Am. J. Public Health 39,* 171 (1949).
2. Kendal, A.P., *Virology 65,* 87 (1975).
3. Compans, R.W., Bishop, D.H.L., and Meier-Ewert, H., *J. Virol. 21,* 658 (1977).
4. Meier-Ewert, H., Compans, R.W., Bishop, D.H.L., Herrler, G., Molecular analyses of influenza C virus, *in* "Negative Strand Viruses and the Host Cell" (R.D. Barry, B.W.J. Mahy, eds.), pp.127-133. Academic Press, New York, (1978).
5. Herrler, G., Nagele, A., Meier-Ewert, H., Bhown, Ajit S., and Compans, R.W., *Virology 113,* 439 (1981).
6. Petri, T., Meier-Ewert, H., Crumpton, W.M., and Dimmock, N.J., *Arch. Virol. 61,* 239 (1979).
7. Palese, P., Racaniello, V.R., Desselberger, U., Young, J., and Baez, M., *Phil. Trans. Roy. Soc. London B 288,* 299 (1980).
8. Hirst, G.K., *J. Exp. Med. 91,* 177 (1950).
9. O'Callaghan, R.J., Gohd, R.S., and Labat, D.D., *Infection and Immunity 2,* 500 (1980).
10. Njoku-Obi, A.N., and Ogunbi, O., *J. Trop. Med. Hyg. 69,* 81 (1966).
11. Gerth, H-J., Bauer, K.H., and Steinitz, H., *Zbl. Bakt. Hyg. I Abt. Orig. A 231,* (1974).
12. Chakraverty, P., *Arch. Virol. 58,* 341 (1978).
13. Meier-Ewert, H., Petri, T., and Bishop, D.H.L., *Arch. Virol. 67,* 141 (1981).
14. Dowdle, W.A., Kendal, A.P., and Noble, G.R., Influenza viruses, *in* "Diagnostic Procedures for Viral, Rickettsial and Chlamydial Infections, 5th ed." (E. Lennette and N. Schmidt, eds.), pp.585-606. American Public Health Association, Washington, D.C., (1979).
15. Clerx, J.P.M., and Bishop, D.H.L., *Virology 108,* 361 (1981).

Part VI
Specific Viral Diseases
B.
Hepatitis Viruses

Chairman R. M. Chanock
Co-Chairman Y. E. Cossart

40

HEPATITIS A VIRUS: A SHORT REVIEW

Ian D. Gust

Virus Laboratory
Fairfield Hospital for Communicable Diseases
Melbourne, Australia

I. INTRODUCTION

In 1973 Steve Feinstone and his colleagues in Bob Chanock's laboratory in Washington reported the detection of 27-32 nm virus-like particles in the faeces of several human volunteers who had been experimentally infected with the MS1 strain of hepatitis A and produced serological evidence that these particles were the aetiological agents.

Similar particles were soon detected in the faeces of patients admitted to Fairfield Hospital, Melbourne, with naturally acquired hepatitis A (Locarnini et al, 1974) and by Cliff Gravelle and his colleagues at the Centre for Disease Control in the faeces of patients involved in a common source epidemic. An exchange of reagents showed that the particles detected by each group were morphologically and serologically indistinguishable.

Over the next few years a number of sensitive and specific serological techniques were developed for detecting hepatitis A virus and total and class-specific antibody directed against it. These included immune electron microscopy, immune adherence haemagglutination, solid-phase radioimmunoassay and enzyme-linked immunosorbent assay. The application of these techniques has provided us with a number of insights into the natural history of the disease.

VIRAL DISEASES IN SOUTH-EAST ASIA
AND THE WESTERN PACIFIC
ISBN 0 12 484820 6

II. LABORATORY DIAGNOSIS

Several specific laboratory tests are now available which can assist physicians or epidemiologists in confirming a diagnosis of hepatitis A. These include detection of HAV particles or antigens in the faeces, detection of a rising titre of specific antibody in sera collected 10-14 days apart, and detection of specific IgM or IgA in acute phase sera or faecal extracts.

Detection of virus particles or specific viral antigens in the faeces is proof that the patient is infected with HAV, however as peak shedding of virus occurs during the late incubation period, shedding may be complete by the time the patient seeks attention. In our experience, virus can be detected in the faeces of about 45% of patients admitted to hospital within a week of the onset of dark urine. The detection rate falls dramatically in the second week and we have never detected particles or specific antigen for more than 21 days (Coulepis et al, 1980a).

The presence of virus in the faeces of a significant number of patients at the time of presentation suggests that they are still potentially infectious and that appropriate care should be exercised in the collection and disposal of their faeces.

Rising titres of anti-HAV can be detected in serum specimens collected 10-14 days apart, provided that the first specimen is obtained early in the patient's illness. Antibody is almost always detectable by the time the patient seeks medical attention and may already have reached peak titre. Thus, although the absence of antibody in a patient's serum precludes a diagnosis of hepatitis A, the absence of a rising titre does not.

To overcome this difficulty, class-specific assays have been developed for detection of hepatitis A specific IgM (Locarnini et al, 1977; Frosner et al, 1979). Some of these assays are so sensitive that traces of antibody can be detected for one to two years after the onset of illness. However, it is possible to adjust the sensitivity of the test so that it will only detect antibody produced in the past two to three months. Hepatitis A specific IgA can be detected in the faeces and serum of some, but not all, acutely infected patients, so that like the detection of specific antigens, it is an unreliable means of confirming the diagnosis (Locarnini et al, 1980).

Thus, of the four alternative systems, the detection of hepatitis A specific IgM is the test of choice as it is always present during the acute stage and early convalescent phase of the illness, and can be performed on a single serum specimen collected as soon as the patient seeks medical attention. Using RIA or ELISA, it is possible to provide a result within 24 hours of the serum reaching the laboratory.

III. CLASSIFICATION

In the past three or four years, the virus has been characterized. Most of this work has been carried out in the laboratories of Yasu Moritsugu, Bob Purcell, Gunter Siegl and our own. This has proved quite difficult because of the need to use human faeces as the source of virus. HAV can be purified from faeces by a series of steps involving differential centrifugation, chloroform extraction, agarose gel filtration, ion exchange chromatography and isopycnic ultracentrifugation (Locarnini et al, 1976).

Particles purified in this way are naked, measure 27-32 nm in diameter, have icosahedral symmetry and, using the Markham rotation technique, have been shown to have 32 capsomers (Siegl, 1981). They have a buoyant density of 1.33-1.34 g/cm^3 and a sedimentation coefficient of 156-160S. When purified HAV is labelled with ^{125}I, disrupted and analysed by discontinuous SDS-polyacrylamide gel electrophoresis, four structural polypeptides have been demonstrated with molecular weights of 30-33,000 (VP1), 24-27,000 (VP2), 21-23,000 (VP3) and 7-14,000 (VP4) daltons (Coulepis et al, 1978, 1980b).

The genome of the virus can be released and examined by electron microscopy or radiolabelled. Studies from Siegl's group and our own (Siegl and Frosner, 1978; Coulepis et al, 1981) indicate that it is composed of a single piece of single-stranded RNA which sediments at 32-35S and has a buoyant density of 1.64 g/cm^3. Its molecular weight has been calculated at 2.25×10^6 when measured under non-denaturing conditions and 2.8×10^6 under fully denaturing conditions. The genome has been shown to have a 40-50 nucleotide sequence of poly-A and to be infectious for cell culture.

This data indicates clearly that HAV should be classified with enteroviruses in the family Picornaviridae.

IV. MODE OF SPREAD

Hepatitis A is an enteric infection and, as such, transmission occurs most readily when there is over-crowding, poor hygiene and inadequate sanitation. It is a particular problem during wars or following natural disasters which disrupt sanitation services and lead to pollution of water supplies.

Water and food borne epidemics have been described when water supplies become contaminated with excrement or food has been prepared by a person with poor hygiene. Most of these outbreaks have been reported from developed countries, where a high proportion of the population is susceptible to infection. The importance of this mode of transmission in developed countries is unknown.

Shellfish may transmit hepatitis A as they are able to concentrate the virus from large volumes of contaminated water. Raw shellfish pose the major threat, as the virus is destroyed by frying (Koff and Sear, 1967).

Although HAV can be detected in the blood transiently during the incubation period of the disease, it is very rarely transmitted parenterally. Outbreaks of blood-borne hepatitis not due to hepatitis B, have usually been shown to be non-A non-B.

V. EPIDEMIOLOGY

Information on the epidemiology of hepatitis A in the region can be obtained both by examining data provided by hospitals and national health authorities and by sero-epidemiological studies.

The quality of the data available from South-East Asia and the Western Pacific is very variable, as there are major differences in the way in which statistics are collected, a great deal of under-reporting of cases and a relative lack of laboratory data.

The importance of laboratory confirmation has been highlighted by the recent demonstration that several large water-borne outbreaks of hepatitis, which had been assumed to be outbreaks of hepatitis A, were due to non-A non-B (Khuroo et al, 1980; Wong et al, 1980). As non-A non-B hepatitis shares epidemiological features with both hepatitis A and B, it is no longer possible to make an aetiological diagnosis on epidemiological grounds alone.

In the South-East Asian region, data is available from Burma, India, Sri Lanka and Thailand (WHO Report, 1977). Although laboratory data is limited, it appears that hepatitis A is endemic in the region and is associated with both sporadic cases and occasional epidemics. Cases occur throughout the year, with some countries reporting a peak during the monsoon period. Most countries reported a peak incidence of disease amongst children and young adults, with males affected more often than females.

Hepatitis is an important cause of morbidity and mortality in the region, e.g. in Burma it accounts for between 1% and 5% of hospital admissions or 18,000 admissions per year. In Sri Lanka the figure is approximately 16,000 admissions. In each country the mortality of patients requiring admission to hospital is alarmingly high, ranging from 1.9% in Sri Lanka to 10% in parts of India, with particularly high rates being observed in pregnant women.

It is important to note that the agent or agents associated with this high mortality have not been identified. This is clearly an area which requires urgent investigation.

A considerable amount of information is available from the Western Pacific region as more than 20 countries or territories supply information to WHO or the SPC on a regular basis. As the region includes large developed countries and tiny island states, hepatitis A is endemic in the area, although the reported incidence which varies from 10-200/100,000 probably reflects differences in the quality of the reporting systems more than the variations in the incidence of the disease.

In recent years a number of cross-sectional studies have been carried out in the region and these have revealed three distinct epidemiological patterns (Gust et al, 1978; Gust et al, 1979).

A. *Patterns of Infection*

1. Hyperendemic. This is a pattern we have recognized in Fiji, New Caledonia, Nauru, Tuvalu, Kiribati, the Cook Islands, Niue, Western Samoa and Tahiti, populations in which there is over-crowding and standards of hygiene and sanitation are poor. Infection is acquired early in life and is usually subclinical. The disease is relatively uncommon except amongst visitors such as tourists, diplomats, missionaries and peace corp workers. Epidemics of hepatitis occurring in these populations and apparently associated with ingestion of faecally contaminated water are unlikely to be due to HAV.

2. *Endemic but Declining.* This pattern is seen in Australia, New Zealand and Japan and is typical of most developed countries. The low prevalence of antibody amongst children and young adults reflects a steady improvement in hygiene and sanitation over the past 40 to 50 years. In Australia this decline in infection rate has been reflected in a decline in hospital admissions, a decline in the prevalence of antibody amongst the adult population and a shift in the age distribution of cases. Whereas a decade ago the majority of cases occurred amongst children, the peak prevalence of the disease is now amongst people aged from 15-29 years.

3. *Previous Epidemic.* This pattern is rare and to date has only been recognized on Ponape (Wong et al, 1978). The pattern occurs following an outbreak which affects virtually 100% of susceptibles in a community. The virus is unable to replicate and disappears from the community. Children born subsequent to the outbreak are not exposed to the virus and hence remain susceptible to infection.

B. Prevalence of Infection

A relatively large number of populations in the Pacific have been investigated and surprisingly pattern *3* has only been encountered on one occasion. There is some evidence that HAV is endemic in a number of these islands. If this is so, there are a number of possible ways in which the virus may survive.

1. *Chronic Carrier State.* In 1952, Capps and coworkers reported transmission of hepatitis to volunteers with faecal extracts collected 5 and 15 months after the onset of illness. Although the illness was clinically and epidemiologically consistent with hepatitis A, it is possible that it may have been non-A non-B hepatitis. Against this data, workers in Australia, the United States, Europe and the Soviet Union have examined the faeces of several hundred patients with naturally acquired hepatitis A and have been consistently unable to detect virus particles or specific viral antigen for more than 3-4 weeks after the onset of illness. Secondly, the fact that hepatitis A only appears to become endemic in institutions with high admission rates suggests that, if a carrier state exists, it must be extremely rare.

2. *Environmental Contamination.* In many of these islands the disposal of faeces is inadequate and contamination of water supplies not uncommon. In several coral atolls, untreated sewage is dumped into the central lagoon. This stimulates a profuse growth of marine life, including shellfish, which are harvested and eaten raw. All of these factors may contribute to persistence of the virus in the population.

3. *Animal Reservoirs.* There has been little systematic attempt to search for animal reservoirs of HAV. Because in many islands dogs play a part in the disposal of human faeces, we obtained sera from a number of animals and examined them for antibody to HAV. Of 64 dogs from two islands tested to date, apparently specific antibody has been detected in nine. It is possible that dogs can become infected with HAV and then transmit the virus to susceptible humans who are in close contact with them. Alternatively we may be detecting antibody to a related canine enterovirus. In any event, we believe that the observation is of interest and worth pursuing.

4. *Repeated Reintroductions.* Perhaps the simplest explanation is to consider the Pacific islands as a single epidemiological entity, rather like the suburbs of a large city. The virus is endemic in the region and even though it may be temporarily absent from one or more places, is likely to be repeatedly reintroduced.

C. Strain Differences

There is no good evidence for the occurrence of different strains of HAV. Second infections in man are unknown, and laboratory animals infected with strains of HAV obtained in one country are resistant to challenge with strains obtained from other countries.

Additional evidence for the existence of a single strain of HAV comes from the effectiveness of normal immunoglobulin in prophylaxis, regardless of the country of origin of the antibody and the ability of serological tests developed in different countries with local reagents to detect infections acquired in other parts of the world.

VI. PREVENTION AND CONTROL

A. *General Measures*

Control of hepatitis A depends upon an understanding of the importance of personal hygiene and developing adequate methods for the disposal of faeces. Teaching children to wash their hands after going to the toilet and prior to eating is a most important factor.

B. *Immunization*

1. Passive. Numerous field trials have demonstrated that normal gammaglobulin (obtained from pools of plasma collected from healthy adults) will confer protection against hepatitis, if it is administered prior to exposure or early in the incubation period of the disease (Yarrow, 1964; Wallace, 1966; Reid, 1971). When given in adequate dose within 1-2 weeks of contact, it prevents illness in 80-90% of those exposed.

As the efficacy of normal gammaglobulin depends upon a high proportion of adults having circulating antibody, batches manufactured in countries where the disease is declining should be monitored to determine whether they contain protective levels of antibody. Batches can be standardized by comparison with an International Reference Preparation of anti-HAV available from the World Health Organization.

2. Active. In recent years, HAV has been isolated in several laboratories and is now growing in primary cell cultures, several cell lines and diploid cell strains.

The best studied strains are those which have been isolated at the Merck Institute in the United States (Provost and Hilleman, 1979). The original strain used in these studies, CR326, was obtained from the faeces of a Costa Rican patient and passaged 31 times in marmosets before it became adapted to growth in a cloned line of foetal rhesus kidney cells. This strain has now been passaged many times, adapted to growth in other tissues and is producing reasonably high titres of virus.

Dr. Purcell's group has isolated another strain from faeces collected from patients with hepatitis in Melbourne, code named HM175. Originally isolated in African green monkey kidney cells, this strain has been passaged about

20 times and appears similar in most properties to CR326 (Daemer *et al*, 1981).

Additional strains have recently been isolated in Europe, Japan and the Soviet Union.

The existence of these strains provides the potential of producing antigens for diagnostic serology and ultimately for the production of vaccines.

Hilleman has already demonstrated that formalin-treated extracts of the livers of marmosets infected with CR326 stimulate the production of anti-HAV in seronegative marmosets and render them resistant to infection. It seems likely therefore, that cell culture derived virus, treated in a similar manner, could serve as the basis of a killed hepatitis A vaccine. It should also prove possible to produce a live vaccine as both CR326 and HM175 appear to become attenuated following on passage.

VII. REPLICATION

The existence of an *in vitro* system for the cultivation of HAV has permitted scientists to study the replicative strategy of the virus and to test the effects of various anti-viral compounds. In our laboratory Stephen Locarnini and his colleagues have studied the replication of HAV in Vero cells and demonstrated the production of at least 11 viral coded proteins, four of which have similar molecular weights to the structural polypeptides, and demonstrated the existence of an intracellular restriction. They have also used this system to demonstrate that the genome of the virus is capable of functioning as its own messenger RNA (Locarnini *et al*, 1981).

Recently Von der Helm and his colleagues (1981) have succeeded in cloning the HAV genome into bacterial plasmids. Two of these clones have expressed small quantities of viral antigens. When this work is confirmed and extended, it may prove possible to use this technique not only to study the genome and gene products, but perhaps to develop a synthetic vaccine.

It seems certain therefore, that we are now on the threshold of the control and possible eradication of one of the last major viral infections of man.

REFERENCES

Capps, R.B., Bennett, A.M., and Stokes, J. (1952). *Arch. Intern. Med. 89, 6.*

Coulepis, A.G., Locarnini, S.A., Ferris, A.A., Lehmann, N.I., and Gust, I.D. (1978). *Intervirology 10, 24.*

Coulepis, A.G., Locarnini, S.A., Lehmann, N.I., and Gust, I.D. (1980a). *J. Infect. Dis. 141, 151.*

Coulepis, A.G., Locarnini, S.A., and Gust, I.D. (1980b). *J. Virol. 35, 572.*

Coulepis, A.G., Tannock, G.A., Locarnini, S.A., and Gust, I.D. (1981). *J. Virol. 37, 473.*

Daemer, R.J., Feinstone, S.M. Gust, I.D., and Purcell, R.H. (1981). *Infect. and Immun. 32, 388.*

Feinstone, S.M., Kapikian, A.Z., Purcell, R.H. (1973). *Science 182, 1026.*

Frosner, G.G., Scheid, R., Wolf, H., and Deinhardt, F. (1979). *J. Clin. Microbiol. 9, 476.*

Gravelle, C.R., Hornbeck, C.L., Maynard, J.E., Schable, C.A., Cook, E.A., and Bradley, D.W. (1975). *J. Infect. Dis. 131, 167.*

Gust, I.D., Lehmann, N.I., and Lucas, C.R. (1978). *J. Infect. Dis. 138, 425.*

Gust, I.D., Lehmann, N.I., and Dimitrakakis, M. (1979). *Amer. J. Epidemiol. 110, 237.*

Khuroo, M.S. (1980). *Amer. J. Med. 80, 818.*

Koff, R.S., and Sear, H.S. (1967). *New Eng. J. Med. 276, 737.*

Locarnini, S.A., Ferris, A.A., Stott, A.C., and Gust, I.D. (1974). *Intervirology 4, 110.*

Locarnini, S.A., Ferris, A.A., Lehmann, N.I., and Gust, I.D. (1977). *Intervirology 8, 309.*

Locarnini, S.A., Coulepis, A.G., Ferris, A.A., Lehmann, N.I., and Gust, I.D. (1978). *Intervirology 10, 300.*

Locarnini, S.A., Coulepis, A.G., Kaldor, J., and Gust, I.D. (1980). *J. Clin. Microbiol. 11, 710.*

Locarnini, S.A., Coulepis, A.G., Westaway, E.G., and Gust, I.D. (1981). *J. Virol. 37, 216.*

Provost, P.J., and Hilleman, M.R. (1979). *Proc. Soc. exp. Biol. Med. 160, 213.*

Reid, D. (1971). *Post Grad. Med. J. 47, 488.*

Report of WHO Inter-regional Seminar on Viral Hepatitis, Kuala Lumpur. (1977).

Siegl, G., and Frosner, G.G. (1978). *J. Virol. 26, 48.*

Siegl, G. (1981). *In* "Viral Hepatitis" (W. Szmuness, H. Alter, and J. Maynard, eds.), Franklin Institute Press, Philadelphia. In press.

REFERENCES

Von der Helm, K., Winnacker, E.L., Deinhardt, F., Frosner, G., Gauss-Muller, V., Bayerl, B., Scheid, R., and Siegl, G. (1981). *J. Virol. Methods 3, 37.*
Wallace, J.M. (1966). *Med. Offr. 116, 282.*
Wong, D.C., Purcell, R.H., and Rosen, L. (1978). *Amer. J. Epidemiol. 110, 227.*
Wong, D.C., Purcell, R.H., Sreenivasan, M.A., Prasad, S.R., and Pavri, K.M. (1980). *The Lancet 2, 876.*
Yarrow, A. (1964). *The Lancet 1, 485.*

41

HEPATITIS B AND NON-A, NON-B HEPATITIS; SOME RECENT DEVELOPMENTS AND UNRESOLVED PROBLEMS

B.P. Marmion
C.J. Burrell

Division of Medical Virology
Institute of Medical and Veterinary Science
Adelaide, South Australia

I. INTRODUCTION

It is a little over a decade since the discovery of an antigen (hepatitis B surface antigen; HBsAg) specific for hepatitis B virus (HBV), and the subsequent identification of the virion itself. During this time spectacular advances have been made in our understanding of the clinical and biological aspects of this virus, so that at the present time a wealth of information is available about the structure of the virus and its genome, and the different clinical responses to infection. Following from this has come the recognition of a previously unsuspected agent or agents not yet identified in virological terms, serologically unrelated to HBV, but capable of producing similar acute and chronic liver injury that is currently designated (in our ignorance) as non-A, non-B hepatitis. It is a tribute to modern immunological and biochemical technology that this has been achieved despite the lack of a suitable cell culture system for propagation of HBV. Parallel with these discoveries has come the rapid widescale application of research discoveries to the routine diagnosis and prevention of hepatitis B infection, in a manner unprecedented in clinical virology. In this highly selective review, we will attempt to highlight some recent information, concepts and practices involving basic knowledge about HBV and NANB and its clinical applications.

VIRAL DISEASES IN SOUTH-EAST ASIA
AND THE WESTERN PACIFIC
ISBN 0 12 484820 6

II. HEPATITIS B VIRUS

Electron microscopy of high speed pellets of serum from individuals infected with HBV reveals three morphological forms of virus-like particles - 22nm spheres, 22 x 50-230nm filaments, and the 42nm double shelled virion (Dane particle). All three forms carry hepatitis B surface antigen (HBsAg), while the latter form contains the DNA genome of the virus, a virion associated DNA polymerase and the hepatitis B core antigen (HBcAg). This internal virion component, and the hepatitis B e antigen which is found free in plasma, are probably differently folded forms of the same polypeptide (Table I).

The genome of hepatitis B virions isolated from patients' serum has been cloned and sequenced by several groups; the genes for HBsAg and HBcAg have been identified, and thus detailed amino acid sequences can now be inferred for these

TABLE I. Structural Features of HBV Components

	HBsAg	HBcAg	HBeAg
Particles			
(i) Spheres (22nm)	+	-	-
(ii) Filaments (22 x 50-230nm)	+	-	-
(iii) Virion - "Dane" particle (42nm)	+	+	+ (after denaturation)
Major polypeptides			
1	23[a]	19.5	19.5
2	27 (glycoprotein)		
Number of antigenic specificities or serotypes	10 (adw_1, adw_2, ayw_1, ayr ...etc.)	1	3
Hepatocyte localisation	Cytoplasm	Nucleus, cytoplasm	Nucleus?

[a] Molecular weight x 10^3

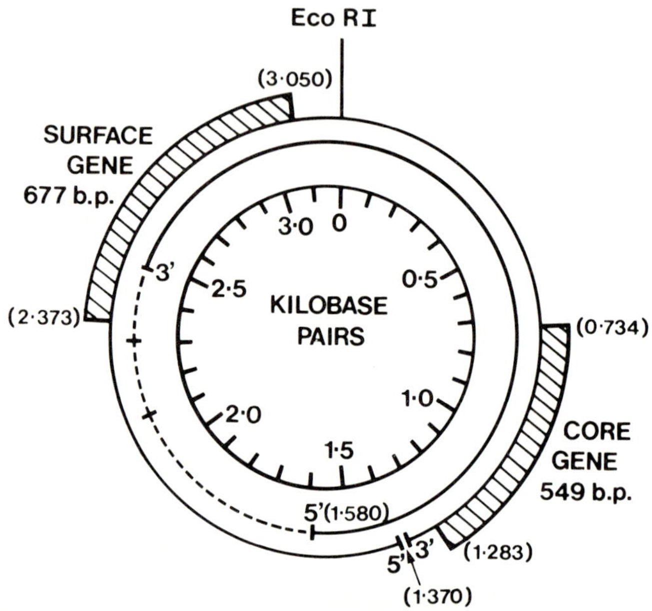

FIGURE 1. Genome of hepatitis B virus

proteins (Figure 1). Two additional open coding regions (designated P (832 amino acids) and X (154 amino acids)) have been noted, although gene products corresponding to these regions have not been described (review; Tiollais, Charnay and Vyas, 1981). A number of groups are attempting to identify short amino acid sequences within the HBsAg polypeptide as the different antigenic determinants of HBsAg, and antisera that react with HBsAg have been produced by immunising animals with short synthetic polypeptides based on different regions of the HBsAg polypeptide sequence (Lerner *et al.*, 1981; Dreesman *et al.*, 1982). Thus the possibility of chemically synthesising an immunogen with potential use as a vaccine is being actively explored.

Recent evidence that infected hepatocytes contain large amounts of single stranded HBV DNA in the cytoplasm rather than the nucleus, suggests that HBV replication is likely to involve a novel strategy unlike that of other small and medium sized eucaryotic DNA viruses (Burrell *et al.*, 1982).

Three different viruses with similar properties to HBV have been recently identified in three different non-primate

TABLE II. *Comparative Properties of Hepadnaviruses Isolated from Different Species*

Property	Man (HBV)	Ground squirrel	Woodchuck	Pekin duck
DNA genome	3182 bp (Gap)	3308 bp (Gap)	3308 bp (Gap)	c3000 bp (Gap)
Virion-associated DNA polymerase	+	+	+	+
Virion:				
Complete	42 nm	47 nm	45 nm	40-45 nm
Core	27 nm	30 nm	27 nm	27 nm
Surface antigen particles	22 nm	15-25 nm	20-25 nm	40-45 nm
	weak cross reaction			Serologically distinct
Polypeptides	P23/27	P22/25	P22/25	?
Replication	Cytoplasmic?	?	?	via RNA Intermediate?
Transmission	Vert., Horiz.	?	?	Vert. (Egg)
Healthy carriers	+	+	+	+
Tissue tropism	Liver	Liver	Liver	Liver (Pancreas)
Chronic liver disease/Hepatoma	+	?	+	?

species (Table II; Summers, 1981) and the term Hepadnaviruses has been provisionally suggested for this group. All four Hepadnaviruses are serologically distinct but in some cases related; the host species range of the non-human viruses has not been fully defined, but there are no reports at present of infection of primates with these non-primate Hepadnaviruses.

TABLE III. Clinical Aspects of HBV Infection

Hepatic	Extra-hepatic
(a) Acute - Anicteric hepatitis - Icteric hepatitis * slow onset * anorexia/nausea * GI/toxic symptoms * variable fever * hepatomegaly * abnormal LFTs * dark urine - Fulminant hepatitis (B + NA, NB synergy)	- Arthritis/arthralgia dermatitis syndrome (10-20% cases) - Polyarteritis nodosa (30-40% HBsAg+) - Infantile papular acrodermatitis * erythematopapular rash * enlarged liver/lymph nodes * age: 80% <2 years * horizontal spread * HBsAg (ayw)/Ig in lesions
(b) Chronic - Chronic persistent hepatitis - Chronic active hepatitis - Cirrhosis - Primary hepatic carcinoma	- Membranous glomerulonephritis - Essential mixed cryoglobulinemia? * vasculitis * glomerulitis * low serum C' * Ig deposition, mixed HBsAg/Danes/Anti-HBs - Polymyalgia rheumatica?

III. CLINICAL ASPECTS OF HBV INFECTION

The clinical features of acute HBV infection are well known and listed in Table III. Mention should be made of the arthralgia/dermatitis syndrome seen in the prodromal phase of 10-20% of patients in some series (occasionally leading to initial presentation in rheumatology clinics), and the infantile papular acrodermatitis syndrome described in Japan but rarely reported elsewhere. The associations (Table III) of HBV with essential mixed cryoglobulinemia and with polymyalgia rheumatica are perhaps less established as ones of cause and effect.

Persistent infection follows approximately 5% of acute infections in adults and a higher proportion of infections acquired in infancy. Two situations involving synergistic infection with HBV and another agent have come to recent attention. (i) The δ agent is a serologically unrelated infective agent that requires coexisting HBV infection to allow its replication. Thus δ infections are seen in some acute HBV infections where δ infection is simultaneously acquired, in some δ-negative HBV carriers who are later infected with δ and in some HBV carriers (often of Italian origin) who also have persistent δ infection. Acute δ infection in a previously healthy HBV carrier can produce a second episode of liver damage (at least in chimpanzees), and HBV carriers with coexisting δ infection are more likely to have ongoing liver damage. Recent epidemiological observations have shown an association between δ agent and HBV in a high-mortality outbreak of hepatitis in Venezuelan Indians (Purcell - personal communication). δ antigen can be detected by immunofluorescence in infected livers, and circulating in serum in a form encapsidated within a coat of HBsAg, and anti-δ antibodies are found in serum of infected individuals (Editorial, 1982). (ii) Analysis of a high mortality outbreak of hepatitis B in a dialysis unit in Edinburgh

TABLE IV. Epidemiological Features of Hepatitis B

Virus in body	*Transmission*
- *Blood and Tissue Fluids Acute or chronic carriage Higher infectivity associated with presence of HBeAg, DNA pol., high titre HBsAg*	- *Skin penetration (++++)*
- *Faeces neg. (HBsAg?)*	- *Mucosal contact (+++) Infection per os, Sexual intercourse*
- *Urine neg. (HBsAg?)*	- *"Respiratory" - No*
- *Saliva pos. (HBsAg+, infectivity+) (Virions: DNA Poly.)*	- *"Enteric" - No*
- *Semen pos. (HBsAg+, infectivity+)*	- *Vertical spread (++)*
- *Sweat/tears (HBsAg+, infectivity?)*	
- *Milk (HBsAg+, infectivity?)*	
- *Amniotic fluid (HBsAg+, infectivity?)*	

suggests that many of the fatal cases were simultaneously infected with HBV and NANB, suggesting a potentiating effect of dual infection on disease severity (Marmion *et al.*, 1982).

IV. TRANSMISSION OF HBV

Epidemiological observations demonstrate that the major routes of infection are (i) skin penetration, (ii) mucosal contact, particularly sexual contact (and particularly among homosexuals), and (iii) vertical transmission from mother to infant. HBsAg can be detected in most body fluids including semen and breast milk, but with the exception of saliva, HBsAg levels are usually low, HBV virions and infectivity are not usually demonstrable, and the role played by virus excretion via these routes in the natural history of the disease is equivocal. Infection may be transmitted by contaminated biting insects in very limited contexts, but this is unlikely to be of major epidemiological significance and there is no evidence for virus replication in arthropods (Table IV).

TABLE V. Vertical Transmission of HBV

- *When mother has acute HB in third trimester:*
  * *High proportion (c 66%) of babies infected: mother's race not significant.*
- *When mother is chronic HBsAg carrier:*
  * *Children of Asian carrier mothers have higher carrier rates than Caucasians.*
- *Predictors of transmission risk:*
  * *Carrier rates in infants born to -*

HBeAg+ mother	*85-95%*
Anti-HBe+ mothers	*40%*
(Taiwan)	

- *Timing of transmission with carrier mother:*
  * *Cord blood/one month postnatal serum specimens often HBsAg negative in babies who later become carriers.*
  * *Antigenemia rates in babies peak around 3 months.*
  * *98% maternal vaginal secretions, 33% amniotic fluids, and 95% gastric aspirates of babies positive for HBsAg.*

Vertical transmission is a major mechanism for maintaining HBsAg carrier rates in high prevalence regions of the world. Transmission is most likely when carrier mothers also show serum HBeAg rather than anti-HBe, and by mothers undergoing acute infection in the third trimester, and is thought to occur at or around the time of delivery (Table V). In a study in the U.K. of infants born to carrier mothers, highest transmission rates were seen in Chinese mothers, while mothers of Caucasian race had the lowest rates; HBeAg was most commonly seen in Chinese mothers, and its presence also correlated strongly with the highest rate of transmission of infection (Derso *et al.*, 1978). Interruption of vertical transmission is a fundamental aspect of any attempt to reduce HBV carriage world-wide (Table VI). Pooled human immunoglobulin containing a high titre of anti-HBs (HBIg) is effective (Beasley *et al.*, 1981) if the first dose is administered as soon as possible after birth (certainly within 48 hours), but supply and logistic factors prevent the widescale use of this approach. Active immunisation (with or without short term cover with HBIg) is more attractive: one study has demonstrated a reduced carrier rate after vaccination in infancy with inactivated HBsAg (Maupas *et al.*, 1981), but the timing and dosage for optimum protection has not yet been defined.

V. HBV AND HEPATOCELLULAR CARCINOMA (HCC)

Recent work has provided a number of converging lines of evidence pointing to a strong association between HBV and HCC (Table VII). The world-wide distribution of rates of HCC closely parallels the distribution of HBsAg carrier rates in

TABLE VI. Interruption of Vertical Transmission of HBV

- *Caesarian section/No breast milk*
  - *No effect in Taiwanese trials.*
- *HBIG (Beasley et al., Taiwan)*
  - *75% protection after 3 doses: at birth, 3 months and 6 months.*
  - *Passive/active immunisation, a common response.*
- *Vaccine*
  - *Vaccination in infancy reduces carrier rate.*

the healthy population in different parts of the world. A higher prevalence of HBsAg in HCC patients than in matched controls has been described for a number of different parts of the world (Hadziyannis, 1980). HBV DNA integrated into tumour cell DNA has been found in a majority of tumours studied, as well as in a number of HBsAg-producing hepatoma cell lines (Shafritz and Kew, 1981; Brechot *et al.*, 1981, Chen *et al.*, 1982; Chakraborty *et al.*, 1980; Edman *et al.*, 1980; Marion *et al.*, 1980; Brechot *et al.*, 1980). Finally, a prospective study of HBsAg carriers and matched controls has established that HBsAg carriers have a 390 fold greater risk of developing HCC, but not other diseases, than controls (Beasley, 1982).

This information provides compelling evidence that HBsAg carriage is a significant risk factor in the development of HCC, and allows the elaboration and investigation of models at the molecular level whereby chronic HBV infection might contribute to the emergence of clones of malignant cells. There is evidence for an incubation period of 20-30 years between acquisition of infection and development of clinical HCC. However, clinical HCC may not be an inevitable outcome of HBV carriage and other genetic and environmental cofactors (e.g., aflatoxin exposure) may also be significant. Of practical value is the observation that high serum α-foetoprotein levels can identify HCC patients sufficiently early for successful surgical intervention (Beasley, personal communication).

TABLE VII. Hepatitis B (HBV) and Hepatoma (HCC)

- *HCC is commoner in areas of high HBsAg prevalence.*
- *HBV markers are commoner in HCC than in controls.*
- *Mothers of HCC patients more often positive than fathers or controls.*
- *In prospective studies HCC was >200 x commoner in HBsAg carriers than in controls.*
- *HCC (and liver) contains free and integrated HBV DNA.*
- *HBsAg +, HCC cell lines have integ. HBV DNA: c 4 genomes per cell.*
- *Related hepadna virus associated with HCC in its host.*

VI. ACTIVE IMMUNIZATION AGAINST HBV

A number of laboratories have purified HBsAg (largely as the 22 nm spherical form) from the plasma of carriers, and after treatment designed to eliminate residual infectivity, have demonstrated the ability of such candidate vaccines to induce an active anti-HBs response in animals or human volunteers. In a recent large scale trial of the best-studied of these preparations in homosexual men, HBV infection was not transmitted to vaccinees, no significant side effects were noted, an anti-HBs response was produced in a majority of vaccinees, and significant protection against HBV challenge was conferred (Szmuness *et al.*, 1980). This vaccine has now been licensed for use in the U.S.A. and is likely to find application in groups at risk of HBV due to their employment (e.g., health workers) or social habits (e.g., drug abusers, homosexuals). However, details of the recommended use for this vaccine have not yet been agreed upon, and these are likely to vary from country to country. An additional potentially very large scale use for this vaccine, is the protection of neonates and infants in high HBV prevalence parts of the world, where infection is often acquired early in life.

Alternative technological approaches for the production of immunogenic material include the synthesis of HBsAg by cloned bacterial or eucaryotic cells containing the appropriate portion of the HBV genome, the large scale production of HBsAg by human hepatoma cells (Wen *et al.*, 1981) and the chemical synthesis of defined polypeptide immunogens capable of inducing an anti-HBs response (see above). The feasibility of all three approaches has been demonstrated, but appropriate largescale studies to demonstrate protection by such candidate vaccines have not been carried out.

VII. NON-A AND NON-B HEPATITIS

The use of specific serological tests to diagnose hepatitis A and B has revealed that a significant proportion of sporadic acute viral hepatitis, and the majority of cases of post-transfusion hepatitis in recipients of HBsAg-negative blood, is not caused by hepatitis A or hepatitis B virus, nor to other infective agents such as Epstein-Barr virus or cytomegalovirus for which specific tests are available. The term non-A, non-B hepatitis is used to refer to infections defined as above, and much current research is aimed at identifying the agent or agents responsible and developing specific serological tests (see Gerety, 1981). A number of publications have claimed to describe specific serological markers for this infection, but in general these have proved unreliable when used to examine coded sera from experimental chimpanzee infections. At least three factors may have contributed to

TABLE VIII. Features of Non-A, Non-B Hepatitis

- *Antigenically unrelated to Hep. A, Hep. B, CMV, EBV, and DELTA.*
- *Incubation periods * 40-103 days: "LONG"*
  *   * 18-50 days: "SHORT"*
- *Commonly anicteric: low mortality.*
- *Chronicity: 20-50% cases have raised LFT for 9-12 months or more.*
- *Chronic sequelae: CAH, CPH, Cirrhosis.*
- *Transmitted by percutaneous and (probably) by non-percutaneous routes.*
- *Now causes 65-90% of post transfusion hepatitis (USA).*
- *Risk with commercial donors 5-20 x that with volunteer donors.*
- *Follows blood products (Fibrinogen, F/VIII, IX).*
- *Comprises 20-40% of "sporadic" hepatitis.*
- *Dialysis-associated outbreaks.*
- *Virus(es) in blood in incubation period, acute disease and chronic carriers.*
- *Several strains * Trans. to chimpanzees (≥3)*
  ** Marmosets (e.g., GB agent)*
  ** "Indian" hepatitis*
- *Evidence of homologous immunity (human volunteers: chimps).*
- *"Virions": Rarely sighted (25-30:32:37 nm)*
- *In hepatocytes - * Cytoplasmic "tubules" and intranuclear antigen/particles (12-20 nm)*
- *Immune complexes, high IgG/IgM ratios present in acute phase illness.*
- *Serological tests: many devised: few confirmed.*

the current lack of success: (i) there is some evidence from sequential infections in chimpanzees and man, from varying incubation periods and from different patterns of liver ultrastructural changes in acute infection, that more than one agent may be involved; (ii) during acute liver injury a number of non-specific, presumably host-coded antigens and their corresponding antibodies may be released to the circulation; (iii) the absolute levels of virus antigen present in the serum during acute infection and of virus antibody during convalescence, may be considerably lower than occurs in hepatitis B infection. In addition, some workers have described HBV-like particles containing antigens reacting with the HBeAg of HBV in some cases of non-A, non-B; when this finding is coupled with the known relationship to HBV of the δ agent (which itself does *not* possess properties consistent with the above definition of NANB), and with the synergistic relationship between HBV and NANB described above, the confusing possibility emerges that in at least some cases of NANB, occult HBV infection may also be involved in some way that is not understood at present.

Some features of NANB infections are listed in Table VIII. Transmission routes, and its particular prevalence among drug abusers, both suggest similar epidemiological features to HBV. Presumptive diagnosis is impossible in situations other than acute viral hepatitis or post-transfusion hepatitis, and in view of the fact that up to 20% of acute HBV infections are HBsAg negative, anti HBcIgM positive, adequate exclusion of HBV infection requires anti-HBc as well as HBsAg testing. Acute infections tend to be clinically milder than HBV, but a much higher proportion of acute infections result in chronic hepatitis than with HBV. Thus it is likely that an unknown proportion of patients presenting with "cryptogenic" cirrhosis or chronic hepatitis may in fact have been infected with NANB. There is no current way of diagnosing NANB in this situation.

VIII. SUMMARY

It is now possible to foresee, more clearly than even several years ago, the eventual realisation of some major goals of hepatitis B research. (i) Reduction to insignificant levels of the risk of acquisition of HBV infection by those at risk due to occupation or social habits. (ii) Reduction of the extent of chronic liver disease due to HBV. (iii) Significant reduction in the world wide incidence of primary liver cancer. (iv) Significant reduction in the enormous human reservoir of HBV. The achievement of these goals will require continuing advances in laboratory and epidemiological research, combined with the will and resources to put such advances into effective action at a national and international level.

Similar success in defining and controlling NANB hepatitis cannot be predicted so readily. Nevertheless, it is likely that approaches used successfully with hepatitis B will eventually yield successful results.

REFERENCES

Beasley, R.P., Hwang, L-Y., Lin, C-C., *et al.* (1981). *Lancet ii,* 388.

Beasley, R.P. (1982). *Hepatology 2,* 21S.

Brechot, C., Pourcel, C., Louise, A., *et al.* (1980). *Nature 286,* 533.

Brechot, C., Hadchouel, M., Scotto, J., *et al.* (1981). *Proc. Nat. Acad. Sci. USA 78,* 3906.

Burrell, C.J., Gowans, E.J., Jilbert, A.R., *et al.* (1982). *Hepatology 2,* 85S.

Chakraborty, P.R., Ruiz-Opazo, N., Shouval, D., and Shafritz, D.A. (1980). *Nature 286,* 531.

Chen, D-S., Hoyer, B.H., Nelson, J., *et al.* (1982). *Hepatology 2,* 42S.

Derso, A., Boxall, E.H., Tarlow, M.J. and Flewett, T.H. (1978). *Brit. Med. J. i,* 949.

Dreesman, G.R., Sanchez, Y., Ionescu-Mattiu, I., *et al.* (1982). *Nature 295,* 158.

Editorial (1982). *Lancet i,* 259.

Edman, J.C., Gray, P., Valenzuela, P., *et al.* (1980). *Nature 286,* 535.

Gerety, R.J. (ed.) (1981). "Non-A, Non-B Hepatitis." Academic Press, New York.

Hadziyannis, S.J. (1980). *Clinics in Gastroenterology 9,* 117.

Lerner, R.A., Green, N., Alexander, H., *et al.* (1981). *Proc. Nat. Acad. Sci. USA 78,* 3403.

Marion, P.L., Salazar, F.H., Alexander, J.J. and Robinson, W.S. (1980). *J. Virol. 33,* 795.

Marmion, B.P., Burrell, C.J., Tonkin, R.W., and Dickson, J.D. (1982). *Reviews in Infectious Diseases,* in press.

Maupas, P., Chiron, J-P., Barin, F., *et al.* (1981). *Lancet i,* 289.

Shafritz, D., and Kew, M.C. (1981). *Hepatology 1,* 1.

Summers, J., (1981). *Hepatology 1,* 179.

Szmuness, W., Stevens, C.E., Harley, E.J., *et al.* (1980). *New Engl. J. Med. 303*, 833.

Tiollais, P., Charnay, P., and Vyas, G.N. (1981). *Science 213*, 406.

Wen, Y-M., Copeland, J.A., Mann, G.F., *et al.* (1981). *Arch. Virol. 68*, 157.

42

FAMILIAL CLUSTERING OF HBsAg IN CHINA

C.B. Liu

Institute of Virology
Chinese Academy of Medical Sciences
Beijing

Y. Lee

Provincial Hygenic and Anti-Epidemic Station
Zhengzhou, Henan

Z.H. Hu

Institute of Bioproducts and Pharmaceutic Control
Beijing

The variable distribution of HBsAg carrier rates in the population is a world-wide phenomenon (4). Viral hepatitis is a common disease in our country. The average HBsAg carrier rate is relatively high (8% by RPHA test) compared to Western countries. Great variation in distribution, however, is observed and there may be as much as five-fold differences between the highest HBsAg carrier rate and the lowest. This unbalanced distribution of HBsAg is not only observed between different provinces and cities but even in different inhabitant groups of the same village (6). Epidemiological investigations indicate that a majority of hepatitis patients and HBsAg carriers have had no history of blood transfusion, surgical injury, or vaccination. We believe that the key factor in the spreading of HBV infection in high-endemic areas is intimate contact between people. Familial activities appear to constitute the major epidemiological factor in HBV infection (1, 3, 8, 9).

VIRAL DISEASES IN SOUTH-EAST ASIA
AND THE WESTERN PACIFIC
ISBN 0 12 484820 6

In collaboration with the health departments of provinces and municipalities we investigated 15,803 families in 1979-1980 in different geographic areas of China, including rural, urban, mountainous and plain regions. The families chosen for this study were composed of at least two generations (parents and children). All blood samples of members of the same family were taken at one time, otherwise they were excluded from this investigation. The presence of HBsAg antigenemia was detected by the reverse passive haemagglutination test. The sensitivity of this is more than 50-100 times that of counterimmunoelectrophoresis.

RESULTS

The overall HBsAg positive rate was 10.54%. HBsAg carriers were found in 31% of families, and 63% of carriers were concentrated in 12% of families. The distribution of HBsAg in families of different size is summarized in Table I.

The phenomenon of familial clustering is very obvious ($p<0.001$) and the frequency of aggregation is 38%. The latter varied directly with the general HBsAg prevalence of the areas. For example, in the rural area of province K., the HBsAg carrier rate was 17.54% and the frequency of familial aggregation was 50.64%. In the rural area of province SH. the antigen carrier rate was 3.62%, while the frequency of familial aggregation was 26.37% (Figure 1).

The prevalence of HBsAg increased with increasing family size. In families with three members, the HBsAg positive rate was 20%, as compared to 47% in families with nine members.

In the rural area, HBsAg positive families was 29% as compared to 22% in the urban area ($p<0.001$), indicating that the HBV infection was heavier in rural areas.

The relationship between HBsAg prevalence of children and the carrier status of their parents was studied. Families were divided into four groups, according to the carrier status of parents as shown in Table II.

The prevalence of HBsAg among children of different groups ranged from 9.2 to 44% ($\chi^2 = 2401$, $p<0.001$). The highest prevalence was found in children of group 1 (both mother and father HBsAg positive) indicating the importance of parents in intrafamilial transmission of HBV. The difference between group 2 (mother only HBsAg positive) and group 3 (father only HBsAg positive) was statistically significant, 38.38% versus 18% ($\chi^2 = 292.7$, $p<0.001$),

TABLE I. Distribution of HBsAg in Families

No. HBsAg positive in families	No. of members in families										Total families
	3	4	5	6	7.	8	9	10	11	12	
0	2636	3035	2427	1479	791	358	132	51	15	11	10953
1	506	800	657	479	307	145	41	33	9	9	2986
2	118	214	252	208	140	59	27	14	8	3	1043
3	27	116	107	102	68	20	18	8	2	1	469
4		25	57	59	40	20	11	5	3		220
5			15	28	25	13	12	4	1		98
6				6	12	6	2	3			29
7							2				2
8						1	2				3
Total families	3287	4190	3515	2379	1383	622	247	118	38	24	15803
Positive families	651	1155	1088	882	592	264	115	67	23	13	4850
(%)	(20)	(28)	(31)	(37)	(48)	(42)	(47)	(57)	(61)	(54)	(31)
Aggregation	18%	31%	41%	46%	48%	0.45%	64%	51%	61%	23%	

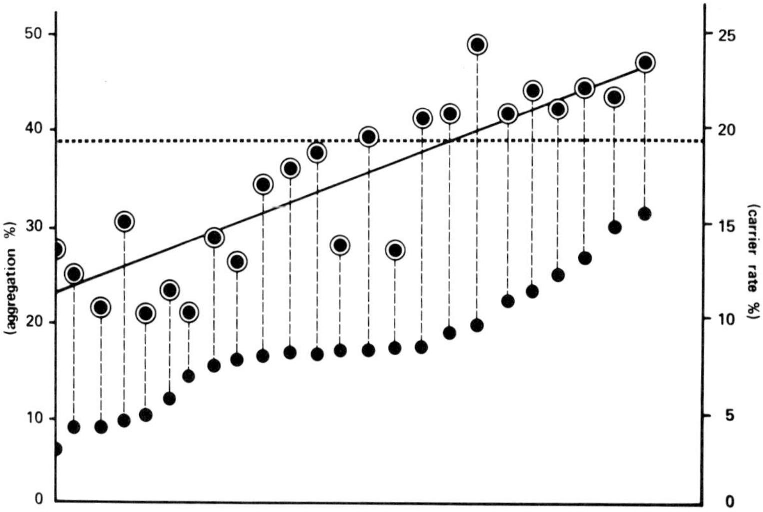

FIGURE 1. The relationship of general HBsAg carrier rate (black points) to the familial aggregation rate (cycle points) in provinces.

TABLE II. Relationship Between HBsAg Carrier Status of Parents and Their Children

Parent Groups			Children		
			No. tested	No. HBsAg positive	%
1	Father +	Mother +	452	199	44.03
2	Father -	Mother +	2697	1035	38.38
3	Father +	Mother -	2979	536	17.99
4	Father -	Mother -	26173	2409	9.20
	Total		32301	4179	12.93

$\chi^2 = 2401$, $p<0.001$
+ HBsAg positive
- HBsAg negative

suggesting that in the formation of familial clustering of HBsAg, mothers played a more important role than fathers. With respect to the transmission of HBV between husband and wife, we investigated 10,000 couples. In only 1.28% were both husband and wife HBsAg positive while in 17.55% only one partner was positive. Thus transmission of HBV between husband and wife is of little importance (3).

COMMENT

We have further confirmed the importance of the familial transmission as a major epidemiologic factor in the spreading of HBV. In a dynamic study of infants born from HBsAg mothers, we found that about 65% of infants became HBsAg positive six months after birth (2). This fact indicates that familial clustering of HBV may be closely related to infection during child birth. Transmission of HBV between husband and wife in hyperendemic areas could be neglected, as the majority of the population have been infected in their early stage of life.

REFERENCES

1. Bogch, J. *et al., Lancet II,* 457 (1973).
2. Keu, M.C. *et al., S. Afr. Med. J. 49,* 1471 (1975).
3. Ohbayashi, A. *et al., Lancet I,* 433 (1977).
4. WHO Collaborative Study on Hepatitis B Progress Report, VIR/cc/77, 15, Geneva.
5. Zhao, H.L. *et al., Act. Academiae Medicinae Sinicae 3,* 179 (1981).
6. Prevention and Treatment of Communicable Disease *4,* (4) 223 (1977).
7. Hu, Z.L. *et al., Chinese J. Epid. 2,* 242 (1981).
8. Zhou, Q.H. *et al., Chinese J. Epid. 2,* (1981).
9. Jong, Q. *et al., Chinese J. Preventive Med. 14,* 235 (1980).

43

HEPATITIS B IN SRI LANKA PRESENTS UNUSUAL FEATURES FOR A TROPICAL COUNTRY

Tissa Vitarana

Medical Research Institute (MRI)
Colombo Sri Lanka

I. INTRODUCTION

There is a higher carrier rate (2% to more than 10%) of HBsAg among adults and children in tropical countries of Asia, Africa and in East Europe (1), while countries of West Europe, North America and Australia have values less than 1%. Chronic liver disease is a problem in Asia and a high proportion of cases (eg: 50%) carry HBsAg. Sri Lanka appears to deviate from this Asian pattern.

II. HBsAg AND ANTI-HBs IN A STUDY IN A DENSELY POPULATED PART OF COLOMBO DONE IN 1975

Forbes, de la Motte and Kono (3) collected blood from 317 persons of different age groups(approximately 50 from each 10 year age group) in a densely populated part of Colombo, the capital, and on testing by RIA found that 5 (1.6%) carried HBsAg and 13 (4.1%) had antibody, so that, in all, 18 (5.7%) had evidence of past infection with HBV. (As four of the HBsAg +ves were from one family and the mother had antibody it is likely that this was due to a recent infection and not to chronic carriage).

VIRAL DISEASES IN SOUTH-EAST ASIA
AND THE WESTERN PACIFIC
ISBN 0 12 484820 6

TABLE I. Detection of HBsAg and Anti-HBs by Radioimmunoassay in a General Population Study of 16 Towns

Age (Years)	No. tested	HBsAg		Anti-HBs		Total	
		No.	%	No.	%	No.	%
½ - 1	10	0	0	0	0	0	0
1 - 4	64	0	0	1		1	1.6
5 - 9	68	0	0	1		1	1.6
10 - 19	151	1	0.6	6	4.0	7	4.6
20 - 39	142	0	0	12	8.4	12	8.4
40 - 59	142	4	2.8	23	16.2	27	19.9
60 +	68	1	1.5	15	22.0	16	23.5
Total	645	6	0.9	58	9.0	64	9.9

III. HBsAg AND ANTI-HBs IN AN AGE-STRATIFIED STUDY DONE IN 1976 OF 16 MAJOR TOWNS IN SRI LANKA

Approximately 50 samples were obtained in each town from all age groups. The sera were tested for HBsAg and anti-HBs by solid-phase radioimmunoassay (RIA) in Melbourne.

HBsAg was detected in 0.9% of sera and anti-HBs in 9.0%, so that 9.9% showed serological evidence of past infection with HBV. The infection appears to be uncommon amongst children and young adults (see Table I). The occurrence of infection with HBV differed considerably from place to place ranging from 2.7% in Galle, in the South, to 22.7% in Tissamaharama, 20.6% in Trincomalee and 18.6% in Batticaloa, all in the East of the island.

IV. HBsAg AMONG BLOOD DONORS

Dr. (Mrs) Nandrani S. de Soysa of the National Blood Transfusion Service, Colombo, tested 1095 blood donors using Reverse Passive Haemagglutination (Auscell, Abbotts) and found 3 positive for HBsAg (0.27%).

TABLE II. Hepatitis B Markers Detected by RIA in Chronic Liver Disease Cases (1980-81)

Marker	No. of cases	+Ves	%
HBsAg	226	12	5.3
Anti-HBs	58	6	10.3
Anti-HBc	49	13	26.5

V. MARKERS OF HEPATITIS B IN CASES OF CHRONIC LIVER DISEASE

A Study of selected cases of chronic liver disease (CLD) was begun in Colombo in February, 1980. Forty nine sera were sent to Dr. D.S.Dane's Laboratory at the Middlesex Hospital Medical School, London, where they were tested by Dr. R.S.Tedder for HBsAg, anti-HBs and anti-HBc by solid-phase RIA. The balance 177 sera were tested for HBsAg at the MRI using RIA (Ausria, Abbotts). Ten of these sera were sent to Dr. D.Burke's Laboratory AFRIMS, Bangkok, for confirmation. The nine sera that were HBsAg negative were tested there for anti-HBs by solid-phase RIA.

The results of the 226 cases studied upto July 1981 are given in Table II. The occurrence of HBsAg was (1) 5.3% among the 226 CLD cases (2) 5.1% among the 117 cirrhotics and (3) 11.1% among the nine primary liver carcinoma cases.

VI. EVIDENCE OF HEPATITIS B INFECTION AMONG THE ABORIGINAL POPULATION IN SRI LANKA.

In a study of the aboriginal population of the South East of the island, ninety seven sera, from all age groups and both sexes, were tested by ID at the MRI and three were positive for HBsAg amd 19 (19.6%) for anti-HBs. By RIA a further two HBsAg positives were detected. Thus the HBsAg carrier rate was 5.2%, and 24.7% in all had evidence of past HBV infection. In contrast among the non-aboriginals of the same area there was one HBsAg positive and no anti-HBs positives among 42 tested by ID.

VII. DISCUSSION

The above findings show that Sri Lanka differs from other Asian and African countries, and resembles U.K., U.S.A. and other temperate countries, in having a HBsAg carrier rate of less than 1%, a very low infection and carrier rate among children, and a HBsAg occurrence of 5.1% in cirrhosis cases and 11.1% in primary hepatocellular carcinoma. However, the later age at which infection occurs in Sri Lanka is probably because of less parenteral drug abuse among the youth and poor sterilization of needles at clinics (diabetes, TB etc.) for the elderly. Social and environmental factors cannot account for the difference in HBsAg carriage as Sri Lanka conforms in most respects with other Asian countries - climate, over-crowding, poor hygiene, dietery habits and cultural and religious practices. The question that must be posed is whether there is some genetic factor responsible. The higher HBsAg carriage and HBV infection among the aborigines and in the east of the island, where inter-marriage with the aborigines in the past is a possibility, and the lower level in the non-aboriginal population in the immediate neighbourhood, tend to support this view. Therefore further studies in Sri Lanka (HLA typing etc.) and abroad eg: in India are certainly indicated.

ACKNOWLEDGMENTS

I acknowledge the help of colleagues at the MRI, the Epidemiology Unit and the hospitals in Sri Lanka, and of Virologists abroad, and thank WHO, SAREC and the NSC, Sri Lanka, for financial assistance.

REFERENCES

(1) Sobeslavsky, O. (1980). Bulletin of the World Health Organization, 58(4): 621-628.

(2) Vitarana, T., Kanapathipillai, M., Gunasekera, H.D.N., Lehmann, N.T., Dimitrikakis, M. and Gust I.D.(1978). Asian Journal of Infectious Diseases 2:247-252.

(3) Forbes, C., de la Motte, P.U. and Kono, R. Personal Communication.

HEPATITIS B VIRUS (HVB) INFECTIONS AND PRIMARY HEPATOCELLULAR CARCINOMA (HC) IN HAWAII AND SOUTH PACIFIC ISLANDS

Arwin Diwan
Nguyen The Thanh
Scott B. Halstead

Department of Tropical Medicine
and Medical Microbiology
University of Hawaii
Honolulu, Hawaii

I. INTRODUCTION

The discovery of Australia antigen, at present referred to as hepatitis B surface antigen or HBsAg by Blumberg (1), and its subsequent association with hepatitis B infection (2,3) has made it possible to answer previously unresolved questions regarding this disease. Seroepidemiological studies show there are approximately 120 million carriers of HBsAg in the world. HBs antigenemia occurs with high frequency in tropical and subtropical countries. World distribution of HBsAg based on the results of population surveys shows the prevalence of HBsAg varies between less than 0.5% in the U.S. and Western Europe, to 1.2% in Central South America, Southern Europe, 1.5% in Japan, 3 to 5% in North Africa and many parts of Asiatic USSR, 7 to 8% in China and 6 to 10% in Central and South Africa and S.E. Asia. The cumulative rate of infections are determined by testing for three Hepatitis B virus (HBV) markers - HBsAg, anti-HBsAg and anti-HBC - which varies between 7 to 10% for the U.S. and Europe (4). Case-control studies in various populations have demonstrated that HBsAg is found more frequently in the sera of PHC patients than in matched controls. Several other observations, such as detection of HBsAg in

VIRAL DISEASES IN SOUTH-EAST ASIA
AND THE WESTERN PACIFIC
ISBN 0 12 484820 6

cell lines derived from PHC, have strengthened the association between PHC and the chronic HBsAg carrier state. HBV may have a major role in the pathogenesis of PHC (5). In this paper we will review our studies of HBV and PHC in the multi-ethnic Hawaiian Island population, and in some of the other Pacific island population.

II. MATERIALS AND METHODS

A. *Serum Specimen*

Seven hundred and ninety-nine serum specimens were obtained in 1970 from residents of the City and County of Honolulu, Island of Oahu, State of Hawaii. This sample represented major racial groups on the Island of Oahu. One hundred and twelve serum samples from American Samoa and 187 serum samples for the Kingdom of Tonga were collected in 1974. Fifty-six sera from Cook Island were collected in early 1970.

B. *Tests for HBsAg and anti-HBsAg*

These were done by commercially available radioimmuno assay (RIA) kits from Abbott Laboratories, Chicago. AUSRIA was used for HBsAg and AUSAB was used for the detection of anti-HBs.

C. *Sub-typing of HBsAg*

This was done by Dr. George Le Bouvier, Yale University School of Medicine.

III. RESULTS

Table 1 shows the prevalence of HBsAg and anti-HBsAg amongst various ethnic groups in Hawaii. The rates of HBs antigenemia varied in various ethnic groups: for Japanese it was 2.5%; Caucasians, 0.5%; Filipinos, 3.8%; and for Chinese, 4.5%. No HBs was detected in bloods from 82 Hawaiian or part-Hawaiian; this was also true for a small sample from Puerto Ricans and Negroes. Samoans on the other hand had a high prevalence of HBsAg (14.3%). Prevalence of anti-HBsAg varied from 6.3 to 12.1% among the 5 major ethnic groups sampled. The anti-HBS rate for Samoans was 28.6%. Overall prevalence rate of HBsAg plus anti-HBs for all populations combined was 11% of the population sampled.

TABLE I. Prevalence of HBsAg and Anti-HBsAg by Race (Residents of Oahu)

Race	HBsAg Pos/Total Tested	Anti-HBsAg Pos/Total Tested	HBsAg Pos + Anti-HBsAg Pos/Total Tested
Japanese	3/122(2.5)*	11/122(9.0)*	14/122(11.5)*
Caucasian	1/217(0.5)	18/217(8.3)	19/217(8.7)
Hawaiian/ Part Hawn.	0/82 (0.0)	10/82 (12.1)	10/82 (12.2)
Filipino	3/78 (3.8)	6/78 (7.7)	9/78 (11.5)
Chinese	5/110(4.5)	7/110(6.3)	12/110(10.9)
Puerto Rican	9/18 (0.0)	1/18 (2.3)	1/18 (5.5)
Negro	0/4 (0.0)	0/4 (0.0)	0/4 (0.0)
Samoan	4/28 (14.3)	8/28 (28.6)	12/28 (43.0)
Other/Mixed	1/140(0.7)	15/140(10.7)	16/140(11.4)
Total:	17/799(2.1)	76/799(9.5)	93/799(11.6)

* *Percent positive.*

When we analysed data by place of birth for the two HBV markers, 66/565 (11.7%) of the Hawaii-born residents were positive, 11/168 (6.5%) born on the continental U.S. were positive and 16/44 (25%) foreign born were positive. Thus, exposure to HBV in Hawaii is intermediate between the U.S. mainland and various Pacific basin countries. Because we found that HBV infection rates for Samoans were very high, we decided to study the prevalence of HBV marker in residents of various Pacific island populations.

Representative samples from American Samoa tested for HBsAg and anti-HBsAg showed the following, 21/112 (18%) samples were positive for HBsAg and 53/104 (51%) of samples tested were positive for anti-HBsAg. Cumulatively, 74/112 (66%) of the population was positive for these HBV markers. Similarly, age stratified samples collected from the Kingdom of Tonga showed that 57/143 (29.5%) were positive for HBsAg, and 122/187 were positive for anti-HBsAg; overall 122/187 (82.5%) had both HBV markers. We also tested limited samples from the Cook Islands; 6/56 (10.3%) were positive for HBsAg and 41/47 (87%) were positive for anti-HBS. Six HBsAg positive sera from Cook Islands were tested for HBsAg; 3 were ayw and 3 were adr.

Our studies have shown that the prevalence of HBsAg differs in various ethnic groups resident in the Hawaiian Islands. In addition, resident populations from American Samoa, the Kingdom of Tonga and Cook Islands have high rates of HBs antigenemia. Age acquisition profiles of HBsAg and of anti-HBsAg suggest that both vertical and horizontal transmission of HBV occurs in these environments. Vertical transmission of HBV from mothers circulating HBs to fetus have been shown in several studies (6,7). HBV is also acquired horizontally by many routes such as parenteral transmission by contaminated needles in drug addiction and tatooing, by the sexual route, and oral-fecal transmission in the institutions for the mentally retarded. Factors influencing horizontal and vertical transmission of HBV in the 3 Polynesian islands remain unstudied.

A. PHC in Hawaii

As can be seen from Table 2, PHC incidence rates are high for Orientals and Hawaiian/part-Hawaiian (Polynesian) population.

TABLE II. Age Adjusted Incidence of PHC per 100,000 Population by Race and Sex (Hawaii) 1973-1977

Race		Male	Female
Japanese	*Oriental*	*7.5*	*2.8*
Chinese	*Oriental*	*10.3*	*3.6*
Filipino	*Oriental*	*13.3*	*4.0*
Hawaiian/ Part Hawaiian	*Polynesian*	*12.6*	*9.7*
Caucasian		*2.9*	*1.9*

* *National Cancer Institute Monograph No. 57, Jan. 1981.*

In order to test the association of PHC in Hawaii to HBsAg, we obtained liver sections from patients with diagnosis of PHC from the Pathology departments of various hospitals in Honolulu. Tissues were obtained for the years 1958-1978. Liver sections from 116 PHC cases were stained by orcein reagent described by Shikata (8). This stain selectively stains HBsAg in the fixed tissue. Table 3 shows the results.

TABLE III. Results of Orcein staining of PHC section 1958-1978 (Hawaii)

Race	*Number of Cases*	*No. Orcein Pos.*	*% Pos.*
Oriental	*81*	*23*	*28.0*
Hawaiian/Part Hawaiian (Polynesian)	*15*	*4*	*26.6*
Caucasian	*13*	*2*	*15.3*
Others	*7*	*2*	*28.5*
	116	*31*	*27.0*

Age and sex matched liver section controls for 116 cases were negative for orcein stain.

B. PHC in Kingdom of Tonga

Although reliable data are not available the general impression among medical personnel in Tonga is that PHC rates are high. One report by Finau (9), found that 13/42 (30%) of biopsy specimen submitted for liver histology from 1970-1979 were diagnosed as PHC. Recent report by Bender and coworkers (10) showed that between January 1979 through July 1980 seven cases of PHC were detected at the Viola Hospital. The diagnosis was confirmed by liver biopsy, either needle biopsy or wedge resection. The age of patients varied from 12-58 years; the mean age was 30.1 years. The youngest PHC found was 12 years of age. The onset of admission for six patients ranged from 2-10 months (mean 5.2 months). The time of admission to death ranged from 8-51 days (mean 25.2 days). Of the 7 patients, 6 were male and 1 female.

IV. DISCUSSION

Our studies show a high prevalence of HBsAg and anti-HBsAg in the multi-ethnic population of Hawaii. HBs antigenemia rates were high in Oriental ethnic groups. Failure to detect HBsAg in the Hawaiian/part Hawaiian sample may have been due to smallness of the sample. The Samoan population in Hawaii showed a high prevalence of HBsAg and anti-HBs. Correspondingly, there is a high infection rate with HBV in the 3 Polynesian islands studied, American Samoa, Kingdom of Tonga and the Cook Islands. This could be due to vertical and/or horizontal transmission. Similar high prevalence of HBV markers have been noted in other S. Pacific Islands (11, 12).

Our studies in Hawaii show that PHC is much more common among the Orientals and Polynesian (Hawaiian/part Hawaiian) populations. HBsAg rates were high in the Oriental populations, and even though there was no HBsAg found in small samples of Hawaiian/part Hawaiian population the exposure to HBV did occur by high prevalence of anti-HBs. Moreover we were able to show presence of HBsAg in the liver section by Orcein stain in a significant number of Oriental and Polynesian cases of PHC in Hawaii. In the Kingdom of Tonga our studies show high exposure to HBV and high prevalence of PHC.

HBV vaccine has been shown to be 90% effective in preventing HBV infection for high risk homosexual population in New York (13). If one wants to study the risk factors for PHC, one of which may be exposure to HBV, the Polynesian island population with genetic homogeneity and endemicity for HBV with limited environmental factors may be ideal to study the risk factors in the genesis of PHC.

This population may also be suitable to study the interruption of post natal HBV transmission which may be responsible for a significant number of HBV infection; and finally, it may be possible to reduce the incidence of PHC if HBV plays a role in PHC.

REFERENCES

1. Bloomberg, B. S., *Bull. NY Acad. Med. 40*, 377 (1964).
2. Bloomberg, B. S., Sutnick, G., and Landown, W. T., *Bull. NY Acad. Med. 44*, 1566 (1968).
3. Prince, A.M., *Proc. Natl. Acad. Sci. U.S.A. 60*, 814 (1968).
4. Sumuzness, W., *Am. J. Pathol. 3*, 629 (1975).

5. Smuzness, W., *Prog. Med. Virol. 24,* 40 (1978).
6. Stevens, C. E., Beasely, R. P., Tsui, J., and Lee, W. C., *N. Eng. J. Med. 292,* 771 (1975).
7. Okada, K., Yamada, T., Miyakawa, Y. and Mayumi, M., *J. Pediat. 87,* 360 (1975).
8. Shikata, T. et al., *Jap. J. Exp. Med. 44,* 25 (1974).
9. Finau, S. A., *NZ. Med. J. 93,* 5 (1981).
10. Bender, T. R., Reinhardt, G. N., Finau, S., Wainwright, M. D., *Second Report to Ministry of Health, Tonga* (1980).
11. Gust, I. D., Lehaman, N. I., Dimitrakis, M., *Jap. J. Exp. Med. 44,* 25 (1974).
12. Wong, D. C., Purcell, R. H., and Rosen, L., *Am. J. Epidemiol. 110,* 237 (1979).
13. Smuzness, W. et al., *N. Eng. J. Med. 303,* 833 (1980).

45

CELL-VIRUS RELATIONSHIPS IN CHRONIC HEPATITIS B; IMPLICATIONS FROM DNA HYBRIDISATION STUDIES[1]

C.J. Burrell
E.J. Gowans
A.R. Jilbert
B.P. Marmion

Division of Medical Virology
Institute of Medical and Veterinary Science
Adelaide, South Australia

I. INTRODUCTION

Recombinant DNA technologies are now making available DNA sequences from many animal virus genomes in much larger quantities than previously possible. This allows the analysis of serum, tissue extracts and tissue sections for virus nucleic acids, so that in the same way that serological reactions have been used for antigen detection, virus genomes and messenger RNA can now readily be detected and quantitated by nucleic acid hybridisation.

Hepatitis B virus (HBV) is the prototype of the provisional hepadnavirus group of animal viruses, which have enveloped virions containing a circular double-stranded DNA genome and multiply significantly in the liver of the infected host; no member of this group has been reliably propagated in tissue culture (Tiollais, Charnay and Vyas, 1981; Summers 1981). In about 5% of acute HBV infections in adults, virus is not eliminated but persists for many years

[1] *This work was supported by a grant from the National Health and Medical Research Council of Australia.*

VIRAL DISEASES IN SOUTH-EAST ASIA
AND THE WESTERN PACIFIC
ISBN 0 12 484820 6

in the liver and serum of the infected individual. Such patients frequently suffer from chronic progressive liver disease, and have a greatly increased risk of subsequently developing primary liver cancer (PLC). Three significant unresolved areas include the molecular mechanism of HBV replication, the mechanism of hepatocyte damage in persistent infection, and the mechanism whereby persistent infection is associated with the production of clones of malignant cells. DNA hybridisation studies by others have established that HBV DNA frequently becomes integrated into the host genome in both tumour and non-tumour areas of persistently infected liver (Shafritz and Kew 1981; Brechot et al, 1981a), and that levels of HBV DNA in the serum correlate in general terms with the degree of presumed virus replication in different patients.

II. IN SITU CYTOHYBRIDISATION

Our group is concentrating on in situ cytohybridisation (Gowans et al, 1981) - tissue culture cells or sections on glass slides are fixed, double stranded DNA within the cells is denatured, and a radiolabelled virus DNA probe (prepared by cloning HBV DNA in E.coli (Burrell et al, 1979; Pasek et al, 1979)) is applied and allowed to hybridise with complementary virus nucleotide sequences within the cell. Finally, the sections are washed to remove unbound probe, and probe bound to individual cells is detected by autoradiography.

Three technical points warrant mention.

A. *Tissue Fixation and Prehybridisation Treatment*

A compromise must be achieved allowing optimal preservation of tissue morphology, optimal retention of nucleic acid molecules within cells, and sufficient cellular disruption to allow access of probe. For example, in this paper we have used conditions under which DNA is retained, but RNA is lost from cells, and hence in these experiemnts virus messenger RNA is not detected.

B. *Sensitivity*

The technique routinely used will detect a minimum of 10 copies of HBV DNA per cell. Cells containing less than this number of copies may still express viral antigens, but will appear negative for HBV DNA by in situ hybridiation.

C. *Specificity*

The specificity of a positive reaction for the nucleotide sequence in question must be rigorously established by the appropriate controls (Gowans et al, 1981), to avoid misleading non specific reactions.

III. RESULTS

We have used a ^{3}H-labelled cloned HBV DNA probe to examine sections of infected human livers as described above, and have obtained new information relating to two of the unresolved areas discussed above (Gowans et al, 1981; Burrell et al, 1982a, 1982b).

A. *Replication of HBV DNA*

1. Infected hepatocytes were often found to contain greater than 10^3 copies of HBV DNA per cell. Pretreatment of sections with DNAase abolished the reaction while RNAase pretreatment had no effect, establishing that the reaction was specific for viral DNA within the cell.

2. HBV DNA was found almost exclusively in the cytoplasm of infected cells.

3. Under conditions designed not to denature intracellular DNA, a significant reaction was still obtained, which was reduced by prior treatment with S_1 nuclease, indicating that much of the cytoplasmic HBV DNA was single stranded.

4. Similar reactions were found using DNA probe fragments representing different regions of the HBV genome; this indicated that single stranded regions were widespread in the cytoplasmic HBV DNA, and were not restricted to that region that is single stranded in the mature virion.

5. Finally, when the same sections were examined for hepatitis B core antigen (HBcAg) by immunofluorescence before in situ hybridisation, cells containing cytoplasmic HBV DNA frequently also contained nuclear or cytoplasmic HBcAg, but the intracellular location of the two markers rarely coincided. This suggested that the bulk of the cytoplasmic HBV DNA being detected was not encapsidated within virus cores.

These findings, taken together suggest that replication of the HBV genome has a significant intracytoplasmic phase. All other small and medium sized DNA viruses of eucaryotes replicate their DNA within the nucleus of the infected cell, making use largely of host DNA synthesising machinery for this function. Our findings indicate that the replication strategy of HBV is likely to be quite different. Recent independent work (Summers 1982) has suggested that the related duck hepadnavirus may replicate via an RNA intermediate in contrast to all other known eucaryotic DNA viruses. Thus it is possible that unique biochemical targets may exist for selective antiviral drugs to suppress HBV replication (Burrell et al, 1982a; 1982b).

B. *Association Between HBV DNA Replication and Hepatocyte Injury.*

Since some individuals may show persistent infection, with hepatocyte expression of HBV antigens, without gross evidence of hepatocyte injury, HBV infection per se has generally been considered not to be cytopathic.. A variety of models for immunologically mediated cell injury have been proposed on the basis of associations between cell injury and various immunological phenomena in different patients (Chisari et al, 1978). We have noted that cells undergoing HBV replication as revealed by in situ hybridisation and defined above, tend to be found in foci that correspond to foci of cells undergoing damage (Gowans et al, 1981; Burrell et al, 1982a). Thus, two types of HBV hepatocyte interaction can be proposed.

1. productive infection, with large amounts of cytoplasmic HBV DNA, associated with cell damage,

2. latent infections where cells containing small amounts of viral DNA, possibly integrated (Brechot et al, 1981b), express viral antigens but need not undergo damage.

IV. SUMMARY

A. *Observations*

1. HBV replication in infected hepatocytes includes a significant cytoplasmic phase.

2. Cells undergoing replicative infection can be focally distributed.

3. Cells undergoing replicative infection show histological evidence of cell damage.

B. *Proposals*

1. A unique cytoplasmic replication strategy for the HBV genome may present unique biochemical targets for antiviral chemotherapy.

2. HBV/hepatocyte interaction may result in either (a) replicative infection, or (b) latent infection with integration and partial genome expression.

3. A cause and effect relationship may exist between virus replication and cell damage in some patients.

4. Those patients with active virus replication might benefit most from withholding of steroids and use of antiviral drugs.

ACKNOWLEDGMENTS

We wish to thank Ken Murray for providing pHBV114 DNA, Ken Jones, Andrew Rogers and Paulin Hall for advice, and Gwen Simmons for skilled technical assistance. Infected liver samples were provided by Robert Hecker, Ian Gust, Graham Williamson, June Halliday, Ann Gillett, Marion Bucens, Pat Mackay and Hector Cameron. Robert Rowland assisted with histological diagnosis.

REFERENCES

Brechot, C., Hadchouel, M., Scotto, J. et al (1981a). *Proc. Natl. Acad. Sci. U.S.A. 78*, 3906.
Brechot, C., Hadchouel, M., Scotto, J. et al (1981b). *Lancet ii*, 765.
Burrell, C.J., Mackay, P., Greenaway, P.J. et al (1979). *Nature 279*, 43.
Burrell, C.J., Gowans, E.J., Jilbert, A.R. et al (1982a) *Hepatology*, in press.

Burrell, C.J., Gowans, E.J., Jilbert, A.R. et al (1982b). Submitted for publication.
Chisari, F.V., Routenberg, J.A., Anderson, D.S. et al. (1978) In "Viral Hepatitis" (G.N. Vyas, S.N. Cohen and R. Schmid, eds.), p. 245. Franklin Institute Press, Philadelphia.
Gowans, E.J., Burrell, C.J., Jilbert, A.R. et al (1981). *J. Med. Virol. 8*, 67.
Pasek, M., Goto, T., Gilbert, W. et al (1979). *Nature 282*, 575.
Shafritz, D.A. and Kew, M.C. (1981). *Hepatology 1*, 1.
Summers, J. (1981) *Hepatology 1*, 179.
Tiollais, P., Charnay, P., and Vyas, G.N. (1981). *Science 213*, 406.
Summers, J. (1982). *Hepatology*, In press.

46

PASSIVE BACTERIAL AGGLUTINATION: A SENSITIVE TEST FOR HBsAg[1]

T. Jacob John
M.S. Rajagopalan

Department of Virology
Christian Medical College Hospital
Vellore, India

INTRODUCTION

Developing countries, where hepatitis B virus (HBV) infection is a major public health problem, require a simple, rapid, inexpensive and highly sensitive method for the detection of HBV surface antigen (HBsAg). Since radio-immuno assay (RIA), enzyme-linked immunosorbent assay (ELISA) and reversed passive haemagglutination (RPHA) require highly purified reagents, we have developed a new method, namely passive bacterial agglutination (PBA). It does not require purified reagents, and is very simple and rapid to perform (3). Here we report the sensitivity of PBA in comparison with counterimmunoelectrophoresis (CIE), a test of moderate sensitivity.

METHODS, RESULTS AND DISCUSSION

The principle of PBA is the agglutination of anti-HBs coated *Staphylococcus aureus* (Cowan I strain) by HBsAg containing serum. The harvesting of bacteria and

[1]*Supported by Indian Council of Medical Research, New Delhi, India.*

VIRAL DISEASES IN SOUTH-EAST ASIA AND THE WESTERN PACIFIC
ISBN 0 12 484820 6

formalinisation have been described previously (2). Antibody coating was achieved by incubating 10% bacterial suspension with pooled human serum containing anti-HBs at 33°C for 30 minutes. Bacteria were then washed and resuspended in phosphate buffered saline (PBS, pH7.4, 0.03M) containing 0.1% sodium azide. The PBA reagent was made by diluting the coated bacteria to 1% suspension in PBS.

Test sera were absorbed with bacteria to remove any staphylococcal agglutinins present. Twenty microlitres each of the absorbed serum and PBA reagent were mixed on a glass slide for 2 minutes and read for agglutination of the bacteria. Confirmation was achieved by blocking the reaction with another batch of human serum containing anti-HBs or a rabbit anti-HBs serum (1).

Sera from 9 asymptomatic HBsAg carriers were titrated by CIE and PBA. The HBsAg titres were 8 to 64 times (mean 30) higher in PBA than in CIE.

Sera from 100 healthy adults were tested by both methods. While one serum was positive in CIE, 7 were positive in PBA. Among 495 sera from patients with liver or renal disease, 66 (13%) were positive in CIE and 217 (44%) in PBA.

Among 22 sera (from the National Institute of Health, U.S.A.) reported to be positive in RIA or ELISA or both, 4 were positive in CIE and 19 in PBA. Thus PBA is a highly sensitive, cheap, simple and rapid test and is suitable for popular use in developing countries.

REFERENCES

1. John, T.J., Shanmugam, R.V., Carman, R.H., and Hill, P.G., *Indian J. Med. Res. 61*, 1489 (1973).
2. Kronvall, G., *J. Med. Microbiol. 6*, 187 (1973).
3. Rajagopalan, M.S., and John, T.J., *Curr. Sci. 50*, 493 (1981).

47

USE OF MONOCLONAL ANTIBODIES IN THE CHARACTERIZATION OF THE ANTIGENIC DOMAINS OF THE HEPATITIS B VIRAL ENVELOPE

Kenneth G. Kenrick

Blood Transfusion Service
Australian Red Cross Society
Sydney, New South Wales

James F. Kelly and Jill S. Stratton

Commonwealth Scientific Industrial Research Organisation
Molecular and Cellular Biology Unit
North Ryde, New South Wales

I. INTRODUCTION

The full amino-acid (a/a) sequences of 25,000 mol.wt. polypeptides (p/p) of adw, ayw and adyw HBsAg subtypes have now been deduced by translation of HBV DNA nucleotide sequences (Valenzuela *et al.*, 1979, Galibert *et al.*, 1979, and Pasek *et al.*, 1979) and short peptides with antigenic (vaccine) promise, corresponding to the hydrophilic sequences of the HBsAg p/p's, have now been synthesized (Lerner *et al.*, 1981, Dreesman *et al.*, 1981, Dreesman *et al.*, 1982). However, the exact sequences which correspond to the a, d, y, w, and r determinants and the epitopes which elicit protective immunity have yet to be identified. To this end we have developed an array of monoclonal antibodies (McAb's) which react with HBsAg.

VIRAL DISEASES IN SOUTH-EAST ASIA
AND THE WESTERN PACIFIC
ISBN 0 12 484820 6

II. PRODUCTION OF MONOCLONAL ANTIBODIES

BALB/c mice were immunized with complexes of HBsAg, (adw and ayw), and human anti-HBs. They were given a tertiary antigen boost 4 days prior to hybridization. Polyethylene glycol was used to fuse spleen cells from each mouse to Sp2/0 myeloma cells (Galfre *et al.*, 1977) using modifications to the classical method of Köhler and Milstein (1975) prescribed by Fazekas de St. Groth and Scheidegger (1980). Supernatants from resultant HAT selected hybridoma cultures were screened for antibody secretion by a two-site immunoradiometric assay (2S-IRMA) (Ling and Overby, 1972). Promising hybrids were subcloned by limiting dilution and stable, high growth types expanded in culture to provide the supernates used in this study and cells for liquid nitrogen storage. 23% of hybrid clones produced detectable antibodies and to date McAb's from subclones of 5 parental clones have been examined in detail.

III. TWO DIMENSIONAL GEL IMMUNODIFFUSION

Culture supernates were tested by the classical gel immunodiffusion method of Ouchterlony (1958) against nine HBsAg preparations classified at the 1975 Paris workshop as distinct virionic phenotypes (Couroucé *et al.*, 1976). The results are summarised in Table 1.

H118 reacts with all HBsAg phenotypes and probably exhibits specificty for the a determinant. H102 exhibits partial immunological identity (PII) with H118 and therefore reacts with portion of the determinant covered by H118. This also applies to H59. H61 exhibits novel specificity evidenced by reactions with 6 sub-types but not ayw1 and adw2. However H61 also shows PII with H118 and therefore binds to some other aspect of the a determinant. The specificity of H94 is similar to that of H61 with which it shows PII.

IV. BINDING STUDIES

Dilutions of hybridoma culture supernates were reacted with HBsAg/adw and free antigen measured by 2S-IRMA. Binding curves for McAb's (Figure 1) produced by representative sub-

TABLE 1. Two-Dimensional Gel Immunodiffusion Analysis of Culture Supernates from Hybridoma Clones Secreting anti-HBS

HBsAg PHENOTYPE**	H59	H61	H94	H102	H118	POLY*
ayW_1	+++	-	-	-	++++	++++
ayW_2	-	++++	++	-	++++	++++
ayW_3	++++	+++	++	++++	++++	++++
ayW_4	+	+	-	+	++	++++
ayr	+	-	-	+	+	++++
adW_2	+++	-	++	+	++++	++++
adW_4	++++	++++	+++	++++	++++	++++
adr	-	+	-	+	++++	++++
adwy	-	++	-	+++	++++	++++

* POLY = POLYCLONAL (Rabbit a/HBs-ad/ay)
+ POSITIVE BY AUTORADIOGRAPHY ONLY
++ TO ++++ = REACTIONS VISIBLE BY UNAIDED EYE
** HBsAg REFERENCE PANEL CLASSIFICATION FROM THE PARIS WORKSHOP 1975.

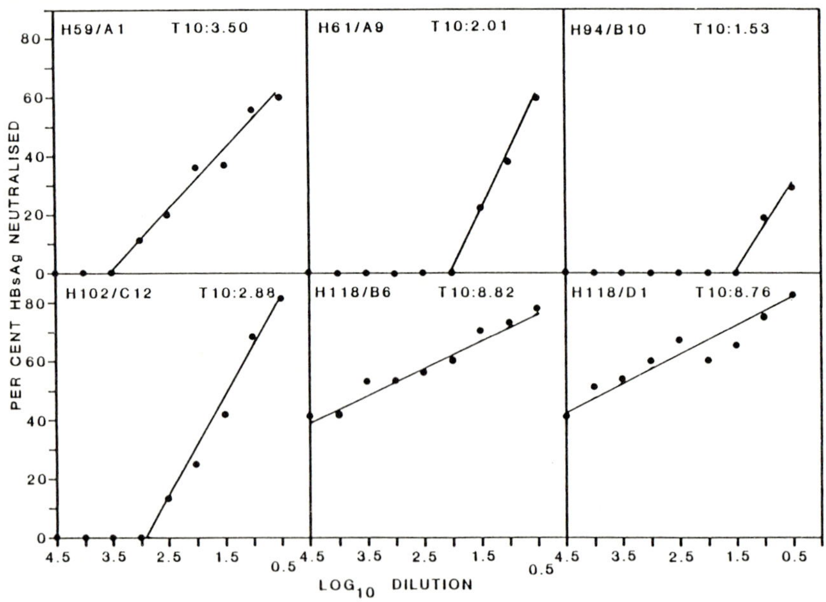

FIGURE 1. Neutralization of monoclonal antibodies with HBsAg/adw.

clones of five clonal families are shown. The slope of each curve reflects antibody affinity, while the point of intersection with the abscissa indicates titre. H118 subclones produce large amounts of antibody while H102 subclones produce fewer antibodies but with the highest affinity of the five clonal types shown.

V. DISCUSSION

Within an HBV phenotype there exists several independant antigenic determinants which together form an antigenic mosaic. Moreover, the existence of an antigenic hierarchy within each antigenic domain is suggested by a/a substitutions predicted from HBV DNA. Now, assuming that mutational embellishment is minimal, then the reactivity range of each McAb would be restricted by the hierarchic station of the epitope which elicited its production in the mouse prior to hydridization. Therefore to derive a clear picture of the antigenic complexity under study, hybridomas should be constructed against all known phenotypes. Furthermore, studies employing an extensive library of McAb's and synthetic p/p's constructed according to a/a sequences translated from HBV nucleotide sequance data, in conjunction with native HBsAg p/p's, should aid the identification of the immunologically relevant HBsAg antigenic determinants. Work is proceeding along these lines.

ACKNOWLEDGMENTS

We wish to thank Dr. A.M. Courouce of the Centre National de Transfusion Sanguine, Paris for generously providing reference materials and also for examining the specificities of our monoclonal antibodies.

REFERENCES

Courouçé, A.M., Holland, P.V., Muller, J.Y., and Soulier, J.P. (1976). *Bibliotheca Haematologica 42*, 1.

Dreesman, G.R., Hollinger, F.B., Sanchez, Y., Oefinger, P., and Melnick, J.L. (1981). *Infect. Immunity 32*, 62.

Dreesman, G.R., Sanchez, Y., Lonescu-Matiu, I., Sparrow, J.T., Six, H.R., Peterson, D.L., Hollinger, F.B., and Melnick, J.L. (1982). *Nature 295*, 158.

Fazekas de St. Groth, S., and Scheidegger, D. (1980). *J. Immunol. Meth. 35*, 1.

Galfre, G., Howe, S., Milstein, C., Butcher, G., and Howard, J. (1977). *Nature 266*, 550.

Galibert, F., Mandart, E., Fitoussi, F., Tiollais, P., and Charnay, P. (1979). *Nature 281*, 646.

Köhler, G., and Milstein, C. (1975). *Nature 256*, 495.

Lerner, R.A., Green, N., Alexander, H., Liu, F.T., Sutcliffe, J.G., and Shinnick, T.M. (1981). *Proc. Nat. Acad. Sci. 78*, 3403.

Ling, C.M., and Overby, L.P. (1972). *J. Immunol. 109*, 834.

Ouchterlony, O. (1958). *Progr. Allergy 5*, 1.

Pasek, M., Goto, T., Gilbert, W., Zink, B., Schaller, H., MacKay, P., Leadbetter, G., and Murray, K. (1979). *Nature 282*, 575.

Valenzuela, P., Gray, P., Quiroga, M., Zaldivar, J., Goodman, H.M., and Rutter, W.J. (1979). *Nature 280*, 815.

48

FALSE POSITIVE RESULTS ENCOUNTERED WITH A RADIO-IMMUNOASSAY FOR HEPATITIS A IgM: OCCURRENCE AND CAUSATION

M. Bucens
G. B. Harnett
G. Pietroboni

State Health Laboratory Services
Queen Elizabeth II Medical Centre
Nedlands, W.A.

The observation that a patient appeared to have remained Hepatitis A specific IgM positive (using the ABBOTT HAVAB-M kit method) for 20 months after the initial clinical Hepatitis A infection led to the finding that false positives occur using this method.

To confirm the occurrence of false positive reactions the sera under investigation were subjected to sucrose density gradient fractionation and the fractions tested by the HAVAB-M assay. The factor producing false positive HAVAB-M results was only present in the IgG containing fractions. False positivity was removed by absorption of sera with Staphylococcal protein A or insolubilized IgG, but was not destroyed by 2-ME treatment.

To define the frequency and distribution of false positive HAVAB-M reactions several patient groups were tested. The results are shown in Table I.

False positive Hepatitis A IgM results were found in 6% of patients who had had a confirmed Hepatitis A infection within the previous 2 years. No false positives were found in other patient groups. False positive patients had a high incidence of RF, but classical RF of the IgM class was not responsible.

VIRAL DISEASES IN SOUTH-EAST ASIA
AND THE WESTERN PACIFIC
ISBN 0 12 484820 6

TABLE I *Distribution of HAVAB-M False Positives*

1. *Patients with previous Hepatitis A*

Months after infection	*No. of patients*	*No. of false positives*
00 - 05	10	-
06 - 10	18	-
11 - 15	32	2
16 - 20	30	4
21 - 25	10	-

2. *Other patient groups*

Clinical condition	*No. of specimens tested*	*No. of false positives*
Acute rubella	10	0
Acute mononucleosis	20	0
Acute CMV infection	5	0
Acute Hepatitis B	11	0
RF± HAV (IgG)	10	0
Seronegative RA	10	0
Haemochromatosis	10	0
Non-HBV CAH	14	0
Blood donors + HAV (IgG)	100	0

It seems possible that the false positive results are due to IgG class rheumatoid-like factors which may bind anti-HAV IgG beads coated with goat IgG.

49

WATER-BORNE EPIDEMICS OF NON A - NON B VIRAL HEPATITIS IN INDIA

Khorshed Pavri, M.A. Sreenivasan, A. Sehgal and S.R. Prasad

National Institute of Virology
Pune, India

INTRODUCTION

Only recently, has it been realised that several epidemics of water-borne hepatitis reported from many parts of India are probably neither due to hepatitis A virus (HAV) nor hepatitis B virus (HBV). The water-borne epidemics of Delhi in 1955-56 and Ahmedabad, 1975-76 were thought to be caused by HAV (1-2). The majority of the cases in these outbreaks were not due to HBV infection (3-2). With the advent of serological tests for HAV in mid-1970s, the sera from Delhi and Ahmedabad were tested and were found to be devoid of specific IgM anti-HAV (4). Around the same time, a non A - non B (NANB) viral aetiology was suspected in another water-borne hepatitis outbreak from Kashmir (5).

RECENT INVESTIGATION OF A WATER-BORNE EPIDEMIC OF HEPATITIS AT KOLHAPUR, MAHARASHTRA

An epidemic of hepatitis at Kolhapur which occurred in February-March 1981 involved a total of 1169 cases. The city is divided into 5 Wards, from A to E. The wardwise incidence of hepatitis ranged from 0.7/1000 to 6.6/1000. The highest incidence was recorded in Ward E where a massive contamination of drinking water with sewage was observed. Overall case fatality rate was around 0.8% (9/1169). The case fatality rate in patients of hepatitis during pregnancy was around 9% (1/11). Although all age groups were involved

VIRAL DISEASES IN SOUTH-EAST ASIA
AND THE WESTERN PACIFIC
ISBN 0 12 484820 6

the largest number of cases occurred in the 11-30 years age group. The male-female ratio was 2:1 except for the 0-5 years age group where the ratio was approximately 1:1. The incubation period was estimated to be 26 days.

Single sera from 53 patients, paired sera from 83 patients and 21 "controls" (collected from healthy persons) were tested by RIA for IgM anti-HAV. Recent infection of HAV was observed in 3 out of 12 children (25%) in 0-10 years age group but none in the older children, adults and controls.

Using HAVAB kit (Abbott) specific IgG antibodies to HAV were detected in all the samples except one control serum from a 3½ years old child. No difference was found in the count rates of the acute and the convalescent sera. There was, however, a marked increase in the count rate for the convalescent serum as compared to the acute serum specimen of the child who was positive for IgM-anti HAV and whose paired sera were available. HBsAg was detected by ELISA in 36 out of 182 patients (12.7%) and in one of the 63 controls (1.6%).

The total serum IgM and IgG were determined by single radial immunodiffusion in 20 acute-convalescent pairs and a similar number of controls. No significant difference between the acute, convalescent and controls was observed for the mean IgM levels. However, there was a statistically significant drop in the mean IgG values from the acute to the convalescent phase samples ($p < 0.01$).

SALIENT EPIDEMIOLOGICAL FEATURES OF WATER-BORNE EPIDEMICS IN INDIA

Nearly 90% of the children acquire antibodies to HAV by the age of 5 years (6). Our data on the sproadic cases of hepatitis at Pune incriminate HAV in hepatitis patients with a mean age of 6.5 and a mode of 5 years only (7). If the water-borne epidemics were due to HAV they would be expected mainly among younger children. In contrast, all the reported outbreaks of NANB hepatitis occurred mainly in older persons particularly those between 15-40 years. The incubation period, as estimated during the Delhi epidemic, was between 18-64 days (mean 40 days). In Kolhapur, however, the serial interval was 15 to 60 days (mean 26 days). In all the epidemics, males were affected more than females (2-3:1). There was, however, no significant sex difference in the 0-5 years age group.

Both in Delhi and Kolhapur, the prodromal phase was short: 2.7 days in Delhi and 3.4 days with a mode of 1 day in Kolhapur. The prodromal symptoms were mainly gastrointestinal and upper respiratory symptoms were uncommon. The overall case fatality rates were estimated to be 0.09% in Delhi, 0.24% in Ahmedabad and 0.8% at Kolhapur which were much less than those generally recorded for sporadic viral hepatitis in major hospitals in India. The exceptions were pregnant women, with rates of 10.5% in Delhi, 9% in Kolhapur and 17.3% in Kashmir. Significant foetal wastage and cholestasis were the prominent features in Delhi. From Australia, there is a report of cholestatic hepatitis also associated with pregnancy and serologically unrelated to HAV (8).

STUDIES ON THE AETIOLOGICAL AGENT

The exact aetiology of these water-borne epidemics remains undetermined. Transmission experiments using chimpanzees and marmosets at Dr. Purcell's Laboratory have provided some evidence for hepatitis in the animals inoculated with the clinical specimens from Delhi and Ahmedabad. Unique histological changes were observed by light microscopy in both the species. These were different from hepatitis caused by other agents. In the case of marmosets, evidence has been obtained for transmission through the 2nd passage but not in chimpanzees. So far, no serological markers have been developed (Purcell - Personal communication). In our laboratory, immune electron microscopic studies were made on the stool samples collected from 22 patients during the acute phase. Initially, the pellets of stool suspensions were screened. In two samples, coronavirus-like particles were seen. Later, immune electron microscopy (IEM) was done using the convalescent sera of the same patients. Coronavirus-like particles but without aggregation were seen in the same two samples. One stool sample showed 27 to 29 nm virus-like particles in an aggregate by IEM alone. However, the particles had no evidence of antibody coating to indicate specific immune aggregation.

CONCLUSIONS

Our studies did not show much difference between the acute and the convalescent serum specimens collected from Kolhapur for specific IgG antibodies to HAV. Strangely, however, there was a statistically significant decline in the total serum IgG value in the convalescent sera as compared to the specimens of the acute phase. These preliminary studies appear to exclude HAV as an agent responsible for the disease. Transmission experiments in animals have also provided evidence suggestive of NANB aetiology.

We now have evidence that NANB hepatitis is endemic in Pune. More than 70% of the sporadic cases and 20-30% of paediatric cases of hepatitis appear to be due to NANB (7). A 5 year survey of hospital records of adult cases of hepatitis, gastroenteritis and enteric fever at Pune indicated a seasonal distribution and the peak for hepatitis followed a few weeks after the peaks observed for the other two disease entities (7). This indicates a probable faecal-oral route of transmission for the majority of the sporadic hepatitis cases.

A puzzling feature is the occurrence of periodic epidemics of water-borne hepatitis in the face of such endemicity. A drop in total serum IgG in the sera of patients of hepatitis at Kolhapur during convalescence and the observation of overt infection mainly in young adults suggest possible involvement of some immune mediated mechanism(s). The possible role of immune complexes or hypersensitive reactions in previously sensitised hosts needs consideration.

REFERENCES

1. Vishwanathan, R., *Indian J. Med. Res. 45* (Suppl.), 1 (1957).
2. Sreenivasan, M.A., Banerjee, K., Pandya, P.G., Kotak, R.R., Pandya, P.M., Desai, N.J. and Vaghela, L.H., *Indian J. Med. Res. 67,* 197 (1978).
3. Pavri, K.M., Niphadkar, K.B. and Sheikh, B.H., *Indian J. Med. Res. 60,* 1575 (1972).
4. Wong, D.C., Purcell, R.H., Sreenivasan, M.A., Prasad, S.R. and Pavri, K.M., *Lancet ii,* 882 (1980).
5. Khuroo, M.S., *Am. J. Med. 80,* 818 (1980).
6. Gandi, B.M., Joshi, Y.K. and Tandon, B.N., *Lancet ii,* 374 (1981).
7. National Institute of Virology, unpublished data.
8. Gust, I.D., Lehmann, N.I., Lucas, C.R., Ferris, A.A. and Locarnini, S.A., *in* "Viral Hepatitis" (Vyas, G.N., Cohen, S.N., Schmid, R., eds), p. 105, Franklin Institute Press, Philadelphia (1978).

50

ACUTE SPORADIC NON-A, NON-B HEPATITIS IN AUCKLAND

Paul N. Goldwater

Section of Microbiology
Department of Pathology
University of Auckland School of Medicine
Auckland

D.G. Woodfield
R.A. Anderson

Auckland Blood Transfusion Centre

M.B. Gill
Sheena Carpenter

Diagnostic Laboratory, Auckland

Acute sporadic hepatitis was studied prospectively in patients referred by their family doctor to a private pathology laboratory for tests of liver function. All patients were symptomatic and had a clinical diagnosis of acute viral hepatitis. Selection of patients on the basis of having alanine aminotransferase (ALT) levels $\geqslant$ 5 times upper limit of normal (40 u/l) was made. Acute and 6 month convalescent sera were tested by RIA (Abbott laboratories) for HB_SAg, Anti-HB_S, HBeAg, anti-HBe, anti-HB_C, HAVAB and HAVAB-IgG and IgM were also performed.

This work was supported by a grant from the Auckland Medical Research Foundation.

VIRAL DISEASES IN SOUTH-EAST ASIA AND THE WESTERN PACIFIC
ISBN 0 12 484820 6

Examination of sera from 94 patients showed that 26 (27%) had acute hepatitis B (HB), 22 (23%) had acute hepatitis A(HA) and 25 (26%) had acute non-A, non-B hepatitis (NANBH). 9 (10%) of patients had Epstein-Barr virus (EBV) associated hepatitis and 1 (1%) had cytomegalovirus (CMV) hepatitis. There were 11 (13%) patients with mixed infections; 8 with HA plus HB, 1 with HB plus EBV, 1 with HA plus EBV and 1 with HA plus CMV. Convalescent sera obtained from 8 patients confirmed acute double infection in 7 of them and indicated an episode of acute HA in one HB_SAg carrier.

Of the 26 HB patients, all were positive for HB_SAg and/or anti-HB_C. Four of the 6 patients positive only for anti-HB_C alone were tested for anti-HB_C-IgM and 2 were found to be negative. Of the 19 of 26 patients tested for HBeAg and anti-HBe, 11 and 3 were positive respectively. 5 were negative in both tests.

9 (36%) NANBH patients had anti-HB_S and 10 (45%) had anti-HAV (IgG only) at the onset of illness. 3 NANBH patients had both these antibodies.

Six month convalescent sera of NANBH patients showed no changes in any of the serological parameters. One NANBH patient showed enzymatic evidence of chronic liver disease (at 6 months).

In our sample of 94 cases of hepatitis, 14(15%) were Polynesians and 58 (62%) were Caucasians. Among the 14 Polynesians, HA was twice as frequent as HB whilst the reverse was true in Europeans. Approximately 30% of the Auckland population are of Polynesian origin.

The sex distribution for HA and NANBH was approximately even but males predominated in the HB group.

The mean age for HA patients was 30 years, for HB 22 years and for NANBH 39 years. No cases of NANBH were detected in children 10 years or younger.

Compared with Health Department figures our study showed that less than 20% of cases of viral hepatitis in Auckland are notified, thus indicating that notification is not an accurate means of assessing disease incidence.

From our study, it is clear that the virus(es) of NANBH must now be regarded as causing a major segment of acute sporadic viral hepatitis cases in New Zealand.

Part VI
Specific Viral Diseases
C.
Enteric Viruses

Chairman I. D. Gust

Co-Chairman B. P. Marmion

51

CONTROL OF POLIOMYELITIS: KILLED OR LIVING VACCINE

John Beale

Wellcome Research Laboratories
Beckenham, Kent

Poliomyelitis has been successfully controlled in most countries where polio vaccines have been widely used (1). The disease remains severe and largely uncontrolled in many developing countries. The WHO Expanded Programme on Immunization has pioneered methods for assessing the incidence of poliomyelitis (2) in these countries based on surveys of lameness, and in various studies they have found that between 50% and 75% of lameness is due to poliomyelitis. The incidence in many countries as varied as Ghana, Kenya, Egypt, The Yemen and Indonesia, have rates which are as high as, or higher than, in the USA in pre-vaccination days. In Indonesia (3) a rate of 9/10,000 was recorded from a lameness survey of the population up to 20 years old. The rate for the 1-3 year old group was 22/10,000, which argues for a recent sharp increase in the incidence of paralytic poliomyelitis. The reasons for the high rate or the increase, if there is a real as opposed to an apparent one, are unclear. The classical view that poliomyelitis is associated with an increased standard of living measurable by a reduced infant mortality rate was persuasively argued by Payne (4). It was assumed that breaking the faecal/oral chain led to slightly later acquisition of infection, and that this was less often under cover of maternally acquired circulating antibodies that prevented clinical disease, but not infection and immunity.

The possibility that other non-polio enteroviruses of human and of animal origin may confer protection against polioviruses has been raised because of the existence of shared antigens. These are usually of the C antigen class as defined by Le Bouvier (5). The case for this view would be strengthened if the rates in urban areas exceed those in rural ones, but on the whole, there is little evidence for this; for example, in Ghana (6). However, Schild has recently reported

VIRAL DISEASES IN SOUTH-EAST ASIA
AND THE WESTERN PACIFIC
ISBN 0 12 484820 6

that some poliovirus C antigen reactive monoclonal antibodies have viral neutralising ability, but this remains type specific. Although the reasons for the increase in incidence of poliomyelitis in developing countries remains obscure, the means of prevention exist.

In many developing countries, living attenuated poliovaccines have proved disappointing in controlling the disease and in producing antibodies to poliovirus (7). Killed poliovaccines were widely used for the control of poliomyelitis after the successful field trial of the vaccine in the U.S.A. (8). The placebo controlled part of this trial gave definitive evidence for the protective power of the vaccine and good correlation between neutralising antibodies at any detectable level and protection. Killed poliovaccine (IPV) was used extensively in the USA and in the late 1950's and early 1960's and achieved an impressive measure of control of the disease. Dissatisfaction with killed poliovaccine in the USA and other countries occurred for a number of reasons. First, there were a number of changes made in the production of killed poliovaccine after the Cutter disaster, in which 250 people suffered from poliomyelitis, 92 of them paralytic as a result of residual living virus remaining in the vaccine (9). These changes resulted in the vaccine being less potent than vaccines used in the Francis trial and in the early studies by Salk (10), for example, his reference vaccine A. The key changes were to extend the period of formalin treatment from 9 days to 12 days, and to institute much more rigorous filtration processes of living virus tissue culture harvest pools, both before and during inactivation. This was to remove cellular debris and clumps in which virus might escape formalin treatment.

Another factor was that, although the vaccine was clearly effective, a number of outbreaks occurred in the sixties in the USA, particularly in poorly vaccinated slum areas of big cities. It was thought that living vaccine would solve these problems, because there was a climate of opinion that only by means of a living vaccine could long-lasting immunity be conferred. Also, since the vaccine is given orally, it was more likely to be accepted. Finally, the acquisition of gut immunity from the vaccine and the possibility of spread of vaccine virus to immunise contacts involuntarily were both likely to impede the distribution of wild polioviruses in the community.

The change to OPV was successfully accomplished in many developing countries, although it has been argued recently (11) that killed vaccine had broken the back of the disease and would have succeeded in the USA, as it did in Sweden, Finland and Holland if it had been persevered with. Moreover, it is argued that killed poliovaccine, after the Cutter incident, is free from the hazards of producing poliomyelitis that persists with OPV (12). The WHO enquiries (13) into persisting paralysis after OPV in many countries in the world show that the risk of paralytic poliomyelitis associated with administration of OPV is real although rare. It is of greater relative importance as the disease becomes more under control; it is worse when monovalent mass immunization is used rather than where routine immunization with trivalent vaccine is employed.

In tropical areas, the performance of living poliovaccine has been less successful than in developed countries. Seroconversion rates have been found to be far inferior in such tropical countries. John and Christopher (7), for example, found less than 50% of children who were triple negative, seroconverted after three doses and five doses were required to achieve 90% conversion (14), and this is impractical. There are many contributing causes of this problem and the exact explanation is uncertain. Vaccine stability is one factor, but in several studies, residual vaccine has been titrated after use and found potent. Moreover, most vaccine is stabilized, usually with Molar magnesium chloride. Maternal antibody has been suggested as a cause of the problem but most studies find that it is of little inhibitory effect. A dietary inhibitor has been suggested by WHO workers in Uganda (15). The most important factor is probably interference from other enteric viruses which are very prevalent amongst children in developing countries. The patterns of interference observed in a detailed study in England show how complex the interactions are (16) but the conclusion that vaccine effectiveness can be impaired is clear.

Routine immunization with trivalent OPV, as used successfully in developed countries, is not a satisfactory means of control of poliomyelitis in developing countries. What, therefore, can be done? There are a number of options. First, to use more doses; as already mentioned, John and his colleagues (14) found that five doses of conventional OPV containing $10^{6.0}$, 5.0 and 5.5 $TCID_{50}$ for types 1, 2 and 3 were required to give more than 90% seroconversion for all three types in the tropics, and such a regime is not practical. Alternatively, monovalent vaccine can be used, either type 1 followed by divalent mixture of types 2 and 3, and then by trivalent vaccine, or all three types as monovalent vaccine given sequentially. These schedules have succeeded in improving the performance of OPV. They need good organisation and mass campaigns in order to ensure that three doses are given to cover all the types satisfactorily to the most susceptible segment of the population. Sampling to ensure good seroconversion is advisable as it can be affected by prevalent enteroviruses. Moreover, the studies of persisting paralysis following OPV showed that trivalent vaccine was less likely to be followed by paralysis than monovalent vaccine (13).

Another approach is to use killed poliovaccine. In studies carried out in Nigeria in 1966 (17,18), it was shown that killed poliovaccine (IPV) given at 3, 4 and 5 months of age with a booster at a year gave a higher percentage of seroconversion than OPV, and also a considerably higher geometric mean titre of neutralising antibodies for the group who had IPV. These results have been rather overlooked until recently for two reasons: first, they came at a time when the trend of informed opinion was against killed poliovaccine, as explained earlier, and also because the results were held up in publication by the Nigerian civil war. The IPV used in the Nigerian work was mixed with diphtheria tetanus and pertussis vaccine, thus protecting against four diseases in one course of injections. Moreover, the IPV was standardised for poliovirus D antigen content and contained 10, 2 and 8 D antigen units of types 1, 2 and 3 respectively (19).

More recently, Dutch workers (20) have introduced a number of technical improvements in the manufacture of killed vaccine. These improvements relate to several stages in vaccine production:

1. Cell Substrate: A technique of trypsinisation which involved perfusion of the monkey kidneys with trypsin increased the yield of primary cells. They also used primary cells passaged a number of times. In order to overcome problems with simian viruses, especially foamy virus revealed by passaging, home bred monkeys were employed. In this way, four passages of primary monkey kidney cells could be made, and one monkey yielded sufficient cells to make a million doses of vaccine.

Another advance has been the proposal to use continuous cell lines. A WHO expert committee has suggested tests for such cell lines on a cell bank system similar to that used for human diploid cell strains. Vaccine prepared according to these proposed methods of control has been described by Montagnon and his colleagues for the Institut Merieux (21), and vaccine made from virus grown in Vero cells is expected to be licensed in France in 1982.

2. Methods of Culture: Van Wezel (22) pioneered the use of "sephadex beads" as carriers for cells to enable adherent dependent cells to be grown in homogeneous culture in large

tanks. In this way, the Dutch group have regularly used 300 litre batches and there is no reason to suppose that 1,000 litres or larger vessels could not be used.

3. Purification and Concentration of Virus: The IPV used in the Nigerian studies already described had been concentrated and partially purified by adsorption and elution from aluminium phosphate and standardised in relation to D antigen content. Van Wezel and his colleagues have introduced purification and concentration before inactivation with formalin, which overcomes the problems of residual virus in formalin-treated vaccines. The methods used have been ultrafiltration to concentrate virus suspension using hollow fibres, followed by purification using gel filtration on sepharose 6B, and then ion exchange on DEAE sephadex. These methods have been shown to remove radiolabelled cellular DNA components by a factor of 10^8. Vaccine prepared in this way can be adjusted for D antigen content and standardised.

Several clinical studies have now been carried out with IPV of different D antigen content in many parts of the world. The results confirm that high levels of antibody, and essentially 100% conversion rates, can be achieved in tropical countries like Mali or Indonesia as well as countries like Finland and Sweden (23). Experiments with different dose levels have shown that a single dose given at one month and a booster six months later is adequate to induce antibodies in all recipients. 40, 4 and 32 D units of R.I.V. (Dutch) vaccine is sufficient for this purpose. Indeed, it is probable that a single dose of such vaccine is all that is required because the dose at six months produces a booster response typical of immunological memory, which would be elicited by natural infection. However, most public health workers would prefer the assurance of circulating antibodies as well as the existence of memory cells.

Melnick (24), who was to have given this talk, has recently presented the advantages and disadvantages of living and killed poliovaccines (Tables 1 and 2) and suggested that a combination of both may be appropriate in some situations, especially in places like the Gaza Strip, which has been disputed territory between Egypt and Israel. In a study there, it was found that there were many cases of poliomyelitis still occurring despite an active campaign of immunization using vaccines. In the period 1973-76 there were 200 cases in the Gaza strip. In 1974 and 1976 the rate for those unvaccinated or with one or two doses of OPV was 3.9 and 4.7 per 1,000 compared with a rate of 0.72 and 0.67 for those who had 3-5 doses of OPV. In an effort to improve the situation a schedule of type 1 monovalent OPV at one month, followed by trivalent OPV plus IPV at 2 months, and trivalent OPV at 5½ and 12 months. This massive effort had some effect on ameliorating the situation and fewer cases have been reported in the first season. It is striking that no child given IPV developed poliomyelitis. However, it is yet early days and it must be doubtful whether the effort can be sustained over several years.

The major disadvantages of IPV listed by Melnick are poor potency, so that there are low seroconversion rates, and a need for repeated booster doses. The present vaccines of high potency seem to have solved this problem. Indeed, Salk (23) has persuasively argued that there is no need for boosters since there is excellent evidence that a single dose of really potent vaccine induces immunological memory and this has been shown to persist; for example, following tetanus toxoid, for several decades.

Another disadvantage is lack of intestinal immunity, hence vaccines do not provide a block against the spread of wild polioviruses. It is clear from direct studies that polioviruses can infect children given potent killed poliovaccine more readily than those immunized with living vaccine (25). Moreover, there is evidence from the field that where OPV is successful, as in England and Wales, it replaces wild polioviruses in the community (26). Nonetheless, killed poliovaccine does limit the spread of polioviruses in the community. This can be observed in a number of ways. It reduces the titre and duration of excretion of viruses (25). It has a herd immunizing effect, as has been well documented by Darrell Salk (11) for the USA. In Sweden the virtual elimination of the circulation of polioviruses in sewage has been recorded by Böttiger and her colleagues (27). The outbreak of poliomyelitis in Holland amongst a strict religious sect refusing vaccination also showed the herd immunity effect because no disease occurred in either immunized or unimmunized members of the general population. Moreover, susceptible pockets of unimmunized individuals in the USA, where OPV is used, could still be infected by co-religionists visiting from Holland.

The next disadvantage is cost. IPV is considered more costly, both on a dose and course basis, and because of the costs of administration of an injectable rather than an oral preparation. This disadvantage can also be challenged. The use of combined vaccines, especially if the two dose schedule for IPV referred to above can be adapted for use with diphtheria and tetanus toxoids, and perhaps pertussis, would enable the cost advantage to lie with killed vaccine. This advantage is likely to be reinforced when the fermenter technology developed in Holland and used there for antigen production is scaled up for industrial manufacture. Moreover, there is scope for improvement in the economies of antigen production since poliovirus C DNA has been cloned (29) and could be used for antigen production as has been successfully achieved for foot and mouth disease virus (30).

The next disadvantage is the growing shortage of monkeys which could threaten the supply of vaccine. As noted already, this disadvantage can be resolved by using cells from home bred monkeys, by using non-tumorogenic cell lines like Vero, or by recombinant DNA technology. Monkeys, on the other hand, remain essential for the neurovirulence testing of OPV, whereas they are not required for the safety testing of killed poliovaccine since it is clear that cell culture safety tests are more sensitive than monkeys for detecting residual virus in formalin treated virus preparations. Moreover, potency testing for IPV can be adequately performed in small animals measuring antibody responses to vaccine containing a predetermined amount of antigen.

The last disadvantage referred to by Melnick is the possibility of a catastrophe if vaccine were released with residual virulent virus in it, as happened in the Cutter incident. This problem is easily resolved by using attenuated strains to make the vaccine.

It would seem, therefore, that the reappraisal of IPV now going on with trials in many developing and developed countries, could well lead to the use of an effective two-dose schedule of immunization against poliomyelitis, diphtheria and tetanus. This programme with killed poliovaccine enables us to dream the impossible dream of eradication of polioviruses from the world. It is at least feasible, because transmission has been halted in some temperate countries and might well be extended more widely with a determined campaign. The work with smallpox has shown what can be done, but the present extent of poliovirus infection is much greater, and the programme of eradication will certainly take more than ten years to accomplish for poliovirus: but the effort is clearly worthwhile.

REFERENCES

1. Beale, A.J., in *"Textbook of Virology"* (A.J. Rhodes and C.E. Van Rooyen, eds.), p. 567. The Williams and Wilkins Company, Baltimore, (1968).

2. LaForce, F.M., WHO document EPI/79/GEN.1, Expanded Programme on Immunization, WHO Geneva.
3. Ulfah, N.M., Parastho, S., Sadjimin, T., and Rohde, J.E. *Int. J. Epidemiol. 10*,171 (1981).
4. Payne, A.M., in *"Poliomyelitis: Third International Poliomyelitis Conference, Rome 1954"*, p. 393. Lippincott, Philadelphia, (1955).
5. Le Bouvier, G.L., *Br. J. exp. Path. 40*, 452 (1959).
6. Ofosu-Amaah, S., Kratzer, J.H., and Nicholas, D.D., *Br. Med. J. i*, 1012 (1977).
7. John, T.J., and Christopher, S., *Am. J. Epidemiol. 102*, 422 (1975).
8. Francis, T. Jr., Napier, J.A., Voight, R.B., Hemphill, F.M., Wenner, H.A., Korns, R.F., Boisen, M., Tolchinsky, E., and Diamond, E.L., in *"Evaluation of the 1954 Field Trial of Poliomyelitis Vaccine. Final Report"*, University of Michigan, Ann Arbor, (1957).
9. Nathanson, N., and Langmuir, A.D., *Am. J. Hygiene, 78*, 16 (1963).
10. Salk, J., *Lancet, ii*, 715 (1960).
11. Salk, D., *Rev. Infect. Dis. 2*, 243 (1980).
12. Salk, D., *Rev. Infect. Dis. 2*, 228 (1980).
13. Assaad, F.A., Cockburn, W.C., and Perkins, F.T., *Bull. WHO 53*, 319 (1976).
14. John, T.J., *Br. Med. J. i*, 812 (1976).
15. Domok, I., and Balayna, M.S., in *Proceedings of the Symposium on Stability and Effectiveness of Measles, Poliomyelitis and Pertussis Vaccines*, p. 45. Yugoslav Acad. Science and Arts, Zagreb, (1976).
16. Gardner, P.S., Wright, A.E., and Hale, J.H., *Br. Med. J. ii*, 424 (1961).
17. Oduntan, S.O., Lucas, A.O., and Wennen, E.M., *Ann. Trop. Med. Parasitol. 72*, 111 (1978).
18. Beale, A.J., *Br. Med. Bull. 25*, 148 (1969).
19. Beale, A.J., *Lancet ii*, 1166 (1961).
20. Van Wezel, A.L., Van Steenis, G., Hannik, Ch.A., and Cohen, H., in *Devel. biol. Standard. 41*, 159 (1978).
21. Montagnon, B.J., Nicolas, A.J., Fanget, B., and Peyron, L., in *Devel. biol. Standard. 47*, 151 (1981).
22. Van Wezel, A.L., *Nature 216*, (1967).
23. Salk, J., van Wezel, A.L., Stoeckel, P., van Steenis, G., Schlumberger, M., Meyran, M., Rey, J.-L., Lapinleimu, K., Böttiger, M., and Cohen, H., in *Devel. biol. Standard. 47*, 181 (1981).

24. Melnick, J.L., in *Devel. biol. Standard. 47*, 265 (1981).
25. Henry, J.L., Jaikaran, E.S., Davies, J.R., Tomlinson, A.J.H., Mason, P.J., Barnes, J.M., and Beale, A.J., *J. Hyg. (Camb). 64*, 105 (1966).
26. Cossart, Y.E., *Br. Med. J. i*, 1621 (1977).
27. Böttiger, M., Mellin, P., Romanus, V., Söderström, H., Wesslen, T., and von Zeipel, G., *Bull. WHO 57*, 99 (1979)
28. Bijkerk, B., in *Devel. biol. Standard. 47*, 233 (1981).
29. Kleid, D.G., Yansura, D., Small, B., Dowbenko, D., Moore, D.M., Grubman, M.J., McKercher, P.D., Morgan, D.O., Robertson, B.H., and Bachrach, H.L., *Science 214*, 1125 (1981).
30. Kitamura, N., Semler, B.L., Rothberg, P.G., Larsen, G.R. Adler, C.J., Dorner, A.J., Emini, E.A., Hanecak, R., Lee, J.J., van der Werf, S., Anderson, C.W., and Wimmer, E., *Nature 291*, 547 (1981).

COMMENTS DURING DISCUSSION

ON POLIO VACCINATION IN TROPICAL COUNTRIES

C. HUYGELEN (BELGIUM) I would like to make a few comments on polio vaccination in tropical countries. First, I believe there is sufficient evidence today that both inactivated and live oral polio vaccine can produce a high level of immunity against the disease. Oral polio vaccine has been used in almost all industrial countries of the world and has led to the virtual disappearance of the disease in those countries. Two countries, Sweden and Finland, have obtained similar results with inactivated vaccine. It must be stressed, however, that in the latter two countries, 100% of the children are receiving a complete vaccination schedule. In the Netherlands where almost all children are immunized with inactivated vaccine, epidemics have occurred from time to time among the members of a small religious minority who refuse all vaccination. The latest one occurred in 1978 and caused 110 cases of polio among this group.

It is generally accepted that oral polio vaccine gives a better herd immunity than inactivated vaccine, because of the high degree of intestinal immunity it induces and also because of its spread to non-immunized contacts.

It has been said that oral polio vaccine is unsuitable for developing countries. The results obtained in several countries in widely separated geographic areas prove that this is not so: Chile, Costa Rica, Singapore, Hong Kong, Fiji, Taiwan, Western Malaysia and others have shown that with a well managed programme using OPV, the disease can be brought under control as effectively as in highly industrialized countries. Even in large tropical countries such as Brazil, vaccination campaigns with OPV have recently been shown to have a dramatic impact on the incidence of polio.

A further remark relates to levels of circulating antibodies; I believe they are a poor indicator of immunity in recipients of live vaccine, because of the insensitivity of the test system and because circulating antibodies are only one aspect of a more general stimulation of the immune system by OPV.

A last comment is related to the cost of inactivated vaccine versus that of live vaccine. Recently, W.H.O. estimated the price of inactivated vaccine to be at least 25 times higher than that of oral polio vaccine.

My conclusion would be that for the time being, inactivated vaccine should be used only in those countries which (a) can afford to pay this high price and (b) can ensure 100% vaccination coverage of their children. Those which cannot meet these two criteria should stay with OPV.

52

VIRAL ENTERITIS
A BRIEF REVIEW

Ian H. Holmes

Department of Microbiology
University of Melbourne
Parkville, Victoria, Australia

I. VIRUSES ASSOCIATED WITH INFANTILE ENTERITIS

After many years lack of success of conventional virus isolation techniques for incrimination of viruses as causes of infantile enteritis, the use of electron microscopy for direct diagnosis has led to the recognition of a number of new agents. They are a disparate group, but they share a high degree of specificity for gut epithelial cells, and most have not yet been adapted to cell culture.

A. *Rotavirus*

1. Morphology. Rotavirus particles are easy to recognize in the electron microscope. Intact particles have a diameter of about 70 nm and a smooth outline. Sometimes flattened tubules with an obvious subunit structure are also seen in specimens, but not all rotavirus strains seem to produce them (Fig. 1). Similar tubules are also produced by certain animal rotavirus strains and they are known to be antigenically related to the virus particles (1). Particles lacking the outer capsid layer are also commonly found in rotavirus preparations. They have a diameter of 60 nm and show the geometrical arrangement of the capsid subunits particularly clearly, especially in the freeze-dried preparations of A. Roseto and his colleagues (2, Fig. 2).

VIRAL DISEASES IN SOUTH-EAST ASIA
AND THE WESTERN PACIFIC
ISBN 0 12 484820 6

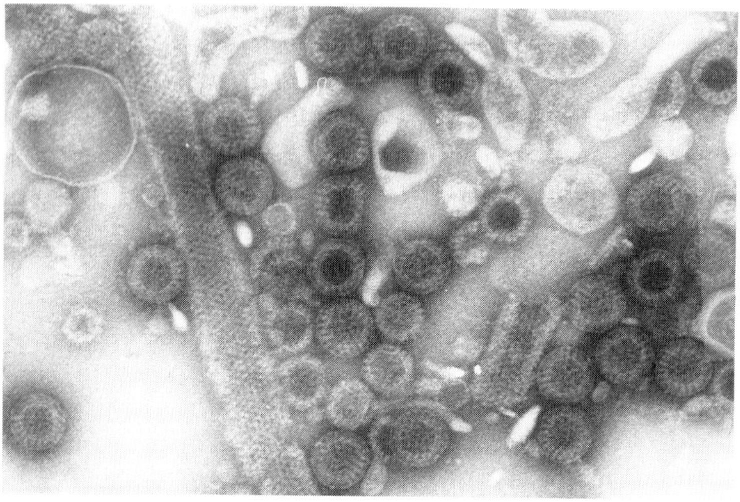

FIGURE 1. Rotavirus particles and virus-associated tubular structures in a stool specimen from Malaysia, kindly provided by Prof. K. Lam, and negatively stained with ammonium molybdate.

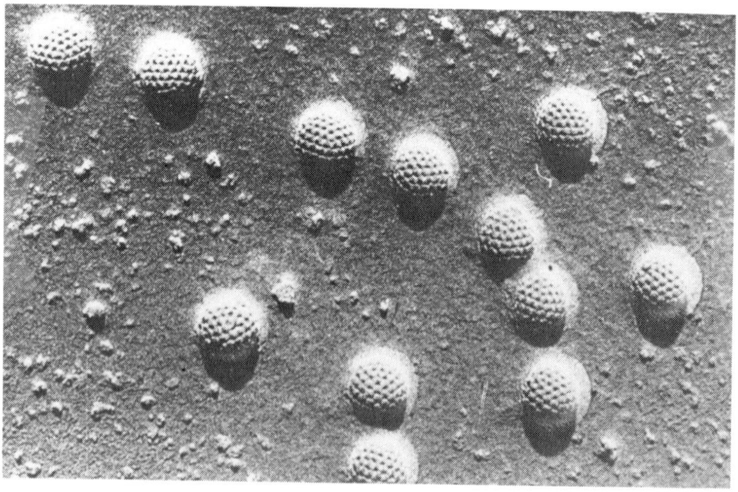

FIGURE 2. Electron microscopy of freeze-dried bovine rotavirus particles, following purification, showing the subunit structure of the inner capsid. Micrograph kindly supplied by A. Roseto (2).

2. *Diagnostic tests.* In faecal samples obtained during the first few days after rotavirus infection, there are generally enough particles to be seen by electron microscopy when slightly diluted samples are negatively stained, without concentration (3). Fortunately for those without ready access to electron microscopes, it is now easier and quicker to use an enzyme immunoassay (ELISA) to detect any variety of rotavirus, since all possess a common antigen, and the results should be at least as sensitive as electron microscopy (4). Both the antisera and the type of plastic used as solid phase in the ELISA are critically important for reproducibility and sensitivity.

It is possible, though fairly laborious, to detect rotaviruses by centrifuging specimens onto monolayers of monkey kidney cells and using fluorescent antibody to detect infected cells after overnight growth (5). The virus in such cultures almost always died out during further passages, until it was discovered that serial passages and plaquing could be achieved if trypsin was present in the culture medium (6, 7). Most animal rotaviruses can be grown fairly readily with trypsin, which is required to cleave one of the structural polypeptides of the virus particle and activate infectivity (8), but cultivation of human strains directly from faeces has been achieved only recently (9, 10). Rotavirus infectivity is best preserved in buffers containing calcium ions (11).

B. *"Small Viruses"*

At least 3 different kinds of viruses with diameters in the range of 28-32 nm have been associated with gastroenteritis, but none are as common as rotaviruses in areas where surveys have been carried out (3). Astroviruses and caliciviruses are recognizable by their morphology in the electron microscope, and the latter group contains the Norwalk agent which can also be detected serologically (12). Norwalk agent was originally found causing sporadic outbreaks of "Winter vomiting disease" in older children and adults in the U.S.A. (13). A recent study in Bangladesh suggests that infections of infants with Norwalk agent can also be common, but generally produce only mild symptoms (R.E. Black, unpublished).

C. *Adenoviruses*

"Enteric" adenoviruses which are difficult to cultivate are moderately common as causes of diarrhoea; the types involved are different from any of the previously recognized 35 human sero-types. They can be diagnosed by electron microscopy or ELISA (14).

D. *Coronavirus-like Particles*

Although conventional coronaviruses are important and well established as aetiological agents of enteritis in pigs and calves, the role of the morphologically slightly different particles shown in Fig. 3 in human diarrhoeal disease remains controversial. Such particles were originally found in the Vellore area of India (15). It has proved difficult to demonstrate that they are viruses, or to detect any serological response to them, but their association with certain outbreaks of diarrhoea is most convincing (16). In some studies they have been found as frequently in asymptomatic controls as in cases, but this may mean that they can cause chronic infections which are well tolerated (3). They appear to be particularly common in faecal specimens from South East Asia and the Western Pacific.

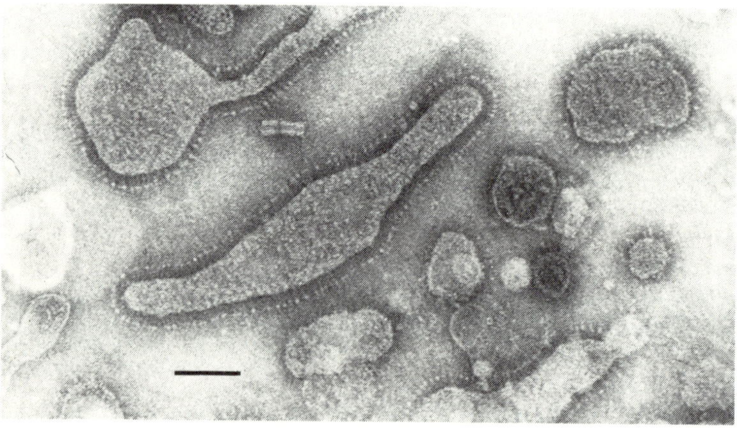

FIGURE 3. Coronavirus-like particles excreted by an Aboriginal infant with acute gastroenteritis in Alice Springs, Central Australia. Micrograph by R.D. Schnagl. Bar = 100 nm.

II. ROTAVIRUS SUBGROUPS, SEROTYPES AND ELECTROPHEROTYPES

A. *Strain Differentiation*

Although as has been mentioned, all rotaviruses have some common antigenic determinants, serological differences are also detectable by ELISA or immune adherence haemagglutination (IAHA) tests (17). The main difficulty has been the production of sera of sufficient specificity, but the availability of cultivable re-assortant strains selected from cells mixedly infected with human and bovine rotaviruses should solve this problem eventually (18).

It is also possible to distinguish strains which will grow at least initially in cell culture by neutralization (19). Recently it has been shown that different antigens on different viral proteins are involved in the two kinds of test, and it has been decided to reserve the term serotype for strains distinguished by neutralization, while the ELISA and IAHA tests distinguish subgroups (20, 17).

The situation may change now that more human rotavirus strains are being cultivated, but currently neither subgrouping nor serotyping is within the reach of most diagnostic laboratories for epidemiological purposes. Although it sounds complicated and does require much work and some special equipment, it has proved to be feasible to distinguish rotavirus strains by extracting their genomic double stranded (ds) RNA and analysing it by polyacrylamide gel electrophoresis (PAGE) (21). The RNA can be extracted directly from faecal specimens, and although only small amounts of many samples remained from earlier electron microscopic investigations S. Rodger and colleagues were able to record "gel patterns" of 188 isolates collected in Melbourne over 6 years. Rotavirus particles always contain 11 segments of ds RNA but various segments of different strains vary slightly in mobility in the gels and by careful comparisons all the isolates could be classified into "electropherotypes", each defined by a different pattern of RNA bands (21, Fig. 4).

B. *Epidemiology of Electropherotypes*

When the dates of isolation of the rotavirus samples and their electropherotypes were correlated, some features of rotavirus epidemiology became evident (Fig. 5).

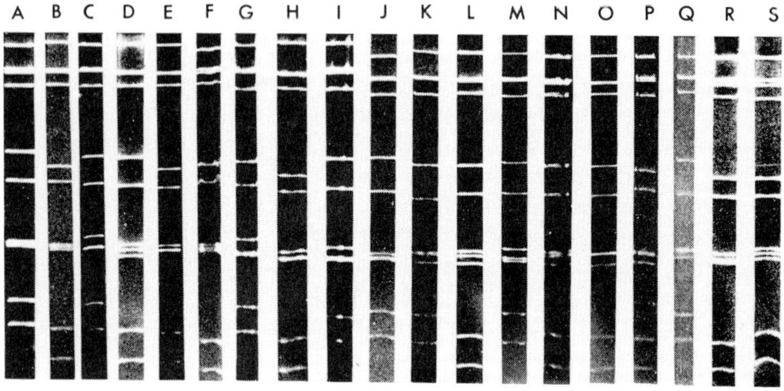

FIGURE 4. *RNA gel patterns of human rotavirus electropherotypes. Electrophoresis was from top to bottom. RNA was stain with ethidium bromide and photographed under ultraviolet light. From (21).*

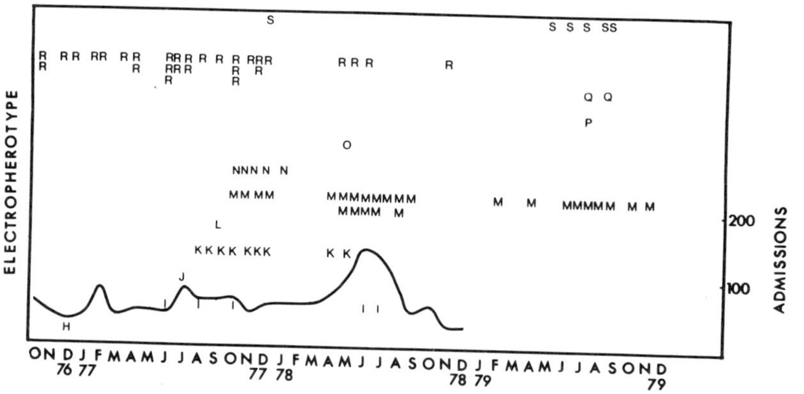

FIGURE 5. *Occurrence of human rotavirus electropherotypes in children admitted to hospital with acute gastroenteritis in Melbourne between mid 1976 and the end of 1979. The solid line shows total numbers of children admitted with acute gastro-enteritis. From (21).*

Samples of a particular electropherotype were generally clustered in time. Only a few examples of some types were found, whereas others obviously represented predominant strains which were common throughout one or two Winter seasons. In some years two predominant electropherotypes coexisted, and from the patterns it could be inferred that they probably represented different subgroups (21).

It it not possible and will probably never be possible to determine serotype by looking at the RNA gel pattern of a rotavirus, but electropherotyping will enable an epidemiologist to group strains which are probably identical so that only a few representatives of each group need to be sent to a reference laboratory for serotyping. Within a particular area, it can also be used to follow the spread of new epidemic strains.

III. CONTROL OF VIRAL DIARRHOEA

While much more work remains to be done, especially in developing countries, before we can be too dogmatic, it is clear that infantile enteritis is a major cause of morbidity and mortality throughout the world, and rotavirus is probably the most important single aetiological agent involved (22). Studies on epidemiology, immunity, vaccine development and treatment are all obviously relevant.

A. Immunity

Serum antibodies indicate past rotavirus infections and can neutralize rotaviruses *in vitro*, but they are not believed to be protective in humans (22). It is believed that local intestinal (secretory) immune responses are most important but a great deal more work is needed in this area, where the veterinarians are far ahead of the paediatricians (3). B. McLean has studied the transfer of antirotaviral immunoglobulins from mothers to their infants and has shown that trypsin inhibitors in breast milk contribute to protection as well as immunoglobulins (23), but she will summarise her own results. A preliminary study of copro-antibody excretion following rotavirus infection suggested that antibodies could only be detected for about 2 months (24, Fig. 6).

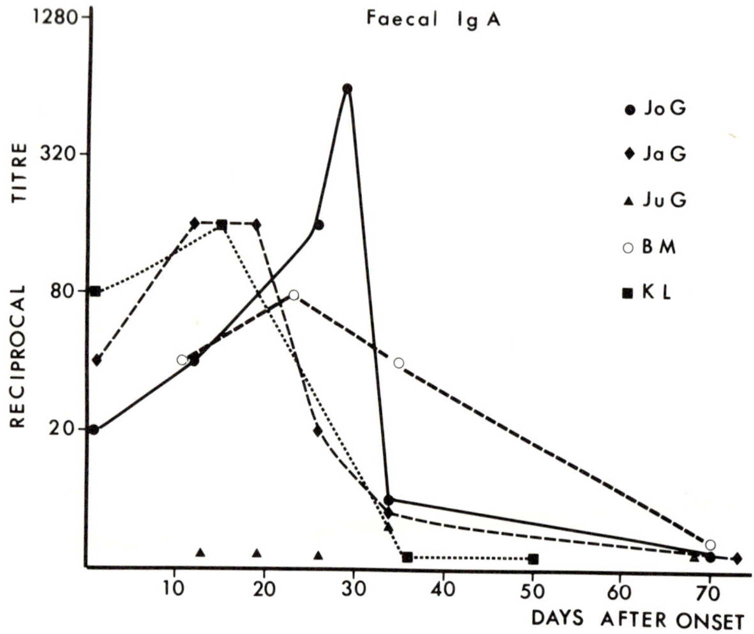

FIGURE 6. Time course of intestinal IgA response following rotavirus infection. JoG aged 2y, JaG 4y, JuG mother, BM 1y, and KL aged 1y. From Sonza and Holmes (24).

B. *Vaccine Development*

There is much interest in the possibility of immunization against rotaviral disease but many problems remain to be overcome. Although a number of serotypes can be distinguished, most antisera show a moderate degree of cross neutralization and it may be possible to immunize infants with a single strain. Recent advances in cultivation of human strains and production of cultivable reassortants will greatly assist this research (18, 9, 10). It is believed that a live, attenuated oral vaccine would be most likely to stimulate the necessary local immunity in the gut (22).

C. *Role of the World Health Organization*

Recognizing the enormous impact of diarrhoeal disease worldwide, the World Health Organization has set up a global programme for Control of Diarrhoeal Disease (CDD). Scientific Working Groups are identifying priorities and supporting much research into diarrhoea caused by bacteria, viruses and parasites, and also drug development and treatment (25). A list of priorities in viral diarrhoea is available from the speaker and those wishing to apply to WHO for support should write to the CDD Programme in Geneva or to the WHO Regional Offices in Manila or New Delhi. Fortunately the same immediate treatment with oral glucose and electrolyte solutions to reverse the effects of dehydration can save lives, whatever the cause of the diarrhoea (26), and other WHO groups are supporting health services' research to find ways to best deliver this therapy. I have tried to indicate some of the aspects of research on rotaviruses in particular on which I believe more work would be useful, to assist this aim of control, but you will be able to define your local priorities much more precisely.

REFERENCES

1. Holmes, I.H., Ruck, B.J., Bishop, R.F., and Davidson, G.P., *J. Virol. 16*, 937 (1975).
2. Roseto, A., Escaig, J., Delain, E., Cohen, J., and Scherrer, R., *Virology 98*, 471 (1979).
3. Holmes, I.H., *Prog. Med. Virol. 25*, 1 (1979).
4. Yolken, R., Wyatt, R.G., and Kapikian, A.Z., *Lancet 2*, 819 (1977).
5. Bryden, A.S., Davies, H.A., Thouless, M.E., and Flewett, T.H., *J. Med. Microbiol. 10*, 121 (1977).
6. Babiuk, L.A., Mohammed, K., Spence, L., Fauvel, M., and Petro, R., *J. Clin. Microbiol. 6*, 610 (1977).
7. Matsuno, S., Inouye, S., and Kono, R., *J. Clin Microbiol. 5*, 1 (1977).
8. Espejo, R.T., Lopez, S., and Arias, C., *J. Virol. 37*, 156 (1981).
9. Sato, K., Inaba, Y., Shinozaki, T., Fujii, R., and Matumoto, M., *Arch. Virol. 69*, 155 (1981).
10. Urasawa, T., Urasawa, S., and Taniguchi, K., *Microbiol. Immunol. 25*, 1025 (1981).

11. Shirley, J.A., Beards, G.M., Thouless, M.E., and Flewett, T.H., *Arch. Virol. 67*, 1 (1981).
12. Greenberg, H.B., and Kapikian, A.Z., *J. Am. Vet. Med. Assoc. 173*, 620 (1978).
13. Dolin, R., Blacklow, N.R., DuPont, H., Formal, S., Buscho, R.F., Kasel, J.A., Chames, R.P., Hornick, R., and Chanock, R.M., *J. Infect. Dis. 123*, 307 (1971).
14. Johansson, M.E., Uhnoo, I., Kidd, A.H., Madeley, C.R., and Wadell, G., *J. Clin. Microbiol. 12*, 95 (1980).
15. Mathan, M., Mathan, V.I., Swaminathan, S.P., Yesudoss, S., and Baker, S.J., *Lancet 1*, 1068 (1975).
16. Clarke, S.K.R., Caul, E.O. and Egglestone, S.I., *Postgrad. Med. J. 55*, 135 (1979).
17. Kapikian, A.Z., Cline, W.L., Greenberg, H.B., Wyatt, R.G., Kalica, A.R., Banks, C.E., James, H.D.Jr., Flores, J., and Chanock, R.M., *Infect. Immun. 33*, 415 (1981).
18. Greenberg, H.B., Kalica, A.R., Wyatt, R.G., Jones, R.W., Kapikian, A.Z., and Chanock, R.M., *Proc. Nat. Acad. Sci. USA 78*, 420 (1981).
19. Beards, G.M., Pilfold, J.N., Thouless, M.E., and Flewett, T.H., *J. Med. Virol. 5*, 231 (1980).
20. Kalica, A.R., Greenberg, H.B., Wyatt, R.G., Flores, J., Sereno, M.M., Kapikian, A.Z., and Chanock, R.M., *Virology 112*, 385 (1981).
21. Rodger, S.M., Bishop, R.F., Birch, C., McLean, B., and Holmes, I.H., *J. Clin. Microbiol. 13*, 272 (1981).
22. Kapikian, A.Z., Wyatt, R.G., Greenberg, H.B., Kalica, A.R., Kim, H.W., Brandt, C.D., Rodriguez, W.J., Parrott, R.H., and Chanock, R.M., *Rev. Infect. Dis. 2*, 459 (1980).
23. McLean, B.S., and Holmes, I.H., *J. Clin. Microbiol. 13*, 22 (1981).
24. Sonza, S., and Holmes, I.H., *Med. J. Aust. 2*, 496 (1980).
25. W.H.O., *Wkly Epidemiol. Rec. 55*, 209 (1980).
26. Mahalanabis, D., Merson, M.H. and Barua, D., *World Health Forum 2*, 245 (1981).

53

POLIOMYELITIS IN CHINA

Ku Fang-chou

Chinese Academy of Medical Sciences
Beijing

Dong De-xiang

Institute of Medical Biology, Chinese
Academy of Medical Sciences, Kunming

Shi Qu-sheng

Anti-Epidemic and Health Station
of Shanghai

Niu Ji-tian

Anti-Epidemic and Health Station
of Henan Province, Zhengzhou

Yang Hong-hui

Anti-Epidemic and Health Station
of Guangxi Autonomous Region, Nanning

The first outbreak of poliomyelitis was documented in China in Nantung prefectural region, Jiangsu province, in 1953. A total of 2,607 cases were reported in 1951-1955. The incidence rate was 32.1 per 100,000 in 1955.

From 1956 on, more cases and outbreaks of this disease were reported, occurring mainly in the big cities, such as Shanghai, Jinan, Nanning, Kunming, Lanzhou, etc.

VIRAL DISEASES IN SOUTH-EAST ASIA
AND THE WESTERN PACIFIC
ISBN 0 12 484820 6

EPIDEMIOLOGICAL EFFECT OF OPV MASS VACCINATION

In Shanghai, OPV was first used in 1960. In the last 20 years, more than 905 of the children born since 1956 have each received 3-5 doses of OPV, and consequently the annual incidence of poliomyelitis in Shanghai has declined steadily. In the last 3 years (1977-1979), the annual average incidence rate has dropped to 0.13 per 100,000.

OPV was first used in Henan in 1962. In 1962-1965, the vaccine was distributed mainly in cities. Only 540,000 doses of each type of OPV were distributed each year. Since 1966 the OPV vaccination program has been expanded steadily and finally covered the whole province in 1970. The annual consumption of OPV reached 5.7 million doses. However, the percentage of OPV vaccination was 40-70% in children in mountainous areas due to ineffective organization. Two big epidemics of poliomyelitis occurred in 1970 and 1974. However, since 1975 when a well organized community campaign of mass vaccination was conducted, OPV reached 10 million doses per year, and the annual incidence of the disease dropped to 0.01 per 100,000 population by 1979, and less than 15 cases were reported.

THE TRANSMISSION OF WILD POLIOVIRUS IN THE COMMUNITY COULD BE CONTROLLED

In the pre-vaccination years of 1961-1962, 24 strains of poliovirus were isolated in Shanghai from 133 healthy children, the isolation rate being 18%. However, after mass vaccination in 1964-1965, only 1 strain of type 2 poliovirus was isolated from 233 stool specimens. In 1973, no poliovirus was isolated, and in 1976, only 2 strains of type 1 poliovirus were found. A similar result was obtained in Tsingtao.

IN THE SUBTROPICAL REGION OF CHINA, OPV CAN ALSO CONTROL POLIOMYELITIS

It is well known that some types of non-polio enteroviruses can interfere with the multiplication of polio vaccine viruses. However, if a mass vaccination program is well organized and conducted to get a maximal number of children vaccinated, a poliomyelitis epidemic can also be eliminated in subtropical regions.

Guangxi, with a population of about 20 million, is located in the subtropical area of China. Apparently healthy children were found to be heavily infected with non-polio enteroviruses, the isolation rate (by monkey kidney cells only) of non-polio enteroviruses being 20.35%. Three severe epidemics of paralytic poliomyelitis occurred in 1957-1973.

OPV was first used in 1960 but still limited to big cities until 1964. The oral vaccination rate was 37-52%. In 1964, an outbreak occurred. Since 1965, OPV has increased to 1.5-2.0 million doses per year. However, due to poor organization, the oral vaccination rate was still very low in rural areas. In 1969-1971, several epidemics occurred in succession.

Since 1972, the Health Department of Guangxi Autonomous Region has made a great effort in strengthening their health network and in conducting training courses for health workers at all levels. In rural areas, barefoot doctors actively took part in distributing OPV. In cities, special teams were set up for propaganda and registration of vaccinees. According to the operation plan all children under 7 years of age in each city or county were to be vaccinated. In 1969-1971, 260,684 children in 13 counties and cities were registered, and 84.5% were vaccinated. The majority of preschool children had received at least one dose of OPV during the 3 year period. Serological studies indicated that a 3-dose OPV vaccination could give a seroconversion rate over 90%. Since 1973, the incidence of poliomyelitis has declined steadily, the annual incidence rate in 1973-1977 being 0.41, 0.29, 0.22, 0.11 and 0.05 per 100,000 respectively. The incidence dropped to 0.02 per 100,000 in 1979.

PRESENT STATUS OF POLIOMYELITIS IN CHINA

During 1972-1974, only Shanghai reported an average annual incidence below 0.50 per 100,000. However, a similarly low incidence was reported by 11 provinces in 1975-1977 and 18 provinces in 1979.

However, several local outbreaks of poliomyelitis have been registered in recent years in some counties where the implementation of vaccination programs was handicapped by the ineffective local health organization, and 10,480 and 5,472 paralytic cases were reported in 1978 and 1979 respectively. The majority of these cases occurred in rural areas. Recently, Sabin wrote: "The problem of elimination of paralytic poliomyelitis from economically underdeveloped countries depends on administrative rather than immunological or epidemiological factors". Our 20-year experience has confirmed his point of view.

Obviously, the key to elimination of paralytic polio-hyelitis from a community is to have a powerful leadership and authority in public health that can provide effective administrational guidance, and measures to train and organize health personnel. Barefoot doctors are indispensable in implementing an effective mass vaccination campaign against poliomyelitis in rural reas of our country.

REFERENCES

Sabin, A.B. (1980). *Bull. Wld. Hlth. Org. 58*, 141.
Ye, S.T. (1959). *Chinese J. Epidemiology 4*, 2.

54

CHANGING PATTERNS OF POLIOMYELITIS IN WEST MALAYSIA (1946 TO 1981)

Dora S.K. Tan

Division of Virus Research
Institute for Medical Research
Kuala Lumpur, Malaysia

I. INTRODUCTION

Although paralytic poliomyelitis had been observed clinically for many years in Malaysia, there had been no laboratory facilities for the confirmation of the disease until 1959, when the Poliomyelitis Unit was set up in the Institute for Medical Research. Since then, studies of laboratory-confirmed cases (1961-81) and notified cases (1946-81) have shown a definite change in the pattern of the disease.

II. RELATIONSHIP OF INFANT MORTALITY RATE TO MORBIDITY

It was shown that in spite of steadily falling infant mortality rates over a period of 25 years (1946 to 1970) poliomyelitis had not assumed epidemic proportions in Malaysia as it had in Singapore in 1958-59 (Table). This was attributed to the fact that Malaysia was less overcrowded and the spread of the poliovirus across the causeway joining the two countries was slow, allowing preventive measures to be taken on time.

Sporadic poliomyelitis in Malaysia was found to affect mainly children below 4 years of age, particularly those aged 6 months to 3 years. The morbidity rate was higher among the Indians than the Chinese and the Malays; higher in males

VIRAL DISEASES IN SOUTH-EAST ASIA
AND THE WESTERN PACIFIC
ISBN 0 12 484820 6

TABLE. Relationship of Infants Mortality Rates with Notified Poliomyelitis Cases, 1946 to 1979

Period	Range of IMR (per 1,000 live births)	Cases per 100,000 pop.
1946 - 50	102 - 81	5.8 - 0.3
1951 - 55	97 - 78	3.7 - 0.6
*1956 - 60	80 - 69	2.9 - 0.7
1961 - 65	60 - 48	4.9 - 0.7
1966 - 70	48 - 42	1.2 - 0.3
1971	39	3.4
1972	38	8.3
1973 - 79	38 - 17	1.2 - 0.4
1980 - 81	N.A.	0.4 - 0

* Poliomyelitis outbreak in Singapore.
N.A. Not available.

than females; and higher in urban than rural dwellers. No seasonal distribution of cases was detectable. However, small peaks were observed every 5 to 8 years in the epidemiological pattern between 1946 to 1970. Of the poliovirus types, type 1 accounted for 77% of all positive isolations, type 2 for 17%, type 3 for 4% and mixed viruses for 2%.

III. POLIOMYELITIS ANTIBODY PREVALENCE

A serological survey for poliomyelitis antibody in children from Kuala Lumpur aged 1 to 7 years in 1966 showed that the immunity status of the children was high and only 12.7% were without antibodies to any one type of poliovirus. The most susceptible group was of Indian children aged 1 year, and the least susceptible, Malay children of the same age. The percentages of children with antibody increased with age. By 4 years of age, more than 90% had antibodies to at least one virus type and more than 40% to all 3 types. However, there was a conspicuously low prevalence of type 3 antibody in all the groups.

IV. THE EPIDEMIC AND MASS VACCINATION

From 1961 through 1970, the predominant causal virus of sporadic poliomyelitis cases was poliovirus type 1. However, in the first half of 1971, a marked increase in poliovirus type 3 isolates was obtained from paralytic cases, threatening to replace type 1 virus. The Ministry of Health was alerted in view of the low immunity status of the child population to type 3 virus and a mass vaccination campaign in W. Malaysia was planned. However, before the campaign could be launched the expected outbreak, which occurred throughout the country, including the rural areas, took place. However, for obscure reasons, the causal agent was not poliovirus type 3 but type 1. In the outbreak the age, sex, racial and urban-rural distributions remained unchanged.

The outbreak started in September, 1971, with the peak in January 1972. Mass vaccination was performed from January to May 1972 followed by routine vaccination in infants throughout the country. A dramatic fall in cases resulted immediately after the campaign but cases started to increase again by 1977.

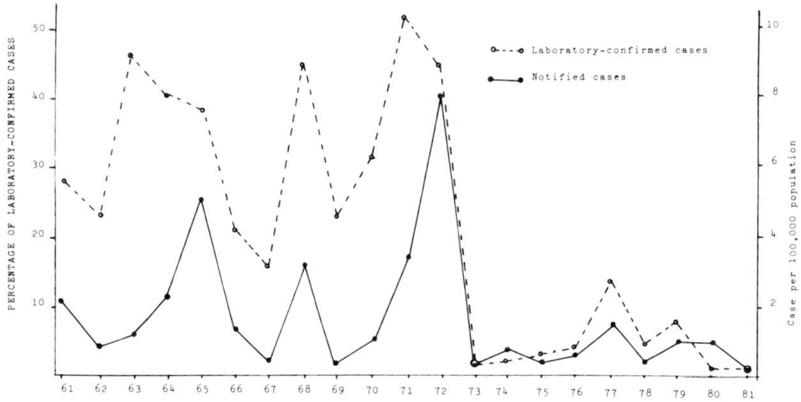

FIGURE. Annual distribution of notified and laboratory confirmed cases of poliomyelitis (1961-81)

An investigation revealed a breakdown in the cold-chain system in the transportation of vaccine to outlying centres. Prompt measures were taken and from 1980 onwards no cases of paralytic poliomyelitis were encountered. The figure shows a close correlation between data from poliomyelitis notifications and laboratory confirmation from 1961 through 1981.

55

ANTIBODY RESPONSE OF INFANTS IN INDIA TO INJECTABLE POLIO VACCINE[1]

T. Jacob John
R. Krishnan
Malati Jadhav
R. Selvakumar

Departments of Virology and Child Health
Christian Medical College and Hospital
Vellore, India

INTRODUCTION

Paralytic poliomyelitis is a major public health problem in India with an incidence rate of about 30 per 100,000 population per year. As in many other countries, only the oral polio vaccine (OPV, Sabin) is used in India, under the Expanded Programme of Immunization (EPI). This vaccine is offered in a routine schedule of 3 doses for primary immunization during infancy and a single booster dose during the second year of life. There is no evidence for any trend of declining incidence of poliomyelitis where OPV is distributed under EPI in India (1). On the contrary, the incidence appears to be on the increase. Vaccine failure is also widely recognised (6). Since an alternative vaccine, namely the injectable poliovaccine (IPV, Salk) is already available, we have commenced studies for the evaluation of its efficacy under Indian conditions. As a first step we have measured the antibody response of infants given 3 doses of IPV. This is a preliminary report of the results obtained on the first 119 infants who have completed the study.

[1] *Supported by the Indian Council of Medical Research, New Delhi.*

VIRAL DISEASES IN SOUTH-EAST ASIA AND THE WESTERN PACIFIC
ISBN 0 12 484820 6

MATERIALS AND METHODS

The Vaccine

IPV incorporated with diphtheria-pertussis-tetanus vaccine into a quadruple vaccine was used. It was manufactured and supplied by the Rijks Institute, Bilthoven, the Netherlands. Each dose (1 ml) contained 20, 2 and 3.5 D antigen units of poliovirus types 1, 2 and 3 respectively. Each infant was given 3 doses of the quadruple vaccine.

The Study Population

Infants from 6 to 45 weeks of age attending our immunization clinic were recruited for the study after obtaining consent from parents. Infants recruited in alternate weeks were assigned to receive vaccine at 4 or 8 weeks interval between doses.

Antibody Measurement

Blood was collected from infants by heel prick before giving the first dose and 4 weeks after the third dose. The paired sera were tested simultaneously for the presence and titres of poliovirus neutralizing antibodies, after serial doubling dilutions starting from 1:8 (3). Virus challenge consisted of 100 median tissue culture infectious doses of poliovirus types 1, 2 and 3. In infants without detectable antibody, the appearance of antibody at any titre was defined as seroconversion. Antibody detected prior to immunization in infants below 6 months was considered to be of maternal origin. In infants with maternal antibody the rate of decline of antibody levels was calculated according to a half-life of 4 weeks. Infants with post-immunization antibody titres 4 or more times higher than the anticipated maternal antibody titres were also considered to have seroconverted.

TABLE I. Antibody Response to IPV

Maternal antibody	Interval between doses	Number of infants showing seroconversion to poliovirus		
		Type 1	Type 2	Type 3
Absent	4 weeks	44/44(100)[a]	47/52(90)	57/63(90)
Absent	8 weeks	29/29(100)	26/26(100)	41/43(95)
Present	4 weeks	25/25(100)	7/17(41)	4/6 (67)
Present	8 weeks	21/21(100)	23/24(96)	6/7 (86)
Both groups	4 weeks	69/69(100)	54/69(78)	61/69(88)
	8 weeks	50/50(100)	49/50(98)	47/50(94)
Both groups	Both groups	119/119 (100)	103/119 (86)	108/119 (91)

[a]No. responding/No. tested, with seroconversion rate as percent within brackets.

RESULTS

The antibody response in 119 infants is summarized in Table I.

Seroconversion to type 1 poliovirus was complete, irrespective of the interval between doses and the presence or absence of maternal antibody. In infants without maternal antibody to types 2 or 3, the response was better when the vaccine was given at 8 weekly intervals, but these differences were not statistically significant. In infants with maternal antibody at the commencement of immunization, seroconversion rates to types 2 and 3 viruses were unsatisfactory when the doses were given at 4 weekly intervals, but were satisfactory when given at 8 weekly intervals. In the case of type 2, this difference was statistically significant ($p<0.01$). In the case of type 3, the difference was not significant.

DISCUSSION

We have evaluated the effect of two factors on antibody response to IPV, namely the presence of maternal antibody and the interval between doses. Seroconversion rates were higher in infants without maternal antibody at the time of giving the first dose of IPV, than in those with maternal antibody, particularly in the case of types 2 and 3 viruses. The adverse effect of maternal antibody on antibody response was shown in an early study of IPV (4). This inhibitory effect could be partly overcome by increasing the interval between doses to 8 weeks. Even with 8 week intervals, the seroconversion rates to types 2 and 3 were higher in infants without maternal antibody than in those with maternal antibody. In an earlier report on a small number of tritypic seronegative infants we had observed better antibody response with 8 weekly intervals than with 4 weekly intervals (2). The influence of the interval between doses on antibody response to IPV has not been recognized earlier (5). In India, the age of highest risk for paralytic poliomyelitis is between 6 and 18 months. Therefore immunization should be completed by 6 months of age. Since a proportion of infants under 6 months may have maternal antibodies, it is important to immunize them with 3 doses at intervals of not less than 8 weeks.

REFERENCES

1. John, T.J., *Indian J. Pediatr. 48*, 565 (1981).
2. Krishnan, R. *et al.*, *Brit. Med. J.*, In press.
3. Lamb, L.H. *et al.*, *Public Health Reports 80*, 464 (1965).
4. Perkins, F.T. *et al.*, *Brit. Med. J. 2*, 68 (1958).
5. Salk, J.E., and Salk, D., *Science 195*, 834 (1977).
6. Sundaravalli, N. *et al.*, *Indian Pediatr. 18*, 539 (1981).

56

VIRAL GASTROENTERITIS ON NORFOLK ISLAND

Alan Murphy
Gary Grohmann

Virology Department
Institute of Clinical Pathology
and Medical Research
Westmead, New South Wales

Michael Sexton[1]

Medical Officer
Norfolk Island

INTRODUCTION

Norfolk Island is situated in the South Pacific some 1600 kilometers ENE of Sydney and approximately 1000 kilometers NNW of Auckland. It is 8 kilometers long and 5 kilometers wide, has a residential population of about 1900 individuals, and is a popular tourist resort. Some 25,000 tourists visit the island each year.

Gastroenteritis has long been a problem and is known amongst the islanders as "the sick and the vomits". In 1978 the incidence was reported as 225/1000 for infants and young children and 384/1000 for older children and adults.

[1] *Present address: 109 Hume Street, Wodonga, Victoria*

VIRAL DISEASES IN SOUTH-EAST ASIA
AND THE WESTERN PACIFIC
ISBN 0 12 484820 6

CLINICAL SYMPTOMS

Clinically the disease is an acute attack of nausea, vomiting, abdominal cramps and diarrhoea usually lasting 24-48 hours and occasionally up to 96 hours. Children up to the age of two years are usually febrile, with diarrhoea sometimes preceded by or accompanied by vomiting. Clinical recovery is complete within seven days. Within family groups, the incubation period varies between 36 and 72 hours. Repeat illnesses occur in the same individual suggesting a number of different organisms are involved or the initial attack does not produce long lasting immunity.

VIROLOGY OF FAECAL SPECIMENS

Bacteriological studies in 1978 and 1979 failed to establish a cause so that in 1980 the virology department of the ICPMR was requested to examine faecal specimens for evidence of viral gastroenteritis. 20% faecal extracts were centrifuged at 3000rpm for 15 mins and the supernatant inoculated into monkey kidney, Hep2 and human embryonic fibroblast cultures. The remainder of the supernatant was ultracentrifuged and the resulting pellets examined by electron microscopy. The results of the first 28 specimens examined are shown in Table I.

TABLE 1. Results of Testing 28 Faecal Specimens by EM

	VIRUSES						
	Rota	Astro	Adeno	Calici	SRV*	None	Total
Adults (17-75 yrs)	3	1	1	1	5	3	14
Children (1-8 yrs)	3	4	-	2	1	4	14
Totals	6	5	1	3	6	7	28

* Small round viruses 22-25 nm in diameter

Viruses were identified by electron microscopy in 21 (75%) of the 28 specimens examined. No viruses were grown in cell culture. These results suggest the illnesses were mainly viral in origin.

WATER SUPPLIES ON NORFOLK ISLAND

Increasing levels of detergents and tracer dye experiments in bore water samples used for domestic purposes suggested waste and sewage contamination as a possible cause for the high level of gastroenteritis on the island. Norfolk Island has no reticulated water supply and stored rainwater is used for most domestic purposes. However due to variable rainfall and limited storage facilities this source is insufficient, particularly for the large hotels, and is supplemented with bore water. There appears to be no shortage of the latter which may come from depths varying from 25ft to 350ft. There are 18 main bores on the island at the present time, and several commercial suppliers of water who distribute, mainly to households, in periods of dry weather. Most of the major hotels are situated on a ridge on the centre of the island and possess their own bores located in nearby valleys. They also discharge waste and sewage into the nearby soil (there is also no reticulated sewage disposal system on the island) or in some cases actually down disused bores. Because the water supplies were suspect, we have, over the past fifteen months tested 32 samples from fifteen water bores.

COLLECTION, CONCENTRATION AND EXAMINATION OF WATER SAMPLES

Water samples were collected from water bores in use on the island and flown to Richmond Air Base by the RAAF. They were then refrigerated until concentrated (usually within 24 hours of receipt). Initially approximately 5 litres of water were collected from five different bores and concentrated to 40-50ml in an Amicon CH4 hollow fibre concentrator. All substances with a molecular weight of greater than 100,000 were retained in the concentrate. The 40-50ml was then ultracentrifuged at 40,000rpm for 2 hours and the resulting pellets examined by electron microscopy and inoculated into cell cultures. Somewhat surprisingly rotaviruses and small round viruses were found in the bore water used by one hotel and small round viruses in that of a second hotel. As only 5 litre samples had been tested a high level of contamination was indicated. A further nine, five litre samples were examined from different sites and a poliovirus type 1 was isolated from two of them. Subsequently 25 litre samples were collected and concentrated, in an Amicon DC10 hollow fibre system, down to approximately two litres. This was then treated the same way as the five litre samples. The results of examining 32 samples are shown in Table 2.

TABLE 2. Results of Virological Examination of 32 Bore Water Samples from 15 Sites on Norfolk Island

Date Collected	No. of Samples	Volume Collected	EM	Cell Culture
Sept. 80	5	5 L	1x Rota 1x SRV	-
Nov. 80	9	5 L	-	2x Polio*
Dec. 80	4	25 L	1x Adeno	2x Polio
Jan. 81	6	25 L	-	2x Polio
Mar. 81	2	25 L	-	1x Polio
Nov. 81	6	25 L	-	2x Adeno**

* Poliovirus isolates were all type 1 vaccine strain
** Adenovirus isolates were serotypes 1 and 5
Bacteriophages were also frequently detected by electron microscopy
1 septic tank effluent sample (4.5 litres) was also examined and rotavirus and poliovirus were detected.

In total three adenoviruses, seven polioviruses, one rotavirus and two small round viruses were found in eleven samples.

DISCUSSION

Normally volumes of 50-100 litres of drinking water need to be examined to successfully demonstrate the presence of viruses. The identification of viruses in five of fourteen 5 litre bore water samples indicates heavy contamination of the water table on Norfolk Island, and provides a logical explanation for the high incidence of gastroenteritis. Most of the larger hotels are grouped closely together and in this area waste water and sewage have presumably overloaded the soil and subsoil. These effluents seep down to nearby valleys where water bores are situated and in some instances it can be fairly said that diluted sewage is being recycled without the benefit of any worthwhile cleansing process. Clearly tourism and its resultant pollution has outstripped the facilities of the island and either the number of tourist should be restricted or adequate sewage disposal provided, together with a system of reticulated water of acceptable standard.

57

THE AETIOLOGY OF PAEDIATRIC DIARRHOEA IN YOGYAKARTA, INDONESIA

Yati Soenarto[1]
Teluk Sebodo
Purnomo Surjantoro
Krisnomurti
Suwardji Haksohusodo
Ristanto
Nurhayati
Jon Rohde

Departments of Child Health, Microbiology, Parasitology, Gadjah Mada University, Yogyakarta, Indonesia

Richard Luke[2]
Norbert Ryan

School of Agriculture, La Trobe University, Melbourne, Australia

Ruth Bishop
Graeme Barnes

Department of Gastroenterology, Royal Children's Hospital, Melbourne, Australia

[1]*Project support: The Rockeffeller Foundation, New York.*
[2]*Project support: Australian Development Assistance Bureau.*

VIRAL DISEASES IN SOUTH-EAST ASIA
AND THE WESTERN PACIFIC
ISBN 0 12 484820 6

I. INTRODUCTION

In Indonesia, the incidence of paediatric diarrhoea is one to two attacks per child per year during the first three years of life (1). Severe diarrhoea with dehydration accounts for approximately one third of all paediatric admissions to hospital in Yogyakarta. Diarrhoea is also a recurrent problem among newborn babies in hospital nurseries (2). This study assesses the relative importance of different enteropathogens in causation of acute diarrhoea.

II. PATIENTS AND METHODS

Faeces were obtained from 407 children aged from one month to 12 years, admitted to Pugeran Hospital, Yogyakarta during June 1978 to June 1979. Two hundred and twenty-one children with acute diarrhoea and 47 control children belonged to families of low socioeconomic level. One hundred and seventeen children with acute diarrhoea and 22 control children were from families of medium-high socio-economic level who could afford private hospital care.

Faeces were also obtained from 86 newborn babies at a rural health centre, and from 39 newborn babies in a Special Care Nursery of an urban hospital.

Faeces were examined in Yogyakarta for bacterial and parasitic pathogens. Portions of all specimens were refrigerated and later flown to Melbourne for identification of viruses by electron-microscopy and of toxigenic coliforms by toxin tests.

III. RESULTS

At least one enteric pathogen was identified in 60% of children with acute diarrhoea. Rotaviruses were the most important aetiological agent identified and were found in 38% of all children with acute diarrhoea. Toxigenic coliforms were isolated from 10% of children, *Salmonella* species from 6.5%, *Shigella* species from 4.6% and parasites (predominantly *Trichuris trichiura*) from 3%. Mixed infections with two or more pathogens were encountered in 8% of children. Parasites were more common in children from families of low socioeconomic level, but socioeconomic level did not influence occurrence of viral or bacterial pathogens.

A. Rotavirus Infection in Paediatric Admissions

Figure is reproduced by permission of the Journal of Clinical Microbiology (3). The number of children admitted to hospital each month with acute diarrhoea is illustrated together with the number excreting rotavirus particles in diarrhoeal faeces. The decrease in admissions in September is due to parental reluctance to permit hospitalisation during the Muslem holy month. Decreased admissions during November and December coincided with the seasonal change from dry to wet conditions. The incidence of rotavirus infection was similar each month except for a decreased incidence during November and December. Socioeconomic level and pre-existing nutritional status did not influence the incidence of rotavirus excretion. Rotavirus infections were more common in children aged six to 24 months than in younger or older children.

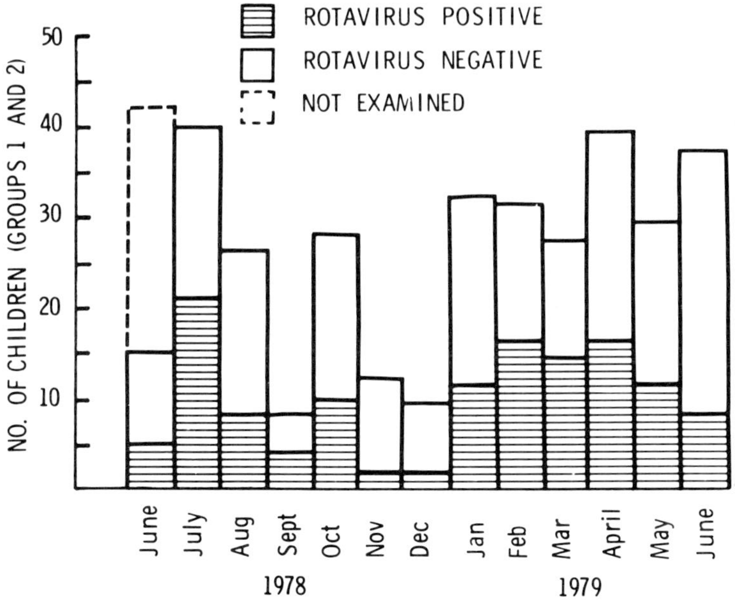

FIGURE 1. Acute gastroenteritis and rotavirus infections in children admitted to hospital, Yogyakarta, Indonesia.

B. Rotavirus Infection in Newborn Babies

Rotavirus infection was identified in 1/42 newborn babies with diarrhoea in a rural health centre and in 1/44 asymptomatic babies. Rotavirus infection was not encountered in newborn babies in hospital. Instead, 47% of these babies with diarrhoea were excreting *Salmonella* species.

IV. CONCLUSION

In Indonesia, rotavirus infection is a major cause of childhood diarrhoea throughout the year, but is an uncommon cause of diarrhoea in newborn babies.

REFERENCES

1. Rohde, J.E., and Northrup, R.S., *in* "Acute Diarrhoea in Childhood" Ciba Foundation Symposium 42 (New Series), p.339. Elsevier Excerpta Medica, North-Holland, (1976).
2. Purnomo, S., Soeprapto, and Marwoto, *Paediatrica Indonesiana 18,* 269 (1978).
3. Soenarto, Y., Sebodo, T., Ridho, R., Alrasjid, H., Rohde, J.E., Bugg, H.C., Barnes, G.L., and Bishop, R.F., *J. Clin. Microbiol. 14,* 123 (1981).

ROTAVIRUS GASTROENTERITIS STUDIES IN INDONESIA

Julie Sulianti Saroso
Iskak Koiman

Ministry of Health
Jakarta, Indonesia

Suharyono

Faculty of Medicine
University of Indonesia, Jakarta

INTRODUCTION

Diarrhoeal disease is one of the most important health problems in Indonesia. It accounts for 20% of admissions in hospital paediatric wards. The incidence rate is around 400 per 1000 population per year with 70-80% occurring in children under five years of age. The number of diarrhoeal episodes in infants begin to increase after the age of 6 months up to 2 years. A child between 1-2 years old may experience 2 diarrhoeal episodes in a year. The majority of cases does not last more than 7 days (1).

After Bishop's report (2), rotavirus associated with acute gastroenteritis in small children has been reported from developing as well as from developed countries with little difference in prevalence (3,4). This suggests that hygiene may not be an important factor in its transmission. Lewis (5) reported respiratory illness preceding the gastroenteritis. All studies showed the highest incidence occurring in children under 2 years of age.

As elsewhere, until recently known pathogens were identified in less than 50% of diarrhoeal cases in Indonesia.

VIRAL DISEASES IN SOUTH-EAST ASIA
AND THE WESTERN PACIFIC
ISBN 0 12 484820 6

This presentation is concerned with rotavirus gastroenteritis studies undertaken by various investigators in Indonesia.

MATERIALS AND METHODS

Faecal specimens were collected from cases with gastroenteritis admitted to hospitals in Jakarta (364 specimens), in Medan (69 specimens) and in Jogyakarta (344 specimens) and from 130 diarrhoeal cases identified in a community longitudinal survey in North Jakarta. Rotavirus was detected by ELISA Standard method except in the first study in the Jakarta Central General Hospital and in Jogyakarta, where specimens were sent to Australia for identification by electron microscopy. In Jogyakarta specimens were collected from diarrhoeal cases of low as well as middle to high socio-economic level. Clinical data were collected from the 48 rotavirus gastroneteritis patients admitted to the CGH in Jakarta during November 1979 until November 1980.

RESULTS AND DISCUSSION

As presented in the table below rotavirus was found in 15 to 47% of the specimens examined. The lowest excretion rate was found in the North Jakarta community study. This may be related to the difference in study population. In all studies the highest incidence occurred in children under 2 years of age with the lowest incidence in this age group in infants under 6 months. Socio-economic level and preexisting nutritional status seemed not to influence the incidence of rotavirus excretion. In Jakarta the excretion rate in bottle-fed children was higher than in children with breastfeeding.

Rotavirus was excreted throughout the year, but two peak rates of rotavirus excretion were noted: one during the dry and one during the wet months. Observations over a longer period are needed to gain a better understanding of the seasonal variation, if any.

The study in the CGH in Jakarta noted that of 48 rotavirus gastroenteritis patients 79% had vomiting, 75% watery diarrhoea, 56% a frequency of diarrhoea 4-10 times a day and 56% concomittant upper respiratory illness. Are the latter symptoms part of rotavirus gastroenteritis? Further observations are recommended.

TABLE I. Occurrence of Rotavirus in Various Gastroenteritis Studies in Indonesia[c]

Source faecal spec.	Period of Study	Method	No. of spec. exam.	No. of pos. spec.	% pos.
CGH Jak.[a]	Nov. 1974 - Jan. 1975	E.M.[b]	19	9	47.4
University Hospital Jogyakarta	June 1978 - June 1979	E.M.	334	126	37.7
CGH Jak. (1)	Aug. 1979 - Oct. 1979	ELISA	52	21	40.4
CGH Jak. (2)	Nov. 1979 - Oct. 1980	ELISA	131	38	29.0
CGH Jak. (3)	Oct. 1980 - July 1981	ELISA	50	10	20.0
Other Hospitals Jakarta	1979 - 1980	ELISA	112	31	26.8
General Hospital Medan	Sept. 1979 - Jan. 1980	ELISA	69	28	40.6
North Jakarta Community	Nov. 1980 - April 1981	ELISA	130	20	15.4

[a]CGH Jak. - Central General Hospital, Jakarta (Rumah Sakit Cipto Mangunkusumo).
[b]E.M. - Electron Microscope.
[c]Data from Suharyono et al. (6), Soenarto et al. (7), Koiman (8) and Sutoto et al (9).

These studies have shown that rotavirus is an important aetiological agent of acute gastroenteritis in children in Indonesia. Findings concerning lower excretion rates in infants under 6 months and in breastfed children support continuation of breastfeeding even when infants suffer from diarrhoea.

Because of the uncertainty of the mode of transmission of rotavirus gastroenteritis and considering its prevalence in developed countries improvements in water supply and refuse disposal may not result in a decline in morbidity of rotavirus gastroenteritis in developing countries. In this connection the development of a vaccine against rotavirus gastroenteritis should be pursued.

CONCLUSION

In all studies on acute gastroenteritis in children undertaken in Indonesia rotavirus was identified when searched for. The highest incidence was found in children under 2 years old.

In view of the findings which were not conclusive, further studies concerning seasonal variation and the importance of respiratory illness in rotavirus gastroenteritis were suggested. Development of a vaccine should be pursued.

REFERENCES

1. Brotowasisto, and Soerachmad, S., Proceedings of 5th Asian Pacific Congress of Gastroenterology, Singapore (1976).
2. Bishop, R. F., Davidson, G. P., Holmes, I. H., and Ruck, B. J., *Lancet,* 1281 (1973).
3. Kapikian, A. Z., Hyun, W. K., Wyatt, R. G., Cline, W. L., Parrott, R. H., Chanock, R. M., Arrobio, J. O., Brandt, C. D., Rodriguez, W. J., Kalica, A. R., and Van Kirk, D. H., *in* "Acute Diarrhoea in Childhood", p. 273, Elsevier, Excerpta Medica, North Holland, (1976).
4. Sengupta, P. G., Sen, D., Saha, M. R., Niyogi, S., Deb, B. C., Pal, S. C., Ibetombi Devi, Sukumar Singh, N., *Trans. Roy. Soc. Trop. Med. Hyg. 75,* 521 (1981).
5. Lewis, H. M., Parry, J. V., Davies, H. A., Parry, R. P., Mott, A., Dourmashkin, R. R., Sanderson, P.J., Tyrrell, D. A. J., and Valman, H. B., *Arch. Dis. Childhood 54,* 339 (1979).
6. Suharyono, Aswitha Budiarso, Gracey, M., Wiharta, A. S., Senduk, J., Koiman, I., and Soeharyono, Paper presented in Fifth Paediatric Congress, Medan (1981).
7. Soenarto, Y., Teluk Sebodo, Rosyid Ridho, Harun Alrasjid, Rohde, J. E., Bugg, H. C., Barnes, G. L., and Bishop, R. F., *J. Clin. Micro. 14,* 123 (1981).

8. Koiman, I., Paper presented in the Eighth SEAMIC Seminar, Singapore (1980).
9. Sutoto, Mochtar, M. A., Karyadi, and Brotowasisto, Paper presented in Gastroenterology Congress, Jakarta (1981).

59

ROLE OF ANTIBODIES, TRYPSIN AND TRYPSIN INHIBITORS IN PROTECTION OF NEONATES AGAINST ROTAVIRUS INFECTION

Barbara S. McLean[1]

The Royal Women's Hospital,
Carlton, Victoria, Australia

I. INTRODUCTION

Rotavirus is a major cause of infantile gastroenteritis, but investigations of the relative protective effect of lacteal secretions and circulating antibody have been so far limited to animals (1). However, a significantly lower incidence of rotavirus infection has been recorded in breast-fed, compared with bottle-fed infants. (2).

Treatment of rotaviruses with trypsin enhances virus production in cell culture (3). It is likely that intestinal trypsin may do so in human infants and that α_1-antitrypsin in human milk, as well as antirotaviral antibody, may be protective.

These possibilities were investigated in a study of 92 infants, 43 of whom were breast-fed, and their mothers (4, 5). An enzyme-linked immunosorbent assay for rotavirus antibody was used (6).

II. CLASSES OF ANTIROTAVIRAL IMMUNOGLOBULINS DETECTED

Antirotaviral IgG was found in all maternal and cord sera tested. Specific IgA, some of which was ScIgA, was present at lower levels in maternal sera only. No antirotaviral IgM

[1] *Supported by 3AW Community Service Trust Fund.*

VIRAL DISEASES IN SOUTH-EAST ASIA
AND THE WESTERN PACIFIC
ISBN 0 12 484820 6

was detected. In lacteal secretions, specific ScIgA was found most frequently and in the greatest quantity. Specific antibody transfer from mother to infant via colostrum and milk is illustrated in Fig. 1.

III. RELATIONSHIP BETWEEN ANTIROTAVIRAL IMMUNOGLOBULIN LEVELS, FAECAL TRYPSIN LEVELS, LACTEAL TRYPSIN INHIBITORY CAPACITY (TIC) AND INCIDENCE OF ROTAVIRUS INFECTION

A. *Antirotaviral Immunoglobulin Levels*

No statistically significant difference was found in levels of any specific antibodies in serum, between infants with or without rotavirus infection. However, the infants of mothers with progressively higher specific ScIgA levels in colostrum and milk were less likely to become infected with rotavirus (Fig. 2). These differences were statistically significant.

B. *Faecal trypsin Levels and Lacteal TIC.*

Breast-fed infants had significantly lower faecal trypsin levels than bottle-fed infants. On day 1 in bottle-fed infants, levels of trypsin were significantly lower in

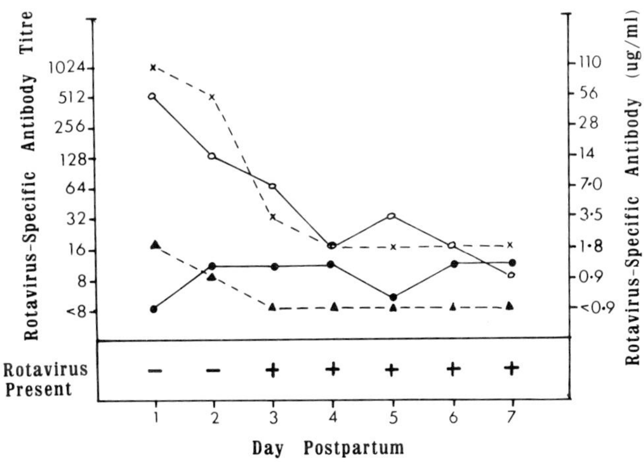

FIGURE 1. Transfer of lacteal antirotaviral immunoglobulins from a mother to her infant. (X) maternal ScIg; (O) maternal IgA; (▲) maternal IgM; (●) IgA in the infant's faeces. From (6).

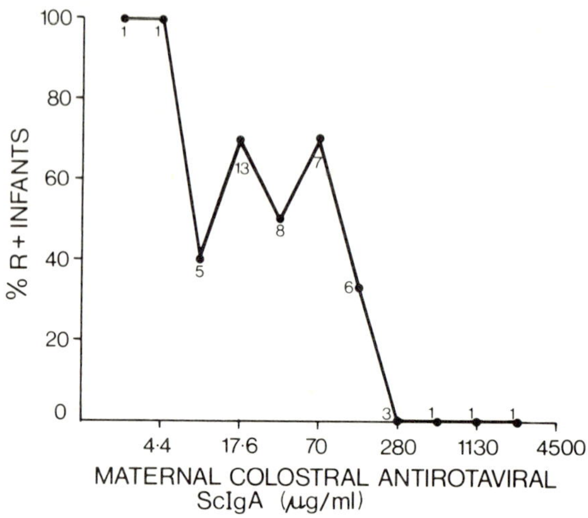

FIGURE 2. Relationship between % rotavirus-positive infants by day 5 post-partum and the specific ScIgA level in their mother's colostrum on day 2. From (5).

stools of uninfected infants than in infants who later became infected. Furthermore, rotavirus-infected breast-fed infants received milk of significantly lower mean TIC than did uninfected breast-fed infants.

C. *Combined Effect of Lacteal TIC and Antirotaviral ScIgA*

To allow for the effect of the other milk factor, matched pairs of breast-fed infants were constructed. Whether matched for mean TIC or specific ScIgA levels, uninfected neonates received milk containing higher levels of the unmatched factor than rotavirus-positive neonates. It was not possible to assess the relative importance of the factors.

IV. PERSISTENCE OF ANTIROTAVIRAL ScIgA, TIC AND α_1-ANTITRYPSIN IN HUMAN MILK

The level of these factors fell progressively over the first 2 months post-partum (Fig. 3). It has been shown that most, if not all the TIC was due to α_1-antitrypsin.

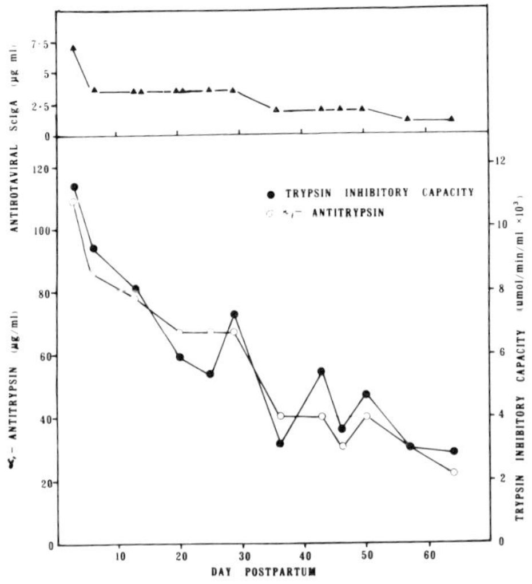

FIGURE 3. Levels of specific ScIgA, TIC and α_1-antitrypsin in a mother's milk to day 64 post-partum.

V. CONCLUSIONS

Both α_1-antitrypsin and antirotaviral ScIgA in milk and colostrum reduce the risk of neonatal rotavirus infection. The duration of this protective effect requires further study in view of the decline in levels of these factors.

REFERENCES

1. Snodgrass, D.R., and Wells, P.W. *Arch. Virol. 52,* 201 (1976).
2. Totterdell, B.M., Chrystie, I.L., and Banatvala, J.E. *Arch. Dis. Child. 51* 924 (1976).
3. Babuik, L.A., Mohammed, K., Spence, L., Fauvel, M., and Petro, R. *J. Clin. Microbiol. 6* 610 (1977).
4. McLean, B.S., and Holmes, I.H. *J. Clin. Microbiol. 12,* 320 (1980).
5. McLean, B.S., and Holmes, I.H. *J. Clin. Microbiol. 13,* 22 (1981).
6. McLean, B.S., Sonza, S., and Holmes, I.H. *J. Clin. Microbiol. 12,* 314 (1980).

EPIDEMIC ROTAVIRUS DIARRHOEA IN KERALA, INDIA

Jayaram Paniker

Department of Microbiology
Medical College, Calicut
Kerala, India

Very large epidemics of acute diarrhoeal disease affecting infants and children have occurred during the months of November to March every year from 1971 in and around Calicut (Lat. 10°N; Long. 75°E) in north Kerala, India. The cases run into several tens of thousands annually. A sample survey in the area identified some 80,000 cases during the epidemic season in 1973-1974. Aetiological studies were unsuccessful till 1976, when all ten stool samples tested in February revealed the presence of rotavirus. Rotavirus has been found in the large majority of faecal samples tested in the epidemic season during each of the five years since then. The incidence of rotavirus infection in children hospitalised with diarrhoea in Calicut has been investigated in two prospective studies.

The first study, from October 1976 to February 1978 was by electron microscopy. Of 3355 children below 5 years hospitalised during the period with acute diarrhoea, 368 (11%) were studied. Faecal samples collected by rectal catheters were examined for bacteria and parasites, and stored frozen for electron microscopy in batches. Rotavirus was detected in 260 (71%) of the specimens overall. It was present during each of the 16 months, but showed a marked seasonal variation, ranging in frequency from a maximum of 100% in November 1976 to a minimum of 27% in May 1977. Other viruses including adenoviruses, astroviruses, caliciviruses, coronaviruses and 23-27 nm small round viruses were detected in 72 (20%) of the samples, with approximately equal frequency in rota positive and negative cases. No seasonal

VIRAL DISEASES IN SOUTH-EAST ASIA
AND THE WESTERN PACIFIC
ISBN 0 12 484820 6

pattern was evident for these viruses, except that adenoviruses were most common in May, when rotavirus was least frequent. Pathogenic bacteria could be detected only in 46 (13%) cases and parasitic infection, including giardiasis and helminths, in 134 (36%).

The second study employed ELISA for detection of rotavirus infection. Faecal samples from children hospitalised for diarrhoea during the 12 month period November 1979 to October 1980 were tested. Of 183 samples tested, 102 (56%) were positive for rotavirus infection. The extent and seasonal distribution of rotavirus infection detected by ELISA were similar to the results obtained by electron microscopy. Rotavirus infection was present throughout the year, ranging in frequency from 92% in January to 6% in April.

The incidence of rotavirus infection was highest in children 6 to 23 months old. The clinical picture of diarrhoea, including the degree of dehydration, mean duration of disease, nature of stools and rate of mortality was not noticeably different in rota positive and negative cases. In both, the mortality was 2%. Vomiting was more common in rota positive patients (92%) than in rota negative patients (69%), and fever less common (47% versus 66%).

Stool samples collected during the epidemic season from 31 children without diarrhoea did not contain rotavirus.

These studies spread over 5 years establish rotavirus as the predominant cause of acute diarrhoea in children requiring hospitalisation in this region, and also demonstrate a distinct seasonal preponderance. This has an important bearing on the proper management of these epidemics. Formerly, oral antibiotics used to be employed widely during these epidemics. This practice had led to extensive dissemination of multiple drug resistance in intestinal bacteria and to epidemics of drug resistant typhoid fever. It has now been shown that prompt oral rehydration therapy may be all that is necessary for the management of rotaviral diarrhoea.

ACKNOWLEDGMENTS

I thank Prof. Minnie Mathen and Prof. V.I. Mathen, Wellcome Research Laboratories, Christian Medical College, Vellore for electron microscopy and Dr. M.R. Saha, National Institute of Cholera and Enteric Diseases, Calcutta for ELISA tests.

61

APPLICATION OF MONOCLONAL ANTIBODIES TO STUDIES OF ROTAVIRUS

Alan Breschkin

National Biological Standards Laboratory
Parkville, Victoria, Australia

Secondo Sonza

Department of Microbiology
University of Melbourne
Parkville, Victoria, Australia

Hybridoma cell lines that produce monoclonal antibodies directed against three rotavirus strains (simian SA11, bovine Northern Ireland calf, and human Wa) have been derived using both NS-1 (non-secretor) and Sp 2/0 (non-producer) murine myeloma cell lines. Hybridoma cell culture fluids were screened for rotavirus antibody using an enzyme-linked immunosorbent assay (ELISA) (McLean et al, 1980) and also in some cases by a radioimmunoassay (RIA) using staphylococcal protein A-coated microtitre plates and ^{125}I-iodinated SA11 rotavirus. The monoclonal antibodies were characterized further by radioimmune precipitation of ^{35}S-methionine labelled viral antigens by the method of Lee et al (1981).

Initially the hybridoma cell lines derived secreted monoclonal antibodies which cross-reacted by ELISA with all three rotavirus strains and are directed against the major inner capsid protein, I_4 (molecular weight 42,000). Two such cross-reactive monoclonal antibodies have been

VIRAL DISEASES IN SOUTH-EAST ASIA AND THE WESTERN PACIFIC
ISBN 0 12 484820 6

successfully used as the capture and enzyme-linked antibodies respectively in a solid-phase ELISA for rotavirus antigen detection.

Several of these monoclonal antibodies directed against polypeptide I_4 have been studied by means of competitive binding to rotavirus-coated microtitre plates. To date we have evidence for two distinct antigenic regions on polypeptide I_4 and presumptive evidence of at least one other region. The two monoclonal antibodies used in the ELISA for rotavirus antigen detection have been shown to belong to different competition binding groups. This combination produces a more sensitive ELISA than using the same monoclonal antibody for both capture and detection.

Recently, several hybridoma cell lines have been derived which react by ELISA to one or two of the rotavirus strains but not to all three. One that is specific for NIC and two that are specific for Wa are directed against polypeptide I_4 and are thus non-neutralizing. However several SA11-specific monoclonal antibodies have been derived which are directed agains the major outer capsid glycoprotein, O_2 (molecular weight 34,000) and show some neutralizing activity by plaque neutralization. We are presently trying to derive similar specific monoclonal antibodies to human Wa rotavirus that should prove valuable in the serological identification of human rotavirus serotypes and subgroups and how these are related to the electropherotypes found by polyacrylamide gel electrophoresis of rotavirus RNA (Rodger et al, 1981).

REFERENCES

Lee, P.W.K., Hayes, E.C., and Joklik, W.K. (1981). *Virology 108*, 134.

McLean, B., Sonza, S., and Holmes, I.H. (1980). *J. Clin. Microbiol. 12*, 314.

Rodger, S.M., Bishop, R.F., Birch, C., McLean, B., and Holmes, I.H. (1981). *J. Clin. Microbiol. 13*, 272.

SEQUENCE DIVERSITY AMONGST HUMAN ROTAVIRUS STRAINS

A.R. Bellamy, J.E. Street, and W.F. Chadderton

Department of Cell Biology
University of Auckland,
Auckland, New Zealand

M.C. Croxson

Virus Laboratory
Auckland Hospital
Auckland, New Zealand.

I. INTRODUCTION

Rotaviruses have been identified as important aetiologic agents of acute gastroenteritis in humans (reviewed by Holmes 1979). They are an important cause of diarrhoeal disease in young children, particularly in developing countries. The number of serological types has not yet been firmly established, but at least three serotypes have been identified (Thouless *et al*, 1981). Variation amongst rotavirus isolates may also be detected by analysis of the viral genomic RNA's on polyacrylamide gels. For example Rodger *et al* (1981) have identified at least nineteen different 'electropherotypes' circulating in Melbourne.

We have investigated the molecular basis for the differences observed in electrophoretic mobility of the genome segments of human rotaviruses. A hybridisation method utilising radioactive copy DNA (cDNA) probes specific for the genome segments of rotaviruses has been used to compare a series of rotaviruses isolated in New Zealand between 1975 and 1980.

VIRAL DISEASES IN SOUTH-EAST ASIA
AND THE WESTERN PACIFIC
ISBN 0 12 484820 6

A. *Northern Blotting of Human Rotavirus RNA's and Synthesis of cDNA Probes*

Methods described by Taylor *et al* (1976) and Alwine *et al* (1979) were applied to RNA's derived from a series of clinical isolates obtained from young children admitted with accute diarrhaea to the Infectious Diseases Ward of Auckland Hospital. Viral RNA purified from faeces by the method of Croxson and Bellamy (1981), was first subjected to electrophoresis on polyacrylamide gels to resolve the various genome segments (Fig.1) and then transferred to freshly converted

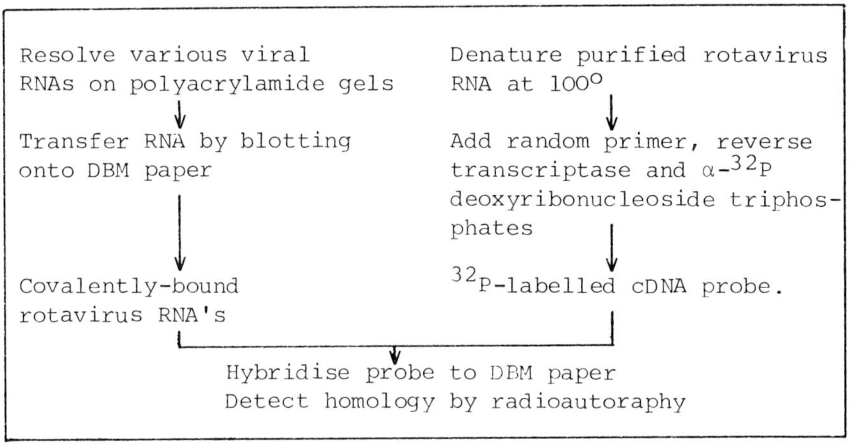

FIGURE 1. Method of analysis of rotavirus strains for sequence relationships.

diazobenzyloxymethyl (DBM) paper by electrophoretic blotting (Stellwag and Dahlberg, 1980). RNA was extracted from the most recent isolate HU/AKL/609/80 by phenol extraction, purified by isopycnic sedimentation on CsSO4, and used as a template for the synthesis of a cDNA probe. The probe, which contained sequences specific for all eleven rotavirus genes, was then hybridised to the blotted genome segments. Homology was detected by radioautography.

B. *Sequence Diversity of Rotaviruses Collected Between 1975 and 1980*

Human rotavirus RNA's resolved by electrophoresis on a polyacrylamide gel are shown in Fig.2a. Genome segments were transferred to DBM paper and hybridised to a cDNA probe specific for the genome of HU/AKL/609/80. Fig.2b reveals substantial sequence diversity: recent isolates demonstrate strong homology with the probe whereas 1978 isolates and one 1975 isolate demonstrate minimal or no homology. No homology is detectable for segment 5 of HU/AKL/78/79, even though other genes show clear evidence for homology

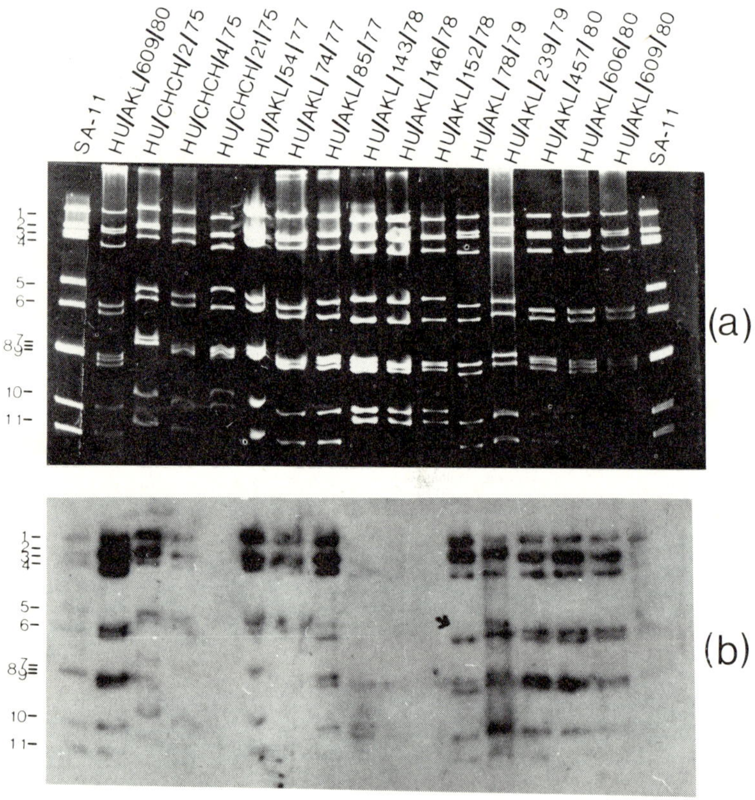

FIGURE 2. Hybridisation analysis of human rotavirus isolates. (a) Ethidium bromide stained acrylamide gel. (b) The gel shown in (a) was blotted onto DBM paper and the cDNA probe specific for HU/AKL/609/80 applied. Homology was detected by radioautography. The arrow indicates the absence of homology to segment 5 of HU/AKL/78/79. Hybridisation was at 52° in 15% formamide and other components as described by Alwine et al (1979). Nomenclature follows Rodger and Holmes (1979).

The distinction between 1978 isolates and the other viruses is also evident when hybridisation is carried out either with a cDNA probe specific for RNA of the cultivable type 2 strain Wa (Fig.3) or with other rotavirus probes (data not shown).

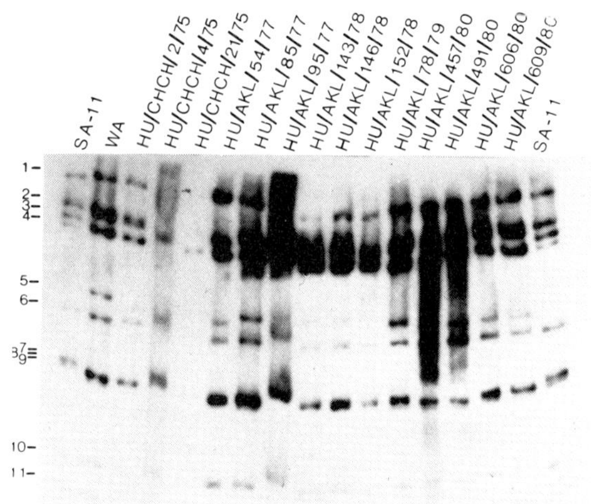

FIGURE 3. Hybridisation analysis of human rotavirus isolates. A cDNA probe specific for the cultivable human strain Wa was applied. Hybridisation was at 52° in 10% formamide.

II. CONCLUSIONS

By analogy with influenza A viruses (Laver and Webster, 1979) rotaviruses might be expected to exhibit antigenic shift due to the known ability of these viruses to interchange genome segments during mixed infections (Kalica *et al*, 1981). The absence of homology between segment 5 of HU/AKL/78/79 and the HU/AKL/609/80 probe supports the notion that segment interchange may play a role in the production of new rotavirus strains. Rotaviruses may also be subject to antigenic drift, a process resulting from the progressive divergence of genes, since some segments which show homology under hybridisation conditions of low stringency, show no hybridisation when the formamide concentration is increased (data not shown). A combination of segment interchange and progressive sequence divergence would thus account well for the great diversity of genome sequence found here.

As a practical application of this work, the immobilisation of rotavirus RNA's on DBM-paper provides the means by which a permanent library of rotavirus genomes could be assembled. Once the genome segments having epidemiological relevance have been identified, new isolates could be compared with previous virus strains. The techniques involved suggest that this approach would be one best suited to a regional virus reference laboratory.

ACKNOWLEDGMENTS

Supported by the New Zealand Medical Research Council, the National Child Health Research Foundation and the World Health Organisation.

REFERENCES

Alwine, J.C., Kemp, D.J., Parker, B.A., Reiser, J., Renart, J., Stark, G.R., and Wahl, G.M. (1979). *Methods in Enzymology 68*, 220.

Croxson, M.C., and Bellamy, A.R. (1981). *Appl. Env. Microbiol. 41*, 255.

Espejo, R.T., Calderon, E., Gonzalez, N., Salomon, A., Martuscelli, A., and Romero, P. (1979). *J. Infect. Dis. 139*, 474.

Holmes, I.H. (1979). *Prog. Med. Virol. 25*, 1.

Kalica, A.R., Greenberg, H.B., Wyatt, R.G., Flores, J., Sereno, M.M., Kapikian, A.Z., and Chanock, R.M. (1981). *Virology 112*, 385.

Laver, W.G., and Webster, R.G. (1979). *Br. Med. Bull. 35*, 29.

Rodger, S.M., and Holmes, I.H. (1979). *J. Virol. 30*, 839.

Rodger, S.M., Bishop, R.F., Birch, C., McLean, B., and Holmes, I.H. (1981). *J. Clin. Microbiol. 13*, 272.

Stellwag, E.J., and Dahlberg, A.E. (1980). *Nuc. Acid. Res. 8*, 299.

Taylor, J.M., Illmensee, R., and Summers, J. (1976). *Biochim. Biophys. Acta 442*, 324.

Thouless, M.E., Beards, G.M., and Flewett, T.H. (1981). *In* Fifth International Congress of Virology W16/05 pg.191.

63

VIRAL EPIDEMIC CONJUNCTIVITIS IN SINGAPORE (1970 - 1980)

Marguerite Yin-Murphy

Department of Microbiology
National University of Singapore

Lim Kuang Hui

Mount Elizabeth Hospital
Singapore

An unusually explosive and extensive epidemic of acute conjunctivitis occurred in September to December 1970 during which 60,118 patients were treated by the Government Out-patient Clinics. The eye affliction was characterised by sudden onset of mild to severe conjunctivitis, lachrymation, pain and a "foreign body sensation", preauricular gland enlargement and chemosis. Small petechial to large blotches of subconjunctival haemorrhage were seen in minority cases. Punctate epithelial keratitis and iritis were rare compared to adenovirus conjunctivitis. Respiratory symptoms which accompanied some cases were of no consequence. Recovery occurred within 2 weeks without sequelae. Steroid and antibiotics had no apparent effect. The causative agent classified as a new antigenic variant of Coxsackievirus A24 is the first human enterovirus known to give rise to an epidemic disease with conjunctivitis as a dominant clinical feature (1-3).

A second epidemic occurred in June to December 1971 during which 38,156 patients were treated. Although the manifestations were similar to those seen in 1970, the causative agent together with isolates from epidemics in Morocco and Japan were classified as a new enterovirus - The Enterovirus Type 70 (4-7).

VIRAL DISEASES IN SOUTH-EAST ASIA
AND THE WESTERN PACIFIC
ISBN 0 12 484820 6

A third epidemic occurred in June to November 1972 when 29,989 cases were treated. The manifestations were similar to those seen during the 1970 and 1971 epidemics. The causative agent in majority cases was however, adenovirus 11 (AV11). E70 was confirmed in a few cases (8).

CA24 was responsible for one other epidemic in June to December 1975 with a record of 60,000 cases (9) and E70 for our last epidemic in July to December 1980 with 48,915 cases recorded (10). CA24, E70, adenovirus types 3, 7, 8, 11 and 19 were implicated in minor outbreaks during inter-epidemic period.

EPIDEMIOLOGICAL AND CLINICAL FEATURES

CA24 gave rise to bigger epidemics than E70. More males than females were affected with an older children and young adult predominancy. The majority contracted infection at home, others at work, schools or from an unknown source. Close contact was an important factor in transmission (10). People of all ethnic and socio-economic groups were affected.

There is no distinctive feature to differentiate epidemics caused by CA24, E70 and AV11. Subconjunctival haemorrhage though striking was seen in only 4-11% cases during our epidemics. Despite recurrences of CA24 and E70 outbreaks, neutralising antibody to both viruses were negative (<1/20) in sera sampled within two days of onset. A few patients had neutralising antibody rises to two viruses namely, CA24 and E70, AV11 and E70, AV19 and E70 (6,8).

ISOLATION, SUSCEPTIBILITY OF CELL LINES AND MICE

CA24 and E70 have been isolated from tears, conjunctival swabs and scrapings, throat swabs and garglings, rectal swabs and faeces. All our CA24 and E70 strains were isolated in Hela. Parallel inoculations into PMK yielded no cytopathogenic agent. Hela sublines however, varied in susceptibility to E70 (2,6,11,12). Higgins (13) reported isolation of several strains of E70 in human embryonic conjunctival, nasal and tracheal organ cultures where parallel inoculations into Hela, PMK, W138 and HEK failed to yield virus.

Strains of CA24 and E70 established in Hela-T26 varied in ability to produce CPE in Vero cells. CA24 strains, namely,

Singapore 24/1970, 65&28/1975, Hong Kong 3751/1971, Bangladesh 1,2,4/1975 and Sri Lanka 75308/1975 could not produce CPE in Vero cultures after three consecutive passes but Bangkok E7/1975, Brunei 4926&4929/1975, Sri Lanka 7518/1975 and Vellore 6852/1978 could. Whereas E70 strains, namely, Singapore 146&32/1971, Hong Kong 3454/1971, Japan 648/1971 and Singapore 57/1972 produced CPE in Vero, Singapore 27/1973 and 1200/1980 could not.

CA24 (Singapore 24/1970) and E70 (Singapore 146/1971) were non-pathogenic for suckling mice tested in Singapore (2,6). Higgins (14) however, reported that the CA24 strain caused stunting of growth and paralysis of mice.

ANTIGENIC VARIATION

Melnick (7) observed that E70 (Singapore 146/1971) established in Hela when passaged in Cynomolgus MK followed by HEL cell cultures became poorly neutralized by homologous monkey antiserum prepared with the virus grown in Hela. This was attributed to a broadening of virus antigen which rendered the virus less neutralizable by antibody raised against the "parent" virus propagated in Hela.

Strains of E70 and CA24 isolated in Singapore and in other Asian countries which we established in Hela-T26 were compared for neutralizability by monkey antisera prepared with E70 (Singapore 146/1971) and CA24 (Singapore 24/1970) grown in Hela in parallel with strains passaged from Hela-T26 to Vero. Invariably, CA24 and E70 strains grown and tested in Hela were neutralized 8 to 32 fold higher than strains passaged and tested in Vero. The neutralizing antibody titres for E70 strains tested in Hela varied between 160 to 1280 compared to 20 to 80 for strains tested in Vero. The titres for CA24 tested in Hela was 80 to 160 compared to 10 to 20 for strains tested in Vero.

OTHER DIAGNOSTIC TESTS

Metabolic-inhibition test in microtitration plates was satisfactorily used for CA24 and E70 investigations (15). Preliminary test on a few sera showed the indirect fluorescent antibody technique to be applicable for serodiagnosis of CA24 and E70 infections.

SUMMARY AND CONCLUSIONS

A review of our study on viral epidemic conjunctivitis from 1970 to 1980 is given.

Ophthalmologists in Singapore were unable to differentiate conjunctivitis caused by CA24, E70 and AV11 clinically. Subconjunctival haemorrhage was seen in only 6-11% of cases during our epidemics compared to 50-100% in some African and Asian countries. This prompted investigators to name the new ocular disease "Acute Haemorrhagic Conjunctivitis" or AHC (11, 16-18). It must, however, be noted that apart from CA24 and E70, AV11 (8,19), AV4 (20) and AV19 (21) have also been implicated in epidemics of AHC where subconjunctival haemorrhage was a prominent feature. We would prefer the term "Picornavirus Epidemic Conjunctivitis" or PEC where an enterovirus etiology is confirmed.

For primary isolation, CA24 and E70 show preference for cells of human to cells of simian origin. Once established in human cell cultures, some strains of CA24 and E70 grow readily in simian cells. It was noted that CA24 and E70 originally grown in Hela when passaged to simian cells undergo antigenic changes which rendered the simian cell-derived virus poorly neutralized by homologous antiserum prepared with the virus grown in Hela.

Micrometabolic-inhibition and indirect fluorescent antibody tests were used for PEC investigations.

ACKNOWLEDGMENTS

We wish to extend our gratitude to doctors in the Government Outpatient Services, the Ministry of Health and Epidemiology Department, Ministry of Environment, for providing us with patients and statistical information. Also to Mrs. Chua Puay Hong for years of dedicated technical assistance.

REFERENCES

1. Lim, K.H., and Yin-Murphy, M., *Singapore Med. J. 12,* 247 (1971).
2. Yin-Murphy, M., *Southeast Asian J. Trop. Med. Pub. Hlth. 3,* 303 (1972).

3. Mirkovic, R.R., Schmidt, N.J., Yin-Murphy, M., and Melnick, J.L., *Intervirology 4,* 119 (1974).
4. Yin-Murphy, M., and Lim, K.H., *Lancet,* 857 (1972).
5. Yin-Murphy, M., and Lim, K.H., *Lancet,* 545 (1973).
6. Yin-Murphy, M., *Southeast Asian J. Trop. Med. Pub. Hlth. 4,* 11 (1973).
7. Mirkovic, R.R., Kono, R., Yin-Murphy, M., Sohier, R., Schmidt, N.J., and Melnick, J.L., *Bull. Wld. Hlth. Org. 49,* 341 (1973).
8. Yin-Murphy, M., and Lim, K.H., *Southeast Asian J. Trop. Med. Pub. Hlth. 5,* 333 (1974).
9. Yin-Murphy, M., Lim, K.H., and Ho, Y.M., *Southeast Asian J. Trop. Med. Pub. Hlth. 7,* 1 (1976).
10. Goh, K.T., Doraisingham, S., and Yin-Murphy, M., *Southeast Asian J. Trop. Med. Pub. Hlth.,* in press.
11. Kono, R., Sasagawa, A., Ishii, K., Sugiura, S., Ochi, M., Matsumiya, H., Uchida, Y., Komeyama, K., and Kaneko, M., *Lancet,* 1191 (1972).
12. Chomel, J.J., Gaudin, O.G., Nejmi, S., and Sohier, R., *Nonv. Presse Med. 2,* 1781 (1973).
13. Higgins, P.G., and Scott, R.J.D., *J. Clin. Path. 26,* 706 (1973).
14. Higgins, P.G., Scott, R.H., Davies, P.M., and Gamble, D.R., *J. Clin. Path. 27,* 292 (1974).
15. Yin-Murphy, M., *Bull. Wld. Hlth. Org. 54,* 675 (1976).
16. Chatterjee, S., Quarcoopme, C.O., and Apenteng, A., *Ghana Med. J. 9,* 9 (1970).
17. Parrot, W.F., *Practitioner 206,* 253 (1971).
18. Pramanik, D.D., *Practitioner 207,* 805 (1971).
19. Tai, F.H., Lin, H.M., Chu, S., Wei, H.Y., and Hierholzer, J.C., *Chinese J. Microbiol. 7,* 79 (1974).
20. Muzzi, A., Rochi, G., Lumbroso, B., Tosato, G., and Barbieri, F., *Lancet 2,* 822 (1975).
21. Taylor, J.W., Chandler, J.W., and Cooney, M.K., *New Engl. J. Med. 292,* 978 (1975).

AN OUTBREAK OF ACUTE MYOCARDITIS ASSOCIATED WITH COXSACKIE A9 VIRUS IN ADULTS

Su Chengqin
Qin Tiansheng
Zhou Dejiu
Chen Chunzhi

Institute of Medical Biology
Chinese Academy of Medical Sciences
Kunming, Yunan, China

In July 1978, two workers in a forest field in Southwestern China died suddenly of unknown cause. A few days later, a number of other workers from the same field complained of headache, weakness, precordial oppression, tachycardia and abnormal ECG with sudden onset. These patients were diagnosed clinically and epidemiologically as acute myocarditis. Faecal and serum specimens were collected from the patients and some of their close contacts for virological and serological studies one and six weeks after the outbreak.

Virus isolation results and the prognosis for 12 patients are shown in Table I. All the patients were adults, male and female. The ECG abnormality lasted at least 6 weeks in half of the patients. Coxsackie A9 virus was isolated from 5 out of 12 patients. In addition, 11 isolates of coxsackie A9 were obtained from 18 contacts (8 adults and 10 children). The total isolation rate was 53.3% (Table II). The highest virus isolation rate was observed from the children contact group (80%), but none of the children were ill. The reason for this is unknown. Coxsackie A9 virus could not be detected six weeks after the outbreak, although other enteroviruses were isolated both from the epidemic and neighbouring non-epidemic forest fields.

A serological study of the 12 patients is shown in Table III. From the serological and virus isolation results,

VIRAL DISEASES IN SOUTH-EAST ASIA AND THE WESTERN PACIFIC
ISBN 0 12 484820 6

TABLE I. Virus Isolation and Prognosis of 12 Patients Suffering from Acute Myocarditis

Case number	Sex	Age (years)	Severity	Virus isolation	Prognosis
1	M	24	Severe	-	Good
2	M	25	Severe	-	Abnormal ECG
3	F	27	Mild	Cox. A9	Good
4	M	28	Mild	Cox. A9	Abnormal ECG
5	M	27	Severe	Cox. A9	Good
6	M	24	Severe	-	Good
7	M	29	Mild	-	Good
8	M	31	Mild	-	Abnormal ECG
9	F	24	Mild	Cox. A9	Good
10	M	24	Mild	Cox. A9	Abnormal ECG
11	F	30	Mild	-	Abnormal ECG
12	M	26	Mild	-	Abnormal ECG

7 patients were diagnosed from laboratory evidence as suffering from coxsackie A9 virus infection.

The virological and serological results from 8 adult contacts are shown in Table IV. Low titre neutralizing antibodies were found in the paired sera of 3 out of 8 contacts, but there was no increase in titre during the epidemic, nor was virus isolated. Virus was isolated from 2 contacts, but they did not exhibit an antibody rise in their paired sera. In one contact, virus was isolated and the contact exhibited a significant rise in titre. All of these contacts were free from symptoms of acute myocarditis, and they may have been healthy virus carriers or suffering from an inapparent infection.

TABLE II. Virus Isolation from the Patients and Their Close Contacts

Group	Number in group	Number of positive Coxsackie A9 isolations	% virus isolation
Patient	12	5	41.6
Adult contact	8	3	37.5
Child contact	10	8	80.0
Total	30	16	53.3

TABLE III. Increase of Neutralizing Antibodies to Coxsackie A9 Virus and Virus isolation in 12 Cases of Acute Myocarditis

Case No.	Acute phase antibody titre	Convalescent phase antibody titre	Coxsackie A9 isolation	Laboratory diagnosis
1	1:10	1:20	-	-
2	<1:5	1:10	-	Cox.A9 infection
3	1:10	1:160	+	Cox.A9 infection
4	1:20	1:20	+	Cox.A9 infection
5	1:20	1:20	+	Cox.A9 infection
6	1:20	1:20	-	-
7	1:40	1:40	-	-
8	1:5	1:40	-	Cox.A9 infection
9	<1:5	1:80	+	Cox.A9 infection
10	<1:5	1:320	+	Cox.A9 infection
11	1:5	1:5	-	-
12	<1:5	1:5	-	-

From the above data, coxsackie A9 virus may have been the causative agent of the outbreak of acute myocarditis in the forest field. This is the first time that coxsackie A9 virus has been associated with acute myocarditis in adults in China.

TABLE IV. Neutralizing Antibody Titres to Coxsackie A9 Virus and Virus Isolation in 8 Adult Contacts

Contact number	Titre in first serum sample	Titre in second serum sample	Coxsackie A9 virus isolation
1	1:5	1:5	-
2	1:5	1:5	-
3	<1:5	<1:5	+
4	<1:5	<1:5	-
5	<1:5	<1:5	+
6	<1:5	<1:5	-
7	<1:5	1:320	+
8	1:10	1:10	-

Part VI
Specific Viral Diseases

D.
Arboviruses

Chairman Natth Bhamarapravati

Co-Chairman I. D. Marshall

65

ARBOVIRUS INFECTIONS OTHER THAN DENGUE IN THE WESTERN PACIFIC AND SOUTH-EAST ASIAN AREAS

R. L. Doherty

Faculty of Medicine
University of Queensland
Brisbane, Queensland

I. INTRODUCTION

Arthropod-borne viruses (arboviruses) cause several major diseases of man in the western Pacific and south-east Asian regions, notably Japanese encephalitis, Murray Valley encephalitis, chikungunya and epidemic polyarthritis, as well as dengue, discussed in a separate chapter. Arboviruses are less prominent in these regions as causes of disease in domestic animals, although bovine ephemeral fever has been important in some countries and bluetongue virus has been described in Japan and Australia. The extensive clinical and research literature on arbovirus disease in Asia and the Pacific was reviewed and summarised by successive World Health Organisation seminars and Pacific Science Congress symposia, and several textbook or monograph treatments are available (1-3). Japanese encephalitis is important over a wide arc of Asia from Siberia through Korea, Japan, mainland China, Taiwan, Indochina to India in the west and Indonesia in the south. Murray Valley encephalitis causes periodic epidemics in Australia and sporadic cases in New Guinea. Chikungunya virus causes dengue-like fever in south-east Asia and antibody distribution suggests its occurrence in Indonesia. Ross River virus is accepted as the cause of epidemic polyarthritis in Australia and New Guinea. Many other viruses have been isolated and are under investigation as possible causes of disease.

VIRAL DISEASES IN SOUTH-EAST ASIA
AND THE WESTERN PACIFIC
ISBN 0 12 484820 6

Early work also defined key problems in the epidemiology of these major diseases, notably the mechanisms of survival between epidemics (e.g. in the case of Murray Valley encephalitis) or over winter (e.g. in the case of Japanese encephalitis in Japan and Taiwan) and the basis for the territorial distribution of arboviruses (e.g. in the apparent boundary between the distributions of Japanese encephalitis and Murray Valley encephalitis viruses).

This paper will not attempt to repeat what is readily available in standard reviews. Instead it will deal in brief and selective fashion with recent additions to our knowledge of these diseases, and attempt to indicate at least some directions of progress.

II. ARBOVIRUSES OF SOUTH-EAST ASIA AND THE WESTERN PACIFIC

There has been a notable increase in the number of arboviruses known in these regions. The 1980 Annual Report on the Catalogue of Arthropod-Borne Viruses, for example, listed 42 viruses as initially isolated in eastern Asia (9 in Japan, 14 in Malaysia, 16 in the eastern U.S.S.R., and 1 each in Cambodia, Singapore and Thailand), 47 in Australia, New Zealand or the Pacific Islands (41 in Australia, 2 in the Philippines and 1 each in Hawaii, New Zealand, Johnston Island and New Guinea), 23 in India and 3 in Pakistan (4). The total list of viruses active in the area is obviously greater as some arboviruses active and important in the regions (e.g. Sindbis, Zika, chikungunya, and Wesselbron) were initially isolated elsewhere. A substantial part of the increase in numbers follows research focussed on specific areas - for example, on island bird-tick-virus ecosystems pioneered by Lvov and colleagues in the eastern U.S.S.R. and extended by others elsewhere, and on biting midges and livestock in Australia. "New" viruses discovered in these studies have been important subjects of research, as possible causes of disease in their own right and also as sources of data for considerations of virus distribution and evolution.

III. DISTRIBUTION OF DISEASE

The incidence and pattern of arbovirus disease have changed in recent years in a number of areas. For example,

Japanese encephalitis was responsible for as many as 8,000 cases a year in Japan in large epidemics of 1924, 1935 and 1948 but for 84 cases with 25 deaths in 1979 and 39 cases with 15 deaths in 1980 (5). In contrast the disease has continued at stable levels in Korea and has shown increased incidence with recurrent epidemics in Thailand (especially in the Chiang Mai Valley), Burma and India where outbreaks from 1973 to 1979 in West Bengal were well documented by Indian workers (6, 7). Murray Valley encephalitis has continued its previous pattern of periodic summer/autumn epidemics in eastern Australia, although the epidemic of 1974 had an unprecedentedly wide distribution involving Central Australia and north and east-central Queensland as well as the traditional Murray-Darling basin of south-east Australia (8). Cases also occurred in that year in north-western Australia and several epidemics have occurred there more recently. Work by Stanley and colleagues suggests that Murray Valley encephalitis virus is now enzootic in the man-made water catchments of the Ord River area, with seasonal epizootic and epidemic spread into the Kimberleys-Pilbara areas, with infection as far south as Geraldton (9). The recent occurrence of chikungunya in Asia, since a series of epidemics in Thailand, Vietnam, Cambodia, Burma and India in the 1960s, has not been well documented. The related Ross River virus has been established as an important cause of epidemic polyarthritis in summer and autumn over much of Australia. Ross River virus made a much publicized irruption into the Pacific with outbreaks in Fiji, Samoa and other islands in 1979 and 1980 (10). The scattered literature does not allow any statement on changes in incidence of endemic tick-borne virus infections such as Kyasanur forest disease, tick-borne encephalitis, or Omsk haemorrhagic fever, but cases continue to occur and come under investigation.

IV. EPIDEMIOLOGY

There has been important progress in studies of the basic epidemiology of several major virus diseases. Early studies by Japanese and American workers on Japanese encephalitis showed the importance of birds, pigs and culicine mosquitoes in the epidemic spread of the virus, but left unsolved the question of how virus survives the temperate zone winter in Japan. Various possibilities, in most cases initially considered for comparable over-wintering problems in North America, were suggested as applicable in Japan: for example, prolonged or recurrent viraemia in poikilothermic animals such as reptiles, and reintroduction of virus from warmer areas by bird movement. In Australia early workers suggested that Murray Valley encephalitis virus survived in northern Australia in cycles involving birds and mosquitoes and was introduced into south-east Australia, where most epidemics have occurred, by the movement of birds at times of abnormal spring rainfall. The discovery by American workers of the importance of transovarial transmission in the mosquito in the survival of California encephalitis virus has led to further examination of this mechanism for other viruses (11). Rosen and his colleagues have demonstrated transovarial transmission of Japanese encephalitis in *Aedes albopictus* and *Aedes togoi* (12). Kay has shown transovarial transmission of Murray Valley encephalitis virus in experimentally infected *Aedes aegypti* (13). Several workers have seen transovarial transmission as a mechanism that might account for such findings as high virus isolation rates from mosquitoes with brief population peaks from the hatching of drought resistant eggs (for example, *Aedes normanensis* in Queensland) and for the survival of Ross River virus in temperate areas (as demonstrated, for example, in its recent discovery in Tasmania) (14,15). Kay points out (13) technical problems in confirming that a mechanism shown to occur in laboratory systems is important under natural conditions, but it can be anticipated that intensive research efforts will be directed to this question.

Studies of the epidemiology of vector-borne diseases such as malaria were facilitated by sets of mathematical models which could be applied to quantitative data. Arbovirus workers have had difficulty in applying similar quantitative approaches to the complex ecosystems with which they deal. Some important recent progress deserves comment. Wada developed mathematical models that related incidence of Japanese encephalitis in an epidemic to various parameters of mosquito population density, age and infection rate (16). He was able to calculate threshold levels of mosquito population at which transmission ceased, and found threshold density particularly sensitive to changes in mosquito survival rate. Kay in Australia attempted to apply Wada's techniques and approach to Murray Valley encephalitis, using a mass of data on mosquito population density, age, infection rate and blood meal origin (17). His conclusions were very tentative because of limitations in knowledge of the vertebrate hosts of the virus and their immunological response, and because his data included only a small number of isolations of Murray Valley encephalitis virus. Nevertheless he found a high correlation between the product of measures of population density and age of *Culex annulirostris* with arbovirus isolation rate at two centres in Queensland in 1974 to 1976. These two studies have obvious relevance to prediction and control of epidemics, and it is to be hoped they will be extended.

Workers on arbovirus epidemiology in Asia and the Pacific have also been influenced by studies of vector competence carried out by Reeves and colleagues in California, with their important relevance to possible genetic control as well as to clearer understanding of the epidemiology of arbovirus disease (18). Tesh and colleagues found geographic strains of *Aedes albopictus* to vary in susceptibility to infection with chikungunya virus (19). Kay found several geographic strains of *Culex annulirostris* to show equal and high susceptibility to Murray Valley encephalitis, but some heterogeneity to Kunjin virus. For that virus colonies of *C. annulirostris* from Mildura, Townsville and Cairns had greater competence than populations from Charleville, Darwin or Brisbane (21).

V. BIOCHEMISTRY

There has been very major progress in the last decade in our understanding of the biochemistry of viruses and virus infection. Research on the arboviruses undoubtedly gained from the availability of a rational classification and nomenclature of viruses based on structural and biochemical characteristics. The gathering together of ungrouped and minor group viruses about which little was known except their exotic names, and their incorporation into defined families and genera must ultimately lead to unifying insights into questions of clinical response, pathogenesis and epidemiology. This process may perhaps be exemplified by the changing concepts we have of the orbiviruses in Australia, allowing discussion of recent bluetongue isolates to proceed in the context of the coexistence of a range of other antigenically and epidemiologically distinguishable orbiviruses in Australia (21). Detailed biochemical studies of virus-coded proteins and nucleic acids are being applied increasingly to intratypic and intertypic virus comparisons (for example, to the distinction between geographically diverse strains of Sindbis virus) (22). Initial studies of arbovirus biochemistry were largely restricted to a small set of laboratory adapted types, not known to cause disease. An important exception to that is the work of Westaway and his colleagues on Kunjin and Murray Valley encephalitis viruses (23,24). Their discovery of internal initiation of translation in those viruses make the flaviviruses among the most interesting of the animal viruses and have yet to be taken into full account in virus classification. Future developments of arbovirus biochemistry, especially with the application of techniques such as monoclonal antibodies and recombinant DNA cloning of defined portions of the genome, clearly have enormous potential for progress in both basic and applied research, for example by providing highly specific diagnostic and survey probes and more highly purified antigens and vaccines.

VI. PATHOGENESIS

Viruses active in the Pacific and south-east Asia pose such classic problems of virus pathogenesis as why viraemic infection may only very rarely cause involvement of target organs such as brain or joints. Recent progress on the pathogenesis of the viruses under review suffers perhaps from comparison with the controversial and provocative findings on dengue haemorrhagic fever discussed elsewhere. However, findings of some interest have been published on the Australian disease, epidemic polyarthritis. Australian workers have, since the isolation of Ross River virus gave them specific diagnostic tests, puzzled over the age and sex distribution of epidemic polyarthritis, with few cases in children and the highest incidence in young adult women (25). This, plus the fact that antibody was detectable in most "acute" sera early in disease, suggested that the actual disease might be caused by the immunological response to infection rather than by infection itself. Fraser, Aaskov and their colleagues have studied a number of cases with results which do not indicate an immunological basis for disease (26,27). Involved joints show a mononuclear cell response, with viral antigen detectable in monocytes and macrophages of some cases early in the course of illness. No cell-associated C3 component of complement or immunoglobulin was detected in any cell type. The authors are cautious in drawing conclusions but the results clearly suggest that epidemic polyarthritis, like rubella, is a direct response to viral infection of joint endothelium, and that the observed age and sex incidence still awaits explanation.

The discovery by Rosen and colleagues of direct inoculation of mosquitoes as a sensitive method of virus isolation (28) may also provide important new information in studies of pathogenesis, especially perhaps in detection and quantitation of viraemia masked to other isolation techniques by antibody. The reported high virus titres in a case of epidemic polyarthritis in a Pacific island outbreak, for example, is in contrast to the difficulty that Australian workers found in isolating viruses from clinical cases of that disease (29)

VII. BIOGEOGRAPHY AND EVOLUTION

As records of virus isolation and serological surveys accumulate, arbovirus workers are inevitably led to consider the origins and evolution of the viruses they study. Theiler and Downs in 1973 analysed the biogeographical distribution of some 279 viruses, known or suspected to be arboviruses (30). Over 240 were restricted to one of the classic zoogeographic regions as defined by Darlington, with the Oriental and Australasian regions, our main areas of concern to-day, accounting for only 56 agents at that time. A paper presented to a Pacific Science Congress in 1966 speculated that the antigenic gradients shown in such virus sequences as West Nile - Kunjin - Murray Valley encephalitis, Sindbis - Whataroa, and chikungunya - Getah - Ross River virus might all result from evolutionary relationships (31). Later it was suggested that viruses of the Simbu and Palyam groups, isolated in Australia and closely related antigenically to viruses in Africa or southern Asia, might, with their vector *Culicoides brevitarsis* and vertebrate hosts, cattle, horses and sheep, have been imported to Australia in the last century (32). Those viruses were contrasted with a number of other Australian viruses unrelated to agents overseas and, by data available at the time, making use of hosts and vectors with long evolutionary associations with the Australian continent. Serious gaps in knowledge made such speculations insecure then, and that insecurity remains in spite of important recent developments. Surveys by Tesh and Kanemitsu confirm the Wallace/Weber lines between the Oriental and Australasian regions as an area of discontinuity for arboviruses as for other biota (33,34).

The discovery of several bluetongue virus types in Australia gave some economic and political urgency to questions about the origins of arboviruses infecting introduced domestic mammals. A first reaction was to see the presence of bluetongue in Australia as being compatible with, although to some extent qualifying, a comment made in 1972 (32) that, if the hypothesis about the introduction of Simbu group viruses with *Culicoides* in cattle into Australia was correct, "then it is clearly a matter of good fortune to Australia that agents of serious veterinary disease were not imported in the same way." Meticulous and extensive studies of the epidemiology of the bluetongue strains in Australia by St George, Standfast, Dyce and colleagues at CSIRO and of their biochemistry by Gorman and his colleagues at QIMR have shown a complex situation which does not fit easily with that simplistic comment. Gorman could find no significant homology by RNA/RNA reassociation between the genome of bluetongue type 20 isolated in Australia and representative serotypes isolated in other geographic regions, and interprets the results as suggesting sequence divergence between geographically isolated viruses and not the recent introduction of the bluetongue virus into Australia (35). The CSIRO workers find that, although *Culicoides brevitarsis* may act as a relatively inefficient vector of bluetongue in Australia, the major vector is likely to be an as yet unnamed *Culicoides* of the subgenus *Avaritia* (36). This would indicate a fortunate finding for Australia, in that *brevitarsis* has a southern range well into the limits of the Australian sheep population, whereas the unnamed *Avaritia* is so far restricted to the north of Northern Territory and Queensland, in keeping with the distribution of antibody in cattle to the bluetongue type 20. More recent work still, with the isolation of two further strains of bluetongue, one antigenically typed as bluetongue type 1, and with antibodies in cattle extending further south, raises further biogeographic problems which must, at some time be addressed (37).

The islands and environs of the Pacific have been important in the history of biogeography and will continue to offer opportunities for students of the arboviruses. It will, for example, be of much interest to monitor the future of Ross River virus in the Pacific islands in which it has recently been epidemic. Will it be possible, for example, to follow the rate of genetic and antigenic change in an isolated island situation? Such data would certainly assist us to interpret findings such as those of

Marshall and his colleagues on the variant of Ross River virus they have detected at Nelson Bay on coastal New South Wales. There are, similarly, opportunities for basic studies of arbovirus survival and variation in the bird/tick ecosystems of the Sea of Okhotsk, the Pacific islands and the sub-antarctic.

VIII. CONCLUSION

I conclude that there has been substantial progress in our understanding of the arbovirus infections of the Pacific and south-east Asia, although major questions of survival and spread remain unsolved and many gaps in our knowledge remain obvious. There has been enormous benefit from the international collaboration and exchange of knowledge that has grown from the establishment by the World Health Organisation of its chain of reference and collaborating centres, and by activities of the American Committee on Arthropod-Borne Viruses which established and maintained the Arbovirus Catalogue and Information Exchange. The most obvious directions in the immediate future are for the explosive growth of basic studies of the biochemistry and immunology of arbovirus infections to be applied to the unsolved questions of pathogenesis and epidemiology.

REFERENCES

1. Beran, G.W., ed. "Viral Zoonoses", CRC Handbook Series in Zoonoses, Section B: Volume 1. CRC Press, Boca Raton (1981).
2. Doherty, R.L., *in* "Infectious Diseases" (P. Hoeprich, ed.), p.919. Harper and Row, Hagerstown, 2nd edition, (1977).
3. Feigin, R.D., and Cherry, J.D., eds. "Textbook of Paediatric Infectious Diseases". W.B. Saunders, Philadelphia (1981).
4. Subcommittee on Information Exchange of The American Committee on Arthropod-borne Viruses, Personal communication, (1981).
5. Okuno, T., *World Health Statistical Q. 31*, 120 (1978).
6. Banerjee, K., Sen Gupta, S.N., Dandawate, C.N., Tongaonkor, S.S., and Gupta, N.P., *Ind. J. med. Res. 64*, 121 (1976).

7. Ming, C. K., Swe, T., Thaung, U. and Lwin, T. T., *S.E. Asia J. trop. Med. publ. Hlth. 8*, 113 (1977).
8. Doherty, R. L., Carley, J. G., Filippich, C., White, J., and Gust, I. D., *Aust. N.Z. J. Med. 6*, 446 (1976).
9. Stanley, N. F., personal communication (1981).
10. Center for Disease Control, *Morbidity and Mortality Weekly Reports 28*, 323 (1979).
11. Beaty, B.J., and Thompson, W.H., *Am. J. trop. Med. Hyg. 24*, 685 (1975).
12. Rosen, L., Tesh, R. B., Lien, J. C., and Cross, J. H., *Science 199*, 909 (1978).
13. Kay, B. H., and Carley, J. G., *Aust. J. exp. Biol. med. Sci. 58*, 501 (1980).
14. Doherty, R. L., Carley, J. G., Kay, B. H., Filippich, C., Marks, E. N., and Frazier, C. L., *Aust. J. exp. Biol. med. Sci. 57*, 509 (1979).
15. Mudge, P. R., McColl, D., and Sutton, D., *Med. J. Aust. 2*, 256 (1981).
16. Wada, Y., Oda, T., Mogi, M., Mori, A., Omori, N., Fukumi, H., Hayashi, K., Mifume, K., Shichijo, A., and Matsuo, S., *Trop. Med. 17*, 111 (1975).
17. Kay, B. H., *Aust. J. exp. Biol. med. Sci. 58*,67 (1980).
18. Hardy, J. L., Reeves, W. C., and Sjogren, R. O., *Am. J. Epidemiol. 103*, 498 (1976).
19. Tesh, R. B., Gubler, D. J., and Rosen, L., *Am. J. trop. Med. Hyg. 25*, 326 (1976).
20. Kay, B. H., Carley, J. G., Fanning, I. D., and Filippich, C., *J. med. Entomol. 16*, 59 (1979).
21. Gorman, B. M., *J. gen. Virol. 44*, 1 (1979).
22. Rentier - Delrue, F., and Young, N. A., *Virology 106*, 59 (1980).
23. Westaway, E. G., *J. gen. Virol. 27*, 283 (1975).
24. Westaway, E. G., *Virology 80*, 320 (1977).
25. Doherty, R. L., Barrett, E. J., Gorman, B. M., and Whitehead, R. H., *Med. J. Aust. 1*, 5 (1971).
26. Fraser, J. R. E., Cunningham, A. L., Clarris, B. J., Aaskov, J. G., and Leach, R., *Aust. N.Z. J. Med. 11*, 168 (1981).
27. Fraser, J. R. E., Tait, B., Aaskov, J. G., Cunningham, A. L., *Aust. N.Z. J. Med. 10*, 597 (1980).
28. Rosen, L., and Gubler, D., *Am. J. trop. Med. Hyg. 23*, 1153 (1974).
29. Tesh, R. B., McLean, R. G., Shroyer, D. A., Calisher, C. H., and Rosen, L., *Trans. R. Soc. trop. Med. Hyg. 75*, 426 (1981).

30. Theiler, M., and Downs, W. G., "The Arthropod-Borne Viruses of Vertebrates", p.341. Yale University Press, New Haven and London (1973).
31. Doherty, R. L., *Jap. J. med. Sci. Biol. 20* (Suppl.), 10 (1967).
32. Doherty, R. L., *Aust. Vet. J. 48*, 172 (1972).
33. Tesh, R. B., Gajdusek, D. C., Garruto, R. M., Cross, J. H., and Rosen, L., *Am. J. trop. Med. Hyg. 24*, 664 (1975).
34. Kanemitsu, M., Taniguchi, K., Urasawa, S., Ogata, T., Wada, Y., Wada, Y., and Saroso, J. S., *Am. J. trop. Med. Hyg. 28*, 351 (1979).
35. Gorman, B. M., Taylor, J., Walker, P. J., Davidson, W. L., and Brown, F., *J. gen. Virol.*, in press.
36. Standfast, H. A., Dyce, A. L., St George, T. D., Cybinski, D. H., and Muller, M. J. in "Arbovirus Research in Australia", Proc. 2nd symposium (T. D. St George, ed.), p.20. CSIRO Division of Animal Health and Queensland Institute of Medical Research, Brisbane (1979).
37. Della-Porta, A. J., McPhee, D. A., Wark, M. C., St George T. D., and Cybinski, D. H., *Vet. Microbiol. 6*, 233 (1980).

66

DENGUE - AN OVERVIEW[1]

Leon Rosen

Arbovirus Program
Pacific Biomedical Research Center
University of Hawaii at Manoa
Honolulu, Hawaii

I assume that most of you are familiar to some extent with the epidemiology and clinical manifestations of dengue and consequently I will use my limited time to review only the significant developments that have occurred within the last five years. In doing so, I will divide the subject matter into four parts. First, epidemiology; second, laboratory technology; third, pathogenesis of severe and fatal disease; and fourth, prevention.

To set the stage, I should like to point out that the four dengue viruses as a group are currently by far the most important viruses transmitted to man by arthropods - whether judged in terms of the number of human infections or the number of human deaths. Moreover, in recent years the incidence of disease caused by these viruses has increased enormously because of increased growth and urbanization of populations in tropical areas and increased frequency and speed of human travel.

EPIDEMIOLOGY

Among recent epidemiologic events in Asia and the Pacific was the introduction of dengue type 4 to Tahiti in 1979 (1) and its subsequent dissemination to a large number

[1]*Supported in part by NIH grants AI 17995 and AI 17953*

VIRAL DISEASES IN SOUTH-EAST ASIA
AND THE WESTERN PACIFIC
ISBN 0 12 484820 6

of other island territories in the South Pacific. This was the first known occurrence of dengue type 4 virus outside of Southeast Asia and was the third dengue serotype introduced and widely disseminated on Pacific islands in the last 10 years. The others were type 2 in 1971 and type 1 in 1974. Other noteworthy events were the large epidemic of dengue type 4 in the Foshan District of Guangdong Province in southern China in 1978 (2) and the epidemics of dengue type 3 in Guangxi Province and Hainan Island, also in southern China, in 1980 (3,4). These were the first known epidemics of dengue in China since World War II.

Turning to the Western Hemisphere, recent events there include the introduction and subsequent dissemination in the Caribbean area and northern South America of dengue type 1 in 1977 (5) and dengue type 4 in 1981 (6). Dengue types 2 and 3 were already present in these areas. The most significant event in the region, however, was the occurrence in 1981 of approximately 400,000 cases of dengue in Cuba with more than 150 deaths (7). This epidemic is said to have been caused by dengue type 2 and represents the first known epidemic of the severe and fatal form of the disease in the Western Hemisphere - though at least one isolated case had been documented previously (8).

Perhaps the most important recent observations on the epidemiology of dengue have been made in West Africa - but this time not in an urban setting. In 1980, approximately 60 strains of dengue type 2 virus were isolated from 4 species of sylvatic mosquitoes generally considered the primary sylvatic vectors of yellow fever in that part of the world (9). These were *Aedes africanus, Aedes luteocephalus, Aedes opok,* and *Aedes* of the *furcifer-taylori* group. The isolates were obtained from mosquitoes captured in the Ivory Coast and in Upper Volta. A previous isolation of dengue type 2 had been made from *Ae. luteocephalus* in Senegal in 1974 (10) but was generally ignored because its unique nature raised the suspicion that it might have been a laboratory error. The new findings on dengue from Africa along with the single isolate of dengue type 4 from a forest-canopy mosquito species (*Aedes niveus* group) in Malaysia (11) lend support to the concept that a sylvatic cycle of dengue, analogous to that of yellow fever, may exist both in Asia and Africa. Thus, *Aedes aegypti*-transmitted dengue, though obviously of importance for human pathology, may, from a biologic point of view, be a relatively new and unimportant phase of the natural history of dengue viruses. It is quite possible, for example, that the 4 dengue serotypes originated in different geographic areas or in association with different mosquito species and now occur together in large urban areas only because of the fortuitous dissemination of a suitable vector, *Ae. aegypti*, and the movement of human populations. It should be remembered that *Ae. aegypti* is of African origin and has been disseminated throughout the world only relatively recently by human activity. It is also pertinent to point out that, in historical terms, humans have lived in large groups in close proximity to one another only relatively recently.

The isolation of dengue viruses from forest mosquitoes does not by itself provide an explanation for the long-term persistence of such viruses unless transovarial transmission occurs in those species or another as yet unknown mechanism exists for viral survival. In many areas of West Africa the populations of forest primates are too small and too isolated to explain the maintenance of virus on the basis of primate transmission analogous to the person to person transmission cycle in large urban areas.

Our laboratory has been working on transovarial transmission of dengue viruses in mosquitoes for the last five years and has demonstrated such transmission for each of the 4 serotypes in *Aedes albopictus* mosquitoes (12). It is of interest that as much as a 10-fold variation in transovarial transmission rates has been observed among different strains of *Ae. albopictus* and variations of comparable magnitude among different strains of the same dengue serotype. Recently, we have turned our attention to studies of transovarial transmission in *Ae. aegypti* and other species of *Aedes (Stegomyia)* mosquitoes incriminated as vectors of dengue. We were surprised to observe very little transovarial transmission in *Ae. aegypti* and much higher rates in some other *Aedes* as compared with *Ae. albopictus*.

TECHNOLOGY

There is a great deal of good news to report with respect to dengue virus technology. As many of you know, in the past dengue viruses have been among the most difficult to isolate and propagate in the laboratory. New developments have changed the situation so that these viruses now are as easy to detect and propagate as almost any other virus. The techniques employed are intrathoracic inoculation of mosquitoes (13), especially the large non-blood-feeding *Toxorhynchites* (14), and the use of cloned mosquito cell cultures, especially the C6/36 clone of *Ae. albopictus* cells (15). The high yield of virus from the latter cells - even when inoculated with unpassaged field material - has made possible the "fingerprinting" of dengue virus RNA (16). The latter technique has already been utilized for epidemiologic purposes and it has been demonstrated that dengue type 2 strains can be subgrouped on the basis of their origin with respect to time and place (17). Finally, with respect to technology I am happy to say that type-specific monoclonal antibodies have been produced for each of the dengue types (18). These can be used in the indirect fluorescent antibody procedure to type dengue viruses either in crushed mosquito tissue or cell cultures. Only those who have struggled with the identification of the cross-reacting dengue viruses in the past can fully appreciate the value of this development.

PATHOGENESIS

As many of you know, there is disagreement about the pathogenesis of the severe and fatal forms of dengue. Basically, the difference of opinion is about whether it is the virus or the host which plays the more important role in determining the clinical expression of infection. More specifically, the divergence of opinion concerns the validity of the sequential infection hypothesis. This hypothesis holds that a dengue infection constitutes a "risk factor" for development of dengue hemorrhagic fever or dengue shock syndrome in the event of a subsequent infection with another dengue serotype. The issue is of more than academic interest because of its relevance to decisions concerning the use of dengue vaccines.

I last had the opportunity to discuss the evidence for the sequential infection hypothesis about 5 years ago and at that time entitled my talk "The Emperor's New Clothes revisited" to indicate my doubt about its validity (19). In the interim, no further epidemiologic studies have been published in support of the hypothesis and, consequently, I have no reason now to be less sceptical than before. One thing that has become clear in the meantime, however, is that a second dengue infection is not a necessary condition for the development of the dengue shock syndrome in persons over the age of 1 year. This has now been documented beyond question for at least dengue types 1, 2, and 3 (20). It has long been known that practically all cases of dengue shock syndrome in persons less than 1 year of age were the result of primary infections. It could hardly be otherwise! Thus, the basic question no longer is, "Can dengue shock syndrome occur with primary dengue infections in persons older than 1 year of age?" but, rather, "Is there increased risk of dengue shock syndrome with a second dengue infection?"

One of the difficulties in evaluating the sequential infection hypothesis is that neither the necessary sequence of dengue serotypes nor the interval between them has ever been specified. Consequently, whenever field observations are made on sequential infections that do not lead to unusual pathogenicity, as they have during many recent island epidemics in the Pacific and Caribbean, it can always be said that the sequence of infecting dengue serotypes or the interval between them were not those which lead to increased pathogenicity.

Those who believe that the sequential infection hypothesis is valid have had the problem of accounting for the fact that practically all cases of dengue shock syndrome in children less than 1 year of age were the result of primary infections. This apparent paradox has now been "explained" by a further hypothesis, that of "immune enhancement" (21). This hypothesis holds that dengue virus replication is enhanced *in vivo*, and pathogenicity consequently augmented, by the presence of either passively or actively acquired antibody of a critical concentration. Dengue shock patients less than 1 year of age presumably have passively acquired maternal antibody and older patients have actively acquired antibody from a previous dengue infection.

It has been shown that when small amounts of flavivirus antibody are added to dengue type 2 virus in cell cultures *in vitro*, an increase in viral yield occurs as compared to control cultures without antibody (22). This occurs with a wide variety of flavivirus antibodies and has not been shown to be more characteristic of, or specific to, the dengue group of viruses. Consequently, if the immune enhancement hypothesis is valid, any prior flavivirus infection, including yellow fever vaccination, could potentially increase the risk of dengue shock syndrome.

One of the factors which led to the development of the immune enhancement hypothesis was the observation that monkeys secondarily infected with dengue type 2 had higher peak viremias than those undergoing primary infections (23). The average duration of the secondary infection type 2 viremias, however, was less than in the primary infections. In the same set of experiments, peak viremias for dengue types 1, 3, and 4 secondary infections were either the same or lower than in primary infections. The average duration of viremias of types 1, 3, and 4 also was less in secondary infections. Although neither we nor others have been able to confirm the observation of an increased magnitude of viremia in secondary dengue type 2 infections, either in lower primates or in man (24,25), it is necessary to consider the possibility that dengue type 2 virus does have greater pathogenic potential than other dengue serotypes. One of the problems of evaluating this question is that dengue type 2 virus is much easier to isolate in the laboratory using mammalian cell culture systems than is either type 1 or 3. Consequently, one cannot rely on previous virus isolation data from severe or fatal cases for an estimate of relative pathogenicity. The situation is now changed with the more sensitive viral isolation techniques which I have mentioned, but they have not been in use long enough for sufficient data to have been accumulated. Of course, it would not be surprising if certain dengue serotypes were more apt to cause severe disease than others - just as the majority of paralytic poliovirus cases were caused by poliovirus type 1 before the advent of vaccination. It is clear at this point, however, that all 4 serotypes of dengue can cause fatal disease, and that large numbers of fatal cases have been caused by dengue types 1 and 3, as well as by type 2.

Before leaving this brief survey of dengue pathogenesis I should like to point out that recent events may have provided unique opportunities to resolve the question of the risk of sequential dengue infections. First, with respect to Cuba, it is known that dengue apparently was absent from 1943 to 1977 - when a dengue type 1 epidemic occurred (26). No cases of dengue shock syndrome were reported during that outbreak. The 1981 epidemic is reported by the Cuban authorities to have been caused by dengue type 2 - presumably exclusively by dengue type 2. It should be relatively simple, even in retrospect, to compare the prevalence of primary and secondary antibody responses in the surviving dengue shock syndrome patients with what would have been expected on the basis of the proportion of the population previously known to have been infected with dengue type 1 in 1977. This approach assumes that yellow fever vaccine has not been used extensively in Cuba and that St. Louis encephalitis or other flavivirus antibodies were not prevalent in the Cuban population. Another approach would be to compare the "fingerprints" of the RNA of the dengue type 2 strains isolated in Cuba with those isolated previously in the Caribbean area and with strains from Asia and Africa. As mentioned earlier, differences have been observed among strains of different geographic origin. Such a study should show whether or not the Cuba type 2 strains were like those previously circulating in the Caribbean which had been relatively innocuous clinically. If so, that would favor the hypothesis that the severe disease in Cuba was the result of an unfortunate sequence and timing of dengue infections. On the other hand, if they did not resemble the previous Caribbean strains, it would suggest that the severe clinical manifestations might have been the result of the introduction of a more virulent strain from outside the Caribbean area.

Another opportunity to obtain evidence on the sequential infection hypothesis may have been provided by the 1978 epidemic in southern China. The published data indicate that this was caused entirely by dengue type 4 virus and that dengue had never occurred in the area previously - at least not in recent years. Although no data on the clinical manifestations of this outbreak have as yet been published, I was told during a visit to China in 1979 that many hemorrhagic cases and a number of deaths occurred. The situation may be a little more complicated in China than in Cuba, however, because of the known prevalence of Japanese encephalitis virus (another flavivirus) in that area. If severe and fatal disease were relatively common during a primary dengue type 4 outbreak however, it would at least establish that sequential dengue infections were not a necessary condition.

Some of you may disagree with my interpretation of data bearing on the pathogenesis of dengue. Obviously, there is not time during a presentation of this type to discuss all the ramifications of the subject. Therefore, I would be very happy to discuss with any of you personally any data which you think are inconsistent with the conclusions that I have drawn.

PREVENTION

As might be expected, there has been considerable interest in the development of a dengue vaccine ever since dengue viruses were first isolated during World War II. Since a very effective vaccine has been available for yellow fever for about 40 years it is natural to wonder why more progress has not been made with respect to dengue. Basically, this has been because dengue viruses were much more difficult to propagate *in vitro* than was yellow fever and, perhaps even more important, because no satisfactory laboratory animal is available to monitor attempts at viral attenuation. This means that all such attempts have to be validated in human volunteers. It is also possible, but impossible to document, that dengue vaccine development has been slowed to some extent by the fear of the sensitization predicted by the sequential infection hypothesis.

Dengue vaccine development has been under way at the Walter Reed Army Institute of Research for the last 10 years and, thus far, work on a single serotype, type 2, has progressed to the point of preliminary trials in man. In my opinion, these trials have been disappointing. In the most recent and extensive test, vaccine was administered in a double-blind study to 99 men and a placebo was given to 49 men (27). Some of the men who received vaccine had previously been immunized against yellow fever and some had not. About 90% of the yellow fever immunes developed detectable neutralizing antibody to dengue type 2 after receiving the test vaccine but only about 60% of the yellow fever nonimmunes did so. More disappointing, however, was the finding that 19% of the men who developed antibody also had illness of great enough severity to warrant absence from work - as compared with 2% of the placebo controls. It is of some interest in relationship to the immune enhancement hypothesis discussed earlier, that the incidence and severity of vaccine-related symptoms were no greater in the yellow fever immune recipients than in those who were not immune. Also, levels of dengue viremia did not differ in the two groups (28). This is consistent with experiments carried out during World War II which showed that prior yellow fever vaccination neither attenuated nor modified experimental dengue infection in man (29). In summary, a vaccine that produced detectable neutralizing antibody in only 60% of subjects without previous flavivirus infection still produced significant illness in about 1 of 6 persons who did develop antibody. Apparently, there is a need for better laboratory markers of virulence for man.

With dengue vaccines obviously not just around the corner, we are left with *Aedes aegypti* control as our primary means of prevention. Most of you from tropical areas know of the problems that this involves. The cooperation of a large segment of the population is relatively easy to enlist during an outbreak of severe and fatal disease. It is almost impossible to maintain in interepidemic periods. Unfortunately, therefore, I think that it is fairly safe to predict that, in view of the increasing growth of urban populations in tropical areas, dengue will be an even more important public health problem in the near future than it is today.

REFERENCES

1. Parc, F., Pichon, G., Tetaria, C., Louis, F., and Laigret, J., *Med. Trop. (Mars.) 41,* 93 (1981).
2. The Collaborating Group for the Prevention and Treatment of Dengue Fever, Foshan, Guangdong, *Acta Microbiol. Sinica 21,* 239 (1981).
3. Wang, S. H., Liu, L. H., Li, X. D., Lin, T. K., Cui, W. Q., Liu, M. T., Yu, Y. X., *Chinese J. Microbiol. and Immunol. 1,* 316 (1981).
4. Li, X. D., Liu, L. H., Qu, X. S., Cui, W. Q., Zhao, G. F., Liu, W. X., Yu, Y. X., Chen, W. Z., Wang, J. H., Zhao, Z. G., Huang, W. Q., Zhang, G. Z., and Liang, F. P., *Chinese J. Microbiol. and Immunol. 1,* 7 (1981).
5. Dengue in the Caribbean, 1977. *Sci. Pub. 375,* Pan American Health Organization, Washington, D.C. (1979).
6. Dengue in the Americas, *Epidemiol. Bull. Pan American Health Organization, 2,* 1 (1981).
7. Dengue fever surveillance in the American region, *Wkly. Epidem. Rec. 56,* 298 (1981).
8. Ramirez-Ronda, C. H., Maldonado, N. M., Rabell, V., Sather, G., and Cline, B. L., *Trop. Geogr. Med., 31* 127 (1979).
9. Digoutte, J.-P., Institut Pasteur, Dakar, Senegal, personal communication.
10. Cornet, M., Robin, Y., Chateau, R., Heme, G., Adam, C., Valade, M., LeGonidec, G., Jan, C., Renaudet, J., Dieng, P. L., Bangoura, J.-F., and Lorand, A., *Cah. ORSTOM ser. Ent. Med. et Parasitol. 17,* 149 (1979).
11. Rudnick, A., *Asian J. Infect. Dis. 2,* 156 (1978).
12. Rosen, L., Shroyer, D. A., Tesh, R. B., Freier, J. E., and Lien, J. C., unpublished data.
13. Rosen, L., and Gubler, D., *Am. J. Trop. Med. Hyg. 23,* 1153 (1974).
14. Rosen, L., *Am. J. Trop. Med. Hyg. 30,* 177 (1981).
15. Tesh, R. B., *Am. J. Trop. Med. Hyg. 28,* 1053 (1979).
16. Vezza, A. C., Rosen, L., Repik, P., Dalrymple, J., and Bishop, D. H. L., *Am. J. Trop. Med. Hyg. 29,* 643 (1980).

17. Grant, J., Rosen, L., Gubler, D., and Trent, D. W., unpublished data.
18. Henchal, E. A., Gentry, M. K., McCown, J. M., and Brandt, W. E., *Am. J. Trop Med Hyg (in press)* (1982).
19. Rosen, L., *Am. J. Trop. Med. Hyg. 26,* 337 (1977).
20. Scott, R. M., Nimmannitya, S., Bancroft, W. H., and Mansuwan, P., *Am. J. Trop. Med. Hyg. 25,* 866 (1976).
21. Halstead, S. B., *Am. J. Epidemiol. 114,* 632 (1981).
22. Halstead, S. B., Porterfield, J. S., and O'Rourke, E. J., *Am. J. Trop. Med. Hyg. 29,* 638 (1980).
23. Halstead, S. B., Shotwell, H., and Casals, J., *J. Infect. Dis. 128,* 15 (1973).
24. Scherer, W. F., Russell, P. K., Rosen, L., Casals, J., and Dickerman, R. W., *Am. J. Trop. Med. Hyg. 27,* 441 (1978).
25. Rosen, L., unpublished data.
26. Mas., P., in *Sci. Pub. 375*, Pan American Health Organization, Washington, D. C., p. 40 (1979).
27. Scott, R. McN., Bancroft, W. H., Hoke, C. H., Jr., Eckels, K. H., Simms, T. E., Jesrani, K. D. T., Summers, P. L., and Russell, P. K., unpublished data.
28. Russell, P. K., Walter Reed Army Institute of Research, Washington, D. C., personal communication.
29. Sabin, A. B., *Am. J. Trop. Med. Hyg. 1,* 30 (1952).

67

WHO ACTIVITIES ON CONTROLLING VECTORS OF ARBOVIRAL DISEASES IN THE WESTERN PACIFIC REGION

L.S. Self

World Health Organization
Regional Office for the Western Pacific
Manila, Philippines

I. INTRODUCTION

Since dengue fever/dengue haemorrhagic fever is the most important arboviral disease in the Region in terms of morbidity and mortality, the information presented here mainly refers to that disease. Other important arboviral diseases are Japanese encephalitis, Ross River fever and, in Australia, Murray Valley encephalitis.

A series of WHO activities have been undertaken in collaboration with Member States. These have involved technical advisory visits, training and strengthening disease vector control programmes with essential supplies and equipment.

II. EXAMPLES OF ACTIVITIES

A. Technical Visits

The WHO epidemiological surveillance team based in Suva has been involved in visiting many countries and territories in the South Pacific to collaborate with national staff in developing surveillance and preventive control activities against vectors of dengue and Ross River fever. Technical cooperation has been provided to several countries during dengue outbreaks, and this includes Fiji, Kiribati, Niue and

VIRAL DISEASES IN SOUTH-EAST ASIA AND THE WESTERN PACIFIC
ISBN 0 12 484820 6

Tonga. A vector control unit has been established in Fiji and also Samoa.

As a result of technical visits and activities in Sabah State, Malaysia, Philippines and Samoa, new methods of vector control involving health education and community participation are being implemented.

B. Consultant Visits

In connection with the rapid detection of dengue viruses by the mosquito inoculation technique, a consultant visited the Philippines, Singapore, Malaysia, Viet Nam, Fiji and Papua New Guinea in 1980 and Papua New Guinea again in 1981. A visit to Tonga was made in 1981 on the competence of Ross River fever vectors.

C. Extrabudgetary-funded Projects

WHO is the executing agency of a UNDP project on preparedness against outbreaks of arboviral diseases in the Pacific. The project helps governments to maintain adequate stocks of insecticides and spray equipment to combat arboviral outbreaks. Countries belonging to this project are Cook Islands, Fiji, Kiribati, Nauru, Niue, Papua New Guinea, Samoa, Solomon Islands, Tokelau, Trust Territory of the Pacific Islands, Tuvalu and Vanuatu. Contributions from the Japan Shipbuilding Industry Foundation have also been used in some countries for emergency vector control. Territories under French and American administration can also collaborate in these activities.

New projects on integrated control of mosquitos were implemented in Fiji and Trust Territory of the Pacific Islands in 1980, utilizing funds donated by the Japan Government. The Australia Government has also made valuable contributions to the regional programme on dengue fever, and this includes training and research on vaccine development.

D. Training

A regional workshop on detecting dengue viruses by the mosquito inoculation technique was organized in 1979. There has been some follow-up in regard to workshop recommendations on establishing a regional dengue reference laboratory.

Training in *Aedes* surveillance and control was given in two intercountry training courses in the South Pacific during February and March 1980. The three-week course in Suva, Fiji, was attended by 30 participants and a similar course was held for French-speaking participants in Papeete, Tahiti, French Polynesia.

The Organization has collaborated with the University of the South Pacific in using its satellite communication network to alert governments in the South Pacific to take preventive measures against vectors of dengue fever and Ross River fever. The satellite network also has been used for training seminars.

In 1980, national courses and workshops on vector control were held in Guam, the Republic of Korea, Tonga and Trust Territory of the Pacific Islands. In 1981, national courses were held in China, Papua New Guinea, Philippines and Trust Territory of the Pacific Islands. This year a regional training course will be supported by the Danish Government and held in Malaysia.

Each year, several national entomologists and health inspectors undertake training abroad on WHO fellowships as part of the overall regional training activities. In 1980, training programmes were arranged for one fellow each from Papua New Guinea and Republic of Korea, two from the Trust Territory of the Pacific Islands, and three each from Laos and the Philippines. In 1981, there was one fellow trained from Fiji, two from the Philippines and seven from Malayasia. In addition, WHO made arrangements to send one participant each from Fiji, Samoa and Tonga to a vector control course and training programme organized in Australia during November 1981.

E. Research

In recent years, the Regional Office has made available grants for studies on the competence of dengue vectors in Fiji, community participation in *Ae. aegypti* control in the Philippines, fish for mosquito control in the Republic of Korea, and two grants on colonization of *Toxorhynchites* mosquitos in Malaysia. Laboratory and field tests with *T. ambioensis, Bacillus thuringiensis* H-14, and *Romanomermis culivorax* have been carried out in Fiji and Samoa. *B. thuringiensis* is also being tested in field trials in several other countries of the Region.

The Tropical Disease Research Programme managed from Geneva has awarded 10 grants on biological control in this Region, which include two scientists from Australia working on *Culicinomyces clavosporus*, a fungal pathogen of mosquitos.

The practical application of most of these research studies is not yet apparent.

From 1965 to 1975, WHO had a research project on control of dengue fever vectors and Japanese encephalitis vectors in Thailand and Republic of Korea. The successful control methods tested there have been widely applied in many countries.

F. *Information*

A WHO Dengue Newsletter has been issued twice a year since 1975. It is widely distributed to health personnel, laboratories and institutions in the South-East Asian and Western Pacific Regions. In 1980, WHO updated their technical guides on the diagnosis, prevention and control of dengue haemorrhagic fever. These guides have proved to be a valuable and popular document.

III. DISCUSSION

The number of dengue fever/dengue haemorrhagic fever cases in the Region appear to be down, except for marked increases in Republic of Viet Nam and China. In both countries, Japanese encephalitis also remains an important public health problem.

More information is needed on incriminating the vector or vectors of Ross River fever in the South Pacific. This information is needed to develop proper preventive vector control strategies based on the bionomics of the vector.

Although many countries now have the capability to immediately respond to an outbreak, excessive time gaps may exist between recognition of outbreaks and control action.

68

THE EXPANDING GAP BETWEEN EPIDEMIOLOGICAL KNOWLEDGE OF ARBOVIRUSES AND THEIR EFFECTIVE CONTROL

William C. Reeves

Department of Biomedical
and Environmental Health Sciences
School of Public Health
University of California
Berkeley, California

The first major discovery relevant to the control of arthropod-borne viral diseases that affect human health was in 1900 when Reed (1901, 1902) reported the classical studies of the Yellow Fever Commission. They reported the transmission of yellow fever from man to man by the bite of Aedes aegypti. These findings were immediately applied by Gorgas (1911) and a program for the control of Ae. aegypti successfully eradicated yellow fever from Cuba where it had prevailed for over 150 years. The secret to control of this major mosquito-borne disease was to find and remove or treat every breeding source of the vector in the domestic environment and thus reduce the vector population well below the level essential to maintenance of the viral transmission cycle. This concept was rapidly extended and yellow fever was controlled and eradicated from the major urban centers of the World where it had prevailed for over a century. Indeed, Ae. aegypti eradication became the focus of a major program of the Rockefeller Foundation led by Soper (1943). The discovery of a jungle and rural cycle of yellow fever in the Americas and Africa (Strode, 1951) extended the epidemiological knowledge of yellow fever and explained the reintroduction of the virus into urban centers where it had been eradicated. The development of an effective vaccine in 1937 (Theiler and Downs, 1973) provided an alternative approach for protection of susceptible individuals, particularly in rural environments where vector control was impractical.

VIRAL DISEASES IN SOUTH-EAST ASIA
AND THE WESTERN PACIFIC
ISBN 0 12 484820 6

The point of the preceding historical review is to emphasize that for over 80 years we have understood the basic epidemiological factors that control the spread of a major mosquito-borne viral disease. In the ensuing period, and particularly in the past 40 years, extensive studies have extended this knowledge to a wide array of arboviruses including the demonstration that prevention and control of epidemics caused by such agents is feasible by vector control although it is extremely expensive.

My concern is that permanent and effective control programs for mosquito-borne viruses are non-existent in most areas even though we continue in a most impressive fashion to add to our epidemiological knowledge of disease associated with mosquito-borne viruses and extend our degree of sophistication regarding the vectors and the causative viruses.

I could use any one of a number of arboviruses to illustrate my concerns further including Japanese B, Murray Valley, Western equine or St. Louis encephalitis. However, the focus of this seminar, and current developments, make dengue fever more appropriate and the above background on yellow fever in its urban cycle serves well as a background.

It has been known since 1902 (Graham), that dengue fever was a viral infection transmitted in an urban cycle by Ae. aegypti. The extension of knowledge in recent years has been rapid and we now know that 4 distinct viruses can cause the disease; that the infection spectrum goes from inapparent infection through febrile illnesses to hemorrhagic fever, shock syndrome and death; and that there are alternative vectors to Ae. aegypti particularly in the Pacific area. None of these important findings have changed the basic concept, that developed from the yellow fever studies, that reduction of the vector populations to levels that cannot support the transmission cycle is the most feasible approach to control. In spite of this knowledge, dengue fevers have continued at endemic or epidemic levels or have been reintroduced repetitively over extensive areas of Asia, the Pacific and Carribean Islands, and South and Central America. Until recently the occurrence of dengue was considered to be a problem primarily for the underdeveloped areas of the World. If this is the case, we can now include parts of Texas and Queensland in that classification based on the reintroduction of dengue virus into those areas and the confirmation that they were receptive because there was an adequate population of Ae. aegypti to support transmission and a susceptible human population was available. Arbovirus epidemiologists were not surprised and had anticipated these developments. The point is there is no concerted effort to carry out the principals of vector control that were established by Gorgas and Soper. An Ae. aegypti control anad eradication program in the United States was making excellent progress in the 1960's (Smith 1967) when the government decided that it was costing too much and wasn't that important. The annual budget in 1968 was 16 million dollars and 2,610 persons were involved. The program was completely abandoned within 2 years and major urban centers in the Southeastern United States now report Ae. aegypti is a major pest. I assume that these are potentially receptive areas for dengue and yellow fever.

A dengue fever epidemic was recently reported in Cuba with over 300,000 cases and 156 deaths. This could not have happened in the early 1900's at the time of Gorgas' successful vector control program. An entomologist who had just returned from Cuba told me he was most impressed by the effectiveness of the island-wide house-to-house search for and eradication of vector sources which was being supplemented by island-wide applications of organophosphorous insecticides. He had no knowledge of the inevitable high cost of the program. I would add that dengue virus infections have remained endemic in Puerto Rico and Southeast Asia since the 1960's in spite of any control effort.

I have expressed concern previously (Reeves 1972, 1980) as have others (Downs 1981), that areas where dengue viruses prevail are potentially receptive to yellow fever. A recent conference on yellow fever (Woodall 1981) reiterated this concern and recommended the use of 17D vaccine in the event of an epidemic. Further study revealed only 7 million doses of the vaccine were available in the World and that this supply probably could not be doubled in the event of an epidemic. That amount of vaccine will not control yellow fever if it is introduced into major urban centers in the Americas, Asia or Africa. Similarly, there is little chance that effective vaccine for other arboviruses will be available in large amounts in the near future.

I do not believe the failure to control dengue, or other major mosquito-borne diseases, is for lack of knowledge on the populations at risk, the causative viruses or which mosquitoes are vectors. The primary problem is that governments and populations in regions where mosquito-borne arboviruses prevail do not give a priority to providing the necessary resources to assure effective surveillance systems for vectors and disease and long-term stable vector control programs. When emergency control programs are instituted in an epidemic, the cost of human suffering is already high as cases have occurred and other individuals are in the incubation period. Such programs are overly expensive, may be ineffective because of insecticide resistance of the vector, and are delayed by endless regulations controlling the use of insecticides and the public's concern over the health significance of insecticide dispersal. When correctly done, area-wide applications of insecticides can effectively kill the older adult females that are infected and this can be done for a sufficient time to break the transmission cycle. An excellent example was control of the St. Louis encephalitis epidemic in Dallas, Texas in 1966 (Hopkins et al. 1975). The problem remained that 145 proven cases of SLE had occurred before the control program had an effect.

To summarize, the factors that contribute to the disparity between epidemiological knowledge and our capacity to control mosquito-borne viral diseases are: (1) a dependence on insecticides rather than source reduction for vector control, (2) legal restrictions on the use of insecticides, lack of a legal basis of water resource management in both urban and rural environments, and economic pressures for the growth of water dependent industries, (3) a limited knowledge of vector behavior essential for control of the adult female population that is transmitting infection, and (4) a low priority by political bodies for funding of control programs due to lack of belief by the public that there is a need for action until an epidemic is in progress. I can only conclude that scientists must make an effort to influence public officials to utilize present knowledge for effective control of arboviral diseases and urge that you become involved in such actions.

REFERENCES

Downs, W. (1981). *Am. J. Trop. Med. Hyg. 30,* 526.

Woodall, J. (1981). *J. Inf. Dis. 144,* 87.

Gorgas, W. (1911). *Wash. Gov. Printing Office Document 822.*

Graham, H. (1903). *J. Trop. Med. London 6,* 209.

Hopkins, C. et al. (1975). *Am. J. Epid. 102,* 1.

Reed, W. (1901). *Med. Record 60,* 201.

Reed, W. (1902). *J. Hyg. 2,* 101.

Reeves, W. (1972). *Am. J. Trop. Med. Hyg. 21,* 251.

Reeves, W. (1980). *Am. J. Trop. Med. Hyg. 29,* 1.

Soper, F. et al. (1943). "The Organization of Permanent Nation-wide Anti-Aedes aegypti Measures in Brazil," Rock. Found. New York.

Smith, J. (1967). *Arch. Env. Health 15,* 137

Strode, G. (ed)(1951). "Yellow Fever," McGraw Hill, New York.

Theiler, M. and Downs, W. (1973). "The Arthropod-borne Viruses of Vertebrates," Yale Univ. Press, New York.

69

ARBOVIRUS-INFECTED HENS ATTRACT MORE MOSQUITOES[1]

Rod Mahon[2]
Adrian Gibbs

Virus Ecology Research Group
Research School of Biological Sciences
Australian National University
Canberra, A.C.T.
Australia

We have examined the possibility that arbovirus-infected hens are more attractive to mosquitoes than healthy ones. Because, if so, transmission of the virus would be enhanced, and, considering the brevity of the viremic phase of most arbovirus infections, such a bias would be of considerable selective advantage to the virus.

In our trials, we used chickens as the vertebrate host, and Sindbis alphavirus (SaV), which in Australia is normally isolated from birds (1) and from the mosquito *Culex annulirostris* (2).

Chickens were infected by a 0.1 ml subcutaneous injection of a chicken-adapted strain of SaV containing 10^5 pfu when assayed on chicken embryo fibroblast monolayers. For each infected chicken, a control bird of similar weight was given a similar injection of inoculum that had

[1]*This research received a grant from the Australian Encephalitis Control Programme of the Australian Department of Health.*

[2]*Present address: C.S.I.R.O., Division of Entomology, Canberra, A.C.T., Australia*

VIRAL DISEASES IN SOUTH-EAST ASIA AND THE WESTERN PACIFIC
ISBN 0 12 484820 6

been UV irradiated to inactivate the virus. A 0.5 ml sample of venous blood was taken from all birds immediately before all experiments, and the titre of SaV determined by plaque formation on CEF monolayers (3). Only the results obtained with birds shown to be infected (>10 pfu/ml serum) are discussed below (>95%), none of the control birds yielded virus.

Two experimental procedures were employed to compare the attraction of mosquitoes to infected and control chickens. In the first, 12-week old chickens were used as 'bait' in mosquito traps. Traps were arranged in pairs, one metre apart; one of each pair containing an infected chicken, the other a control bird. At dusk the traps were placed along the margin of Barren Box Swamp near Griffith, N.S.W. At dawn, the *C. annulirostris* mosquitoes captured were counted. Table I presents the number of occasions that the infected bird or the control bird attracted more mosquitoes. The number of occasions that the trap containing the infected bird captured more mosquitoes was significantly greater than the null hypothesis, i.e. that they should be at random.

TABLE I. Comparison of infected versus healthy chickens as mosquito 'bait'[b]

	Viremic >healthy	Healthy >viremic	p
1980 (3 trials)	8	3	-[a]
1981 (1st trial)	11	5	-
1981 (2nd trial)	16	5	<0.01
	35	13	

Source	d.f.	Deviance	χ^2
1:1 ratio overall	1	10.08	<0.001
Homogeneity of expts.	2	0.20	-
Total	3	10.28	

[a] -, $p > 0.05$

[b] for safety, chickens were isolated, at all times, from mosquitoes by two spaced layers of wire gauze

In the second series of experiments, we examined the feeding preference of *C. annulirostris* caged with an infected and a control chicken. In these trials, birds paired and inoculated as in the first experiments were given a 0.2 ml intraveneous injection of $NaCrO_4$ (33 μg/ml) in saline at the time of SaV inoculation (i.e. 24 hr before the trials). One bird from each pair was chosen, at random, to receive the chromate in the form of ^{51}Cr (7.5 x 10^8 counts/min/ml).

Pairs of chickens were enclosed in a 40 x 40 x 40 cm cage, into which, at dusk, 50-150 *C. annulirostris*, captured while seeking a blood meal, were introduced. At dawn, engorged mosquitoes were collected, and gamma emission identified those that contained ^{51}Cr-labelled red blood cells. Dual feeding (on both chickens) was a potential source of bias, however in our experiments this did not appear to be significant as, overall, about half the engorged mosquitoes contained ^{51}Cr. The results of the 13 trials (Table II) show that the bias exhibited by mosquitoes

TABLE II. Comparison of infected and healthy chickens as blood sources to Culex annulirostris

Total fed	No. fed on viremic birds	No. fed on healthy birds	p
28	24	4	<0.05
8	6	2	-
10	6	4	-
9	3	6	-
3	1	2	-
26	21	5	<0.05
7	3	4	-
10	4	6	-
6	3	3	-
7	5	2	-
10	7	3	-
3	1	2	-
14	12	2	<0.05
141	96	45	

Source	d.f.	Deviance	$p(\chi^2)$
1:1 ratio overall	1	18.88	<0.001
Homogeneity of expts.	12	23.20	<0.05
Total	13	42.08	

towards feeding on the infected bird was statistically highly significant, although the heterogeneity between experiments was also significant. Inspection of the data shows that the feeding bias was greatest when the number of mosquitoes feeding was large, perhaps indicating that there was some form of 'activation', similar to the effect of CO_2 on mosquitoes (4).

Thus two types of experiments demonstrated that mosquitoes are attracted to infected chickens. We have attempted to determine the cause of this bias. Several factors are known to be important in the host-seeking behaviour of mosquitoes. The most important cues utilised by mosquitoes are thought to be CO_2, body odour and warm, moise convection currents rising from the host. We suspected that the most likely stimulus that would be modified by a viral infection would be body temperature. However, we have found no consistent difference in the body temperatures of infected and healthy birds. Similarly, we found no consistent increased output of water vapour, or CO_2 by infected birds. We also failed to detect qualitative or quantitative changes in the mass spectrometer profiles of liquid N_2-trapped volatiles expired by infected and healthy chickens.

Thus the reason for the feeding bias, which is at least 2:1, remains unexplained, however there is little doubt that such a bias would have important consequences on the course of epidemics. In temperate regions, minimum threshold densities of mosquitoes required to sustain an epidemic would be reached earlier in the season and persist for a longer period than would otherwise be the case. At the height of the epidemic, the excess of mosquitoes above that minimum would ensure that the epidemic is of greater intensity. Our results also cast doubt on the value of using tests on mosquito feeding preferences to try to understand arbovirus ecology, unless virus-free mosquitoes are tested with infected vertebrates and *vice versa*.

REFERENCES

1. Liehne, C.G., Stanley, N.F., Alpers, M.P., Paul, S., Liehne, P.F.S., and Chan, K.H., *Aust. J. Exp. Biol. Med. Sci. 54*, 505 (1976).
2. Doherty, R.L., *Aust. J. Exp. Biol. Med. Sci. 55*, 103 (1977).
3. Cooper, P.D., *in* "Methods in Virology" (Maramorosch and Koprowski, eds.) Vol. III, p. 243. Academic Press (1967).
4. Gillies, M.T., *Bull. Ent. Res. 70*, 525 (1980).

EPIDEMIOLOGY OF DENGUE IN FIJI

J.U. Mataika
J.A.R. Miles[1]

Wellcome Virus Laboratory
Tamavua Hospital
Suva, Fiji Is.

INTRODUCTION

Dengue fever in Fiji in the last 6 years appeared to occur more frequently around Suva, the capital of Fiji. It may indicate that the dengue virus has not totally disappeared from the community in the last few years but has continued to survive.

Dengue virus infections in Fiji have been recorded in 1885, 1930 and 1943-44. Serological evidence due to age differences in prevalence suggested that there might have been another epidemic in 1905. After 1950, there was no epidemic until March, 1971, when cases of dengue type 2 occurred in the highly susceptible population. An epidemic of rubella occurred concurrently. Dengue cases peaked in July when 740 were notified. The total cases notified up to April 1972 were 3,111 and a limited number of notifications continued to 1973. A few haemorrhagic cases were seen at the Suva Hospital. No deaths were reported due to dengue (1).

In January 1975, type 1 dengue started in Suva and soon exploded to epidemic proportions. From January to July, a total of 16,203 cases were notified from all over Fiji. By age, the highest percentage of persons reporting illnesses were in the 10-19 and 20-29 year old groups. The lowest percentages were in those below 10 years.

[1]*Present address: c/- Lake Hawea, New Zealand.*

VIRAL DISEASES IN SOUTH-EAST ASIA
AND THE WESTERN PACIFIC
ISBN 0 12 484820 6

There was a slight preponderance of males in all ethnic groups. In a survey carried out during the epidemic in Suva by Health Inspectors, out of 226 persons who reported clinical dengue, 27 (12%) reported some form of severe bleeding. There were more than 12 deaths reported in the Suva area. Serology indicated about 45% were primary infections and about 42% were secondary (2).

No cases of dengue were reported in 1977 and 1978. In 1979, there were 10 serologically proven cases and all were from the Suva area.

In early 1980, dengue was again active in Fiji and it was still active in mid-May. Cases were reported from Labasa in November. The cases were mild with very few haemorrhagic complications. The virus was not isolated but was confirmed serologically. Positive cases in Suva appeared to be concentrated in the Nasinu/Nadera area about 5 miles north east of Suva. Later, cases were found in the Tamavua/Nausori areas.

In 1981, a small outbreak of dengue type 4 occurred and was confined to the Suva locality especially in the Samabula area. The first case was in early April and the cases peaked in mid-May. Three cases were admitted to Suva Hospital with haemorrhagic fever, and one child died in shock.

SUVA

The capital of Fiji in 1974 had a population of 103,000. The present population is about 127,000. This has brought with it social changes, with overcrowding and the springing up of temporary shelters and housing projects in and around Suva.

Population Movements

There is a continuous flow of people from villages to the next village, and from village to townships and back again, especially during the Christmas and New Year periods. In one instance, 50 people (20%) were counted leaving a village of 250 inhabitants and about 50 new residents settled in within the space of 3 months. There may be a parallel here of the "walk about" phenomenon in Australia.

The building of new roads has opened up new areas and settlements in the interior of the two main islands of Vitilevu and Vanualevu.

The ferrying and passengers between the two main islands has grown in number in the last three years.

Six new airfields have been constructed in the smaller islands in the Eastern group, including Rotuma Island.

Improvements in communications and especially air traffic from South-East Asia has enabled individuals to travel within the incubation period of the disease to receptive areas in the Pacific including Fiji.

Vectors

Aedes aegypti is the important vector of dengue in Fiji. *Aedes rotumae*, another efficient vector, is confined to Rotuma Island. There are two other vectors, *Aedes polynesiensis* and *Aedes pseudoscutellaris*, but their efficiencies are low.

Aedes aegypti, a domestic mosquito, is common throughout the year in Suva. Monitoring of this mosquito during the last 3 years showed Breteaux indices to be persistently high, between 40% and 90%. At Nadi, however, in dry periods between May and October, the Breteaux indices may be low to nil. The average rainfall at Nadi in 1980 was 130.25 mm whereas in Suva it was 328.5 mm.

CONCLUSION

Dengue virus appears to survive at least in Suva where there is a persistently high *Aedes aegypti* population throughout the year. Travelling brings in susceptible hosts from villages and pools of infection from overseas.

We continue to monitor the *Aedes aegypti* population in the main centres. Primary Health Care at village level is being stepped up in all divisions in Fiji.

REFERENCES

1. Maguire, T., Macnamara, F., Miles, J., Spears, G., and Mataika, J., *J. Hyg. (Camb) 69,* 287 (1971).
2. Reed, D., Maguire, T., and Mataika, J., *Amer. J. Trop. Med. Hyg. 26,* 784 (1977).

71

CELL-MEDIATED IMMUNE RESPONSES IN MICE INFECTED WITH DENGUE-4 VIRUS

T. Pang
P. Y. Wong
S. Devi

Department of Medical Microbiology
University of Malaya,
Kuala Lumpur, Malaysia

R. Pathmanathan

Department of Pathology
University of Malaya,
Kuala Lumpur, Malaysia

I. INTRODUCTION

Little is known about cell-mediated immunity (CMI) to dengue viruses. Earlier studies have reported evidence of CMI (1), but others conclude that CMI does not develop in dengue-infected animals (2). Halstead's immune enhancement hypothesis of dengue haemorrhagic fever/dengue shock syndrome (DHF/DSS) also suggests the probable involvement of CMI in the pathogenesis of DHF/DSS (3). In light of this we have studied the induction of CMI in dengue-infected mice as measured by the delayed-type hypersensitivity (DTH) reaction.

II. MATERIALS AND METHODS

The following viruses were used: dengue virus type 1 (DEN-1): Hawaii, DEN-2: TRIN 1751, DEN-3: H87, DEN-4: H-241

VIRAL DISEASES IN SOUTH-EAST ASIA
AND THE WESTERN PACIFIC
ISBN 0 12 484820 6

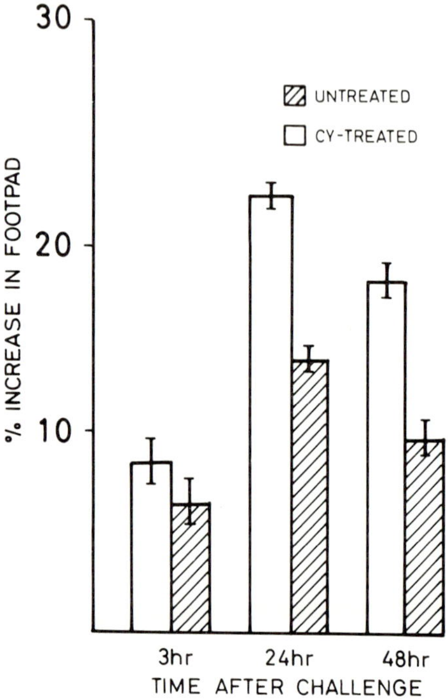

FIGURE 1. DTH to DEN-4 virus and Japanese encephalitis (JE) virus: Nakayama. Mice were immunized subcutaneously with DEN-4 and DTH measured at various times thereafter by challenging the left footpad with DEN-4 and the right footpad with normal mouse brain antigen. Footpad thickness was measured 24 hrs later.

III. RESULTS

Significant DTH to DEN-4 virus was detected which was maximal 24 hrs after challenge (Fig. 1) and was enhanced by cyclophosphamide pre-treatment (Fig. 1). Maximum response was noted 6 days after infection with an optimum sensitizing dose of 10^7 PFU/mouse. DTH was also enhanced by Freund's incomplete adjuvant. Histology of test footpad revealed a predominantly mononuclear cell infiltrate 24 hrs after challenge. Fibrin deposition was also noted. DTH reactivity

TABLE 1. Transfer of DTH reactivity

Cells/serum transferred[a]	24 hr footpad increase (% ± S.E.)
Immune spleen cells	20.0 ± 0.7
Normal spleen cells	4.4 ± 0.4
Immune serum	8.2 ± 0.8
Normal serum	4.3 ± 0.5
Donor mice	24.1 ± 1.2

[a] 5×10^7 spleen cells or 0.5 ml serum injected i.v.

was transferable to normal mice by immune spleen cells but not by immune serum (Table 1). DTH was apparently specific for DEN-4 as significantly lower responses were seen when DEN-1, DEN-2, DEN-3 and JE viruses were used as challenge antigens in DEN-4-infected mice. Also, infection of mice with DEN-4 induces a transient immunosuppression of CMI indicated by a significantly reduced DTH response to an unrelated antigen, sheep red blood cells (SRBC). Preliminary results indicate that transfer of DTH T cells may result in early, increased mortality in dengue-infected mice.

IV. DISCUSSION

The results indicate that CMI is elicited in response to infection with DEN-4 in mice. The data satisfies most of the criteria for a classical DTH response. To the best of our knowledge, these results represent the first report of an _in vivo_ DTH response to dengue virus infection in mice.

However, the true role of DTH in protection and/or pathogenesis in viral infections is far from clear. T cells mediating DTH reactions (T^{DTH}) are of importance in protective immunity to herpes (4) but can also produce severe pathological consequences as has been shown with influenza. It has been proposed (4) that DTH reactions are vital in recovery from primary infection but that once other arms of immunity (e.g. antibody production) are activated then DTH responses could be superfluous or even damaging e.g. following reinfection with a virus. In relation to the

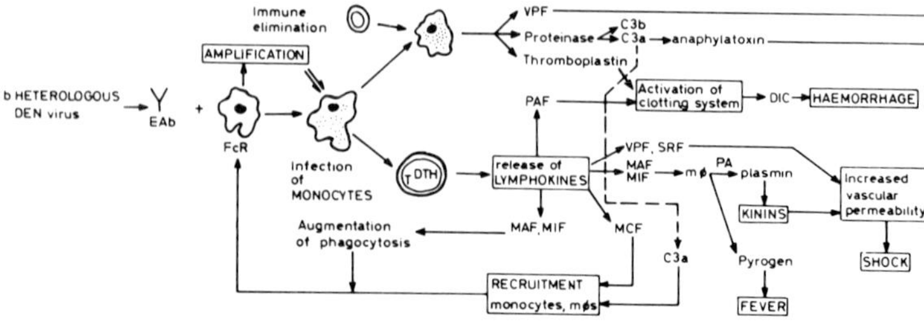

FIGURE 2. Systemic DTH in the pathogenesis of DHF/DSS

pathogenesis of DHF/DSS, it is possible, for example, that the CMI response against dengue-infected monocytes as proposed by Halstead (3) is mediated by T^{DTH} cells. An alternative possibility which we wish to propose is that dengue-infected monocytes act as antigen-presenting cells to T^{DTH} memory cells. This could then result in a *systemic DTH reaction* in which these activated T cells release a variety of lymphokines (5) which in turn produces the symptoms of haemorrhage and shock seen in DHF/DSS (Fig. 2). Further studies to elucidate the true role of T^{DTH} cells in dengue virus infection are in progress.

REFERENCES

1. Nagarkatti, P.S., D'Souza, M.B., and Rao, K.M. *J. Immunol. Methods 23,* 341 (1978).
2. Chaturvedi, U.C., Tandon, P., Mathur, A., and Kumar, A. *J. Gen. Virol. 39,* 293 (1978).
3. Halstead, S.B. *Bull. W.H.O. 58,* 1 (1980).
4. Nash, A.A., and Gell, P.G.H. *Immunol. Today 2,* 162 (1981).
5. Cohen, S., Pick, E., and Oppenheim, J.J. "Biology of the Lymphokines", Academic Press, New York, (1979).

72

GENETIC ANALYSIS OF STRAIN VARIATION IN DENGUE TYPE 2 VIRUSES

Peter J. Walker
Stephen T. Garrett
Barry M. Gorman

Queensland Institute of Medical Research
Herston, Queensland, Australia

Donald S. Burke

Armed Forces Research Institute of Medical Science
Bangkok, Thailand

I. INTRODUCTION

Dengue viruses are a major cause of childhood disease in many countries of south-east Asia and the western Pacific region. In most individuals, symptoms of dengue disease are relatively mild but, in its more severe forms, the infection is characterized by acute haemorrhage and shock which, if untreated, can be fatal. The severity of dengue disease is clearly influenced by the immunological status of the host. Dengue haemorrhagic fever/dengue shock syndrome (DHF/DSS) occurs most frequently as a result of a second or subsequent infection or in the presence of declining maternal antibody (1). However, several studies have reported that severe dengue disease can also occur during primary infections (2,3) suggesting that other factors may influence the course of infection. Genetic differences between virus strains could have a role in determining disease severity.

Four types of dengue virus have been identified by serological methods and all have been associated with both severe and mild disease. Vezza *et. al.* (4) have shown that ribo-

VIRAL DISEASES IN SOUTH-EAST ASIA AND THE WESTERN PACIFIC
ISBN 0 12 484820 6

TABLE 1. Dengue-2 Strains Used in This Study

Strain	Geographic origin	Severity of disease
New Guinea C	New Guinea 1944	Dengue fever
Trinidad 1751	Trinidad 1953	Dengue fever
SP7-259	Manila 1966	DHF
SP7-264	Manila 1966	DHF
SP7-422	Manila 1966	DHF
T-80D	Bangkok 1980	DHF
T-80E	Bangkok 1980	DHF/DSS
T-80G	Bangkok 1980	DHF
T-80H	Bangkok 1980	DHF/DSS
T-80J	Bangkok 1980	DHF

nuclease T_1 fingerprints of each serotype are related but quite distinct. We have used T_1 fingerprints to examine the nature and extent of structural variation amongst strains of a single dengue virus serotype with the view of identifying subtypes which may have different virulence characteristics.

The strains of dengue-2 virus used in this study are shown in Table 1. The viruses were obtained from New Guinea, Thailand, the Philippines and Trinidad from patients with mild and severe forms of disease. Each virus was grown in cultured mosquito cells (*Ae. albopictus* clone C6-36) and purified from infected cell culture fluid by polyethylene glycol precipitation and density gradient centrifugation. RNA was extracted from purified virions and digested with guanosine-specific ribonuclease T_1. RNA was either radiolabelled with inorganic phosphate in culture or 5'-end labelled *in vitro* using polynucleotide kinase. The fingerprints were generated by two-dimensional gel electrophoresis of the digestion products and visualized by autoradiography.

II. VIRUSES ISOLATED AT DIFFERENT GEOGRAPHIC LOCATIONS

Dengue-2 viruses from New Guinea (New Guinea C strain, 1944), Trinidad (1751 strain, 1953), the Philippines (264 strain, 1966) and Thailand (T-80H strain, 1980) were compared. Fingerprints of 3 of these strains are illustrated in Figure 1. Each virus generated a distinctive fingerprint. The New Guinea strain displayed little similarity to the Trinidad and Thailand isolates but shared a number of large distinctive

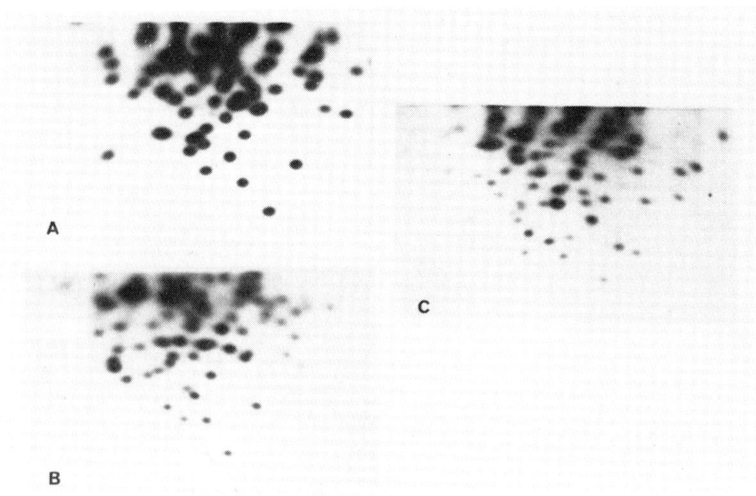

Figure 1. T_1 fingerprints of the RNA of selected dengue-2 strains from A. *New Guinea, 1944* B. *Philippines, 1966* C. *Thailand, 1980*

oligonucleotides with the 1966 Philippine strain. The results indicate that substantial genetic diversity exists within the serotype and demonstrate the value of T_1 fingerprinting for distinguishing closely related dengue viruses.

III. VIRUSES ISOLATED DURING A SINGLE DENGUE EPIDEMIC

During the summer of 1966, a large dengue epidemic occurred in Manila. Of almost 10,000 reported cases of DHF, 2.6% were fatal (5). Three isolates of dengue-2 virus recovered from DHF patients during that epidemic were kindly provided by Dr A. Rudnick for use in this study. The strains produced fingerprints that were very closely related. For example, 46 large T_1 oligonucleotides examined in strain 264 were also detected in strain 259. Only 3 large oligonucleotides in strain 264 and 4 in strain 259 were not shared. Strain 422 shared a similar close relationship with each of the other isolates. These results appear to provide evidence of genetic drift in dengue-2 strains during the 1966 epidemic. It is not yet known if these variants were circulating concurrently.

IV. VIRUSES ISOLATED FROM A DHF ENDEMIC AREA

Thirty-nine strains of dengue-2 virus isolated in Bangkok during 1980 are being examined by the T_1 fingerprinting method. The set of viruses includes approximately equal numbers from patients with classical dengue fever, dengue haemorrhagic fever and DHF with shock (Table 1). Five strains have been analysed to date. Three were isolated from patients with mild DHF and 2 from patients with shock syndrome. The viruses fell into two groups. Strains T-80D, T-80E, T-80G, and T-80J shared similar but distinct fingerprints. For example, strain T-80D shared 31 of 42 large oligonucleotides with T-80E and 30 with T-80G. Strain T-80H, however, generated a fingerprint that was quite different from those of the other Bangkok strains. This virus appears to represent a different subtype of dengue-2 which was circulating in the endemic area. A representative of each subtype was isolated from individuals with dengue shock syndrome indicating that each has a potential to produce severe disease.

V. CONCLUSIONS

The T_1 fingerprinting method has revealed in dengue-2 viruses a level of genetic diversity that was not evident from previous serological studies. The virus appears to exist as a number of distinct subtypes, each of which is represented by a set of structural variants. Viruses of two distinct subtypes from a single endemic location have been isolated from DHF patients. It is conceivable that the genetic diversity illustrated by these strains could be reflected in their virulence characteristics.

REFERENCES

1. Halstead, S.B., *Bull. W.H.O. 58*, 1 (1980).
2. Rosen, L., *Am. J. Trop. Med. Hyg. 26*, 337 (1977).
3. Gubler, D.J., Reed, D., Rosen, L. and Hitchcock, J.C., *Am. J. Trop. Med. Hyg. 27*, 581 (1978).
4. Vezza, A.C., Rosen, L., Repik, P., Dalrymple, J. and Bishop, D.H.L., *Am. J. Trop. Med. Hyg. 29*, 643 (1980).
5. Venzon, E.L., Rudnick, A., Marchette, N.J., Fabie, A.E. and Dukellis, E., *J. Philippine Med. Assn. 48*, 297 (1972).

73

ANTIBODY MEDIATED ENHANCEMENT OF DENGUE VIRUS YIELDS IN MOUSE MACROPHAGES USING HUMAN SERA

James S. Porterfield
Mary Jane Cardosa
J.S. Malik Peiris

Sir William Dunn School of Pathology
University of Oxford
Oxford, England

Donald S. Burke

Armed Forces Institute of Medical Research
Bangkok
Thailand

INTRODUCTION

Hawkes (1964), and Hawkes & Lafferty (1967) first described the phenomenon of antibody mediated enhancement of viral replication, but substantially greater enhancement was demonstrated by Halstead and his colleagues when they studied the replication of dengue viruses in human or primate mononuclear cell preparations in the presence and absence of antiviral antibody (Halstead et al., 1973; Halstead et al., 1976; Halstead & O'Rourke, 1977). They showed that enhancement was mediated by the IgG portion of immunoglobulin, and that the phenomenon could be demonstrated only in host cells which carry receptors for the Fc portion of immunoglobulin (Halstead & O'Rourke, 1977).

In Oxford, we have been interested in the possible uses of continuous lines of macrophage-like cells as hosts in which to explore the enhancement phenomenon. Although we

VIRAL DISEASES IN SOUTH-EAST ASIA
AND THE WESTERN PACIFIC
ISBN 0 12 484820 6

were at first unable to detect dengue virus replication in any of the macrophage-like cells we used, we were able to show that the flavivirus West Nile virus (WNV) replicated in P388D1 and J774.1 cells, which are of mouse origin, and in U937 cells, of human origin, virus yields being enhanced in all three lines by low concentrations of antiviral antibody. (Peiris & Porterfield, 1979, 1981). One of the mouse macrophage-like cell lines, P388D1 cells, formed monolayers in which WNV and several other viruses induced lytic plaques, enabling enhancement to be quantitated by a direct antibody dependent plaque enhancement (ADPE) assay. (Peiris & Porterfield, 1981).

In our initial studies with dengue viruses we had used a mouse brain preparation of the Tr. 1751 strain of dengue virus type 2, whereas Halstead & O'Rourke (1977) had used the 16681 strain of the same serotype, propagated in monkey kidney cells. We received the 16681 strain from Professor Halstead, and sent him the P388D1 cells, and both laboratories were able to show that this strain of dengue virus not only replicated, but showed enhanced yields in the presence of antiviral antibody. Unfortunately, no cytopathic effect was produced, so that it was necessary to use a two stage technique in which virus yields from infected P388D1 cells were titrated by plaque formation in the PS line of pig kidney cells by previously described methods (Madrid & Porterfield, 1969).

MATERIALS AND METHODS

Paired sera from Thai children in whom a diagnosis of dengue virus infection had been established on laboratory criteria were received from Bangkok. The clinical diagnosis was dengue haemorrhagic fever (DHF) in some cases, dengue shock syndrome (DSS) in others, uncomplicated dengue fever, or "pyrexia of unknown origin, presumed dengue fever".

Details of the method of titrating enhancing antibodies against West Nile virus have been described (Peiris & Porterfield, 1981). For dengue virus tests, serial 10-fold dilutions of the serum under test were made from 10^{-1} to 10^{-6} in Leibovitz L15 medium with 3% heat inactivated foetal calf serum (HIFCS) (56°C for 30 minutes), and the dengue 2 strain 16681 was diluted in the same medium. Equal volumes, 100µl each, of dilute antibody and virus were mixed in individual wells of Linbro 6x4 multi-well plates and were incubated for 30 minutes at 37°C, after which P388D1 cells (0.5 ml of a

TABLE 1. Enhancing antibody titres against West Nile and dengue type 2 viruses of paired sera from Thai children with primary or secondary dengue virus infections

Infection	Enhancement titres*				HI titres	
	West Nile virus		Dengue 2 virus		Dengue 2 virus	
	Acute	Conv.	Acute	Conv.	Acute	Conv.
Primary	<10	10^3	10	10^5	<10	80
"	<10	10^2	<10	10^3	<10	80
"	<10	10^2	<10	10^3	<10	40
"	<10	$5x10^2$	<10	10^3	<10	20
"	<10	$5x10^2$	<10	10^3	<10	160
"	<10	10^2	10	10^3	<10	40
Secondary	$5\ 10^4$	10^4	$>10^6$	$>10^6$	5120	>10240
"	10^5	$5x10^4$	$>10^6$	$>10^6$	>10240	>10240
"	10^4	$5x10^4$	$>10^6$	$>10^6$	5120	5120
"	10^4	$5x10^4$	10^5	$>10^6$	2560	>10240
"	10^4	10^5	10^5	10^6	1280	1280
"	10^4	$5x10^4$	10^5	$>10^6$	1280	1280

*Reciprocal of serum dilution

suspension containing $5x10^5$ cells per ml) were added and the preparations reincubated. Four hours later a further 0.5 ml of L15 medium containing 10% HIFCS was added, and incubation was continued for 5 or 6 days. At this time, supernatant fluids were removed from individual wells and viral infectivity was titrated in PS cells, using duplicate or triplicate PS wells for each well of P388D1 cells. Dengue virus plaques were stained after 5 or 6 days of incubation of PS cells, using naphthalene black stain.

RESULTS

P388D1 cells were infected with 16681 virus at different multiplicities of infection (m.o.i.) and virus yields were determined at different time intervals by titration in PS cells. At m.o.i. of 0.04 and 0.004, in the absence of dengue antibody, virus was first detected on day 4, and rose to maximal yields on day 8, after which levels declined. When cells were infected at m.o.i. of 0.05 in the presence of human dengue immune serum at a dilution of 1:200 (50% plaque reduction neutralisation titre 1:160), maximal yields occurred on day 5, and were about 20-fold higher than yields from controls infected at the same multiplicity without antibody.

Paired sera from 6 children who had had primary dengue infections, and from another 6 children who had had secondary type infections (as determined by the pattern of their haemagglutination inhibition responses) were tested in P388D1 cells against both West Nile and dengue virus type 2, with the results which are shown in Table 1. Acute phase sera from primary dengue subjects showed no enhancing antibodies against either virus over a range of serum dilutions from 10^{-1} to 10^{-6}, whereas convalescent sera from these children enhanced both viruses, with titres against dengue virus being higher than those against WNV. When sera from secondary dengue infections were examined, it was found that acute and convalescent sera from all 6 children enhanced both viruses to high titres, all the convalescent sera enhancing dengue virus to titres in excess of 10^{-6}. In the WNV tests, enhancement spanned the range of serum dilutions from 10^{-1} to the end point for any particular serum, but in the D2 tests all the secondary dengue convalescent sera showed a marked prozone, with no virus being detected at 10^{-1} and 10^{-2} serum dilutions, presumably because neutralisation occurred at these dilutions.

Further tests with more paired human sera from virologically confirmed dengue cases have given essentially similar results. There is some evidence that D2 enhancement titres may be lower in sera from patients from whom D2 virus was isolated than in sera from children who had type 1 virus infections.

REFERENCES

Halstead, S.B., Chow, J.S. and Marchette, N.J. (1973). *Nature (Lond.) New Biol.* *243*, 24-26.

Halstead, S.B., Marchette, N.J., Chow, J.S. and Lolekha, S. (1976). *Proc. Soc. Exp. Biol. Med.* *151*, 136-139.

Halstead, S.B. and O'Rourke, E.J. (1977). *J. Exp. Med.* *146*, 201-217.

Hawkes, R.A. (1964). *Aust. J. Exp. Biol. Med.* *42*, 465-482.

Hawkes, R.A. and Lafferty, K.J. (1967). *Virology* *33*, 250-261.

Madrid, A.T. and Porterfield, J.S. (1969). *Bull. W.H.O.* *40*, 113-121.

Peiris, J.S.M. and Porterfield, J.S. (1979) *Nature (London)* *282*, 509-511.

Peiris, J.S.M. and Porterfield, J.S. (1981) *J. Gen. Virol.* *57*, 119-125.

SPONTANEOUS IN VITRO DENGUE ANTIBODY PRODUCTION BY MONONUCLEAR LEUKOCYTES FROM PATIENTS WITH DENGUE HEMORRHAGIC FEVER

Ananda Nisalak
Donald S. Burke
Michael A. Ussery

Department of Virology
Armed Forces Research Institute
of Medical Sciences, Bangkok, Thailand

I. BACKGROUND

Marchette et al (1979) noted that after in vitro cultivation of 10^6 DHF mononuclear leukocytes per milliliter, weak hemagglutination inhibiting activity could be found in some culture supernatant fluids. We recently developed a highly sensitive "antibody capture" solid phase radioimmunoassay for detecting immunoglobulin class specific antibodies to flavivirus antigens capable of detecting as little as 50 picograms of high-specific activity antibody in 50 microliter volumes (Burke and Ananda, 1982). We applied this assay to detect IgM and IgG dengue antibodies in supernatant fluids of cultures of unstimulated human leukocytes.

II. METHODS

Mononuclear leukocytes were separated from fresh heparinized blood by the Ficoll-hypaque density flotation method and washed exhaustively (7 times with RPMI 1640 containing 10% FBS) until wash supernatants were devoid (less than 10 nanograms per ml) of IgM and IgG for at least 2 washes. Cells

VIRAL DISEASES IN SOUTH-EAST ASIA
AND THE WESTERN PACIFIC
ISBN 0 12 484820 6

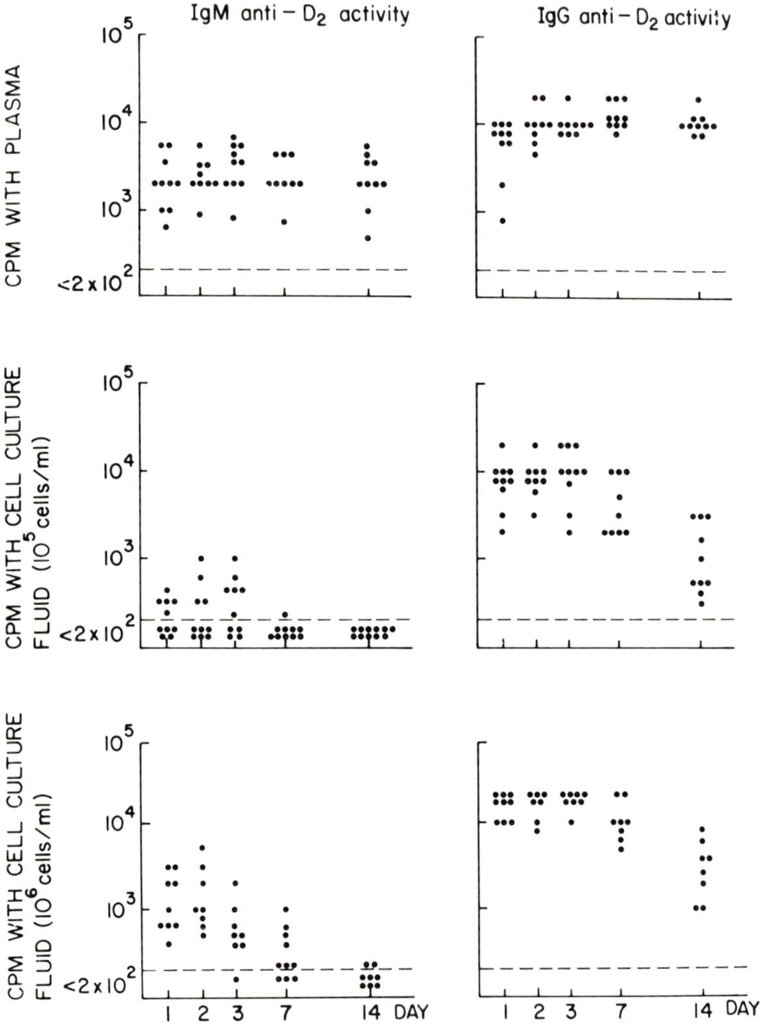

FIGURE 1. Antibody capture radioimmunoassay IgM and IgG anti-D2 activity in plasma and supernatant fluids of cultures of mononuclear leukocytes obtained from DHF patients on days 1, 2, 3, 7, and 14 after hospital presentation.

were diluted to 10^5 or 10^6 per ml and cultured in flat-bottomed screw-capped 1 dram glass vials at 37° in 5% CO_2 in RPMI 1640 with 10% FBS. Mitogens or dengue antigens were not added. Supernatant fluids were collected at 72 hours by centrifugation and stored frozen until testing. Cells were obtained on days 1, 2, 3, 7, and 14 after hospital presentation from ten DHF patients and on day 1 from nine control febrile patients who were subsequently serologically proven not to have acute dengue infections. All DHF patients showed a typical secondary or anamnestic serum antibody response by standard dengue hemagglutination inhibition serology. Plasma specimens were tested at a 1:100 dilution and cell culture fluids at a 1:4 dilution for IgM and IgG D2 antibodies by the "antibody capture" radioimmunoassay technique.

III. RESULTS (SEE FIGURE 1)

IgM and IgG anti-D2 activity was detectable in all DHF patient plasma specimens tested. Detection of IgM anti-D2 activity in cell culture supernatant fluids was dependent in the number of cells cultured; with more cells antibody was more regularly detected. IgM anti-D2 production was greatest by cells taken on day 2. IgG anti-D2 was readily detected in all cell culture fluids with either 10^5 or 10^6 cells per milliliter. Production of IgG anti-D2 decreased by day 14. Neither IgM nor IgG anti-D2 activity was detectable in the culture fluids of leukocytes taken from non-dengue febrile control patients. Phosphate buffered saline, fetal bovine serum, and normal human serum all lacked both IgM and IgG anti-dengue activity (less than 200 CPM in both assays).

REFERENCES

Burke, D., Nisalak, A. (1982). *J. Clin. Micro.*, in press.

Marchette, N., Halstead, S., and O'Rourke, T., McNair Scott, R., Bancroft, W., and Vanopruks, V. (1979). *Inf. and Immun.* 24, 47.

75

MONOCLONAL ANTIBODIES TO DENGUE-4 VIRUS

T. Pang
S. Devi
R.A. Pereira
S.K. Lam

Department of Medical Microbiology,
University of Malaya,
Kuala Lumpur,
Malaysia

I. INTRODUCTION

Monoclonal antibodies promises to be extremely useful in the detailed antigenic characterization of dengue viruses. Such information may be invaluable in understanding relationships between various dengue serotypes, in identifying antigens involved in disease pathogenesis and in vaccine development. We describe the production of monoclonal antibodies to dengue-4 (DEN-4) virus.

II. MATERIALS AND METHODS

BALB/cJ mice were immunized with DEN-4 (H-241) and immune spleen cells fused with NS-1 myeloma cells according to standard protocols. Hybrids were selected in HAT medium and supernatants assayed for activity by complement fixation test (CFT) and immunofluorescence on infected AP-61 mosquito cells. Cloning of positive hybrids was done by limiting dilution.

VIRAL DISEASES IN SOUTH-EAST ASIA
AND THE WESTERN PACIFIC
ISBN 0 12 484820 6

TABLE I. Monoclonal Antibodies to DEN-4 Virus

Clone No.	Immunofluorescence vs AP-61 cells[a]	CFT vs DEN-1	DEN-2	DEN-3	DEN-4	JE
1-3	NT	-	-	-	+	NT
4-18	NT	-	-	-	+	-
19	NT	+	-	+	+	-
20	NT	+	+	-	+	-
21-33	+	-	-	-	-	-
34	+	NT	NT	NT	NT	NT
Immune serum	+	+	+	+	+	+

[a]AP-61 cells infected with DEN-4 virus. NT = not tested

III. RESULTS AND DISCUSSION

Several factors which influence fusion efficiency were investigated. Inclusion of Freund's incomplete adjuvant with the immunizing dose and use of macrophage feeder layers significantly increased hybrid frequency. Multiple immunizations with DEN-4 was not necessary. Reactivity patterns of several of these monoclonal antibodies are shown in Table I. Characterization of the antibody produced by clone 23 showed it to be IgG1. No biological activity has been detected with antibodies produced to date.

Results indicate that most hybrids produced antibodies specific for DEN-4 (Table I). In contrast, immune serum was broadly cross-reactive (Table I). Some clones were also detected, however, which secreted antibodies reacting with other dengue serotypes (e.g. clones 19, 20; Table I). These antibodies may, in fact, be more useful for diagnostic purposes than antibodies with more restricted specificity. Also, many clones positive by immunofluorescence were negative by CFT (Table I) which may reflect reactions with different antigens. Antigenic specificity of these monoclonal antibodies and also their apparent lack of biological activity are currently under investigation.

76

INCIDENCE OF ARBOVIRAL DISEASES AND THEIR CONTROL IN NEW CALEDONIA, WALLIS AND FUTUNA

P. Fauran
G. Le Gonidec

Institut Pasteur
Noumea, New Caledonia

Epidemiological studies on arboviral diseases affecting populations of New Caledonia, Wallis and Futuna islands, showed the incidence of four different serotypes during the last ten years.

Dengue type 2 was imported into New Caledonia in September 1971 and was later responsible for a large outbreak that ended in August 1972. About 25,000 persons were affected, some by haemorrhagic forms, with at least one fatal case. This serotype was never found again in the research area.

Dengue type 1 appeared in Noumea, in March 1975, and affected some people of Ouvea island in July. This virus has probably been responsible for the epidemics recorded in New Caledonia during the Second World War (1941-1942). After control measures, only imported cases were seen in Noumea till March 1976; then, the virus transmission became apparent again and lasted till October 1978, causing about 3,000 clinical cases (572 confirmed by laboratory examination) in New Caledonia, 400 in Futuna and 20 in Wallis. One fatal case of encephalitis associated with dengue 1 infection was observed in Noumea.

Dengue type 4 was first isolated in March 1979, from imported cases detected in Noumea. After sporadic manifestations, an outbreak developed in 1980 (537 confirmed cases - 60 virus isolations). Transmission of this serotype also affected the population of Wallis (October 1979) and Futuna (January, 1980).

VIRAL DISEASES IN SOUTH-EAST ASIA
AND THE WESTERN PACIFIC
ISBN 0 12 484820 6

Ross River virus was discovered in November 1979 by isolation from sera of patients of Futuna. Laboratory examinations proved that RR virus was also transmitted later in Wallis (2 cases) and in New Caledonia (31 cases).

Research on arthropod vectors showed that *Aedes aegypti* in urban areas of New Caledonia and *Aedes polynesiensis* in Futuna were naturally infected during the outbreaks.

To control arboviral diseases, surveillance of suspected cases is exercised continuously by the Institut Pasteur laboratory in Noumea; blood specimens are tested for virus isolation and for antibody titrations. As soon as one case is discovered, investigations are made on mosquito breeding places and adults biting man or at rest, inside and around the premises of the patients.

Temephos is used for focal treatment (1-2 mg/l). Cold aerosols of insecticide are sprayed to destroy adult forms: malathion ULV from 1975 to 1978 and deltamethrin ULV in isophorone from 1979. Aerial sprayings of the whole infected area are performed, when necessary, at 8-10 days interval.

77

ROSS RIVER VIRUS IN THE SOUTHWEST PACIFIC

F. J. Austin
T. Maguire

Medical Research Council
of New Zealand
Virus Research Unit
University of Otago
Dunedin, New Zealand

I. INTRODUCTION

Since Ross River (RR) virus was first isolated in 1963 from Aedes vigilax mosquitoes collected in Townsville, Australia(1), accumulated evidence has clearly associated it with epidemic polyarthritis in man(2). Virus isolations and serological surveys indicate that until 1979 the virus was active only in Australia(2,3), West Indonesia, Papua New Guinea and the Solomon Islands (4, Table I).

TABLE I. Neutralizing antibody in human sera collected before 1979

Locality	*Number tested*	*Number with antibody*	
Papua New Guinea	*572*	*195*	*(34%)*
Solomon Islands	*458*	*31*	*(7%)*
Vanuatu	*206*	*1*	*(0.5%)*
Fiji	*743*	*2*	*(0.3%)*
Kiribati	*164*	*1*	*(0.6%)*
Tonga	*47*	*0*	
Niue	*175*	*0*	
Cook Islands	*92*	*0*	

VIRAL DISEASES IN SOUTH-EAST ASIA
AND THE WESTERN PACIFIC
ISBN 0 12 484820 6

II. DISEASE OUTBREAKS

In April 1979 cases of polyarthritis with rash were recognized on Viti Levu, the main island of Fiji (5,6). The isolation of RR virus from acute sera of two clinical cases and serological evidence identified the outbreak as epidemic polyarthritis caused by RR virus infection. During the next few weeks the disease spread through virtually all of the Fijian Islands in an epidemic which is estimated to have caused 30,000 clinical cases.

In August cases of polyarthritis began to appear in American Samoa (7). Serological tests confirmed recent RR virus infections and RR virus was isolated from a patient's serum. During 1979 and 1980 confirmed cases of RR virus infection occurred in Wallis and Futuna Islands and New Caledonia (P. Fauran and G. Le Gonidec, personal communication), Tonga and the Cook Islands (8). Imported cases were recognized in Australia, New Zealand and continental United States.

III. VECTORS

The most important RR virus vectors in Australia are *Ae. vigilax* and *Culex annulirostris* (9). *Ae. vigilax* occurs in an area bounded by Papua New Guinea in the north and Fiji in the east, while the distribution of *Cx. annulirostris* extends north to Kiribati and east to the Cook and Society Islands (10). Although all RR virus infections have occurred within the range of one or both of these mosquitoes, in many areas they are an insignificant part of the mosquito fauna and are unlikely to have been important vectors there. During the Cook Islands outbreak RR virus was isolated a number of times from *Ae. polynesiensis* (8) which is distributed in a band between latitude 8° and 20°S extending from longitude 170°E to 130°W.

Several groups of workers have been studying the vector competence of *Ae. polynesiensis* and other indigenous Pacific mosquitoes and some of their results are reported at this meeting.

IV. NON-HUMAN VERTEBRATE HOSTS

In Australia RR virus antibody has been detected in the sera of a number of different animals and it is believed that mammals may play some role in the ecology of the virus there(9). RR virus antibody was found in rat, dog, pig, cattle and chick sera during the Samoan and Cook Island epidemics(8,9). Tests on pig sera collected in Fiji before, during and after the epidemic there indicated that although pigs did become infected with RR virus during the epidemic and may have played a part in its spread, there was no evidence of pre-epidemic infection of these animals, nor was there any evidence that the virus is continuing to survive in them.

V. ROSS RIVER VIRUS IN NEW ZEALAND

When it was recognized that RR virus was probably being imported into New Zealand by viraemic individuals arriving from epidemic areas the possibility of indigenous mosquitoes becoming infected and causing secondary infections was considered. A study of the vector competence of two anthropophilic mosquitoes revealed that although both *Ae. australis* and *Ae.notoscriptus* can be infected with RR virus by feeding, only *Ae. australis* is able to transmit it. An antibody survey of 954 human sera from areas of high mosquito activity gave no indication of secondary spread of the virus in New Zealand.

VI. DISCUSSION AND CONCLUSION

An important question in relation to the Fijian epidemic is whether it was caused by the introduction of RR virus at that time or by a perturbation of an established host-virus relationship which had previously not caused excess clinical disease.

Serologically the viruses isolated in Fiji and Samoa are indistinguishable from the RR virus prototype(6,7). Retrospective serology revealed that prior to the epidemic there were a few people with low levels of RR virus neutralizing antibody in their serum, possibly due to a previous virus introduction which caused small ephemeral foci of infection which failed to survive. The appearance of the first cases near the international airport and the rapid spread of the infection suggests that the epidemic was caused by the introduction of RR virus into a population with minimal immunity.

The only way in which mosquito-borne arboviruses can be introduced naturally into a new area is by the entry of infected vectors or viraemic vertebrate hosts. Since the proportion of infected vectors at the height of an epidemic is only about 2% (8) even suboptimal spraying of incoming aircraft would probably prevent the entry of an infected vector. However the potential for viraemic individuals to carry arboviruses to new areas is well known. One might speculate therefore that RR virus was introduced into Fiji early in 1979 by a viraemic person arriving at Nadi International Airport. The subsequent spread to adjacent island groups could well have been due to viraemic people travelling from Fiji.

Although RR virus caused clinical disease in a number of Pacific countries in 1979 and 1980, some areas with susceptible populations and fauna containing known and potential vectors are still at risk of incursion by RR virus.

REFERENCES

1. Doherty, R. L., Whitehead, R. H., Gorman, B. M., and O'Gowen, A. K., *Aust. J. Sci. 26,* 183 (1963)
2. Doherty, R. L., *Progr. Med. Virol. 17,* 136 (1974)
3. Clarke,J. A., Marshall, I. D., and Gard, G. *Amer.J. Trop. Med. Hyg. 22,* 543 (1973)
4. Tesh, R.B., Gajdusek, D. C., Garruto, R. M.,Cross,J. H. and Rosen, L., *Amer. J. Trop. Med. Hyg. 24,* 664 (1975)
5. Thomson, K. D. B., Austin, F. J., Maguire, T., and Miles, J. A. R., *N.Z. Med. J. 90,* 30 (1979)
6. Aaskov, J. G., Mataika, J. U., Lawrence, G. W., Rabukawaqa , V., Tucker, M. M., Miles, J. A. R., and Dalglish, D. A., *Amer. J. Trop. Med. Hyg. 30,* 1053 (1981)
7. Tesh, R. B., McLean, R. G., Shroyer, D. A., Calisher, C. H., and Rosen, L., *Trans. Roy. Soc. Trop. Med. Hyg. 75,* 426 (1981)
8. Rosen, L., Gubler, D. J., and Bennett, P. H., *Amer. J. Trop. Med. Hyg. 30,* 1294 (1981)
9. Doherty, R. L., *Aust. Vet. J. 48,* 172 (1972)
10. Belkin, J. N., in *"The Mosquitoes of the South Pacific" vol 2,* pp. 38, 263. University of California Press, Berkeley and Los Angeles (1962)

78

VECTORS OF ROSS RIVER VIRUS: AN OVERVIEW

B.H. Kay

Queensland Institute of Medical Research
Brisbane, Australia

J.A.R. Miles

Wellcome Virus Laboratory
Suva, Fiji

D.J. Gubler

C.D.C., San Juan Laboratories
San Juan, Puerto Rico

C.J. Mitchell

C.D.C. Vector Borne Diseases Division
Ft Collins, U.S.A.

I. GEOGRAPHIC DISTRIBUTION OF ROSS RIVER VIRUS

From its isolation in 1963 from Townsville, until the clinical outbreaks throughout the south-west Pacific in 1979 - 80 (1,2,3), Ross River virus (RR) was considered primarily Australian with extension into Papua New Guinea region (4,5). Given suitable vectors in recipient nations, RR could be spread even further, especially by viraemic international air travellers. In the previous paper, Frank Austin indicated that both *Aedes australis* and *Ae notoscriptus* from New Zealand were at least susceptible to infection with RR. Prior knowledge of potential vectors, therefore, will expedite control strategies by directing operations only against those species known to be capable of transmission.

VIRAL DISEASES IN SOUTH-EAST ASIA
AND THE WESTERN PACIFIC
ISBN 0 12 484820 6

II. DEFINING THE VECTORS

Three modes of transmission, mechanical, biological and transovarial have been described for RR in mosquitoes (6,7). Our consideration will be limited to biological transmission, in which the virus replicates in the vector following ingestion and is transmitted after a suitable extrinsic incubation period (EIP), via the salivary glands to susceptible vertebrates.

Generally the best vectors are those species which are (i) easily infected (ii) capable of transmitting virus efficiently after a relatively short EIP (iii) abundant (iv) long-lived and (v) feeding commonly on the amplifier vertebrate hosts. In Australia, it is generally accepted that RR has mammalian, especially rodent and marsupial amplifiers (8,9), but in the South Pacific, serological data from American Samoa suggest a man-mosquito cycle with animals less frequently infected (2,3).

A. *Virus Isolations From Mosquitoes*

In Australia, RR has been isolated from 5 genera of mosquitoes, *Culex annulirostris*, *Aedes vigilax*, *Ae normanensis*, *Ae theobaldi*, *Anopheles amictus* (s.l.), *Mansonia uniformis* and *Coquillettidia linealis* (4,9,10), suggesting wide susceptibility. Of these *Cx annulirostris* and *Ae vigilax* are considered to be principal vectors. RR was also isolated from *Ae polynesiensis* during the Rarotonga outbreak (3).

B. *Experimentally-Infected Mosquito Species*

Laboratory experiments to determine vector competence have been done either using viraemic animals as blood donors or, alternatively, by feeding virus suspensions in blood via cotton pledgets or animal skin membranes. Such feedings, employing 4 different strains of RR, have facilitated comment on an additional 10 species (Table 1).

Although many of the differences in competence between geographically-isolated species e.g., *Ae aegypti* from Townsville, Jakarta and Fiji may be real ones, differences in methodology and virus strain used preclude quantitative comparison. However, some specific differences in vector competence were noted in individual studies.

TABLE 1. Summary of data on oral infection of mosquitoes with Ross River virus, using different infection methods.

	Species	Locality	Efficiency[a] of		Ref.
			Inf.	Trans.	
Ae	vexans	Tonga	P	P	BK
	oceanicus	"	+		"
	vigilax	Redcliffe	4.5[b]	G	(7)
	aegypti	Townsville	4.9	G	(11)
	"	Jakarta	G	F	(16)
	"	Fiji	E	F	DG
	"	"	G	P	JM
	albopictus	Hawaii	E	G	CM
	polynesiensis	Cook Is.	G	+	(16)
	"	Am. Samoa	E	G	"
	"	Fiji	E	G	JM
	pseudoscutellaris	"	P	P	"
	tongae tabu	Tonga	F	P	BK
	funereus	Redcliffe	+		(12)
Cx	annulirostris	Brisbane	G	P	(13)
	"	Fiji	E	F	JM
	quinquefasciatus	Tonga	R		BK
	"	Florida	R		(16)
	"	Brisbane	P		(14)
	"	Cairns	R		"
	"	Kowanyama	P		"
	"	Charleville	P		"
	"	Darwin	P		"
	"	Mildura	P		"
	sitiens	Tonga	P		BK
Cq	xanthogaster	Brisbane	+		(15)
Ma	uniformis	Brisbane	+		"

Infection (Inf.) and Transmission (Trans.) data grouped generally as follows:

a. Refractory (R), Poor 1-25% (P), Fair 26-50% (F), Good 51-75% (G), Excellent >75% (E), in response to virus dosage >$\log_{10}$ 3.5 suckling mouse LD_{50}/mosquito.

b. Virus dose in $\log_{10}$ suckling mouse LD_{50}/mosquito required to infect 50%.

In Fiji, *Ae polynesiensis* and *Cx annulirostris* showed greater susceptibility to infection than either *Ae aegypti* or *Ae pseudoscutellaris*. Although these species transmitted when first tested experimentally at 7-8 days, poor survival of *Ae polynesiensis* and *Ae pseudoscutellaris* contrasted with that of *Ae aegypti* over a 21 day EIP. The rapid development of RR in *Ae vigilax* which transmitted from 4 days after ingestion (6,7), contrasted with Fijian *Ae polynesiensis* which may have an extended EIP. When tested 13-14 days after ingestion, Samoan *Ae polynesiensis* were more efficient RR vectors than were *Ae aegypti* from Jakarta. However, that *Ae aegypti* engorged more readily than did *Ae polynesienses* even after prolonged starvation may enhance the potential of *Ae aegypti* even further (16).

In general, Tongan culicids tested were poorly susceptible to the 2 different pools used. This may, in fact, partly explain why RR entered Tonga without causing an epidemic. However more study of these mosquitoes is necessary. That the common day-biting *Stegomyia*, *Ae tabu* is partly autogenous would lessen the potential of this species.

The limited evaluation of *Ae albopictus*, an Asian dengue vector, suggests high competence. Extensive evaluation of the cosmopolitan peridomestic *Cx quinquefasciatus* suggest almost no potential at all.

III. CONCLUSIONS

There are several important points evident from this overview:

(a) Because 18 of the 19 species considered in this or the previous paper have some potential as vectors, control strategies should be developed not only from viral susceptibility and transmission data but also from entomological considerations of abundance, longevity in relation to EIP and of man-vector contact.

(b) *Aedes (Stegomyia)* spp., particularly *Ae polynesiensis* and other *Scutellaris* group mosquitoes plus *Ae aegypti* are likely to be important for the following reasons: (i) they are the predominant group numerically (ii) these mosquitoes are noted man-biters, indoors and outdoors and breed in a variety of artificial e.g. tyres, drums, rainwater tanks, or natural containers e.g. crab holes, coconut husks (iii) dengue type IV transmitted by *Stegomyia* group mosquitoes was occurring at the time of the South Pacific epidemic polyarthritis outbreak (iv) serological data indicate a man-mosquito cycle with *Ae polynesiensis* a suspect on epidemiological grounds, in both American Samoa and Rarotonga (2,3).

(c) Because man may act as an amplifier host prior to onset of symptoms and because cosmopolitan species such as *Ae aegypti* and *Ae albopictus* are efficient vectors, RR potentially could become a widespread public health problem throughout Asia and other parts of the World.

REFERENCES

1. Aaskov, J.G., Mataika, J.U., Lawrence, G.W., Rabukawaqa, V., Tucker, M.M., Miles, J.A.R. and Dalglish, D.A. (1981). *Am. J. Trop. Med. Hyg. 30*, 1053.
2. Tesh, R.B., McLean, R.G., Shroyer, D.A., Calisher, C.H. and Rosen, L.(1981). *Trans. R. Soc. Trop. Med. Hyg. 75*, 426.
3. Rosen, L., Gubler, D.J. and Bennett, P. (1981). *Am. J. Trop. Med. Hyg. 30*, 1294.
4. Doherty, R.L. (1977). *Aust. J. Exp. Biol. Med. Sci. 55*, 103.
5. Kanamitsu, M., Taniguchi, K., Urasawa, S., Ogata, T., Wada, Y. and Sulianti Saroso, J. (1979). *Am. J. Trop. Med. Hyg. 28*, 351.
6. Standfast, H.A., Fanning, I.D., van Kammen, A. and Steen, M.A. (1969). *Annu. Rep. Qd Inst. Med. Res. 24*, 7.
7. Kay, B.H., *Aust. J. Exp. Biol. Med. Sci.* (in press).
8. Doherty, R.L. (1972). *Aust. Vet. J. 48*, 172.
9. Gard, G., Marshall, I.D. and Woodroofe, G. (1973). *Am. J. Trop. Med. Hyg. 22*, 551.
10. Marshall, I.D. (1979). *In* St George, T.D. and French, E.L., Arbovirus Research in Australia, *Proc. Second Symp., CSIRO-QIMR*, p 47.
11. Kay, B.H., Carley, J.G., Fanning, I.D. and Filippich, C. (1979). *J. Med. Entomol. 16*, 59.
12. Kay, B.H., Carley, J.G. and Filippich, C. (1977). *J. Med. Entomol. 13*, 451.
13. Kay, B.H., Carley, J.G., Fanning, I.D. and Barrow, G.J. (1976). *Annu. Rep. Qd Inst. Med. Res. 31*, 12.
14. Kay, B.H., Fanning, I.D. and Carley, J.G. *Am. J. Trop. Med. Hyg.* (in press).
15. Kay, B.H., Carley, J.G., Barrow, G.J., Walker, P.J. and Fanning, I.D. (1972). *Annu. Rep. Qd Inst. Med. Res. 27*, 8.
16. Gubler, D.J. (1981). *Am. J. Trop. Med. Hyg. 30*, 1303.

DIAGNOSIS OF JAPANESE ENCEPHALITIS BY DETECTION OF IgM AND IgG VIRUS SPECIFIC ANTIBODIES IN CEREBROSPINAL FLUID BY "ANTIBODY CAPTURE" IMMUNOASSAY

Donald S. Burke
Ananda Nisalak
Michael A. Ussery

Department of Virology
Armed Forces Research Institute
of Medical Sciences, Bangkok, Thailand

I. IMMUNOGLOBULIN M (IgM) IN ACUTE JE

Edelman et al (1979) demonstrated that virus specific IgM antibodies are detectable in sera obtained early in the illness of most patients with acute JE and that these antibodies disappear within a few months. Recently we devised an "antibody capture" solid phase radioimmunoassay (Burke and Ananda, 1982) for measuring IgM JE serum antibodies (JE IgM ACRIA, see figure 1). By substituting goat anti-human gamma chain for anti-human mu chain we also performed a modified assay to detect IgG class antibodies against JE virus (JE IgG ACRIA).

II. KINETICS OF "ANTIBODY CAPTURE" TYPE IMMUNOASSAYS

As performed by us, all available antibody capture sites (goat anti-mu or gamma chain molecules) attached to the solid phase are occupied at test sample immunoglobulin concentrations in excess of 1 microgram per milliliter. Therefore, when biological fluids with class specific immunoglobulin concentrations in excess of this level are assayed, the CPM ultimately bound to the solid phase are

VIRAL DISEASES IN SOUTH-EAST ASIA
AND THE WESTERN PACIFIC
ISBN 0 12 484820 6

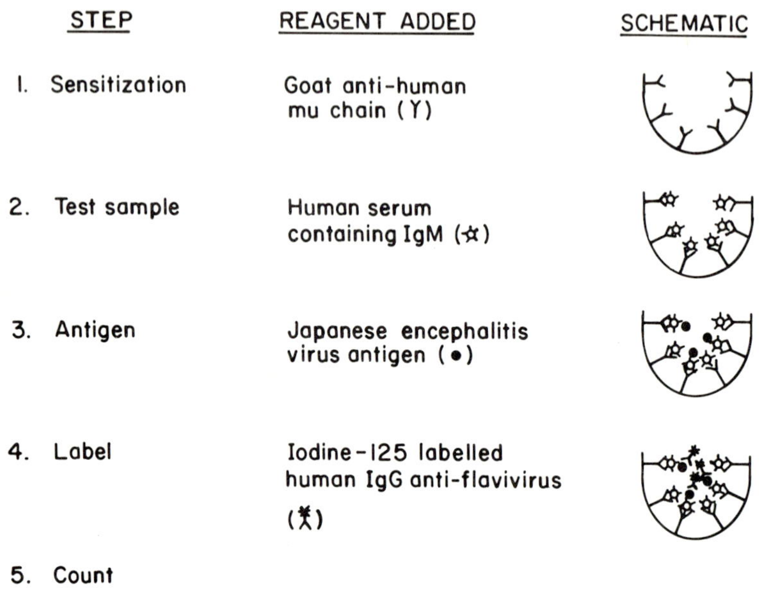

FIGURE 1. Schematic diagram of steps in the JE IgM antibody capture radioimmunoassay (JE IgM ACRIA)

proportional to the fraction of the total immunoglobulin molecules of that class with anti-JE activity, rather than to the absolute number of JE specific immunoglobulin molecules in the sample. Both IgM and IgG concentrations in CSF specimens from patients with inflamatory diseases of the central nervous system typically are greater than 1 microgram per milliliter (Gill and Brody, 1979). Thus the CPM obtained by JE ACRIA reflect the relative specific antibody activities of serum and CSF. This is demonstrated in figure 2 where the JE IgG ACRIA activities and total IgG concentrations of serial dilutions of acute serum and CSF from a representative JE patient with a secondary (anamnestic) flavivirus antibody response are shown.

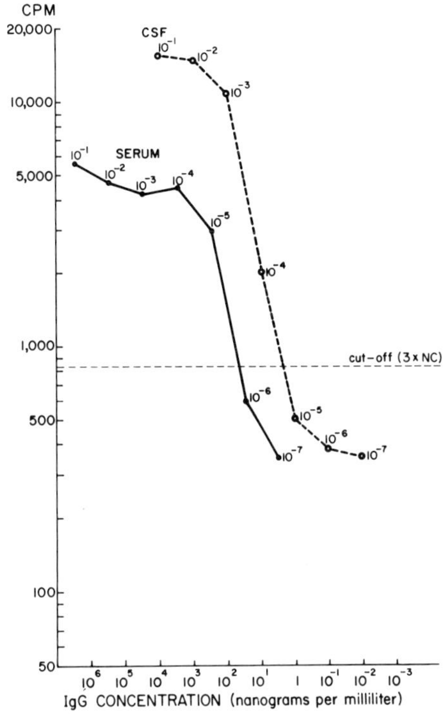

FIGURE 2. Counts per minute bound to the solid phase in the JE IgG ACRIA with varying dilutions of acute serum and CSF from a representative case of acute encephalitis.

III. MEASUREMENT OF JE ANTIBODIES IN PATIENT SERUM AND CSF SAMPLES

Eleven of twelve patients with JE infections subsequently proven by hemagglutination inhibition (HAI) serology had JE IgM ACRIA antibodies in the acute CSF specimen (geometric mean titer=1:2500) as compared to none of eight patients with acute encephalitis proven not to be due to JE. Specific IgM anti-JE activity (units/ug) was greater in CSF than in simultaneous sera specimens in all eleven positive cases by a mean factor of more than four fold (range 1.4 to 13). Among seven patients with broadly reactive HAI seroresponses typical of persons previously exposed to other flaviviruses, six had high levels of JE IgG ACRIA antibodies in their acute phase cerebrospinal fluid (GMT=1:26,000), while in five patients experiencing their first flavivirus infection, JE IgG ACRIA antibodies were either absent (one patient) or weakly reactive (four patients, GMT=1:3,200). Specific IgG anti-JE activity was greater in CSF than in simultaneous sera specimens in eight of the nine positive cases measured (range 1.3 to 24 fold).

IV. CONCLUSION

The antibody capture solid phase immunoassay approach is uniquely well suited to detect virus specific antibodies of defined immunoglobulin class in CSF.

REFERENCES

Burke, D., and Nisalak, A. (1982). *J. Clin. Micro.* in press.
Edelman, R., and Pariyanonda, A. (1979). *Amer. J. Epidemiol. 98,* 29.
Gill, D., and Brody, M. (1979). *Arch. Dis. Child. 54,* 961.

80

PROTECTION AGAINST LETHAL SINDBIS VIRUS INFECTION WITH SPECIFIC MONOCLONAL ANTIBODIES[1]

G. A. Cole
A. L. Schmaljohn

Department of Microbiology
School of Medicine
University of Maryland
Baltimore, Maryland, U.S.A.

J. M. Dalrymple

Virology Division
U. S. Army Medical Research Institute
of Infectious Diseases
Fort Detrick, Frederick, Maryland, U.S.A.

I. INTRODUCTION

Antibodies are known to play an important role in specific immunity to alphaviruses. Recovery from infections with these viruses is associated usually with the appearance of circulating specific antibodies, particularly those that neutralize virus infectivity *in vitro*, and resistance to infection can be transferred passively with immune serum containing neutralizing (NT) antibodies. In some cases, however, one infecting alphavirus will induce protective immunity to another with which it shares antigenic determinants, but to which cross-reactive NT antibodies are undetectable (1, 2). This type of immunity has been attributed to a cellular mechanism mediated possibly by

[1]*This work was supported by USPHS grant NS17741 and by the U.S. Army R&D Command.*

VIRAL DISEASES IN SOUTH-EAST ASIA
AND THE WESTERN PACIFIC
ISBN 0 12 484820 6

cross-reactive cytotoxic T lymphocytes which have been demonstrated during certain alphavirus infections of mice (3, 4). However, the findings to be presented here and elsewhere (5) favor the possibility that humoral immunity to alphaviruses can be mediated by antibodies that lack NT activity and react exclusively with virus-infected cells.

We have prepared monoclonal antibodies to the AR339 strain of Sindbis virus (SV), the prototype of the *Alphavirus* genus, to investigate relationships between their protein specificity, NT activity and ability to passively protect mice against infection. Since SV is of low virulence for mice, protection was assessed using a neuroadapted variant (NSV) of SV that produced paralysis and fatal encephalitis when given intracerebrally (i.c.) to adult C57BL/6J mice (5).

II. PROTECTION BY NEUTRALIZING MONOCLONAL ANTIBODIES

Sindbis virus contains two envelope glycoproteins, E1 and E2, and an internal nucleocapsid protein (NC). As predicted by earlier studies using monospecific antisera (6), most monoclonal antibodies having NT activity were specific for E2 (7); a single anti-E1 antibody also neutralized SV, indicating that viral envelope determinants involved in neutralization are not restricted to E2. No NT activity was exhibited by anti-NC antibodies.

All antibodies that neutralized NSV (80% plaque-reduction in the presence of added complement) also prevented paralysis and/or death (Table I) when given intraperitoneally (0.1 ml of ascitic fluid) 24 hours before i.c. challenging mice with 1000 plaque-forming units (PFU) of NSV. Consonant with the general observation that alphavirus-NT antibodies are type-specific (6, 8), antibodies that neutralized SV, but not NSV, were non-protective even though these two viruses are very closely related. However, in no case did antibodies bind to either virus without neutralizing it. All protective anti-E2 antibodies were able to mediate complement (C')-dependent lysis of NSV-infected BHK-21 cells as measured by ^{51}Cr-release (5).

Taken together, these results suggested that, in addition to their neutralizing virus directly, antibodies specific for E2 determinants might effect virus elimination *in vivo* indirectly by mediating lysis of infected host cells.

Table I. Passive protection by antibodies that neutralize NSV and/or lyse NSV-infected cells

Antibody and Specificity	Log_{10} antibody titer[a]				Passive protection against NSV challenge[b]	
	Neut.		Cytolysis		%	%
	SV	NSV	SV	NSV	Paralysis	Mortality
49-E2	5.0	3.0	≥4.0	3.0	10	3
50-E2	5.0	3.0	≥4.0	3.0	0	0
10-E2	5.0	<1.0	≥4.0	<1.5	100	100
33-E1	3.0	3.0	3.5	3.5	0	0
7-E1	<1.0	<1.0	2.0	3.0	0	0
16-E1	<1.0	<1.0	3.0	3.0	0	0
38-E1	<1.0	<1.0	2.0	3.0	0	0
1-E1	<1.0	<1.0	2.5	3.0	12	4
3-NC	<1.0	<1.0	<1.5	<1.5	100	100

[a]*Highest antibody dilution effecting ≥80% plaque reduction in NT assay or ≥10% virus-specific cytolysis in Cr-51-release assay.*
[b]*Excess antibody (0.1 ml ascitic fluid) given intraperitoneally 24 hours before i.c. challenge with 1000 PFU NSV.*

III. PROTECTION BY NON-NEUTRALIZING MONOCLONAL ANTIBODIES

With the exception mentioned above, monoclonal antibodies specific for E1 neutralized neither SV nor NSV but (as represented in Table I) most were found to be protective *in vivo*. The fact that these antibodies shared with protective anti-E2 antibodies the ability to mediate C'-dependent lysis of NSV-infected cells *in vitro* suggested a common mechanism of action *in vivo*. However, we have been unable to reduce the protective capacity of antibodies to either E1 or E2 in mice decomplemented by treatment with cobra venom factor (data not shown).

The general failure of anti-E1 antibodies to exhibit NT activity is not simply the result of their recognizing determinants on the "wrong" glycoprotein. Current evidence suggests that these determinants are not expressed on the surfaces of intact virus particles. As measured in a solid-phase ELISA, antibodies specific for E1 and E2 bound to plastic-adhering proteins of detergent-disrupted purified SV (Table II). However, only those having NT activity could be

Table II. Failure of non-NT anti-E1 antibodies to bind intact virus

Antibody and Specificity	ELISA titer (Log_{10})	% Inhibition of binding by:	
		Intact SV	Disrupted SV (Triton X-100)
49-E2	4.8	97	97
50-E2	4.1	99	90
10-E2	5.0	95	95
33-E1	4.3	84	96
7-E1	4.0	0	93
16-E1	5.2	0	94
38-E1	4.3	0	96

inhibited from binding by previously mixing them with an excess of intact (infectious) virus. A comparable inhibition of non-NT antibodies was obtained only by mixing them with detergent-disrupted SV (Table II, Schmaljohn *et al*, manuscript in preparation).

That non-NT anti-El antibodies did not recognize infectious SV was indicated further by their failure to reduce virus infectivity in the presence of C' or polyvalent anti-mouse Ig antibody, both of which augmented the activity of NT antibodies (data not shown).

In sum, these results provide compelling evidence that certain El determinants appearing on the plasma membranes of infected cells, when incorporated into nature virions become inaccessible to antibodies, presumably because of steric or conformational changes in El that occur during virus maturation. Containment of infection *in vivo* by antibodies to these determinants must, therefore, be mediated through binding to El on infected host cells. While, theoretically, antibody-binding alone could prevent the completion of viral morphogenesis (9); an adjunctive role for other host elements such as C' or Fc receptor-bearing cells cannot be excluded.

IV. CONCLUSIONS

The collective data from this study point to a clear relationship between the glycoprotein specificity of monoclonal antibodies to SV and the site(s) of their protective action *in vivo*. Thus far, all antibodies to E2 have been found to neutralize virus infectivity and bind to determinants common to the surfaces of both virions and infected cells. As a general rule, antibodies to El lack NT activity because their binding is restricted to determinants on infected cells; infectious virions possess these same determinants but they are inaccessible to antibody. While the NT activity of these antibodies *in vitro* can account for at least one of the ways in which they protect *in vivo*, the mechanism(s) of protection by antibodies binding exclusively to virus-infected cells are more speculative and have been alluded to above. How the Ig isotypes of protective antibodies (which in Tables I and II were G2a or G2b) may either limit or amplify their functional capabilities is discussed elsewhere (5). Since a number of monoclonal antibodies to the El (but not the E2) glycoprotein of SV have been found to cross-react serologically with other members of the same alphavirus subgroup (7) we anticipate, in future studies, their being able to mediate a corresponding cross-protection *in vivo*.

REFERENCES

1. Casals, J., *Am. J. Trop. Med. Hyg. 12*, 587 (1963).
2. Porterfield, J. S., in "The Togaviruses: Biology, Structure, Replication" (R. W. Schlesinger, ed.), p. 13. Academic Press, New York, (1980).
3. Müllbacher, A., Marshall, I. D., and Blanden, R. V., *Scand. J. Immunol. 10*, 291 (1979).
4. Peck, R., Brown, A., and Wust, C. J., *J. Immunol. 123*, 1763 (1979).
5. Schmaljohn, A. L., Johnson, E. D., Dalrymple, J. M., and Cole, G. A., *Nature* (1982) in press.
6. Dalrymple, J. M., Schlesinger, S., and Russell, P. K., *Virology 69*, 93 (1976).
7. Dalrymple, J., Cole, G. A., Jahrling, P., Johnson, E., and Harrison, S., *Abstr., 5th Int'l. Cong. Virology*, p. 301 (1981).
8. Karabatsos, N., *Am. J. Trop. Med. Hyg. 24*, 257 (1975).
9. Bracha, M. and Schlesinger, M. J., *Virology, 74*, 441 (1976).

81

SUPERINFECTION IMMUNITY AND THE GEOGRAPHICAL DISTRIBUTION OF TOGAVIRUSES[1]

Mary Davey[2]
Rod Mahon[3]
Adrian Gibbs

Virus Ecology Research Group
Research School of Biological Sciences
Australian National University
Canberra, A.C.T.
Australia

Some of the mosquito-borne encephalitis group of flaviviruses are distributed sympatrically (e.g. Murray Valley encephalitis (MVEfV) and Kunjin flavivirus (KfV), both in Australia), others parapatrically (e.g. MVEfV and Japanese B encephalitis flavivirus (JefV)) and other allopatrically (e.g. MVEfV and West Nile flavivirus (WNfV)). Sabin (1952) demonstrated that *Aedes aegypti* mosquitoes infected with dengue flavivirus (DfV) resisted subsequent infection with yellow fever flavivirus (YFfV), and, noting the absence of YFfV from areas of the world where DfV causes epidemics, suggested that "the introduction of yellow fever virus into a dengue epidemic area may find enough mosquitoes relatively refractory to the yellow fever virus to prevent the establishment of yellow fever into the same area".

[1]*This work was supported by a grant from the Australian Encephalitis Control Programme of the Commonwealth Department of Health.*

[2]*Present address: Department of Obstetrics and Gynaecology, Royal North Shore Hospital, Sydney, N.S.W., Australia*

[3]*Present address: Division of Entomology, C.S.I.R.O., Canberra*

VIRAL DISEASES IN SOUTH-EAST ASIA AND THE WESTERN PACIFIC
ISBN 0 12 484820 6

We have examined this idea further using variants of MVEfV and KfV obtained from persistently infected *Aedes albopictus* cells, that had been subcultured every week for 45 weeks. The variants were called M-mp and K-mp, respectively; their replication was temperature sensitive, and their virions antigenically slightly different from type isolates of the viruses (J. Casals, pers. comm.).

Adult *Culex annulirostris* were injected with 0.3 μl of virus-free medium or a suspension (10^2 pfu/individual) of one or other of the variants, and then seven days later with a similar inoculum of either MVEfV, KfV, JEfV or WNfV.

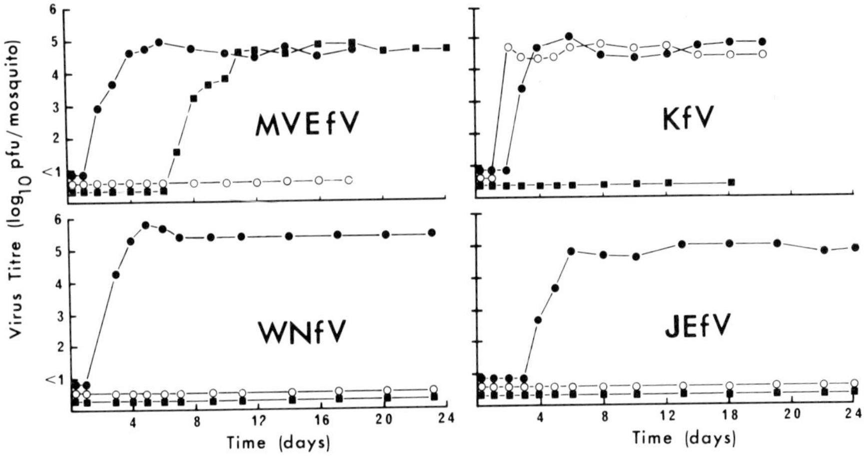

FIGURE 1. Concentration of four flaviviruses in mosquitoes after challenge inoculation. Seven days before challenge, the mosquitoes were injected with virus-free medium (●), M-mp (○) or K-mp (■); the mp isolates did not produce plaques at the temperature used for the bioassay.

The assays (Fig. 1) showed that all viruses grew normally in virus-free mosquitoes; KfV, JEfV and WNfV failed to grow in K-mp infected mosquitoes; MVEfV, JEfV and WNfV failed to grow in M-mp infected mosquitoes; but KfV grew in M-mp infected mosquitoes, and MVEfV grew, though tardily, in K-mp infected mosquitoes. Thus the sympatrically distributed viruses did not interfere, or did so ephemerally, whereas the allopatrically or parapatrically distributed ones interfered. Similar results were obtained using cultured *A. albopictus* cells, rather than mosquitoes.

TABLE I. Togavirus interference in mosquitoes or their cultured cells

		Second (challenge) virus								
		alphaviruses				flaviviruses				
		EEE	RR	SF	S	JE	K	MVE	WN	YF
First virus: alphaviruses	SF-ts		+	++						
	S			–						
	S-sp	+			+					
	WEE	–								
First virus: flaviviruses	D									+
	D-2							–		
	JE							+		
	K-mp			–		++	++	+	++	
	M-mp					++	–	++	++	
	WN			–					++	

++ *complete interference,* - *no interference.*
\+ *partial interference, such as slowed growth or increased lag period, or interference only in certain conditions.*

Names - Eastern Equine Encephalitis, Ross River, Semliki Forest, Sindbis and Western Equine Encephalitis alphaviruses; Dengue, Japanese Encephalitis, Kunjin, Murray Valley Encephalitis, West Nile, Yellow Fever flaviruses; -ts, temperature sensitive; -sp, small plaque; -mp, multiple passage. Sources of information (1-10).

The published reports of togavirus interference (Table 1) are very incomplete. However, none show interference between an alphavirus and a flavivirus, and, with one unconfirmed exception, all report that strains of one virus interfere completely. There is also some evidence that interference within togavirus subgroups is correlated with antigenic relatedness, and that sympatrically distributed viruses do not interfere.

REFERENCES

1. Sabin, A.B., *Am. J. Trop. Med. Hyg. 1*, 30 (1952).
2. Altman. R.M., *Am. J. Trop. Med. Hyg. 12*, 425 (1963).
3. Chamberlain, R.W., and Sudia, W.D., *J. Infect. Dis. 101*, 233 (1957).
4. Davey, M.W., Mahon, R.J., and Gibbs, A.J. *J. Gen. Virol. 42*, 641 (1979).
5. Davey, M.W., Mahon, R.J., and Gibbs, A.J., in preparation.
6. Lam, K.S.K., and Marshall, I.D., *Am. J. Trop. Hyg. Med. 17*, 625 (1968).
7. Peleg, J., *Ann. N.Y. Acad. Sci. 266*, 204 (1975).
8. Regnery, R.L., *Ph.D. thesis*, A.N.U. Canberra,(1976).
9. Rozeboom, L.E., and Kassira, E.N., *J. Med. Ent. 6*, 407 (1969).
10. Stollar, V., and Shenk, T.E., *J. Virol. 11*, 592 (1973).

Part VI
Specific Viral Diseases

E.
Other Zoonotic Viruses

Chairman C. A. Mims

Co-Chairman E. L. French

82

RABIES: ITS PATHOGENESIS PREDICTS ITS ECOLOGIC ENTRENCHMENT

Frederick A. Murphy

College of Veterinary Medicine and Biomedical Sciences
Colorado State University
Fort Collins, Colorado, USA

The ancient scourge, rabies, must still be regarded as a most important disease of man, a disease measured not only in terms of statistical morbidity/mortality comparisons with other diseases, but also in terms of individual suffering and public hysteria. Similarly, the importance of animal rabies must be measured in terms of costs of control, loss of livestock production and impact upon fragile wildlife populations. Within the geographic scope of this Seminar we see the harsh contrast between the rabies-free status of Australia, New Zealand, Japan, Antarctica, Hong Kong, Singapore, and many islands of the Pacific including Hawaii, Fiji, New Caledonia and Samoa, and the rabies-entrenched status of Indonesia, Thailand, the Philippines, India, Pakistan and other places where the incidence of the disease may be similar but reporting is incomplete.

I. THE VALUE OF RABIES EXCLUSION - THE BURDEN OF RABIES CONTROL

The rabies-free status of an area is no guarantee against future problems -- the virus is not excluded from any area by specific ecologic limitations. This point becomes quite clear if we extrapolate from our knowledge of the natural history of the virus in well-studied problem areas. The key to deriving value from such extrapolation lies in distinguishing simple, single-host ecosystems from complex, interactive multiple-host systems. It would be naive to extend principles drawn from ecologically simple fox rabies episodes in Europe, mongoose rabies episodes in the Caribbean, or arctic fox rabies episodes in the northern polar regions, to areas which are more like those where overlapping transmission patterns occur. The potential for rabies virus to

VIRAL DISEASES IN SOUTH-EAST ASIA
AND THE WESTERN PACIFIC
ISBN 0 12 484820 6

become entrenched in Australia must be judged differently from that of Great Britain, Switzerland or small tropical islands. Perhaps those concerned about the reintroduction of the virus into Great Britain can be optimistic--after all, it was eliminated in 1903 by the rather simple means of controlling the movement of dogs (stray animal control, importation control) (5). However, there is no evidence that rabies virus ever was present in fox or other wildlife populations of Great Britain in the nineteenth century, and it remains a fact that rabies has never been eliminated from a complex, multiple-host ecosystem involving wildlife. Even in instances where comprehensive control programs have been put in place, there have been reintroductions and extensions. For example, within the past ten years rabies occurred on the island of Guam, and despite what should have been adequate regulatory activity, the virus reached the island's feral deer population (via a feral carnivore reservoir) where it engendered a substantial eradication campaign. Extension of this ecologically simple example to the larger islands of the Pacific immediately stretches our imagination concerning the capabilities and resources of available disease control agencies.

It must be clear that efforts to maintain the rabies-free status of a country or area are worth the costs and efforts. A recent report of the costs associated with the identification of a single rabid dog in California is enlightening (6). Although the dog bit only three persons, investigation resulted in the identification of 70 persons who also required post-exposure treatment. In addition, a stray dog control program was instigated and special clinics were set up in the area to vaccinate dogs. This episode, in which no person or other animal developed rabies, generated costs totalling (in U.S. dollars) $105,790 ($92,650) for human treatment, $4,190 for 2,000 dog vaccinations, $8,950 for stray animal control). This episode was of typical magnitude, but in Amsterdam in 1962, an episode stemming from a primary dog case (and involving five human deaths) resulted in post-exposure treatment of more than 500 people, immunization of 650,000 pets, and incredible costs.

Just as it must be clear that maintenance of a rabies-free status is worthwhile, so it must also be clear that where rabies is present, control programs to minimize human exposure are a public obligation. Rabies control involves 1) specific control of animal movement (stray dog control, especially), 2) immunization of dogs (and cats), 3) public education, 4) surveillance based upon reliable laboratory diagnosis, 5) and, in many cases, programs to interrupt wildlife transmission cycles. A primary intention must be to eliminate dog rabies, that is, to prevent spillage of virus from other reservoir host cycles into a dog-to-dog transmission cycle which presents maximum human and livestock risk.

Control of rabies will become increasingly difficult. In this time of rapid transport of animals (including illegal transport), quarantines may not prevent all movement of virus within and between rabies-endemic areas. Publicly supported control programs must be backed up with research on the many aspects of the natural history of the virus which, on the one hand lead to its entrenchment, and on the other hand represent its vulnerability to human intervention. We need to know more about 1) *the virus*, its genetics and its antigenicity; 2) *the disease*, its pathogenesis in relation to host immune responsiveness; 3) *the transmission cycle*, its variability in various reservoir hosts; and 4) *the population dynamics of host species* which influence the behavior and movement of the virus in natural settings. Each of these aspects impacts on disease control considerations; taking one of these as an example, the following section focuses on pathogenetic characteristics which underscore ecologic entrenchment of the virus.

II. THE PATHOGENETIC BASIS FOR VIRUS TRANSMISSION

Most warm-blooded animals are susceptible to rabies virus infection, and with rare exceptions, the infection ends in death. This outcome circumvents the development of any degree of "herd immunity" which would otherwise be a major influence upon the movement, persistence, and reintroduction of the virus in reservoir host populations. If the lethality of rabies infection in the individual animal is a key to the behavior of the virus in whole populations, then the question of why the infection is so lethal has added interest.

Following the deep introduction of the virus by the bite of a rabid animal, initial virus replication occurs in striated muscle cells at the site (8-10). This infection can serve as an amplifying source of virus for assualt on the peripheral nervous system; it may also be the site of sequestration of virus during long incubation infections. Long incubation infections are a key to entrenchment of virus where transmission would otherwise be interrupted by a shortage of susceptible animals caused by a rabies epizootic and/or a seasonal breeding pattern.

Deep in muscles the peripheral nervous system is exposed in neuromuscular spindles (the sensory proprioceptors made up of modified muscle cells wrapped in unmyelinated nerve endings). In our studies of street rabies in hamsters, spindles were the second tissue to become infected; we, therefore, concluded that these exposed nerve endings were more important entry sites into the nervous system than were motor nerve endings. Recently, Tignor and his colleagues showed that motor end plates are important sites for nervous system invasion; they found that cholinesterase positive sites (i.e., motor plates) serve as specific receptors for rabies virus present in extracellular space and that the attraction of virus to these sites may be inhibited by neurotransmitter blocking agents (14).

Other nerve endings may play a role in rabies virus entry into the nervous system. The olfactory end organ (neuroepithelial cells exposed to the body surface and extending directly to the olfactory bulb of the brain) in the nares is easily infected via intranasal instillation of virus. This is the key to the efficient aerosol transmission of virus in bat caves and the entrenchment of virus in some colonial species of bats (1). The many epithelial and subepithelial sensory nerve endings of the skin and mucous membranes may serve as yet another entry site for virus when exposed by superficial abrasion. Virus amplification at such sites may occur through epithelial cell infection. Superficial abrasion has been the route of virus entry in human rabies cases and probably is the key to transmission between animals in the absence of fury.

The entry of virus into nerve endings begins a phase in which neuronal infection and centripetal passive axoplasmic movement of virus genome leads to invasion of the central nervous system in the spinal cord and later in the brain (11). The slow course of rabies movement to its ultimate target organ, the brain, would seem to provide opportunity for a full spectrum of host defenses to come to bear. Nonspecific inflammatory response should be stimulated by trauma at the bite site. Specific humoral and cell-mediated immune responses are easily stimulated by virus proteins in model systems, but in the real disease, host defenses are a failure. The key seems to be that very little virus antigen is presented to trigger host response: 1) there may be very little virus delivered into the bite site; 2) there may be very little virus budded early from plasma membranes of infected muscle cells (and in the absence of cytopathic changes virus budding upon internal membranes of muscle cells would be trapped); 3) there may be very little virus budded from the plasma membranes of infected peripheral nerve axons and most of such virus would be permanently trapped beneath myelin sheaths; and 4) there may be very little virus budded early from plasma membranes of central nervous system neurons (here, too, in the absence of cytopathic changes most virus would be trapped) (Figure 1). In addition, because most rabies antigens accumulate in the immunologically sequestered environment of the central nervous system, free from most lymphocyte trafficking and lymphatic drainage, the triggering problem is compounded. So, the host response to rabies infection has reason to be delayed and of minimal intensity until too late to matter. This is what happens in natural infections--in man and in animals, neutralizing antibody and inflammatory infiltrations are usually absent at the time of the onset of encephalitic signs, and reach substantial levels only at the time of death. Whether the disease has an immunopathologic basis, or not, does not matter in an ecologic sense.

Following the entry of virus into the central nervous system, usually in the spinal cord, an ascending wave of neuronal infection and neuronal dysfunction occurs--this is seen clinically as ascending paralysis and experimentally as an ascending wavefront of immunofluorescent virus antigen or infectivity titer. A consistent topographic localization of this wavefront of infection within the brain is the most likely cause of specific clinical signs including fury. At the stage when ascending infection has reached the limbic system but not the neocortex, neuronal dysfunction correlates with alertness, loss of natural timidity, aberrant sexual behavior and agressiveness (4). Of course, one of the most remarkable aspects of this infection pattern is that it has become a necessity for the transmission and survival of the virus. In those species in which infection does not involve a furious phase, the topographic pattern and speed of the ascent of virus seems to differ.

As if the necessity for this precise pattern of infection in the brain were not remarkable enough, consider the added necessity that for transmission to occur, virus must be delivered into saliva at the same time as the animal becomes furious. In order to accomplish this, the infection, which until this point has been narrowly neuronotropic (muscle excepted), broadens to involve mucous acinar epithelial cells of the salivary glands. This infection site, initiated from nerves entering the glands, is very productive, delivering in some reservoir host species up $10^6 ID_{50}$/ml of saliva. One more remarkable attribute of the infection is that, although in the nervous system most virus buds upon internal membranes

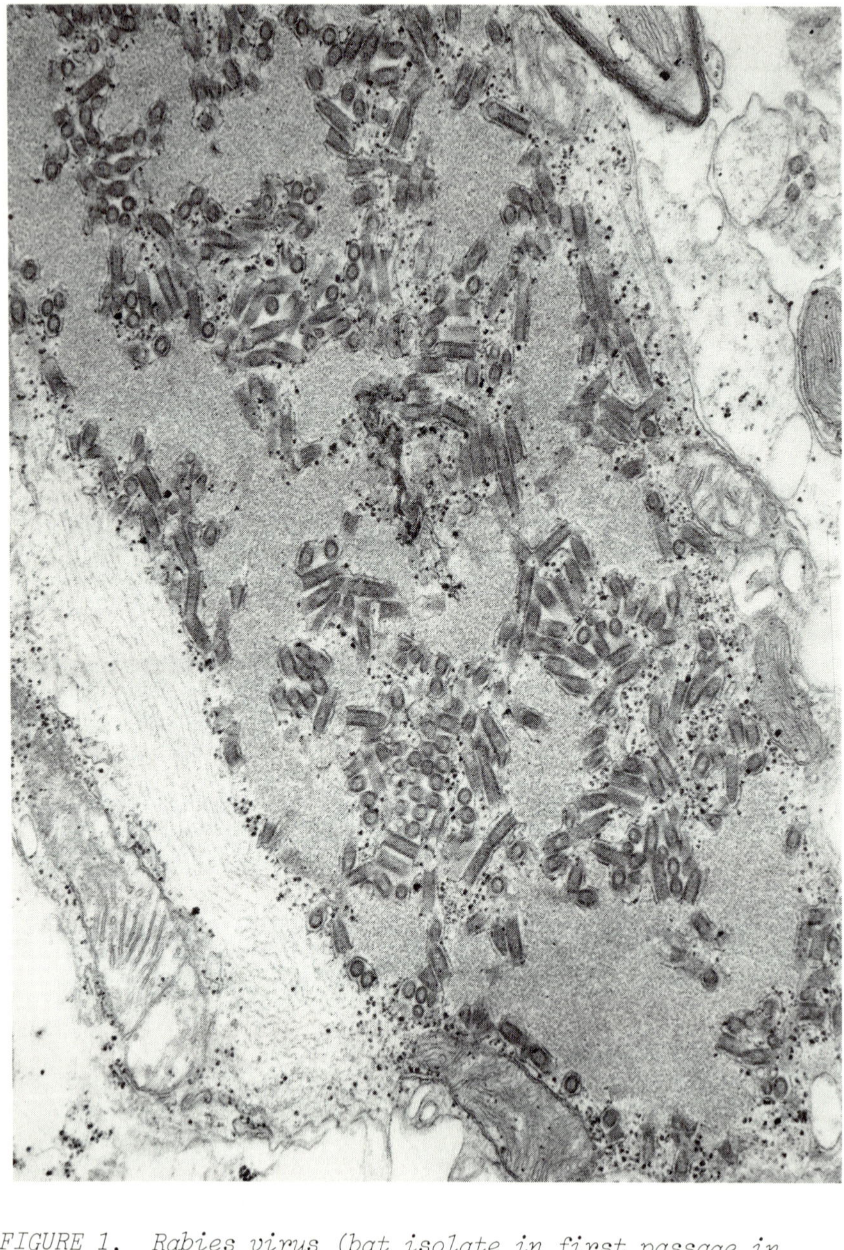

FIGURE 1. Rabies virus (bat isolate in first passage in mouse brain) trapped within cytoplasm of brain neuron in association with massed viral nucleocapsid inclusion material (X35,000).

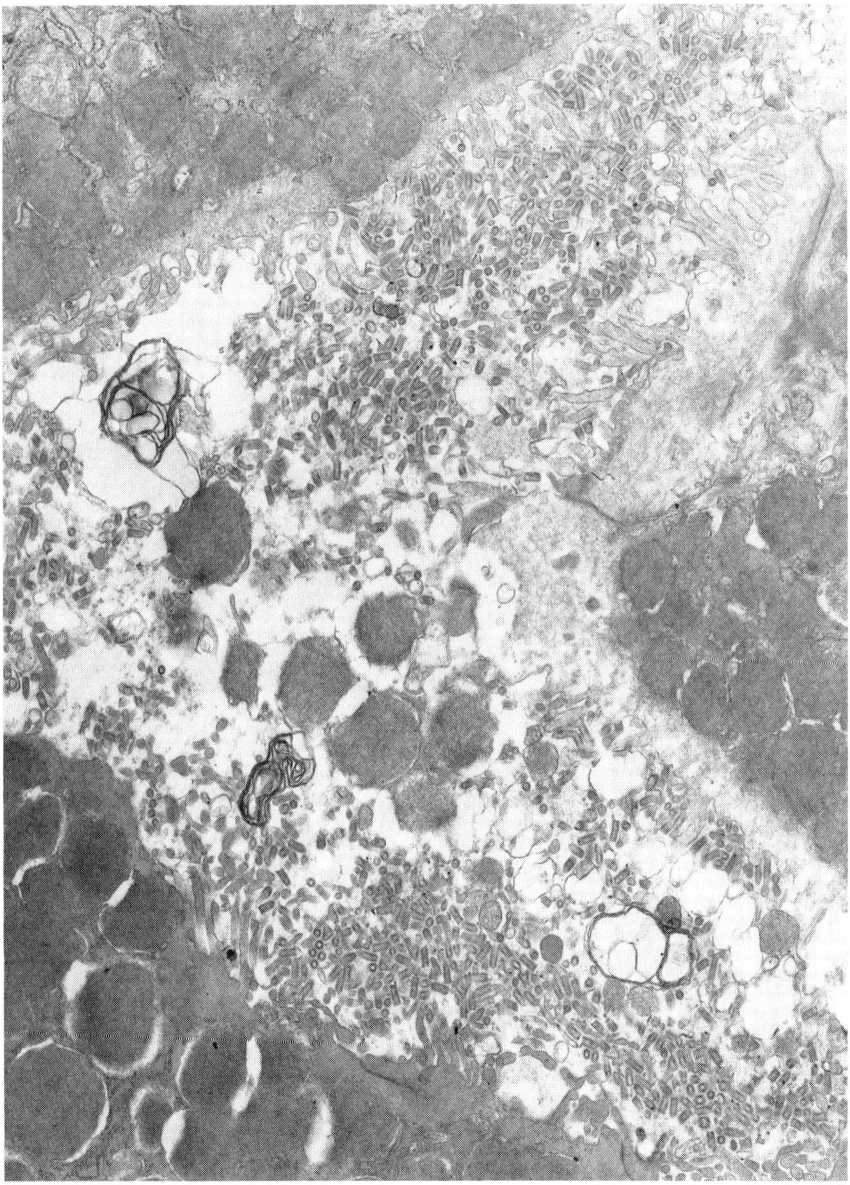

FIGURE 2. Rabies virus in fox salivary gland. This accumulation of virus within the lumen of a terminal salivary duct is a result of viral budding from the plasma membrane of mucous acinar cells (X20,000).

of infected cells and is thereby trapped, in the salivary gland nearly all virus buds upon apical plasma membranes of mucous cells from where it is freely delivered into saliva by normal secretory flow (2) (Figure 2). Late in infection, other tissues and organs are infected via the centrifugal neural spread of viral genome, but it is difficult to attribute any important aspect of the natural history of the virus to infection and dysfunction anywhere other than in the nervous system, muscles and salivary glands.

Consideration of all of the elements of rabies pathogenesis may tempt the conclusion that virus survival in nature is tenuous--this temptation might be reinforced by similar consideration of the ecologic hurdles faced by the virus. But this is not the case in fact--within its diverse econiches, there is regular transmission, virus perpetuation, and *entrenchment*. In reality, the same elements of rabies pathogenesis and ecology which predict tenuous survival probabilities may be interpreted as the bases for ecologic entrenchment. This subject drifts too easily from an evolutionary adaptation theme into teleology.

III. RABIES ENTRENCHMENT VERSUS CONTROL

The pathogenetic pattern of rabies virus infection is the same in all reservoir host species which have been studied (with the possible exception of *derringue*--rabies in vampire bats). Despite its complexity, this pattern has allowed the virus to adapt to host societies as diverse as those of the skunk in the United States, the mongoose and meerkat in South Africa, and the jackal and pariah dog in Asia. Rabies in bats reflects diverse adaptation too; the virus survives in insectivorous bats in North America, vampire bats in South America, dog-faced bats in Thailand. In Africa, bats have even yielded the first viruses (Lagos bat and Duvenhage viruses) which are rabies-like, but antigenically quite distinct (13). The ecologic significance of this antigenic variation is not certain, but the whole question of whether vaccine strains should be adjusted to better match street strains is currently under review in several countries.

Few experimental studies have been undertaken to test the reservoir host potential of unique fauna. In 1966, R. J. Morahan of the Commonwealth Serum Laboratories, Australia, took to the Center for Disease Control, United States, sugar-gliders (*Petaurus brevicepts*) and cuscus (*Phalanger orientalis and maculatus*) from New Guinea (7). Following street virus inoculation, all of these animals developed rabies and half of them shed virus in their saliva. It was concluded that similar species in Australia would most likely also be susceptible, but that Australasian marsupials do not have other necessary attributes to make them successful rabies vector species (3). Certainly, this study begs the question of whether other unique Australasian species, especially carnivorous species, might possess all necessary attributes for entrenchment of virus, once it was introduced. More studies are needed.

Failings in rabies control programs in some parts of South-East Asia, as in many other parts of the world, stem simply from lack of financial resources. This is seen in the most recent *WHO World Survey of Rabies* (15) as an incongruity between large numbers of cases (human and animal) reported, small numbers of doses of vaccine used, and minimal availability of diagnostics. WHO provides excellent information on the elements of rabies control programs, but there is need to reduce the cost of each element to its minimum. Perhaps the cost of animal movement control, quarantine, surveillance and public education cannot be affected, but surely we can lower the cost of immunization (of man and domestic animals) and of diagnostics, and surely we can bring the controversial subject of wildlife immunization to a safe and efficacious reality.

Finally, given the nature and magnitude of rabies assaults upon the many places in the Western Pacific where the virus has thus far been excluded, the question must be asked whether plans for handling an introduction would work. For example, would the "Plan for the Eradication of Rabies" of the Australian National Health and Medical Research Council (12), which looks so good on paper, be implemented effectively? This general question leads to further specific questions concerning each program element--from reference diagnostic confirmation to vaccine availability and usage. Hopefully, in each rabies-free area, answers to such questions are sought as part of ongoing exercises and reviews. A rabies epizootic is no place to find that the plan is outdated, resources inadequate, and expertise unavailable.

ACKNOWLEDGMENTS

The author wishes to express thanks to Dr. George M. Baer, Dr. Ian M. Parsonson, and Mrs. Ann Beruff for their help with this paper.

REFERENCES

1. Constantine, D. G., Emmons, R. W., and Woodie, J. D., *Science 175*, 1255 (1972).
2. Dierks, R. E., Murphy, F. A., and Harrison, A. K., *Amer. J. Pathol. 54*, 251 (1969).
3. French, E. L., and Geering, W. A., Service Publication (Animal Quarantine) No. 11, Australian Government Publishing Service (1978).
4. Johnson, R. T., in "Rabies" (Y. Nagano and F. Davenport, eds.), p. 59, University Park Press, Baltimore (1971).
5. Kaplan, C., "Rabies, The Facts", Oxford University Press, Oxford (1977).
6. Morbidity and Mortality Weekly Report *30*, 527 (1981).
7. Morahan, R. J., unpublished study (1966).
8. Murphy, F. A., *Arch. Virol. 54*, 279 (1977).
9. Murphy, F. A., and Bauer, S. P., *Intervirol. 3*, 256 (1974).
10. Murphy, F. A., Bauer, S. P., Harrison, A. K. and Winn, W. C., Jr., *Lab. Invest. 28*, 361 (1973).
11. Murphy, F. A., Harrison, A. K. Winn, W. C. Jr., and Bauer, S. P., *Lab. Invest. 29*, 1 (1973).
12. National Health and Medical Research Council of Australia, Report of 87th Session of the Council, Australian Government Publishing Service (1979).
13. Shope, R. E., Murphy, F. A., Harrison, A. K. Causey, O. R., Kemp, G. E., Simpson, D. I. H., and Moore, D. L., *J. Virol. 6*, 690 (1970).
14. Tignor, G. H., and Smith, L., Proceedings of Fifth International Congress of Virology, Strasbourg (1981).
15. WHO World Survey of Rabies XVIII (for years 1976-77). Publication 79.187, World Health Organization, Geneva (1979).

83

HAEMORRHAGIC FEVERS

K. M. JOHNSON

U.S. Army Medical Research Institute of Infectious Diseases, Fort Detrick, Maryland

In historical perspective it is not so long ago that haemorrhage was prescribed by physicians as a principal therapy for most acute infectious diseases. Today we rightly view this sign as an ominous and life-threatening complication of a disease group of viral infections caused by only some of the 100-odd RNA membrane-limited agents which infect man. The viruses in question are zoonoses. They have diverse ecological life cycles, produce clinical syndromes which also appear to differ significantly, and are, in my opinion, still dimly understood pathogens. Except for yellow fever, which was only perceived to be the prototypic haemorrhagic fever virus after the fact (1), definitive prevention or control has not been achieved for any of these diseases. Furthermore, only two of these agents, dengue and Hantaan, are known to occur in South-east Asia and the Western Pacific regions. Why then should we bother today? Although the context is different, I believe that Rene Dubos provides a solid reason in his recent book entitled "Celebrations of Life" (2). His third chapter is entitled "Think Globally, but Act Locally." That dictum should be dear to every person engaged in the study of geographically subscribed zoonotic infection. In that spirit I wish to pursue two main theses; knowledge concerning viral haemorrhagic fever is today largely descriptive and rather fragmented, and, that situation is about to change dramatically.

VIRAL DISEASES IN SOUTH-EAST ASIA
AND THE WESTERN PACIFIC
ISBN 0 12 484820 6

I. THE DESCRIPTIVE BASELINES

Although a certain sense of frustration rides constantly with the excitement resident in the minds of all who have worked seriously with these viruses, it is important to remember that recognition of these agents is a very recent process. William Osler's 1892 textbook of medicine makes no mention of the syndrome (3). He devotes chapters to the then clinical entities of yellow fever, dengue, typhoid (very long and detailed) and dysentery. After working on haemorrhagic fever in rural Latin America and Africa, I am easily persuaded that his text is still the basis for much of the practice of medicine in these regions. As shown in Table 1, nearly all of the haemorrhagic fevers and their etiologic viruses were discovered in the last 40 years. Why? Of the many factors responsible I believe that three are the most noteworthy:

a. the redoubling of human populations since World War II in pertinent areas of the world with attendant human perturbation of ecosystems containing these viruses;

b. the global use of antibiotics and anti-malarials which serve both as clinical screen to reveal nonbacterial

TABLE 1. Chronology of Discovery: Viral Haemorrhagic Fevers (HF) and Their Etiologic Agents

Syndrome	*Year described*	*Agent*	*Year isolated*	*Geography*
HF with renal syndrome	*1911*	*Hantaan*	*1976*	*Euro-Asia (Beyond?)*
Dengue HF	*(1928)*	*Dengue*	*1907*	*Asia, Cuba*
	1954	*Types 1 & 2*	*1945*	
		Types 3 & 4	*1960*	
Omsk HF	*1945*	*OHF*	*1947*	*USSR*
Kyasanur Forest disease	*1957*	*KFD*	*1957*	*India*
Argentine HF	*1953*	*Junin*	*1958*	*Argentina*
Bolivian HF	*1958*	*Machupo*	*1963*	*Bolivia*
Lassa Fever	*1969*	*Lassa*	*1969*	*W. Africa*
Marburg disease	*1967*	*Marburg*	*1967*	*Africa*
Ebola HF	*1976*	*Ebola*	*1976*	*Africa*
Rift Valley fever	*1975*	*RVF*	*1930*	*Africa*
Congo-Crimean HF	*1944*	*C-CHF*	*1966*	*Euro-Asia Africa*

acute infections and an an important suppressive filter to permit *in vivo* and *in vitro* isolation of viral agents, and

c. the explosive development of a global technology which permits and promotes rapid international travel and instant communication.

Does this recent history mean that we have now completed the list of viral haemorrhagic fevers? I think not, and perhaps the best example is that of Rift Valley fever virus (RVFV) described in 1930, studied continuously since that date, but only recognized as a cause of haemorrhagic disease in 1975 (4) and then explosively so in Egypt in 1977 (5, 6). Does it mean that the rate of discovery of new agents will decline? I think so, because I am confident that none of these viruses is in fact a novel recent mutant, and because there are so few remaining ecosystems which man has not penetrated in significant sentinel numbers.

Now let us examine briefly our knowledge base concerning the existing viruses.

II. DISEASE OCCURRENCE AND EPIDEMIOLOGICAL PARAMETERS

A summary of cardinal features is provided in Table 2. Note that the estimated annual occurrence of the various haemorrhagic fevers varies over a range of at least three orders of magnitude. It is to be emphasized, in addition, that these figures are in many instances just poor guesses of the real state of affairs, with very serious under-estimation of the toll in human morbidity and mortality. None of these diseases is officially reportable in the eyes of the World Health Organization and in many instances such official status would matter little, because the surveillance systems and specific diagnostic tools required simply are not available in the places where the syndromes occur. This is a pernicious, pressing, and frustrating situation.

Action in every area of human endeavor can be fairly said to be definable as a function of problem perception. Where are we if we cannot even count the cases? Table 3 makes the case with stark eloquence. During 1977 when prospective study of acute febrile illness was maintained in two rural hospitals in eastern Sierra Leone, it was discovered that Lassa virus was the single greatest cause of such morbidity in this tropical locale and the most important cause of death among all patients admitted to the medical wards.

We do know a fair amount concerning the epidemiology of most of the viral haemorrhagic fevers. Most occur in rural

TABLE 2. Incidence and Epidemiological Summary of Viral Haemorrhagic Fevers, Part A

Syndrome	Annual incidence	Incubation (days)	Case pattern
HFRS	2,000-10,000	14-30	Forest-Farm Urban (Asia)
CHF	50-500	2-7	Pastoral
OHF	< 20	3-8	Pastoral (trapping)
KFD	100-1,000	3-8	Forest-Pastoral
AHF	200-3,000	7-14	Maize harvest
BHF	0-15	7-14	Rural homes
LF	2,000-20,000	7-15	Rural homes
DHF	5,000-50,000	2-5	Urban (children)
MBG	Sporadic	5-12	Rural, Nosocomial
EBO	Sporadic (600 in 1976)	5-16	Rural, Nosocomial
RVF	10-10,000	2-6	Pastoral

Part B

Syndrome	Seasonal pattern	Vertebrate host	Arthropod vector
HFRS	Spring-fall-winter	Field mice *Rattus*	None proven ? Ectoparasites
CHF	Summer	Domestic animals	Ticks (*Hyaloma*), others
OHF	Spring-summer-winter	Domestic animals, muskrats	Ticks (*Dermacentor*)
KFD	Spring	Domestic animals, monkeys	Ticks (*Haemophysalis*)
AHF	Fall	*Calomys* rodent	None
BHF	Fall	*Calomys* rodent	None
LF	Continuous (spring peak)	*Mastomys* rodent	None
DHF	Summer-fall (wet)	Man	Mosquitoes (*Aedes*)
MBG	None	Unknown	Unknown
EBO	None	Unknown	Unknown
RVF	Summer (epidemic)	Domestic animals	Mosquitoes (epidemic) Unknown (maintenance)

TABLE 3. Lassa Fever in Adult Medical Services of Two Hospitals, Sierra Leone, 1977[a]

Parameter	Number (% of total)			
	Panguma		Segbwema	
Admissions	711		2,067	
Lassa	93	(13)	123	(6)
Febrile admissions	175		301	
Lassa	93	(53)	123	(41)
All deaths	41		78	
Lassa	12	(29)	23	(30)
Lassa case fatality = 16.3%				

[a]Center for Disease Control, Special Pathogens Branch, Virology Division.

environments. Many are vector-borne and we have identified the important arthropods, be they mosquitoes or ticks. But the maintenance vector(s) for RVFV have not been elucidated (7), nor has the question of arthropod vectoring of Hantaan virus been clearly settled (8). Chronic infection of, and environmental contamination by, specific small rodents appears to represent the essential means for transmission of arenaviral infections to man (9, 10). But we are still completely ignorant of either reservoir or vector of the devastating African Marburg and Ebola viruses. Furthermore, work on these two, as well as the pathogenic areanviruses and the Congo-Crimean haemorrhagic fever virus (C-CHF), is greatly impeded by their documented natural and/or laboratory communicability which dictates expensive maximum containment facilities for safe manipulation and a certain sense of chronic anxiety in countries far removed from endemic areas concerning the possible exotic introduction of these viruses.

III. CLINICAL FEATURES AND PATHOGENESIS OF VIRAL HAEMORRHAGIC FEVERS

Some of the striking characteristics of these diseases are set out in Table 4.

TABLE 4. *Clinical Variability in Pathophysiology of Viral Haemorrhagic Fevers*

Syndrome	Bleeding	Hepatitis	Pneumonitis	Encephalitis	Nephritis	Altered immune response
HFRS	± to ++	±	++	-	++++	?
CHF	+++[a]	+++	±	-	±	-
OHF	+	±	+++	++	-	-
KFD	+	±	+	++	-	-
AHF	+	±	±	++[b]	±	+++[c]
BHF	++	±	±	++[b]	±	+++[c]
LF	+	+++	++	±	+	+++[d]
DHF	++	+	++	±	±	+++[e]
MBG	+++[a]	++++	++	±	±	-
EBO	+++[a]	++++	++	±	±	-
RVF	+++[a]	++++	-	++	±	-

[a] Disseminated intravascular coagulation demonstrated or highly suspect.
[b] Encephalopathy without direct viral damage.
[c] General humoral suppression.
[d] Split humoral response.
[e] Pathological immune enhancement suspected.

Judgments are relative, descriptive only, and refer to the most severe clinical syndromes associated with infection. I am impressed by the diversity of pattern and by our collective general ignorance of the real mechanisms which underlie the phenomena which have been recorded. It is clear that pulmonary and encephalitic manifestations are important in the tick-borne flavivirus syndromes of OHF and KFD which are caused by close antigenic relatives of the Euro-Asian tick-borne encephalitis virus. One also is impressed with the evidence for significant acute liver damage observed in Marburg, Ebola, Lassa, C-CHF and RVFV infection as well as the apparent reticuloendothelial localization of pathology in dengue, Junin, Machupo and Hantaan syndromes.

In addition, it is noteworthy that there are major differences in infection-serious disease ratios among these viruses. Marburg, Ebola and C-CHF produce severe illness with high frequency, dengue, Lassa, and RVFV with low frequency, while the others are either intermediate in virulence or are not yet well studied.

In all cases I submit that we do not yet understand the how nor the why of these patterns. Although the observations are few, the data strongly suggest that Marburg-Ebola infections produce classical severe disseminated intravascular coagulation (11, 12). But we know not how this happens, nor why it apparently does not occur regularly in fatal infections with dengue or the arenaviruses. Dengue haemorrhagic fever may have something to do with secondary infection (13). But that thesis is not yet generally accepted (14), much less elucidated. In all of the syndromes, moreover, it is probably fair to say that only limited progress has been made to date in the struggle to sort out the fascinating and complex virus-host interactions which occur. We can surmise that many of these agents attack cells which are important in host defense against any foreign antigen. In so doing they complicate the assessment of response to specific viral invasion. Sophisticated dissection of both cellular and humoral immune functions, very probably modulated by as-yet undiscovered host genetic factors, is in its infancy.

To understand this situation we must be aware that many of the haemorrhagic fevers occur where facilities for detailed investigation of cases are scarce. It has required several years of painful effort, for example, to learn that fatal Lassa virus infections are marked by higher viremia and greater chemical hepatitis than are experienced by survivors (Table 5). This is a splendid clue, indeed it represents perhaps the first such demonstration for any systemic viral disease of man. Sadly the means to exploit this observation are not available in Sierra Leone. It also should

TABLE 5. Hospital Admission Values for Blood, Virus and Selected Chemical Parameters as Function of Outcome, Sierra Leone, 1978-79

Outcome	*No.*	*SGOT*	*No.*	*BUN*	*No.*	*Viremia$_{10}$/ml*
Survival	*89*	*171*	*70*	*24*	*104*	*2.1*
Death	*41*	*923*	*16*	*43*	*46*	*4.1*

If SGOT $<$ 150 and viremia $<$ 4.0, 22/25 survived;
if SGOT $>$ 150 and viremia $>$ 4.0, 17/18 died.

be mentioned that we do not have good animal models for most of these diseases. Monkeys and sometimes guinea pigs appear to be useful in the study of the arenaviruses, Marburg and Ebola viruses (15-19), and in-bred laboratory rats provide reasonable simulation of the varying responses in man to infection by RVFV (20). But no animal reproduces the dengue shock syndrome, and there are as yet no good systems for study of Hantaan or C-CHF viruses.

IV. THE NEAR TERM PROMISE

By now the reader may be verging on boredom. Do not succumb. Things have never been better, and real progress is imminent. Let me be specific. In the first place several new maximum containment laboratories have been or are being built. These are listed in Table 6. These resources, some of them outfitted with the "space-suit" configuration which permits virtually all modern technology to be used (Figure 1), mean direct increase in scientific work on haemorrhagic fevers. The next consideration is the fact that we are making strides in the understanding of the basic molecular anatomy of all of these viruses. Three are arenaviruses, three others are flaviviruses, two and possibly a third, Hantaan, are bunyaviruses (21, 22), and Marburg and Ebola viruses have now been shown to be at least first cousins of the Rhabdoviridae (23, 24). Virionic proteins for all of these agents have been or can now be isolated and purified, and the nucleic acids of these or close relatives have been

TABLE 6. Maximum Containment Laboratories of the World

Country	*Institute*	*Year*
USA	*Fort Detrick, Maryland*	*1955*
	CDC, Atlanta, Georgia	*1969*
UK	*Porton Down, Wiltshire*	*1962*
Belgium	*Inst. Trop. Medicine, Antwerp*	*1978*
South Africa	*Nat. Inst. Virology, Johannesburg*	*1979*
USSR	*Inst. Polio. & Encephalitis, Moscow*	*1981*
Japan	*Nat. Inst. Health, Tokyo*	*1981*
Canada	*Ontario Pub. Health Laboratories, Toronto*	*1982 (Const)*
Australia	*CSIRO, Geelong*	*1982 (Const)*

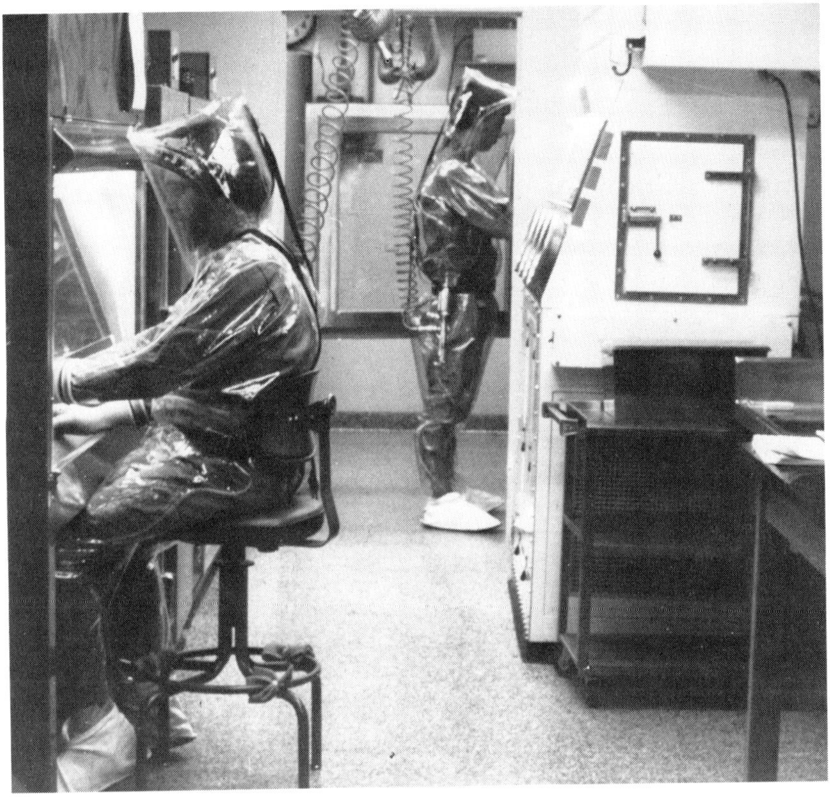

Figure 1. Suited maximum containment laboratory, CDC, Atlanta, Georgia. Workers are protected by positive-pressure suits with independent remote source of breathing air. Primary containment of aerosols is achieved by use of filtered vertical laminar flow work stations. The ultracentrifuge is contained in an explosion-proof laminar flow hood. A full range of spohisticated equipment is available, and animals as large as monkeys can be studied.

at least partially characterized. We know that the middle-sized RNA segment of bunyaviruses codes for the surface glycoproteins (25), and that the small genomic segment of arenaviruses directs synthesis of the three major virionic structural polypeptides (26-28).

We now possess powerful new tools; endonucleases which yield molecular fingerprints useful for epidemiologic and other purposes. This method permitted documentation of the biologically amazing fact that near-simultaneous premier epidemics of Ebola virus disease in adjacent Zaire and Sudan were caused by distinct agents, rather than by dissemination of a single agent as originally surmised (29, 30). We can make monoclonal antibodies; this approach has already yielded completely type-specific dengue reagents and antibodies capable of distinguishing closely related viruses of the Lassa complex (31, 32). More are on the way, including important specific cell markers which will permit a new order of precision in study of viral pathogenesis. We are beginning to make real progress in the development of specific and eventually inexpensive binding immunoassays (cf, the paper by Dr. Halonen in this Seminar). One can honestly predict the imminent cloning to expression of pertinent genetic material of many of these viruses; transcription by plasmid insertion in *Escherichia coli* has already been achieved for Pichinde, a nonpathogenic arenavirus (33). It is now conceptually feasible to begin working on eventual identification and synthesis of the critical immunogenic antigenic sites of many if not all of the haemorrhagic fever viruses, and various approaches for enhancing immunogenicity of defined antigens are under active investigation (34-36).

Finally, mention must be made of several highly encouraging non-molecular events. These are the recent clear exposition of the phenomenon of immune enhancement of infection *in vitro* by certain flaviviruses (see paper by Porterfield et al., this Seminar), the classical demonstration that passive antibodies are highly effective in the treatment of haemorrhagic fever caused by Junin, and by inference Machupo, virus (37), the further attenuation of Junin virus and its possible field testing as vaccine within a year (38), and the emerging epidemiology of Hantaan virus as parasite of urban and laboratory *Rattus*. which poses the distinct chance that the virus may have a truly global distribution (for details see papers of D. C. Gajdusek and H. W. Lee et al. in this Seminar).

What does all this mean? To me, at least, these omens foretell that more laboratories around the world will be active in haemorrhagic fever research; that we will begin to close some basic information gaps in diagnosis, epidemiology, and pathogenesis of infection by use of more specific, more sensitive, and more inexpensive assays for infection and its consequences; and that we are likely to be able to produce safe and effective vaccines to relieve us of much of the need for present Andromeda-style biosafety facilities as well as the burden of morbidity and mortality caused world-wide by these diseases.

How shall we best accomplish these goals? Be keeping in contact and minding our individual and regional knitting. By remembering with Dubos that "In most cases, however, the manifestations of diversity are more important in everyday life than are generalizations derived from uniformity, because they provide the materials out of which individual persons create what they prize most - the uniqueness of their own individuality and of their place." This student of zoonotic infections murmurs a fervid amen.

REFERENCES

1. Dennis, L. H., Reisberg, B. E., Crosbie, J., Crozier, D., and Conrad, M. E., *Br. J. Haematol. 17*, 455 (1969).
2. Dubos, R., "Celebrations of Life," McGraw-Hill, New York, 1981.
3. Osler, W., "The Principles and Practice of Medicine," D. Appleton & Co., New York, 1892.
4. Van Velden, D. J. J., Meyer, J. D., Olivier, J., Gear, J. H. S., and McIntosh, B., *S. Afr. Med. J. 51*, 867 (1977).
5. Laughlin, L. W., Meegan, J. M., Strausbaugh, L. J., Morens, D. M., and Watten, R. H., *Trans. R. Soc. Trop. Med. Hyg. 73*, 630 (1979).
6. Meegan, J. M., in "Contributions to Epidemiology and Biostatistics" (T. A. Swartz, M. A. Klingberg, and N. Goldblum, eds), vol. 3, p. 100. S. Karger, Basel (1981).
7. McIntosh, B. M., and Jupp, P. G., in "Contributions to Epidemiology and Biostatistics" (T. A. Swartz, M. A. Klingberg, and N. Goldblum, eds), vol. 3, p. 92. S. Karger, Basel (1981).
8. Lee, H. W., Lee, P. W., Baek, L. J., Song, C. K., and Seong, I. W., *Am. J. Trop. Med. Hyg. 30*, 1106 (1981).
9. Johnson, K. M., Webb, P. A., and Justines, G., in "Lymphocytic Choriomeningitis Virus and Other Arenaviruses" (F. Lehmann-Grube, ed.), p. 241. Springer-Verlag, Berlin (1973).
10. Monath, T. P., *Bull. WHO 52*, 577 (1975).
11. Havemann, K., and Schmidt, H. A., in "Marburg Virus Disease" (G. A. Martin, and R. Siegert, eds), p. 34. Springer-Verlag, New York (1971).

12. Gear, J. S. S., Cassel, G. A., Gear, A. J., Trappler, B., Clausen, L., Meyers, A. M., Kew, M. C., Bothwell, T. H., Sher, R., Miller, G. B., Schneider, J., Koornhof, H. J., Gomperts, E. D., Isaacson, M., and Gear, J. H. S., *Br. Med. J. 4,* 489 (1975).
13. Halstead, S. B., *Am. J. Epidemiol. 114,* 632 (1981).
14. Rosen, L., *Am. J. Trop. Med. Hyg. 26,* 337 (1977).
15. Eddy, G. A., Scott, S. K., Wagner, F. S., and Brand, O. M., *Bull. WHO 52,* 517 (1975).
16. Walker, D. H., Johnson, K. M., Lange, J. V., Gardner, J. J., Kiley, M. P., and McCormick, J. B., *Am. J. Pathol.* in press (1982).
17. Simpson, D. I. H., Bowen, E. T. W., and Bright, W. F., *Lab. Anim. 2,* 75 (1981).
18. Jahrling, P. B., Hesse, R. A., Eddy, G. A., Johnson, K. M., Callis, R. T., and Stephen, E. L., *J. Infect. Dis. 141,* 580 (1980).
19. Bowen, E. T. W., Platt, G. S., Simpson, D. I. H., McArdell, L. B., and Raymond, R. T., *Trans. R. Soc. Trop. Med. Hyg. 72,* 188 (1978).
20. Peters, C. J., and Anderson, G. W., Jr., in "Contributions to Epidemiology and Biostatistics" (T. A. Swartz, M. A. Klingberg, and N. Goldblum, eds), vol. 3, p. 21. S. Karger, Basel (1981).
21. White, J. D., Shirey, F. G., French, G. R., Huggins, J. W., Brand, O. M., and Lee, H. W., *Lancet 1,* in press (1982).
22. McCormick, J. B., Sasso, D. R., Palmer, E. L., and Kiley, M. P., *Lancet 1,* in press (1982).
23. Kiley, M. P., Regnery, R. L., and Johnson, K. M., *J. Gen. Virol. 49,* 333 (1980).
24. Regnery, R. L., Johnson, K. M., and Kiley, M. P., *J. Virol. 36,* 465 (1980).
25. Bishop, D. H., *Curr. Top. Microbiol. Immunol. 86,* 1 (1979).
26. Bishop, D. H., Beaty, B. J., and Shope, R. E., *Ann. N.Y. Acad. Sci. 354,* 84 (1980).
27. Leung, W. C. Hernish, D., Ramsingh, A., Dimock, K., and Rawls, W. E., in "Replication of Negative Strand Viruses" (D. H. L. Bishop, and R. A. Compans, eds), p. 51. Elsevier/North Holland Biomedical Press, Amsterdam (1981).
28. Vezza, A. C., Cash, P., Jahrling, P., Eddy, G., and Bishop, D. H. L., *Virology 106,* 250 (1980).
29. Cox, N. J., McCormick, J. B., Johnson, K. M., and Kiley, M. P., *J. Infect. Dis.,* in press (1982).
30. International Commission, *Bull. WHO 56,* 271 (1978).

31. Henchal, E. A., Gentry, M. K., McCown, J. M., and Brandt, W. E., *Am. J. Trop. Med. Hyg.*, in press (1982).
32. Buchmeier, M. J., Lewicki, H. A., Tomori, O., and Johnson, K. M., *Nature 288*, 486 (1980).
33. Ramsingh, A., and Leung, W. C., in "5th International Congress Virology," p. 372. Strasbourg (1981).
34. Sanchez, Y., Ionescu-Matiu, I., Dreesman, G. R., Kramp, W., Six, H. R., Hollinger, F. B., and Melnick, J. L., *Infect. Immun. 30*, 728 (1980).
35. Chedid, L., Carelli, C., and Audibert, F., *J. Reticuloendothel. Soc. 26*, 631 (1979).
36. Edelman, R., Hardegree, M. C., and Chedid, L., *J. Infect. Dis. 141*, 103 (1980).
37. Maiztegui, J. I., Fernandez, N. J., and DeDamilano, A. J., *Lancet 2*, 1216 (1979).
38. Barrera-Oro, J., and Eddy, G. A., unpublished observations (1982).

84

HEMORRHAGIC FEVER WITH RENAL SYNDROME (KOREAN HEMORRHAGIC FEVER, EPIDEMIC HEMORRHAGIC FEVER, NEPHROPATHIA EPIDEMICA): A NEWLY RECOGNIZED ZOONOTIC PLAGUE OF THE EURASIAN LANDMASS WITH THE POSSIBILITY OF RELATED MUROID VIRUS NEPHROPATHIES ON OTHER CONTINENTS

D. Carleton Gajdusek

Laboratory of Slow, Latent, and Temperate Virus Infections, National Institute of Neurological and Communicative Disorders and Stroke, National Institutes of Health, Bethesda, Maryland

The recent isolation of the virus causing Korean hemorrhagic fever (KHF), now called the Hantaan virus, from the lungs of the natural reservoir, the wild mouse *Apodemus agrarius*, has launched a new era in the study of hemorrhagic fevers with renal syndrome (HFRS) throughout the world. It has made possible the demonstration that the widespread HFRS of Eastern Sibera and the epidemic hemorrhagic fever of 19 provinces of China are caused by the same virus. It has also made it possible to determine that the cases of HFRS in man in European Russia (Tula and Yaroslav fevers) and the nephropathia epidemica (NE) of Scandinavia are caused by serologically related virus(es) which are distinguisable serologically from the Hantaan virus, and to discover the antigen of NE and HFRS in European Russia in the lungs of the natural reservoir voles, *Clethrionomys glareolus* and *Microtus* sp.

Similarly, the HFRS of the Balkan countries, recognized clinically in Hungary, Czechoslovakia, Bulgaria, Romania, Yugoslavia and Greece, has been shown to be caused (in Yugoslavia and Greece, thus far) by an agent serologically resembling that of NE of Scandinavia. Thus, HFRS viruses are causing viral nephropathy across much of the European

VIRAL DISEASES IN SOUTH-EAST ASIA AND THE WESTERN PACIFIC
ISBN 0 12 484820 6

landmass, in the form of a hemorrhagic disease of great clinical severity with 5% to over 20% mortality in East Asia and in a much milder form of nonhemorrhagic nephropathy and low mortality in Scandinavia, and perhaps in both forms in the Balkan countries and European Russia. Urban forms of the disease have also been identified: a form carried to man by infected laboratory rats throughout Japan, where the laboratory-bred white rats, *Rattus norvegicus*, are silently infected carriers, and a form carried to city dwellers as a mild nonhemorrhagic acute febrile nephropathy by infected commensal rats in cities in Japan and Korea.

The availability of serological tests for both KHF (Hantaan) virus and NE virus has led to the recognition that

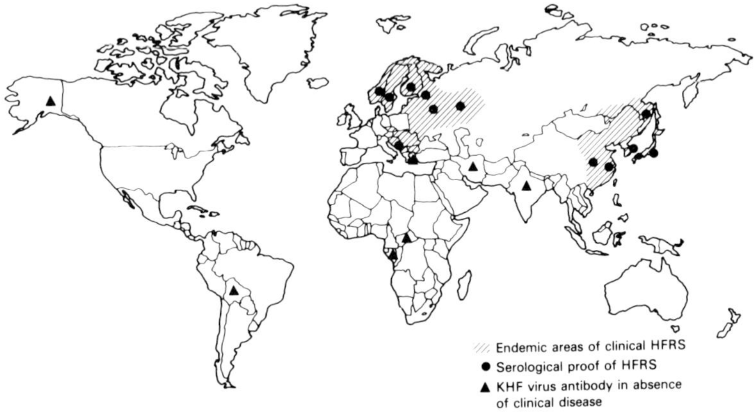

FIGURE 1. World distribution of hemorrhagic fever with renal syndrome. Locations where serological study of human convalescent serum has proved serological relationship to Hantaan virus and where serology of human serum has demonstrated such specific antibody but where the clinical disease has not yet been recognized are shown.

this newly defined group of Bunyamwera-like viruses of rodents is present throughout the world, in seaport and other urban rats in a form serologically resembling the KHF virus, and in laboratory rats in Japan, while different but serologically related viruses are apparently present in wild rodents in the Americas.

THE TERMINOLOGY OF VIRAL HEMORRHAGIC FEVERS

The viral hemorrhagic fevers are characterized by bleeding in a significant portion of patients. They are caused by a diverse array of RNA-containing viruses belonging to the flavivirus, arenavirus, nairovirus and probably the Bunyamwera virus groups. Yellow fever, caused by a mosquito-borne flavivirus, although described over a century ago, clearly belongs in the group of viral hemorrhagic fevers.

The disease which brought this designation and classification to Western European and American medicine was epidemic hemorrhagic fever, now called Korean hemorrhagic fever, and it is this disease and diseases caused by serologically related Bunyamwera-like viruses which we now call hemorrhagic fever with renal syndrome (HFRS). Since urban cases of HFRS acquired from contact with commensal rats in Korea and Japan and nephropathia epidemica of Scandinavia rarely show any bleeding phenomena although they are caused by serologically closely related viruses, the term hemorrhagic fever used for these clinical entities is misleading. All known diseases caused by virus related to the KHF virus (Hantaan virus) are characterized by a proteinuria and azotemia in most patients. The virus is carried to man by excretions and aerosols, probably from infected respiratory droplets, from healthy rodent carriers who excrete the virus in their lungs, in saliva, and in urine. All these unaffected rodent carriers belong to the suprafamily *Muroidea* and the genera *Apodemus, Clethrionomys, Microtus* and *Rattus*. Thus, I have, in consultation with Dr. Robert Traub, recently suggested the name *muroid virus nephropathies* to replace the name HFRS for all diseases caused by this newly defined group of viruses carried to man by healthy rodents of the suprafamily *Muroidea* and belonging to the families *Muridae* (genera: *Apodemus* and *Rattus*) and *Cricetidae* (genera: *Clethrionomys* and *Microtus*).

HISTORICAL BACKGROUND

"Hemorrhagic fever" was a term which came into general use in Western medicine only since the period of the Korean War when an infectious disease, new to Western medicine, often accompanied by a bleeding syndrome, appeared among United Nations troops and was designated epidemic hemorrhagic fever. Subsequently, the Korean disease was often referred to as Korean hemorrhagic fever (KHF). During investigation of this new illness, Western physicians became aware of the existence of a whole group of hemorrhagic fevers which had been described in the Soviet Union during the previous decade, and which were usually distinguished by prefacing the term "hemorrhagic fever" with the geographic locality in which the syndromes were observed. Thus, Crimean hemorrhagic fever, Far Eastern hemorrhagic fever, Uzbekistan hemorrhagic fever, Central Asian hemorrhagic fever, Yaroslav hemorrhagic fever, and numerous other such terms entered the medical literature. Subsequent investigation established that these designations encompass a number of distinct nosological entities; the viral etiological agent of each of these has been isolated. All are caused by RNA-containing viruses, but they belong to several different taxonomic groups. Unfortunately, the already ambiguous designation, "hemorrhagic fever" was later applied to yet other distinct disease entities which have been encountered in the Philippine Islands, Thailand, Singapore, Argentina, Bolivia and elsewhere. Moreover, to confuse matters further, the name "epidemic hemorrhagic fever", at first applied specifically to the Korean disease, was used by *Index Medicus* and in other medical indices to include a variety of other infections caused by viruses belonging to very different groups than that causing the Korean disease.

The simple designation "hemorrhagic fever" would best be applied to no single disease entity. Instead, it conveniently describes a syndrome, common to a number of diseases, the rule in some, and the rare exception in others. In many infections an increase in capillary permeability, associated often with small ruptures of capillaries, can produce petechiae and even more extensive cutaneous hemorrhages; and, should this phenomenon extend to other organs, petechial hemorrhages, or more severe extravasations of blood into the urinary or gastrointestinal tract, the endocrine and cardio-respiratory systems, and central nervous system, and other tissues of the body may occur. At times this syndrome may give rise to massive bleeding and produce symptoms of hemoptysis or hematemesis, hematuria or gastrointestinal bleeding, uterine hemorrhage, epistaxis, conjunctival hemorrhage, and ecchymoses. Thus, among the common infectious diseases, hemorrhagic syndromes, which could be properly designated hemorrhagic fever, may appear in typhoid fever, chickenpox, rubella, or measles and are not uncommonly encountered in infectious mononucleosis and infectious hepatitis. Furthermore, all the viral and rickettsial diseases which have occasionally caused thrombocytopenia may lead to a hemorrhagic syndrome which might be so designated. The pathophysiology of the bleeding phenomena in the common infectious diseases of childhood and that in the hemorrhagic fevers are apparently in no way different: capillary changes and/or thrombocytopenia play a role in each. The diseases which have been called hemorrhagic fever *per se*, with appropriate geographic prefixes, have, in general, had only a greater incidence of the hemorrhagic syndrome than is to be expected in the usual exanthems of childhood, but even in the classical Omsk hemorrhagic fever or in epidemic KHF bleeding phenomena are not invariable and are only encountered in a portion of the cases. The best clinical physiological studies have been made on HFRS and on dengue hemorrhagic fever syndromes and even in these it has not been possible to demonstrate direct cytopathological effect of the viruses on capillary endothelium or on platelet-producing cells. In both of these diseases the increased capillary fragility is accompanied by leakage of protein-rich fluid from the vascular bed which leads to an acute shock syndrome, and yet the direct action of the virus on any cell groups has not been shown to cause these phenomena. It would be better to designate the symptom complex described above as the *hemorrhagic syndrome* and to restrict the use of the term "virus hemorrhagic fever" to those virus diseases in which the hemorrhagic syndrome attains a high incidence: of these, the earliest defined and most widespread is epidemic hemorrhagic fever itself, now grouped under the term "hemorrhagic fever with renal syndrome", or, as I now propose in order to encompass its nonhemorrhagic forms of low virulence, "muroid virus nephropathies".

THE NEW ERA OF HFRS RESEARCH

In 1976 Ho Wang Lee and Pyung Woo Lee in Seoul, Korea, finally resolved the impasse that had resulted from failure to isolate the virus causing any of the forms of HFRS. They found that the lungs, and no other organ, of wild-caught *A. agrarius* collected in the endemic areas of Korea, contained antigen which reacted in a virus-like pattern in an immunofluorescent (IF) test with convalescent and not with early acute phase sera of patients with KHF. They succeeded in demonstrating with this IF antibody test seroconversion of antibody-free *A. agrarius* after inoculation with suspensions of such antigen-positive lung tissue and also with whole blood collected early in the acute phase of KHF from patients. These seroconverted *A. agrarius* also developed KHF antigen in their lungs. Subsequently the virus has been adapted to Fischer and Wistar laboratory rats and to nude mice and also to A-549 (human lung carcinoma cells) and Vero-E-6 (cloned African green monkey kidney cells) continuous cell lines, and all of these adapted virus lines provide sources of antigen for IF tests. The infected cells have permitted good electronmicroscopic visualization of the KHF virion, which has now been called Hantaan virus. The virion has been shown to have a Bunyavirus-like structure, but the tripartite RNA-virus genome of this group has not yet been demonstrated for Hantaan virus. An ELISA test has been developed for the Hantaan virus using A-549 or Vero-E-6 infected cells, and blocking antibody tests using the ELISA test or IF antibody system are providing a new sensitive method for antibody estimation. Neutralization tests can also be done with the Hantaan virus by inoculating susceptible rats with the rat-adapted virus.

The NE virus of Scandinavia has been successfully demonstrated in the lungs of *Clethrionomys glabreolus* caught in the endemic regions, and it has been successfully passed into seronegative *C. glabreolus*, causing development of specific antibody and the appearance of the antigen in their lungs, but it has not been possible to maintain the virus in serial passages. Infected cell lines have also failed to retain antigen.

The viruses produce no CPE in any infected cells, and none of the susceptible rodents develop clinical disease. Thus there is no laboratory model for assessing virulence of strains.

Sera from East Asian cases of HFRS give much lower IF antibody titers with the NE antigen than with the homologous (Hantaan virus) antigen, whereas sera from Scandinavian and European Russian patients give only 2-, 4-, or 8-fold lower titers with the Hantaan virus antigen than with the homologous NE antigen. This partial one-way cross is however not shown when Scandinavian sera are used in blocking tests against the Hantaan virus (KHF) antigen by either ELISA or IF techniques or in neutralization tests using the rat-adapted strain of Hantaan virus. In such tests Scandinavian sera demonstrate no neutralization and no blocking antibody.

Sera from Yugoslavian patients with HFRS have behaved like the sera from Scandinavian NE patients. However, one Yugoslavian serum demonstrates a pattern seen only with the KHF human sera (i.e., very much lower IF antibody with NE antigen than with KHF antigen), suggesting that perhaps both viruses are present in the Balkans.

Occasional Scandinavian *Clethrionomys* sera and some Yugoslavian human sera show almost equal titers to both NE and KHF antigens, usually 2-fold higher to KHF. This is a pattern not previously seen either in the East Asian patients or in classical NE patients, and brings up the possibility of yet a third serotype of the HFRS viruses.

HEMORRHAGIC FEVER WITH RENAL SYNDROME (EPIDEMIC HEMORRHAGIC FEVER, FAR EASTERN HEMORRHAGIC NEPHROSO-NEPHRITIS)

In the spring of 1951, United Nations troops near the fighting front in Korea began to appear on sick call with chills and high fever, prostration, and anorexia, severe retroorbital headache, generalized muscle and joint pains, vomiting, a flushed face, and diverse hemorrhagic manifestations including petechiae, ecchymoses and scleral hemorrhages. Laboratory examination often revealed leukocytosis and marked proteinuria. The unusual and dramatic subsequent course of this severe, often fatal illness with cardiovascular instability, shock, and renal failure soon convinced physicians, who had first suspected leptospirosis, allergic and idiopathic thrombocytopenia, purpura, leukemia, infectious mononucleosis, hemorrhagic smallpox, and lower nephron-nephrosis, and other renal disorders, that they were dealing with an infection hitherto unknown to the Western world.

By the end of the year 1951 this illness had taken the lives of fourscore of some 1,000 men who had contracted it. By the end of 1952 another thousand cases had been seen in Korea; all nationalities of United Nations troops, including South Korean, were affected. Cases continued to occur in 1953 and 1954, after hostilities ceased, and over 3,000 cases in all occurred in the United Nations forces. The disease continued to be diagnosed in troops and in the civilian population in subsequent years and soon became the major infectious disease problem of the Korean army, which took over surveillance of the Demilitarized Zone, and it was recognized more and more frequently in the civilian population in locations further and further south in Korea than the area of its endemicity recognized during the war. Although mortality was at first well over 10%, it dropped to about 5% with improved methods of medical care, resulting from better understanding of the disease and with recognition of milder forms of the illness.

In 1932 the Russians observed a new disease along the lower Amur River basin in the southeastern part of the Soviet Far East. Thereafter, yearly outbreaks of the illness occurred in the valley of the Amur which forms the boundary between Manchuria and the Soviet Union and in the valleys of its tributaries. Shortly after, across the Amur, along its Manchurian tributaries, the Japanese Army encountered cases of this disease among its troops. Research teams from both nations studied the disease independently, without knowledge of each other's work, established its infectious (a probably virus) etiology, and made extensive clinical and epidemiological studies. Both Russian and Japanese workers succeeded in producing typical disease in human volunteers by intravenous injection of blood and urine from patients early in their illness. Serial passage in man was also successful, and experimental infection so produced conferred immunity to subsequent rechallenge with the agent. They could not, however, establish the disease in experimental animals. The Russian expeditionary team was in the Far East in 1939 and 1940; the Japanese studies dated from 1936 to 1942. The Russians called the disease by various names, including: Churilov's disease, Far Eastern nephroso-nephritis, epidemic hemorrhagic nephroso-nephritis. The Japanese, before settling on epidemic hemorrhagic fever (ryokosei shukketsu netsu) used a number of names based on geographic locations of their cases: Erhtaokiang disease (Nidoko fever), Heiho fever, Hulin (Korin) fever, Kokko (Kokuo) fever, Manchurian hemorrhagic fever, Songo (Sunwu) fever, and Tayinshan disease. American medical literature quickly settled on the term epidemic hemorrhagic fever, whereas the Russian authors tended to use the term hemorrhagic fever with renal syndrome in later years, instead of their earlier preferred epidemic (Far Eastern) hemorrhagic nephroso-nephritis.

During the Korean War the American Army Medical Service established a Hemorrhagic Fever Center near Uijongbu, close to the region in which the largest number of cases occurred in South Korea, and all suspected cases of the disease were evacuated by helicopter to the Center's hospital where a careful investigative program, aimed at the best treatment of the disease and at other research on it, was conducted.

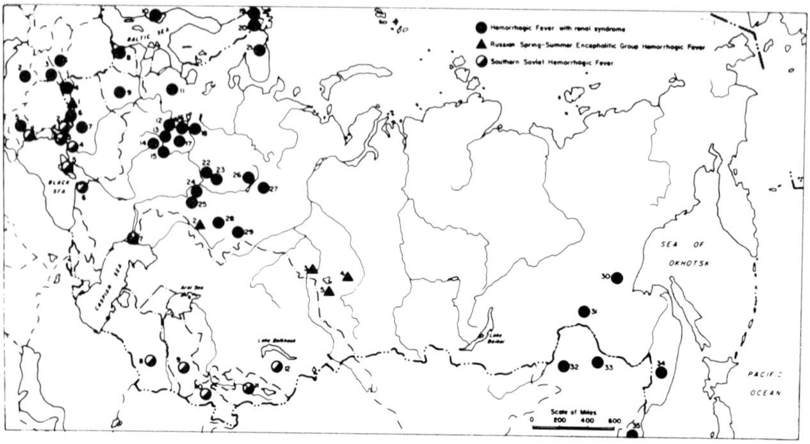

Hemorrhagic fever with renal syndrome:
1. Czechoslovakia
2. Yugoslavia
3. Hungary
4. Transcarpathia
5. Bulgaria
6. Moldavskaya SSR
7. Southwestern Ukraine
8. Kaliningradskaya Oblast
9. Belorusskaya SSR
10. Sweden
11. Novgorodskaya Oblast
12. Kalininskaya Oblast
13. Moskovskaya Oblast
14. Tulskaya Oblast
15. Ryazanskaya Oblast
16. Yaroslavskaya Oblast
17. Vladmirskaya Oblast
18. Kostromskaya Oblast
19. Northern Norway
20. Northern Finland
21. Murmanskaya Oblast
22. Mariyskaya ASSR
23. Udmurtskaya ASSR
24. Tatarskaya ASSR
25. Kuybyshevskaya Oblast
26. Permskaya Oblast
27. Sverdlovskaya Oblast
28. Bashkirskaya ASSR
29. Chelyabinskaya Oblast
30. Khabarovskiy Kray
31. Amurskaya Oblast
32. Inner Mongolia (Tuliho), China
33. North Manchuria, China
34. Primorskiy Kray
35. North and South Korea

Southern Soviet hemorrhagic fever:
1. Bulgaria
2. Moldavskaya SSR
3. Izmail'skaya Oblast
4. Khersonskaya Oblast
5. Crimean Peninsula
6. Tamanskiy Peninsula
7. Astrakhanskaya Oblast
8. Turkmenskaya SSR
9. Uzbekskaya SSR
10. Tadzhikskaya SSR
11. Kirghizskaya SSR
12. Kazakhskaya SSR

Russian spring-summer encephalitis group hemorrhagic fever:
1. Bukovina
2. Orenburgskaya Oblast
3. Omskaya Oblast
4. Novosibirskaya Oblast
5. Zapadno-Barabinskiy Steppes

FIGURE 2. Map of the Soviet Union and adjoining regions showing natural endemic foci of hemorrhagic fever with renal syndrome (black circles), Southern Soviet hemorrhagic fever (half-shaded circles) and Russian spring-summer encephalitis group hemorrhagic fever (black triangles) as we knew the situation in 1962. Numbers associated with the 3 symbols refer to the above.

American efforts, more extensive than earlier Russian and Japanese attempts, likewise failed to establish the disease in any of a wide range of experimental hosts, including chimpanzees and monkeys and continuous and primary animal and human cells in tissue culture.

During the resettlement of Korean farmers into the former combat zone, evacuated during hostilities, cases of the disease were first observed in the civilian Korean populace. A few cases, mild in nature and short in duration, were even seen in children less than 10 years of age. No evidence was found to suggest that a part of the population had acquired resistance to the disease through prior residence in the area in which it was known to occur.

In 1958 and 1959 Soviet physicians established that the clinical, pathologic and epidemiologic features of hemorrhagic fever which they had been studying in the Yaroslav Oblast along the Upper Volga River, and in the Urals of European Russia was actually HFRS and recognized that it was also the same disease which they had previously called Tula fever: 915 cases of this disease, with 5 deaths, had been reported from 1930 to 1934 in and around Tula. Thus, Tula fever is the oldest described hemorrhagic fever in the Soviet Union. The demonstration that HFRS was occurring over a wide range of European Russia, westward to the Urals, northeastward to the Murmansk Oblast, and south-westward to Hungary, Czechoslovakia, Bulgaria, Romania and Yugoslavia strengthened the suspicion that nephropathia epidemica of northern Scandinavia was the same disease. Furthermore, the likelihood that between the Far Eastern foci in the Soviet Far East, northern China (Manchuria), and Korea, and the foci in Europe, further foci would be found appeared great. In 1959, Chiu and colleagues reported HFRS in Inner Mongolia in the Chinese People's Republic. The new revelation that since 1963 the disease has been a major problem in southern and central China as well, and that by 1981 it was recognized in 19 provinces of China, confirmed our earlier predictions that the disease would be found widespread in Europe and Asia.

EPIDEMIOLOGY

Incubation period of the disease may be as brief as 1 week or as long as 6 weeks. It is usually 10 to 25 days. Incubation period in experimental transmission of the disease to man by intravenous inoculation was 12 to 16 days. There

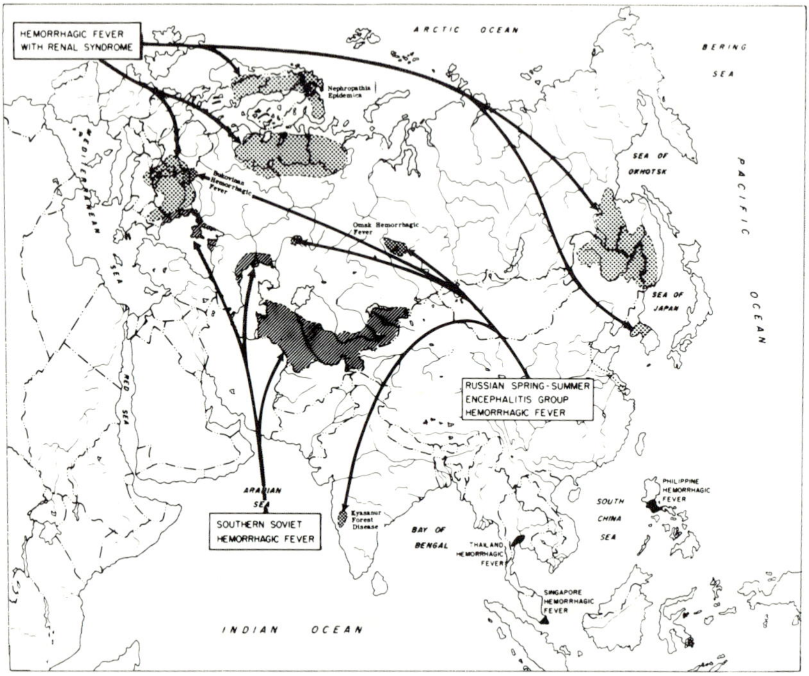

FIGURE 3. Map of the Eurasian land mass and adjoining regions showing location of endemic foci of viral hemorrhagic fevers. Hemorrhagic fever with renal syndrome includes Korean, Soviet Far Eastern (epidemic hemorrhagic nephrosonephritis), Yaroslav, and Ural hemorrhagic fever, as well as the nephropathia epidemica of Norway, Sweden, and Finland. The Russian spring-summer encephalitis group hemorrhagic fevers include Omsk hemorrhagic fever and the related Kyasanur Forest disease and Bukovinan hemorrhagic fever. Under the term Southern Soviet hemorrhagic fever, the clinically and epidemiologically similar entities occurring in Bulgaria, Romania, Czechoslovakia, Crimea, and adjacent Black Sea areas, Soviet Central Asia, and Transcaucasia are grouped together. These are now known collectively as Crimean hemorrhagic fever and the virus causing these is the same as the Congo virus, a nairo virus of Africa. The map, drawn in 1962, reflects our knowledge of the situation two decades ago, and should be compared with Figure 1, as we know the situation today.

have been several deaths from the disease in the United States in military personnel who have returned to America during the long incubation period of their disease; the first case seen in the United States was in November 1953 in Kansas City, Missouri, and he recovered, and a fatal case has occurred as recently as late 1981 in Honolulu, Hawaii.

In Korea and parts of the Soviet Far East the disease has occurred with two peaks per year, with the majority of cases occurring in late spring to early summer and again in autumn. Sporadic cases occur throughout the year. No secondary cases or evidence of person-to-person transmission have been seen and no nursing or medical personnel caring for patients have developed the disease. However, many investigators working on the disease, particularly those handling infected rodents, have developed HFRS. The first clearcut evidence that HFRS infections were contracted by the respiratory route stems from the large outbreak of laboratory infections in Moscow in 1962 with 83 affected laboratory workers. A more recent epidemiological study of infections in medical research laboratories in Japan indicated a respiratory route of infection of laboratory workers working in contact with enzootically and silently infected commercially reared white Wistar rats. Studies of outbreaks in China also led to the conclusion that most infection was by contaminated aerosols. Clinical and epidemiological studies in Scandinavia, Hungary, the Soviet Far East and Korea failed to directly incriminate the respiratory route of infection. Urine and feces, contamined foodstuffs, aerosols, arthropod vectors, especially ectoparasites such as mites and chiggers on infected rodents, were usually thought to be the sources of human infection; however, it is now evident that infection occurs most often by the respiratory route from contaminated aerosols produced by asymptomatically infected reservoir rodents. Whether saliva and respiratory droplets - the only secretions from which the virus has been isolated - are the only source of such aerosol contamination remains to be proved. Finally, high titer antigen has been found only in the lungs of infected wild mice (*A. agrarius*), voles (*C. glabreolus*), wild rats (*R. rattus* and *R. norvegicus*), and laboratory rats of the Wistar strain in Japan; other tissues contain lower concentrations of antigen as demonstrated by immunofluorescence. In experimentally infected white rats (Wistar and Fischer strains) and athymic nude mice the virus also appears in highest concentration in the lung. The virus has been isolated only from lung, saliva, throat washings, and blood of human patients; no other tissue or secretion has been found to be infectious. In naturally and experimentally infected rodents the virus has not been isolated from feces or urine, but it has been obtained regularly from lung, saliva, and acute phase blood.

CLINICAL COURSE

The clinical description of epidemic hemorrhagic fever is based largely upon observations of military cases during the Korean War. The few Korean children with the disease who have been studied have suffered rather mild forms. The disease varies greatly in its severity, yet the majority of recognized cases follow a fairly typical course. Although occasionally the illness is so mild as to make the diagnosis difficult, all patients exhibit proteinuria and many show petechiae and some degree of hemoconcentration, hypotension, and renal failure. Only about one fifth of the patients exhibit such severe consequences as shock, serious hemorrhages, and marked fluid and electrolyte imbalances. The clinical course and the important laboratory features of a case of moderate severity are summarized diagrammatically in Figures 4 and 5. The disease is conveniently, if rather arbitrarily, divided into five phases: febrile, hypotensive (shock), oliguric, diuretic, and convalescent.

PATHOLOGY

On postmortem examination of patients dying in shock during the hypotensive phase, rarely after the eighth day, large quantities of protein-rich, gelatinous retroperitoneal edema are found. The kidneys are swollen and on section reveal a pale cortex overlying an extremely congested, frequently hemorrhagic medulla. At times areas of necrosis are found in the center of the medullary pyramids. Glomeruli and convoluted tubules are usually normal, except for protein-containing material in their lumens. Tubules of the loop of Henle and collecting tubules are surrounded by dilated and engorged vascular spaces and extravasated blood. A distinctive feature of the renal lesion is hemorrhage in the junctional zone. There may be resulting extensive necrosis of tubular epithelium with gross rupture of many tubules, as Oliver and MacDowell have beautifully shown by microdissection. Hemorrhages in the right atrium of the heart and

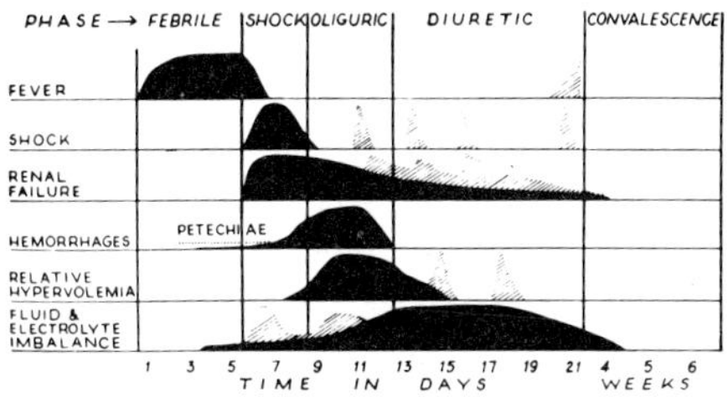

FIGURE 4. Schematic course of certain clinical manifestations in severe hemorrhagic fever with renal syndrome (epidemic hemorrhagic fever in Korea). The height of the black areas represents the intensity of the symptom complexes listed along the right. The cross-lined areas represent occasional additional patterns seen in very severe cases.

congestion with infarctlike necrosis of the anterior lobe of the pituitary gland extending into the infundibulum are discovered in patients dying after the ninth day of the disease. Although foci of hemorrhage have been found in the pars intermedia and posterior lobe of the pituitary and in the hypothalmus above the infundibulum, no necrosis is seen in these structures. Less often, similar congestion and hemorrhages and occasionally necrosis in the submucosa of the gastrointestinal tract and in the adrenal glands are seen, and rarely the islands of Langerhans of the pancreas are similarly affected. No thrombi or other evidence of vascular occlusion is found. All these findings support the assumption that the basic lesion is capillary damage manifested by dilatation, engorgement, diapedisis of erythrocytes, and capillary rupture.

PROGNOSIS

Survivors, with the exception of those who have had central nervous system hemorrhages, usually recover completely without any apparent sequelae. Deaths occur in the

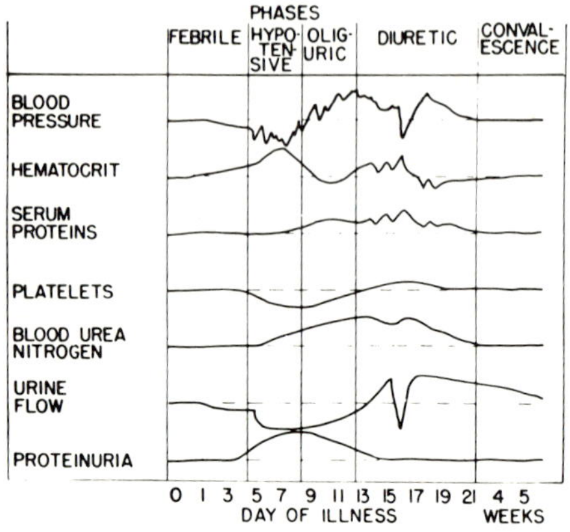

FIGURE 5. Schematic course of certain laboratory measurements in severe hemorrhagic fever with renal syndrome.

hypotensive, oliguric and diuretic phases at about the same frequency in each. No single finding is of great prognostic value in individual patients; however, protracted or recurrent shock, high fever, and persistent hemoconcentration are all ominous features. After techniques for early diagnosis; relatively nontraumatic evacuation; and prompt, adequate treatment were developed, the case fatality rate among United States Armed Forces personnel dropped to 5%. Recent observations of the disease in the Korean civilian populace indicate that the fatality rate is not considerably higher in the primitive villages in spite of the lack of modern medical care. In China, however, the disease has usually been severe and mortality has usually been above 5% and at times over 20%. During different years mortality in the European outbreaks has ranged from 1% to 7 to 8%. Although urine-concentrating power may not return completely until 3 to 4 months after the illness, and a few patients suffer mild loss of renal reserve probably compatible with normal duration of life, most patients regain normal kidney function. Some hypopituitarism has also been reported as a sequel in a rare patient.

85

RECENT PROGRESS OF KOREAN HAEMORRHAGIC FEVER RESEARCH

Ho Wang Lee
Luck Ju Baek
Pyung Woo Lee[1]

Department of Microbiology
Korea University Medical College
Seoul, Korea

Karl M. Johnson

US Army Medical Research Institute
of Infectious Diseases
Frederick, Maryland

Korean haemorrhagic fever (KHF) with its diverse clinical symptoms occurs in many parts of the world(1,2). A serological test for diagnosis of this disease is now available and the etiologic agent of KHF was named Hantaan virus after the Hantaan river which runs near 38th Parallel between South and North Korea(3,4).

I. INTRASPECIFIC TRANSMISSION OF HANTAAN VIRUS IN THE RODENT APODEMUS AGRARIUS, RESERVOIR OF KHF IN THE RURAL ENDEMIC AREAS OF KOREA

It has been hypothesized that KHF can be transmitted by ecto-parasites harbored by various field rats. The only

[1] *Present address: NINCDS, NIH, Frederick, Md.*

VIRAL DISEASES IN SOUTH-EAST ASIA
AND THE WESTERN PACIFIC
ISBN 0 12 484820 6

positive report supportive of this view so far published was that by Kasahara et al (5) who were able to induce the disease in monkeys by inoculation of a saline suspension of 203 *Laelaps jettmari Vitzthum* obtained from 40 *Apodemus agrarius*. However, to date this finding has yet to be confirmed by independent investigators though many attempts have already been made.

We have demonstrated for the first time that large quantities of virus are excreted in the saliva, in the urine and in the feces from infected *Apodemus agrarius* (6).

The infected *Apodemus* mice excrete the virus in saliva and the feces for a period of one month and in the urine for 2 years at least as shown in Table 1. Horizontal transmission of the virus between *Apodemus* mice was demonstrated as non-infected *Apodemus* mice caged together with infected *Apodemus* for several days acquired infection beginning 10 days after inoculation of the virus into the first animal. Results were not different when ecto-parasitized and clean animals were used in these experiments. The main route of infection in *Apodemus* mice is through the respiratory tract and infection can be transmitted via the saliva, urine or feces of infected *Apodemus* mice. Transmission of the virus among house rats and experimental animals remains to be studied.

TABLE I Quantitative Infectivity in Excreta and Organs of *Apodemus agrarius coreae* Infected with 1,000 ID_{50} of Hantaan Virus

Excreta & organs	*Apodemus* -log ID_{50}/ml or g. on days after virus inoculation												
	7	9	12	15	25	35	45	85	141	181	360	489	650
Blood	1.0	2.4	1.9	≧0.5									
Saliva		≦2.1	2.6	3.9	3.6	2.2	≦2.1						
Urine		1.8	3.8	3.8	4.1	2.2	1.8	2.8	2.3	2.1	1.8	2.8	1.8
Feces		≦1.5	2.5	3.3	3.0	1.8	≦1.5						
Lungs			n.t.	8.7	n.t.				1.2	≦1.2			
Kidneys			n.t.	7.2	n.t.								
Liver			n.t.	6.7	n.t.								
Submaxillary & parotid glands			n.t.	8.2	n.t.								
Lacrimal glands			n.t.	5.6	n.t.								

n.t. : not titrated

II. EPIDEMIC CYCLES OF KHF

There are three epidemiologic types of KHF according to the outbreaks and the reservoir host of the disease.

1. *Rural Type:* The reservoir for KHF in rural areas of Korea, China and probably in the Eastern parts of the USSR as well is Apodemus species (3). These rodents live only in the field but will invade houses during the snowing season. Cases of the rural type occur in the endemic rural areas and annually there are two seasonal peaks when incidence of the disease is high. The victims are primarily farmers and soldiers stationed in the field.

2. *Urban Type:* The reservoir is house rats. There were many cases of KHF reported in metropolitan areas of Seoul in individuals who have never been outside of the city limits and who had histories of contact with house rats (7); 130 cases of KHF were reported also among residents of urban areas of Osaka City in Japan (8). Cases of the urban type occur throughout the year but tend to appear more in fall and winter seasons. Urban rats captured in Seoul and four nearby Korean cities were found to have immunofluorescent (IF) antibodies reactive with Hantaan virus. Antibodies were detected in 13 percent of sera from 477 R. norvegicus and 11 percent of 47 R. rattus. Hantaan viral antigen was found in pulmonary tissues of 42 animals and Hantaan virus strains were recovered from 23 rats. Wistar rats were qualitatively much more sensitive than Apodemus agrarius rodents for isolation of virus strains from wild rat tissues. Wistar rats inoculated with one of these strains had virus in lung and spleen for at least 75 days (9). These results document the existence of an urban cycle for Hantaan virus, previously suspected on the basis by the occurrence of sporadic urban human cases of KHF, and suggest that Rattus-borne Hantaan virus may be widely distributed in urban centers of Asia or elsewhere.

3. *Experimental Animal Type:* The reservoir is colonized rats. There were 21 outbreaks of KHF among personnel of animal rooms of medical centers in Korea and in Japan since 1976, and no. of victims that were 130. These cases may occur at any time of the year, but a series of outbreaks occured during the winter season when the air is dry in the animal rooms(10, 11).

ACKNOWLEDGMENTS

This work was supported in part by grant no. DAMD17-81-G-9482 from the U.S. Army Medical Research and Development Command, Frederick, Md.

REFERENCES

1. Gajdusek, D. C., J. Pediat. 60. 851 (1962).
2. Lee, H. W., Lee, M. C., and Cho, K. S., Pract. Therap. 2, 15 (1980).
3. Lee, H. W., Lee, P. W., and Johnson, K. M., J. Infect. Dis. 137, 298 (1978).
4. Information Exchange Subcommittee, Karabatsos, N. ed. Box 2087, Ft. Collins, Co 80522.
5. Kasahara, S., Kitano, N., Kikuchi, H., Sakyuama, M., Kanazawa, K., Nezu, N., Yoshimura, M., and Kudo, T., J. Jap. Pathol. 34, 3 (1944).
6. Lee, H. W., Lee, P. W., Baek, L. J., and Song, C. K., J. Trop. Med. & Hyg. 30 1106 (1981).
7. Lee, H. W., Bark, D. H., Baek, L. J. Choi, K. S., Whang, Y. N., and Woo, M. S., Korean J. Virol. 10, 1 (1980).
8. Tamura, M., Biken J. 7, 79 (1964).
9. Lee, H. W., Baek, L. J., and Johnson, K. M., J. Infect. Dis. (Submitted for publication).
10. Umenai, T., Lee, H. W., Lee, P. W., Saito, T., Toyoda, T., Hongo, M., Yoshinaga, K., Nobunaga, T., Horiuchi, T., and Ishida, N., Lancet, 1914 (1979).
11. Lee, H. W., Kawamata, J., and Tamura, T. (In preparation)

COMMENTS DURING DISCUSSION

ON A POSSIBLE MILDER FORM OF EPIDEMIC HAEMORRHAGIC FEVER

C.M. CHU (CHINA) In addition to the severe form of epidemic haemorrhagic fever (EHF) transmitted mainly by *Apodemus agrarius*, there may be a milder form of the same disease, possibly transmitted by *Rattus norvegicus*. Two outbreaks were investigated in 1981, one in Henan in Central China and the other in Shanxi in North China. The disease is characterized by fever and haemorrhagic manifestations, but is much milder and lacks the stages of shock, anuria and diauria. Epidemiologically, many patients had no history of contact with wild rodents and multiple cases often occurred in the same households where *Rattus norvegicus* was the main rodent species. These features are all different from those of EHF. After the isolation of EHF agents both in *Apodemus* from disease-free areas and in A539 cells, sera from these patients were tested retrospectively against EHF antigens by immunofluorescence and were found to be positive with fairly high titres. The lung specimens of about 10% of *Rattus norvegicus* captured around the patients' households were positive for EHF antigen by the immunofluorescence test. Cross serological tests with sera from typical cases of EHF and from the mild form of disease against antigens prepared from the lungs of *Apodemus* and of *Rattus* respectively did not reveal significant antigenic differences. It appears, therefore, that this disease is caused by a less virulent EHF virus and *Rattus norvegicus* may be the reservoir host. These results will be reported by Dr. Song and his colleagues from our institute at a WHO workshop to be held in Tokyo.

86

FLEXIBLE FILM ISOLATORS IN RESEARCH, DIAGNOSIS AND TREATMENT OF VIRAL HAEMORRHAGIC FEVERS

B.A. Page-Roberts
G.J. Smallridge

Vickers Medical, Basingstoke, U.K.

P.C. Trexler

University of Surrey, Guildford, U.K.

INTRODUCTION

Viral haemorrhagic fevers carry a risk of nosocomial infection, and pose serious occupational and environmental health hazards as no vaccines are available.

Isolation is therefore important to contain the threat of virus infection from haemorrhagic fever patients and from infective laboratory material. Increased awareness of the risks associated with these viruses has necessitated wider deployment of facilities for biohazard containment.

PATIENT ISOLATORS

Patient isolation systems based on the 'Trexler' principle have been in use for several years, for isolation of infected patients during treatment in hospital and during transportation. These systems are based on the flexible film principle. The patient is surrounded by an air-tight flexible plastic enclosure through which air enters and leaves via high efficiency filters. The pressure inside the

VIRAL DISEASES IN SOUTH-EAST ASIA AND THE WESTERN PACIFIC
ISBN 0 12 484820 6

isolator is maintained slightly below atmospheric, to prevent escape of contaminated air in the event of the envelope being punctured. A bed isolator has been produced for treatment of the patient in hospital, together with aircraft and stretcher transit isolators which facilitate transport of the patient over long distances by air, or shorter distances by road. These isolator systems have been in use for some time and have proved to be both practical and effective.

LABORATORY ISOLATION SYSTEMS

We have designed flexible film laboratory isolators to meet the performance criteria of the British Standard for Class III microbiological safety cabinets for a variety of laboratory applications.

Laboratory Diagnosis and Management of Infected Patients

Patient management laboratory tests provide important information to clinicians treating a seriously ill patient, but such tests cannot normally be performed on haemorrhagic fever patients because of the risk of infection. An isolator has been developed which provides facilities for both patient management and differential diagnostic tests.

A small protable isolator has also been designed which may be used for limited diagnostic tests, in the hospital isolation facility, or in the field.

Virology

Virological studies make varying demands for microscopy facilities as well as requiring different proportions of incubator and working space. A number of isolator modules have been developed, having facilities for inverted, transmitted light or fluorescence microscopy, incubators and working space. Appropriate modules may be assembled into an 'isolator line' with the facilities required.

CONCLUSION

Flexible film isolators have been used successfully for a number of years for isolation of infectious disease patients. In the laboratory, rigid microbiological safety cabinets are the usual means used for biohazard containment. Whilst effective, these cabinets have the disadvantages of expense, ergonomic inconvenience and requiring a prolonged installation and commissioning period. Flexible film isolators have been developed for laboratory use and have been shown to be safe in independently performed tests. These isolators have also proved to be ergonomically convenient and may therefore be a preferable alternative in several applications.

AUSTRALIA AND ARENAVIRUSES

Geoff Gard

Department of Primary Production
Darwin, Northern Territory

Robert Begg

Conservation Commission of the Northern Territory
Darwin, Northern Territory

Jordi Casals

Yale Arbovirus Research Unit
New Haven, Connecticut

Arenaviruses have not been recorded as occurring naturally in Australia. Table 1 has been compiled from the International Catalogue of Arboviruses (1) and lists 8 of the 10 documented arenaviruses, their natural reservoirs and the cited isolation rate. The usual reservoir of Lymphocytic choriomeningitis virus is the house mouse *(Mus musculus)* but LCM has been recovered from a variety of species including man, monkeys, dogs, field mice, hamsters and guinea pigs. The tenth arenavirus, Tacaribe, will not be discussed here because it is a virus of bats.

With two exceptions, all of the species listed in Table 1 are rodents of the family Cricetidae, the New World rats and mice. These two exceptions are *Mus musculus* and *Mastomys natalensis*, members of the family Muridae, to which all of Australia's rodents belong. *Mus musculus* is very rare in the monsoonal northern quarter (Top End) of the Northern Territory. *Mastomys natalensis* is now included as a subgenus of the genus *Rattus*. The only endemic species of this genus

VIRAL DISEASES IN SOUTH-EAST ASIA
AND THE WESTERN PACIFIC
ISBN 0 12 484820 6

TABLE 1. Rodent Reservoirs of Arenaviruses

Virus	*Natural reservoir*	*Number isolations / Number tested*
Amapari	*Oryzomys capito*	*124/918*
	Oryzomys goeldii	*5/41*
	Neacomys guianea	*97/1095*
Junin	*Calomys laucha*	*4/36*
	Calomys laucha	*1/28 pools*
	Mus musculus	*10/33 pools*
	Akodon arenicola	*1/13 pools*
Lassa	*Mastomys natalensis*	*18/109*
Latino	*Calomys callosus*	*3/8; 14/119; 1/35*
Machupo	*Calomys callosus*	*2/6*
Parana	*Oryzomys buccinatus*	*3/4*
Pichinde	*Oryzomys albigularis*	*45/230; 7/32; 2/8*
	Thomasomys fuscatus	*1/173*
Tamiami	*Sigmodon hispidus*	*9/294; 28/912*
	Oryzomys palustris	*1/149*

in the Top End of the Northern Territory are *R. colletti* and *R. tunneyi*.

Early in 1981 fourteen *R. colletti* sera and nine *R. tunneyi* sera were examined at YARU for arenavirus antibody. Using an indirect immunofluorescence test with antimouse conjugate, two of the *R. colletti* sera reacted with LCM antigen to dilutions of 4 and 8. These sera did not react with uninfected cells or with Tacaribe, Pichinde, Junin or polyvalent Ebola-Lassa - Marburg antigens. None of the 21 other sera showed any reactions.

Complement-fixation tests with the 23 sera against LCM and normal brain antigens were meaningless. Sera that were not negative were non-specific or anticomplementary.

The dusky rat *(R. colletti)* is found on the subcoastal plains of the monsoonal north of the Northern Territory. They form the dominant component of the small mammal fauna of these plains, with only the grassland melomys *(Melomys burtoni)* and the common planigale *(Planigale maculata)* also occurring. The Dusky rat is often rare in occurrence but is sometimes sufficiently numerous to be regarded as a pest. Localised peaks in numbers result from (non-breeding) adults refuging onto the higher levee banks of the coastal rivers during annual flooding of the plains. Most females become pregnant immediately after the monsoonal rains (April) and young are recruited into the population around June (2).

The grassland melomys is a tropical rodent restricted to coastal northern Australia. They are usually found in a wet, forested or swampy habitat and are good climbers, constructing spherical nests in trees. The common planigale is one of the smaller Dasyurid marsupials and is found in all mainland states except Victoria.

In the study area where the dusky rats were collected the grassland melomys is not uncommon but the common planigale is rare. The trapping methods used heavily favoured the collection of dusky rats.

Most of the arenaviruses listed in Table 1 have been recovered from rodent kidney or tissue pools containing kidney and all of the viruses plaque in Vero monolayers, some without laboratory adaptation. We elected to attempt recovery of the putative Northern Territory arenavirus by inoculation of sera and kidney homogenates of dusky rats onto Vero monolayers and examining for plaques 14 days later, 4 days after staining the monolayers with neutral red. To date 111 mature dusky rats and 1 common planigale have been examined without any plaques being obtained.

Future virus recovery will be attempted from further collections of dusky rats, especially foeti and newborn, and from grassland melomys. In addition, some inocula will be passaged in Vero and BHK cells before plaquing is attempted in case the putative virus requires laboratory adaptation before plaquing.

REFERENCES

1. Berge, T.O. (ed.), *International Catalogue of Arboviruses* (2nd edition), U.S. Department of Health, Education and Welfare, Publication No. (CDC) 75-8301, (1975).
2. Redhead, T.D., *Aust. J. Ecol. 4*, 115 (1979).

88

RABIES IN THAILAND

Prasert Thongcharoen
Chantapong Wasi
Lersuang Chavanich

Department of Microbiology
Faculty of Medicine Siriraj Hospital, Mahidol University
Bangkok

Siriwan Sirikawin

Bamrasnaradul Infectious Hospital
Ministry of Public Health
Bangkok

Rabies is an endemic disease causing a serious health problem in Thailand. Although control measures for rabies were started in 1913, approximatley 200 to 300 cases of human rabies have been reported and about 60,000 to 80,000 people are treated for post-exposure rabies prophylaxis each year. Dogs are the main vectors but cats are also responsible for transmitting the diseases to man. Wildlife rabies are less important in Thailand. Between 1966 and 1969 the SEATO Medical Research Laboratory reported 14 rabies-positive bats out of 483 samples caught from several areas of Thailand (1). The 1969 investigation by Smith *et al.* on rabies among rodents and small mammals found that 37 out of 1,037 samples (3.6%) were positive for rabies. The highest rate (7.9%) was found in *Bandicoota indicus* (2). A 1976 study on rabies in bats and small rodents by Swasdikosol *et al.* found negative results in more than 400 animals (3).

Stray dogs in Bangkok and some other cities harboured from 0 to 3% the rabies virus and as shown by other

VIRAL DISEASES IN SOUTH-EAST ASIA
AND THE WESTERN PACIFIC
ISBN 0 12 484820 6

investigators about 15-19% of them showing positive antibody for rabies, possibly occurring from abortive rabies infections or other reasons (3-7).

PROPHYLAXIS

Before 1978, there were three types of rabies vaccine available: i.e. Semple (5% sheep brain, NTV); suckling mouse brain (2% suspension, SMB); and duck embryo vaccine (DEV). Semple vaccine produced locally has been supplied throughout the country. Most rabies patients neither had rabies vaccination nor received adequate treatment (1). Between 1961 and 1970, 59,597 people receiving NTV reported neurological complications at the rate of 1:400 and rabies deaths occurred after a complete series of vaccine in 1:2,000 (8).

For animals, locally produced 25% sheep brain vaccine, imported live-attenuated chick embryo vaccine and inactivated tissue culture vaccine have been available. However, the number of domestic animals which have been immunized is still very small.

TABLE I. Local and Systemic Reactions after HDCV Vaccination

	Pre-exposure		*Post-exposure*	
	Number	*%*	*Number*	*%*
Local at injection site	*3*	*2.80*	*6*	*1.56*
Tenderness	*1*		*1*	
Pain	*2*		*3*	
Itching	*0*		*2*	
Systemic (mild)	*1*	*0.93*	*21*	*5.45*
Generalized itching	*0*		*5*	
Fever	*1*		*5*	
Hives	*0*		*1*	
Paresthesia	*0*		*3*	
Circumoral paresthesia	*0*		*2*	
Headache	*0*		*3*	
Palpitation	*0*		*1*	
Generalized muscular pain	*0*		*1*	
Total No. of reaction	*4*	*3.73*	*27*	*7.01*
None	*100*	*96.27*	*358*	*92.99*

Inactivated human diploid cell vaccine (HDCV) has been licensed in Thailand since 1978. In our study, approximately 500 persons receiving the vaccine as both pre- and post-exposure prophylaxis have been investigated at Siriraj Hospital. Local and systemic reactions were mild (Table 1). Neutralizing antibodies were demonstrated in some cases on the seventh day (after receiving two injections of vaccine, 1.0 ml subcutaneously on day 0 and day 3). The mean antibody titer in the HDCV group was much higher than those receiving NTV, SMB and DEV (Fig. 1). All persons receiving post-exposure treatment were followed up for between 1-2 years. No serious complications or rabies death occurred in our study group.

MONOCLONAL-ANTIBODY STUDY

In collaboration with P. Sureau in Paris, antigenic types of rabies virus have been studied, using antinucleocapsid hybridoma monoclonal antibodies and the indirect immunofluorescent technique applied to brain impressions prepared from the original brain specimen. Fifty-one dog brains from Thailand were able to be separated into three subgroups: four isolates negative with antibody 111-14; 17 isolates negative with 389-2; but positive with 111-14; and 30

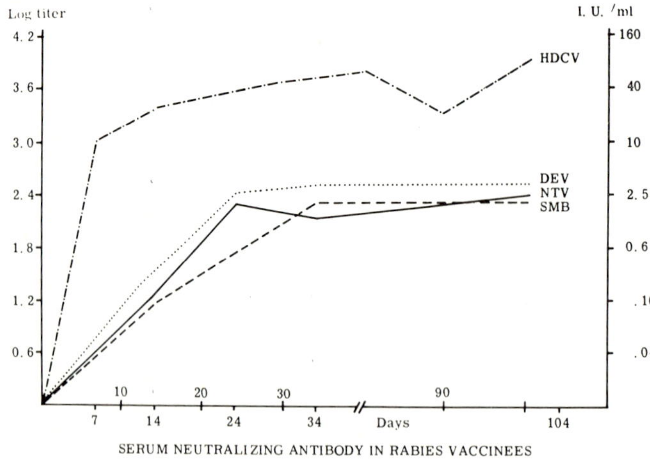

FIGURE 1. Antibody responses after different kinds of vaccine.

isolates positive with both. This preliminary report confirmed that nucleocapsid antigens of rabies virus in Thailand had different patterns of geographical distribution from some other countries (Table 2).

HUMAN-TO-HUMAN TRANSMISSION

It has long been questioned whether human-to-human transmission of rabies could occur naturally. In our records there were two instances concerning this matter. Two babies born from rabid mothers did not contract the infection vertically (9). The first case was noticed in 1972. The mother of a boy, aged 43 years old, was bitten by a dog on the knee 18 days before delivery. Two days after giving birth she showed symptoms and signs of rabies and died 4 days later. Neutralizing antibody determinations of the infant's sera obtained at birth and again one year later were below 1:5 on both occasions. The second boy was born in 1975 by caesarean section at Siriraj Hospital from a rabid mother, 43 years of age. She was bitten on the left calf by a dog almost 3 months before her illness. She received 14 injections of Semple vaccine starting three days after the bite. She came to the hospital with typical symptoms and signs of rabies. Caesarean operation was performed on her last day two hours before she died. Autopsy findings confirmed that she had rabies infection. These two boys are presently in a good health.

The second instance appeared in 1981. Two patients died of rabies after receiving corneal transplantation. The first case, a woman 41 years of age, who died 22 days after

TABLE II. Monoclonal Antibody Study on Antigenic Types of Viruses

Origin of Isolates	*Monoclonal Antibodies*					
	111-2	*103-7*	*590-2*	*111-14*	*389-2*	*120-2*
Tunisia	+	+	+	+	+	+
Madagascar	–	+	+	–	–	–
Thailand	+	+	+	–	–	–
"	+	+	+	+	–	–
"	+	+	+	+	+	–
France	+	+	–	+	+	+
"	+	–	–	+	+	+

keratoplasty. The second case, a 25-year old man, who died 33 days after the same type of surgical operation. Both patients received corneal grafts from the same donor, a 16-year old boy, who died with the provisional diagnosis of respiratory disease, but careful retrospective pathological examination revealed Negri's bodies. These were the third and the fourth reported cases in the literature (10). From these reports, control measures and selection of the donors for corneal grafts should be carefully considered.

CONTROL MEASURES

In the future more attention to control measures for rabies must be paid by the health authorities. The Rabies Control Act is now under amendment. Mass vaccination programmes for domestic animals, especially dogs and cats, will be strengthened. More laboratory services for rabies must be established in rural areas. Health education for the public has now been undertaken both by the governmental and private sectors. Other means including the slaughter of stray dogs and antifertility procedures are also being undertaken. The production of animal vaccine to meet the local need is another one of these strategies.

REFERENCES

1. Thongcharoen, P., *in* "Rabies (in Thai)" (P. Thongcharoen, ed.), p.214 & 271. Aksornsmai Press, Bangkok, (1980).
2. Smith, P.C., Lawhaswasdi, V., Vick, W.E., and Stanton, J.E., *Nature 217,* 954 (1968).
3. Swasdikosol, S., Unpublished data (1979).
4. Thongcharoen, P., Charoenrath, M., Panpatana, P., and Wasi, C., *J. Med. Ass. Thailand 55,* 537 (1972).
5. Spertzel, R.O., Morris, J.H., and Lawhaswasdi, K.L., *SEATO Med. Res. Lab. Ann. Rep.,* 291 (1966).
6. Ratanarapee, S., Wasi, C., Chavanich, L., Puthavathana, P., Chattuchai, K., and Thongcharoen, P., *J. Med. Ass. Thailand 65,* 33 (1982).
7. Yasmuth, C., Nelson, K.E., Laima, T., Supavadee, C., and Thaiyanant, P., *J. Med. Ass. Thailand,* In press (1982).
8. Phong-Aksara, S., *Roy. Thai. Army Med. J. 24,* 303 (1971).
9. Sirikawin, S., *in* "Rabies (in Thai)" (P. Thongcharoen, ed.) p.266. Aksornsmai Press, Bangkok, (1980).

10. Thongcharoen, P., Wasi, C., Sirikawin, S., Boonthai, P., Bedavanij, A., Dumavibhat, P., Chantarakul, N., Eungprabbanth, V., Puthavathana, P., Chavanich, L., and Tantawachakit, S., *Morb. Mort. Wkly Rpts 30*, 473 (1981).

89

RABIES IN MALAYSIA

Dora S.K. Tan

Institute for Medical Research
Kuala Lumpur, Malaysia

Rabies is a public health problem in Malaysia along the Malaysia-Thai border where the disease is introduced through dogs crossing over from Thailand. The infection has been successfully contained in that area only because of an "immune-belt" established in 1954, before which Malaya (as the country was known at that time) was highly endemic for rabies.

The immune belt stretches 30-50 miles south of the Malaysian-Thai border and includes the entire state of Perlis and parts of the states of Kedah, Perak and Kelantan (Figure 1). Within this area, continual compulsory vaccination and registration of dogs, and destruction of stray and unlicensed dogs, are maintained.

The effective maintenance of the belt is essential to rabies control in Malaysia. This was evident when in 1970 a major epidemic of rabies occurred and spread rapidly throughout Perlis and Kedah because of heightened communist activities along the border which hampered the effective maintenance of stray dog control.

The outbreak involved 11 human cases (one of whom died), 4 dogs and 1 cat. The brain specimens of the human case, the cat and dogs were examined by the immunofluorescent technique (IFT), the Seller's staining method, histopathology and mouse inoculation. All 6 specimens were negative in the three microscopic tests but yielded evidence of infection by mouse inoculation. The inoculated mice were all unequivocally confirmed positive by each of the 3 microscopic tests.

VIRAL DISEASES IN SOUTH-EAST ASIA
AND THE WESTERN PACIFIC
ISBN 0 12 484820 6

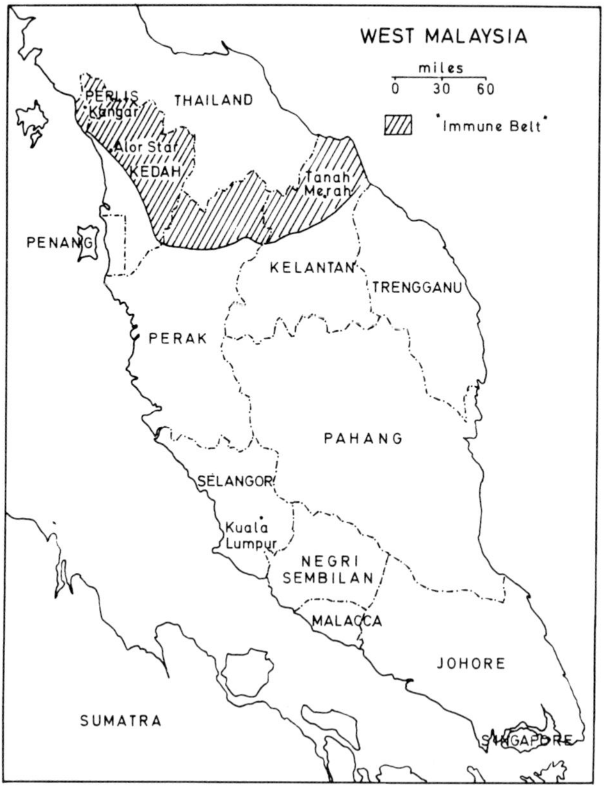

FIGURE 1. Map of West Malaysia.

As these observations were rather perplexing, the WHO Regional Office in Manila was consulted and Dr. G.W. Beran, a WHO consultant on rabies was sent here to assist in clarifying the situation. Dr. Beran found no fault with the laboratory techniques and concluded that it was a changed property of the virus strains which was responsible for the unusual laboratory observations (1). He also conducted some experiments in dogs with the Malaysian virus strains at the Siliman University Medical Centre, Phillipine, and reported: "The long incubation periods in the dogs, especially 105 days, were quite amazing. This is especially unique in that the clinical period is then very short *and* the experimental animals are loaded with Negri bodies and FA antigen." (2).

The 1970 epidemic lasted for 3 months. Since then, sporadic cases have been occurring in the "immune belt" at the attack rate of 1 to 5 dogs and 0 to 2 human cases annually. Furthermore, 50% of the brain specimens examined still behaved in the same manner as did the 1970 strains.

In view of the delay in obtaining results due to this phenomenon, the brain specimens, if negative by IFT, are inoculated into suckling mice as well as adult mice. From day 3 to day 6 of inoculation, the brain specimens of 2 suckling mice are examined daily by IFT. In this way, rabies can be detected earlier than if only adult mice are employed.

The author would appreciate it if readers would inform her of any similar experience with the rabies virus. It is possible that the atypical 1970 virus might have emerged as a variant strain through the continual co-existence during the past two decades of 2 live rabies viruses; the Flury LEP strain on the Malaysian side of the border and street rabies virus on the Thai side. It would seem that the co-existence of these 2 types of rabies virus in dogs is a unique situation prevalent only along the Malaysian-Thai border.

REFERENCES

1. Tan, Dora S.K., Abd. Wahab Mohd Ariff, Mohd Noordin Keling, and Beran, G.W., *Med. J. Malaysia 37*, 107 (1972).
2. Beran, G.W., Personal communication, (1972).

Part VI
Specific Viral Diseases
F.
Viruses of Veterinary Importance

Chairman F. A. Murphy

Co-Chairman W. A. Snowdon

90

VIRUSES OF VETERINARY IMPORTANCE AN OVERVIEW

E.L. French

P.O. Box 141
Mount Eliza, Victoria

The first four days of this Seminar on Viral Diseases in South-East Asia and the Western Pacific have been devoted, almost entirely, to considerations of viruses infecting human beings. Today we began by considering some zoonotic diseases but again largely those aspects affecting human health. In the remaining time between now and the closing session we need to consider not only the "Viruses of Veterinary Importance", but also the effects that virus diseases of livestock have on human populations in South-East Asia and the Western Pacific area.

Although there are many large cities in some areas of South-East Asia, a very large proportion of the area is given over to subsistence farming organized on a family or village basis.

Ruminants have an important role in the socio-economic life of farmers in South-East Asia. Animals are a source of protein; they provide traction and transport and are a kind of savings account to provide for marriages, religious festivities and unforeseen circumstances.

Foot and Mouth Disease

Perhaps the most important disease of livestock in South-East Asia is Foot-and-mouth disease (FMD), not because it causes the death of many animals, but because of its debilitating effects upon those that recover, and because of the restricting effect it can have on the trade movement of

VIRAL DISEASES IN SOUTH-EAST ASIA
AND THE WESTERN PACIFIC
ISBN 0 12 484820 6

animals between countries and areas. Its importance is probably reflected in the fact that three of the seven papers to be given in this session on "Viruses of Veterinary Importance" are directed toward some aspect of FMD.

Foot-and-mouth disease is an acute febrile disease of cloven footed animals with vesicle formation in the mouth, on the feet, on the teats and in the rumen. In young animals, particularly pigs, the virus causes muscular lesions. Man is only occasionally infected: FMD should not be confused with hand, foot and mouth disease in human beings which is caused by Coxsackieviruses A5, 6, 10, 16 and Entero 71. Foot-and-mouth disease is caused by a very small Picornavirus with a single stranded RNA core contained within a protein coat which consists of 32 capsomeres forming a symmetrical icosahedral capsid with a diameter of about 23nm. It has a relatively narrow range of pH stability, being most stable between pH 7.4 and 7.6, and is rapidly destroyed on the acid side of pH 6 or on the alkaline side of pH 9.5. Survival of the virus at adverse pH is favoured by increased salt concentration. The virus is resistant to external influences and can remain viable for long periods in the environment, on clothing and in carcases, particularly in glandular organs and lymph nodes.

Seven main serological types of the virus are recognized - the original European types O, A and C, the South African Territories types SAT 1, SAT 2 and SAT 3 and ASIA 1. Within these major types, considerable antigenic variation occurs with more than 60 sub-types within the seven major types. These sub-types may be of importance primarily for the selection of virus strains for use in vaccines for control of outbreaks of this disease. Field strains vary considerably in virulence, and the severity of the disease in the field may be influenced by the immune status of the population of animals and their nutritional state: fat animals are often more severely affected than lean animals.

The clinical picture of FMD can range from severe lesions in the mouth and on the feet, with inappetence, loss of condition, a marked drop in lactation, abortion, severe lameness with sometimes loss of the horny covering of the hoof, to a mild syndrome in which lesions may escape notice by being almost entirely limited to a superficial erosion of the epithelium of the mouth. Secondary bacterial infections are the most damaging feature in the later stages of the disease. Mastitis, with consequent drop in milk supply in dairy animals, and the prolonged loss of condition in fattening cattle are the most serious economic sequelae. Sudden death due to myocarditis is associated with FMD infection in young animals particularly pigs.

Although FMD has been under study for decades, it is only recently that knowledge of the epizootiology and natural history of the disease has become available. The main mode of spread of FMD is via respiratory aerosols. The usual primary site of infection and initial replication of virus is in the cells of the mucous membrane of the throat. Less frequently, infection is through abrasions in the mucous membranes or skin as a result of contact with contaminated materials such as food stuffs (including unsterilized meat products), clothing, fomites, birds, etc. After the initial infection the replicated virus is transported to the sites of predeliction where visible lesions develop, e.g. tongue and the interdigital space. FMD mainly affects ruminants and swine, but many rodents are susceptible and hedge-hogs can act as reservoirs of infection. Oesophageal-pharyngeal fluid collected by use of a cup-probang has been shown to contain FMD virus before, during, and after the appearance of clinical signs and lesions of the disease. By this technique, recovered animals have been shown to harbour virus in their throat area for varying times (6-24 months in cattle, 4-6 months in sheep and goats but only during the clinical phase in pigs). The quantity of virus excreted in the respiratory aerosol of pigs is many times greater than the virus content of aerosols from other species. Pigs are considered to be dangerous multipliers and spreaders of the virus, and cattle, because of their great susceptibility, are the indicators of the presence of the virus. Lactating cows infected with FMD virus excrete the virus in their milk, and aerosols of infected milk created while transferring milk from the farm to milk tankers facilitated the spread of the disease in at least one recent outbreak in the United Kingdom.

The European types O, A and C are widely distributed in Europe, South America, and Asia with types O and A occurring more frequently than type C. The Asia 1 type virus was first observed in Pakistan in 1957 and has subsequently been found in Hong Kong, Thailand, Burma, India, Afghanistan, Iran, Syria, Israel, Lebanon, Turkey and Jordon. At present the only South-East Asian country that is free of FMD is Singapore where the last outbreak was recorded in 1973, and the disease eradicated by a slaughter and compensation policy within three weeks. Control by mass vaccination has brought the type O FMD virus, that has been present in Indonesia since about the middle of the nineteenth century, under control.

There are three recognized methods of control of FMD in the field:

(a) eradication by slaughter of clinically infected and all incontact susceptible animals with subsequent quarantine and surveillance of animals in the area,

(b) mass vaccination over an extended period,

(c) a combination of both methods in which the affected herd is destroyed and vaccination of all susceptible animals that may have come in contact with infected animals.

Vaccination with the inactivated virus established an immunity for a period not greater than four to six months, but repeated vaccination enhances the duration of immunity. Attenuated live virus vaccines have been tried, but generally are not considered to be as safe as the inactivated vaccine.

Rinderpest

This highly infectious disease of ruminants and pigs is caused by a virus of the *Morbillivirus* subgroup of the paramyxoviruses, and shares antigens with other members of the group, e.g. canine distemper and human measles viruses. The disease is characterized by fever, necrotic stomatitis and gastroenteritis. The introduction of a very effective, attenuated tissue culture grown vaccine has brought the disease under control in Africa and its eradication from South Africa.

It is still endemic in parts of Asia, but although not eradicated, it can be controlled by mass vaccination. The main host species are cattle, buffalo and pigs, but deer, camel, sheep and goats can be infected. Transmission is principally by direct contact and, to a lesser degree, indirectly from virus-laden nasal discharge, urine or faeces. Variation in innate resistance to rinderpest virus has been described. Cattle reared on the Indian plains are much more resistant than cattle bred in the Himalayan valleys. Egyptian buffaloes react only mildly to infection, whereas Thai buffalo are severely affected. Infections in Asiatic pigs are clinically manifest, but in European-type pigs the infections are clinically inapparent. Carrier animals, if they exist at all, are rare.

From formerly being a much dreaded disease of cattle called "cattle plague", rinderpest is now fairly well under control by means of vaccination programmes, but it can still break out and cause wide-spread stock losses as demonstrated when a major pandemic swept through the Middle East from Afghanistan to the Mediterranean in 1969, and the disease lingered on into 1973.

Rabies

This dreaded zoonotic disease has been dealt with in earlier papers today. It is necessary to emphasize, however, that rabies, quite apart from its human public health aspects, can be the cause of serious economic loss of cattle in endemic areas. Of the countries of South-East Asia, only Malaysia and Singapore have succeeded in eradicating rabies by an intensive campaign of vaccination and destruction of dogs.

Bovine Malignant Catarrh (BMC)

This disease has been described as a clinico-pathological entity and occurs sporadically world-wide, although epizootics of it have been reported in both deer and cattle. Two varieties of the disease appear to exist, viz. the African cases caused by a herpesvirus, and an almost identical disease occurring outside of Africa. In Africa the herpesvirus cycles silently in wildebeest and possibly sheep being transmitted congenitally and probably by direct contact. Infection of domestic cattle is believed to occur through contact with parturient and new-born wildebeest and hartebeest. There is an apparent seasonal incidence and African herdsmen have learned empirically not to drive cattle over the grazing areas where wildebeest are calving. The disease is not contagious between acutely ill and healthy cattle. The herpesvirus associated with this African form of the disease can be isolated in tissue cultures of bovine thyroid cells and is often highly cell-associated. The virus can be readily transferred to susceptible cattle by intravenous inoculation and to rabbits by intracerebral inoculation. Recovered animals become carriers of the virus. Virus neutralizing antibody develops and persists throughout the life of the affected animal, but its significance is unknown.

Outside of Africa an identical clinico-pathological disease occurs, but the herpesvirus associated with the African disease appears not to be associated either aetiologically or serologically with this condition. Work in Australia, the USA and the United Kingdom has tended to confirm the association of sheep with outbreaks of BMC in these countries.

Recently, a cell-associated, syncytium producing *Morbillivirus* has been isolated by workers in the USA and northern Ireland from typical cases of BMC but its significant association with BMC is uncertain at this stage. It seems likely on epidemiological, clinical and pathological evidence that this disease is present in South-East Asia wherever both sheep and cattle are run together.

At present the only method of control is to avoid running sheep and cattle in close proximity particularly during the lambing season. Buffalo are very susceptible to this disease as are the various strains of local cattle in Asia.

Mucosal Disease-Virus Diarrhoea

This disease has long been recognized in the USA, Australasia and Europe, and most likely it is present in most areas of South-East Asia. With the availability of more veterinary virology diagnostic laboratories in this area, this, and a number of other diseases of livestock, will be recognized.

The causal agent is a non arthropod-borne togavirus which is now classified as a *Pestivirus* along with the swine fever or hog cholera agent. It is an RNA virus of about 30-80 nm in diameter. The virus naturally infects cattle, buffaloes, sheep, goats, pigs, deer and wallabies, but in not all species with clinical effects. In cattle MD virus causes either an acute or a chronic disease. The acute disease bears some gross pathological resemblance to rinderpest. The chronic disease in some cases appears to be the result of intra-uterine infection of the foetus with MD virus. Foetuses that survive these intra-uterine infections usually have high titre virus in their blood at birth and no detectable neutralizing antibody.

These congenitally infected animals usually survive for up to 6-18 months of age exhibiting a chronic wasting syndrome and they provide foci of infection for susceptible young cattle.

Breeding ewes brought into contact with cattle chronically infected with MD virus become infected with the virus, but exhibit no clinical signs of infection. However, if the virus crosses the placenta, depending on the particular stage of gestation at which this occurs, the foetus may be aborted, born with a hairy birth coat and cerebral damage, or be born as a weak lamb that fails to thrive. Hence, pregnant ewes should not run with young cattle, particularly if there are some "poor-doers" among these and showing the chronic wasting syndrome associated with MD infection. The congenitally infected lambs shed virus from the nose and throat and should be destroyed as soon as possible.

The similarities between chronic MD infections in cattle and sheep, and the congenital rubella syndrome in human beings have been noted and provide an interesting piece of comparative virology, pathology and medicine.

Swine fever (Hog Cholera)

This disease has occurred wherever pigs are raised in South-East Asia. It is caused by a *Pestivirus* which shares a common group antigen with the MD virus detectable by gel-diffusion or complement fixation. There is also some evidence that infection of pigs (asymptomatic) with MD virus protects them from virulent swine fever (SF) virus. The disease is spread by direct contact, or indirectly by contaminated feed, fomites or environment. The classical disease presents as an acute infection with a high temperature, reddening of the skin, diarrhoea with, in 90% of cases, death in 3-13 days. There is a low virulent form of the disease, with a much reduced mortality rate, but with intra-uterine infections giving rise to chronically infected piglets that are stunted and fail to thrive. Classical Swine fever must not be confused with African Swine fever which, although it produces a similar clinical and pathological picture, is caused by a medium sized DNA virus, whereas SF is caused by a small RNA virus.

The Arthropod-borne Virus Diseases Affecting Animals in S.E. Asia

1. *Bovine Ephemeral Fever.* This disease is caused by a *Vesiculovirus* of the *Rhabdoviridae* family. In Australia it is endemic in the far north, tropical area of the country, and epizootics occur from time to time when climatic and other environmental conditions bring about the spread south of the presumed vectors, i.e. (*Culicoides* spp.) and possibly some mosquitoes, e.g. (*Culex annulirostris*). The disease is characterized by fever of short duration with stiffness in the joints and muscle pain. There is often a severe drop in milk supply of lactating cows, and bulls and fat cows are more severely affected than other cattle. There is only a

small mortality rate, usually associated with recumbency due to muscle pain and weakness followed by hypostatic pneumonia. This disease certainly has been recognized in cattle and buffalo in Malaysia, but almost certainly it is present wherever suitable carrier animals and vectors of the disease are present in South-East Asia.

2. *Japanese encephilitis infection in horses and pigs.* These conditions are caused by the same Flavivirus that causes Japanese B encephalitis in man in various parts of South-East Asia. The main recognized vectors are *Culex tritaeniorhynchus* and *C. gelidus*. In horses there is fever and clinical signs of encephalitis. The reaction may be peracute, acute, or subacute with the mortality rate usually being less than 25%. In pigs adult animals show no clinical evidence of infection, but pregnant sows may abort or produce mummified foetuses, still born, or weak piglets at term. Piglets up to six months of age that are naturally infected show encephalitis, sudden death, or a short syndrome of fever, ataxia, tremor, leading to coma and death or to recovery. The infected pig has a high titre viraemia following infection, and consequently is a potent source of virus to infect the arthropod-borne vectors which in turn carry the virus to other susceptible hosts including man and horses.

The prophylactic vaccination of horses at risk is recommended using a tissue culture grown, inactivated vaccine. This vaccine has not been very successful in the prevention of still-births in sows, and attempts are being made to develop a safe, live vaccine for use in pigs.

3. *Bluetongue.* Bluetongue is a non-contagious disease of sheep caused by an *Orbivirus* of the family *Reoviridae* that is carried by *Culicoides* spp. Cattle, goats, camels and deer can be infected but rarely show overt clinical signs of infection. These are the reservoir hosts, while sheep are the definitive hosts, but there are breed differences, e.g. indigenous African sheep rarely show any clinical signs of disease but can be infected with antibody production. Bluetongue has been recognized in Africa since 1905, Cyprus (1924), Turkey (1944), Israel (1951), USA (1952) Iberian Peninsula (1956), Pakistan (1960) and India (1964). The isolation of type 20 from captured field insects in Australia in 1975 was the first isolation of the virus in the Southern Hemisphere.

There are at least 20 serological types of this double-stranded RNA virus which all share a common group antigen detectable by gel-diffusion, complement fixation and immunofluorescence tests. There is great variation in the virulence of the different types and strains of the virus. In Australia, despite the isolation of at least three serological types of bluetongue virus from insects or cattle, no overt disease has been seen in either cattle or sheep. This may be related to the distribution of vectors of the virus in relation to the distribution of sheep and cattle in Australia. This disease has a fascinating and complicated natural history which is only now beginning to be understood by research workers in Australia, the USA and Africa. The factors involved include the ecology of the various vectors, the interaction of various host animals, and selective pressures on antigenic and virulence variations in the viruses.

4. *Ibaraki virus.* Ibaraki virus, which causes a bluetongue -like disease of cattle in Japan, has been shown to be closely related, if not identical, to the Alberta strain of the virus causing enzootic haemorrhagic disease of deer in the USA. This virus was first isolated from infected cattle in Japan and a similar virus has recently been isolated from the blood of a healthy cow in the Northern Territory of Australia. The isolation was made in the course of routine collections of blood for virus isolations, and not because of any overt disease problem. There is a strong likelihood that, if similar investigations were undertaken in other parts of South-East Asia to the immediate north of Australia, Ibaraki virus would be isolated, since antibody to this virus has been detected in cattle blood collected in Indonesia and Taiwan.

5. *Akabane and related simbu serogroup bunyaviruses.* These viruses, some of which have been shown to be associated with severe outbreaks of congenital malformations (e.g. arthrogryposis and hydranencephaly) will be dealt with in the paper by Dr. I.M. Parsonson and his colleagues later today. Again ecological factors play an important part in the epizootiology of these viruses and it is becoming clear that these viruses may well be more widely distributed than is realized.

Other Recognized Virus Diseases of Livestock

1. Aujesky's disease which is caused by a porcine herpesvirus is known to be present in parts of South-East

Asia principally in pigs, but cattle and rodents can be infected with this virus.

2. Bovine rhinotracheitis is caused by a bovine herpes virus and is very likely present over most of South-East Asia wherever European type cattle have been introduced.

3. Parainfluenza type 3, adenovirus, reovirus and syncytial virus infections of cattle and sheep are likely to be present and these viruses await laboratory isolation and identification.

4. Sheep Pox, Goat Pox and Contagious Pustular Dermatitis (CPD) are infections caused by poxviruses that have been described in India for Sheep Pox and Goat Pox, and in South-East Asia for CPD. These diseases can be controlled by vaccination programmes using live virus vaccines.

Jembrana Disease

This is a rinderpest-like disease of cattle and buffaloes first recognized in the Jembrana district of Bali, Indonesia. An estimated 60,000 animals, including domesticated bantengs, buffaloes and cattle were killed by this disease over a three year period. There is an apparent age-related, innate resistance, in that animals over two years of age rarely die of the disease. The aetiology of this disease is uncertain, but the available evidence points to the implication of an, as yet, unidentified rickettsia. The disease, and its clinical pathology, resembles somewhat the tick-borne fevers of Africa and elsewhere (Ondiri disease of East Africa caused by *Ehrlichia [Cytoecets] ondiri*, and benign tick-borne fever caused by *Ehrlichia phagocytophilia)*. The study of this disease presents a challenge to both local and consultant virologists and pathologists in Indonesia.

Avian Virus Diseases

Poultry-raising, both in village and more intensive systems, is practised in most of South-East Asia. Poultry provides an additional protein source, both as poultry meat and as eggs. Mainly ducks and chickens are raised, and practically the whole known range of avian virus diseases have been recognized in poultry in South-East Asia.

Newcastle disease and avian influenza have been actively studied in these areas and control of these diseases by vaccination has been practised extensively.

CONCLUSION

There is a need to upgrade both the genetic quality of the flocks in most places as well as the animal husbandry and disease control programmes to improve the productivity of the important sources of animal protein.

There can be little doubt that the control of infectious diseases of livestock generally, and virus diseases in particular, could improve the standard of living of people in most parts of South-East Asia and the Western Pacific.

Australia and Australian scientists, through programmes organized by the Australian Development Assistance Bureau, and financed by the Australian Government, have been contributing for some years to these objectives. A substantial proportion of this aid has been directed towards food and agricultural needs of the developing countries of South-East Asia. The recently established Australian Centre for International Agricultural Research contracts with Australian institutions to undertake research in agricultural science and animal health and disease in South-East Asia.

Whatever the immediate problems (and there are many) that need attention, in the long run it will be an understanding of the ecological and natural history aspects of infectious diseases of both animals and man that will pave the way for improved standards of living and well-being of our friends and neighbours in South-East Asia and the Western Pacific. Perhaps our deliberations in this symposium may kindle a light to show the way to this objective.

91

TOWARDS A GENETICALLY ENGINEERED FOOT-AND-MOUTH DISEASE VACCINE

Fred Brown

Animal Virus Research Institute,
Pirbright, Woking, Surrey, U.K.

I. THE DISEASE

Foot-and-mouth disease is the most economically important virus disease of farm animals. Cattle, pigs, sheep and goats are susceptible and the loss of productivity following infection, which is usually estimated at 25%, makes it a disease of major importance. The problem is worldwide and no country can be considered safe because of the ease with which the disease can spread. Countries such as Australia, Japan, New Zealand, North America and the United Kingdom, which are free from the disease, owe this position to their geographical isolation, the application of strict quarantine measures and the restriction of imports. In those countries where the disease does not normally occur, animals that become infected are slaughtered. This 'stamping out' policy is favoured in those countries because it is cheaper than vaccination and also because it reduces the chances of a carrier state being established.

II. CONTROL BY VACCINATION

Countries where the disease is endemic attempt to control it by vaccination. This has been highly successful in Europe but less so in other parts of the world. For effective vaccination there are several problems to be overcome. In the first place, the virus exists as seven distinct sero-

VIRAL DISEASES IN SOUTH-EAST ASIA
AND THE WESTERN PACIFIC
ISBN 0 12 484820 6

types, O, A, C, Southern African Territories types SAT1, SAT2 and SAT3, and Asia 1. The antigenic difference between them is such that an animal which has recovered from infection with a virus of one serotype is still fully susceptible to the other serotypes, although it is immune to re-infection with virus strains of the same serotype. Sub-types also exist within each serotype; in practical terms the result of this variation is that, when the level of immunity is low, such as exists, for example, several months after vaccination, infection with virus from another sub-type can occur although protection would be afforded against the homologous virus. This means that not only must vaccines against all seven serotypes be available but in addition there is often the need for vaccines against antigenic variants within an individual serotype.

Secondly, the virus to be used for vaccine production must be capable of growing to high enough titre, preferably in tissue culture cells, to provide sufficient antigenic mass to ensure that immunity is achieved when the inactivated preparation is inoculated. This can usually be achieved with most virus strains but several examples are known where it has been impossible to obtain sufficient antigenic mass for effective vaccine production.

A third problem arises with some virus strains which, although growing to sufficiently high titre, do not afford protection after inoculation of the inactivated preparation. Early work by Brown and his colleagues (5,6) had shown that the major immunizing antigen in virus preparations was located on the 146S intact virus particle. The 12S particles and the empty 75S particles had less than 1% of the activity of the 146S particles. Subsequent work by Rowlands, Sangar and Brown (13) showed that by preserving the integrity of the 146S particles by fixation with formaldehyde, the immunizing activity of a 'poor vaccine strain' could be improved 50 fold. Similar observations with the empty particles (14,15) led to the conclusion that the low activity of these particles was due to their instability after inoculation.

III. NATURE OF THE ANTIGEN PRODUCING NEUTRALIZING ANTIBODY

The most important observation regarding the antigenic activity of the 146S particle came from experiments with trypsin. It had been known for several years (4) that trypsin decreased the infectivity of the virus and work by

Wild and Brown (18) showed that the immunizing activity was also severely reduced. The enzyme treated particles did not form complexes with IgM antibody. However, the morphology of the treated particles was indistinguishable from that of the untreated virus although the surface charge was altered. Further analysis of the alterations taking place on the virus particle required a more detailed examination of its structure and composition. The virus particle is spherical, with a diameter of 25nm. It contains one molecule of a single-stranded RNA, mol. wt. c. 2.6 x 10^6 and four major polypeptides VP1, VP2, VP3 and VP4. There are 60 copies of each of these polypeptides and their mol. wt. are c. 24,000 for VP1, VP2 and VP3(3) and c. 10,000 for VP4. Polyacrylamide gel electrophoresis showed that only VP1 was affected when the virus particles were treated with trypsin (19) suggesting that this polypeptide has an important role in eliciting the immune response. This supposition was supported by the important observation of Laporte and his colleagues in 1973, which was later confirmed by several other groups, that VP1 isolated from virus particles also has immunizing activity (1,8,12).

The level of activity of the isolated VP1 is very low compared with that of the intact virus particle. The implication of this observation is that the configuration of the protein is of major importance in determining its immunogenicity.

The low immunizing activity of the 12S protein sub-unit, which is a pentamer consisting of 5 copies of each of the three polypeptides VP1, VP2 and VP3, lends support to the concept that the configuration of VP1 is of considerable importance in determining its immunizing activity.

IV. GENETIC ENGINEERING OF A VACCINE

Despite the low immunizing activity of VP1, several groups of workers in Europe and the U.S.A. are investigating the possibility of producing the protein by recombinant DNA technology (2,9,10). Progress in this field has depended on a knowledge of the location of VP1 on the genome and this has been provided by the biochemical mapping experiments described during the last five years (7,16).

The genome of the virus has a polyadenylic acid tract containing about 50-100 residues at the 3' end of the molecule and a polycytidylic acid tract, containing 100-250 residues depending on the particular isolate, about 400

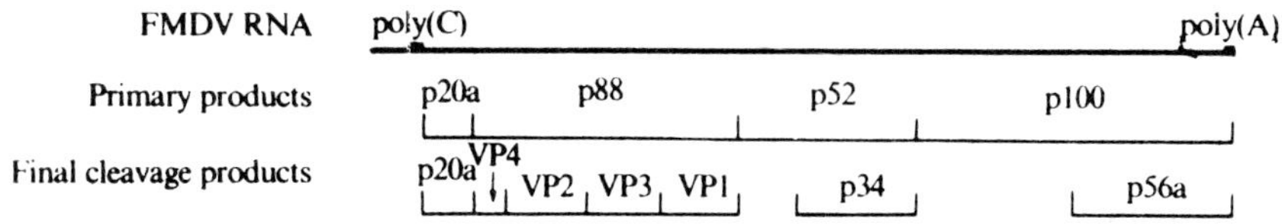

FIGURE 1. Biochemical map of foot-and-mouth disease virus. The immunizing polypeptide is associated with polypeptide VP1.

nucleotides from the 5' end (Figure 1). The 5' end of the RNA terminates in a uridylic acid residue linked covalently to the tyrosine residue of a protein, mol. wt. c. 4 x 10^3. The synthesis of the virus proteins proceeds by uninterrupted translation of the genome, starting at the 3' side of the polycytidylic acid residue (17), and the polyprotein thus produced is then processed by a series of proteolytic cleavages (Figure 1). The first series of cleavages, which give rise to the primary products, are probably mediated by host cell enzymes whereas the subsequent cleavages of the primary products probably involve virus-specified enzymes.

Mapping of the gene products has been greatly facilitated by the presence of a single ribosome binding site near the 5' end of the genome. Consequently interruption of ribosome initiation with pactamycin followed by labelling of the induced proteins with radioactive amino acids and measurement of the specific radioactivity of the separated proteins has allowed the positions of their coding regions on the genome to be determined (Figure 1).

The structural proteins are derived from P88 and polypeptide VP1 is located about 2,500-3,500 nucleotides from the 5'-end of the genome. Using oligo (dT) as primer, DNA molecules complementary to different regions of the virus genome have been synthesised by the use of reverse transcriptase and then converted to double stranded molecules. The DNA molecules corresponding to the regions of the virus RNA coding for the immunizing polypeptide have been inserted into expression vectors and the protein has been obtained in high yields. The work of the Genentech-Plum Island group has shown that 1-2 x 10^6 copies of the immunizing polypeptide can be produced per bacterial cell (9). However, the biological activity of this engineered protein is no higher than that of VP1 isolated from virus particles. Although it is possible to protect animals by two inoculations, each of 140 μg of the expressed protein, protection can be afforded by a single inoculation of 1-5 μg of inactivated virus particles. This great difference in biological activity leads me to the conclusion that the activity of the genetically engineered protein must be increased by several orders of magnitude before it can be regarded as a potential commercial product. Experiments are in progress to determine whether the configuration of the expressed protein can be manipulated to provide greater immunogenicity.

ACKNOWLEDGMENTS

The work described in this paper was largely performed by many past and present colleagues in the Biochemistry Department at Pirbright. Their names appear in the reference list and I am grateful to them for their contributions to the molecular biology of foot-and-mouth disease virus. I hope the paper provides a good example of the amount of background information required before genetic engineering of a virus component can be contemplated and undertaken.

REFERENCES

1. Bachrach, H.L., Moore, D.M., McKercher, P.D., and Polatnick, J., *J. Immunol. 115,* 1636 (1975).
2. Boothroyd, J.C., Highfield, P.E., Cross, G.A.M., Rowlands, D.J., Lowe, P.A., Brown, F., and Harris, T.J.R., *Nature 290,* 800 (1981).
3. Boothroyd, J.C., Harris, T.J.R., Rowlands, D.J., and Lowe, P.A., *Cell,* In press (1982).
4. Brown, F., Cartwright, B., and Stewart, D.L., *J. Gen. Micro. 31,* 179 (1963).
5. Brown, F., and Crick, J., *J. Immunol. 82,* 444 (1959).
6. Brown, F., and Newman, J.F.E., *J. Hyg. 61,* 345 (1963).
7. Doel, T.R., Sangar, D.V., Rowlands, D.J., and Brown, F., *J. Gen. Virol. 41,* 395 (1978).
8. Kaaden, O.R., Adam, K.-H., and Strohmaier, K., *J. Gen. Virol. 34,* 397 (1977).
9. Kleid, D.G., Yansura, D., Small, B., Dowbenko, D., Moore, D.M., Grubman, M.J., McKercher, P.D., Morgan, D.O., Robertson, B.H., and Bachrach, H.L., *Science 214,* 1125 (1981).

10. Küpper, H., Keller, W., Kurz, C., Forss, S., Schaller, H., Franze, R., Strohmaier, K., Marquardt, O., Zaslavsky, V.G., and Hofschneider, P.H., *Nature 289,* 555 (1981).
11. Laporte, J., Grosclaude, J., Wantyghem, J., Serge, B., and Rouze, P., *C.R. Acad. Sci. Paris 276,* 3399 (1973).
12. Meloen, R.H., Rowlands, D.J., and Brown, F., *J. Gen. Virol. 45,* 761 (1980).
13. Rowlands, D.J., Sangar, D.V., and Brown, F., *Arch. ges. Virusforsch. 39,* 274 (1972).
14. Rowlands, D.J., Sangar, D.V., and Brown, F., *J. Gen. Virol. 26,* 227 (1975).
15. Rweyemamu, M.M., Terry, G., and Pay, T.W.F., *Arch. Virol. 59,* 69 (1979).
16. Sangar, D.V., Black, D.N., Rowlands, D.J., and Brown, F., *J. Gen. Virol. 35,* 281 (1977).
17. Sangar, D.V., Black, D.N., Rowlands, D.J., Harris, T.J.R., and Brown, F., *J. Virol. 33,* 59 (1980).
18. Wild, T.F., and Brown, F., *J. Gen. Virol. 1,* 247 (1967).
19. Wild, T.F., Burroughs, J.N., and Brown, F., *J. Gen. Virol. 4,* 313 (1969).

92

FOOT AND MOUTH DISEASE VACCINE PRODUCTION IN INDONESIA

H.M. Geysen

Commonwealth Serum Laboratories
Parkville, Melbourne

As a result of the importation of dairy cattle, Foot and Mouth Disease (FMD) virus was introduced into Indonesia by the Dutch in 1887 at Malang, a town in eastern Java. Once introduced the disease spread rapidly east and west, and in the next two years had spread to the western end of the island of Java. By 1911 FMD was endemic in the central most populated islands of Java, Madura, Bali and Lombok. Documentation about the severity of the disease for the period up until the 1950's is sparse, but indicates that regular outbreaks continued to occur throughout this time. In 1956, the FAO funded a project to establish an FMD vaccine production facility at Surabaya, east Java. A new laboratory was constructed and equipped to produce vaccine by the Frenkel method, i.e., virus production in freshly collected tongue tissue. This project failed to produce significant quantities of vaccine, and the laboratory fell into disuse.

During the middle 70's, a time when the incidence of FMD was on the increase, Australia undertook to provide aid to Indonesia under the Colombo Plan agreement as follows:

(1) To provide for the immediate establishment of a vaccination programme by the purchase of vaccine from the U.K., and by the provision of the necessary equipment for its transport to, and use in the field.

(2) To refurbish the original FAO project building, and provide the equipment and facilities for FMD vaccine production by virus culture in BHK suspension cells, the so-called simplified process as developed at the Animal Virus Research Institute, Pirbright. This process was deemed to be the most suitable for implementation in Indonesia.

VIRAL DISEASES IN SOUTH-EAST ASIA
AND THE WESTERN PACIFIC
ISBN 0 12 484820 6

Vaccination of cattle was started in 1974/75, in Bali and the eastern end of Java with over one million doses. Coverage was increased in subsequent years, as the campaign moved to include central and east Java. The effect of this concerted effort was a rapid decrease in the incidence of the disease, with the last confirmed positive case of FMD occurring in late 1979 in south central Java. The rapid control of the disease by vaccination can be attributed to both the well-established veterinary service which exists in the central islands of Indonesia and the limited cattle movement associated with normal Indonesian animal husbandry.

With the completion of the laboratory in late 1979, commissioning of the vaccine production plant and associated equipment was begun. By the middle of the following year, it was producing trial batches of vaccine. By 1981, the total Indonesian requirement for the continuation of the vaccination campaign was being produced at Vetma, Surabaya.

While it is clear that the immediate implementation of the vaccination programme was extremely successful in controlling the disease, the success of the second phase of the project, namely the continued production of vaccine, is still to be determined. Direct external support of the production facility, both financial and in the form of aid-expert assistance, ceased at the end of 1981. Production of additional vaccine for at least two more years is required to complete the vaccination campaign in all areas. It is also intended that vaccine suitable for a strategic reserve will be produced, as well as possibly some vaccine for export to other countries in the ASEAN region.

Several speakers have in the past few days commented on the problems attending work in the biological field in developing countries. I would now like to identify and briefly comment on the difficulties experienced over the past two years of working in Indonesia to establish the FMD vaccine production facility described above:

(1) Maintenance and repair, particularly of specialised instruments, and the ready accessibility to spare parts, is a recurrent problem. That this will become worse is obvious, as more sophisticated machines are replacing the older manual versions faster than service facilities are being set up in developing countries.

(2) Access to specialised and routinely used chemicals, reagents, diagnostics and other biological materials, e.g., vaccine strains and cell lines, is difficult. Whilst it can be said that the delays experienced, and the often poor condition of biological materials on arrival, are in no small way due to inflexibility of bureaucracies which exist in

developing countries, Aid Agencies themselves slow the establishment of service and supply organisations in these parts of the world. The usual practice of Agencies to stipulate that where possible, aid project equipment and supplies should be purchased in the donor country does not encourage competition by equipment manufacturers or supply agencies to establish outlets or service facilities in these countries. It would seem to me to be much better in the long term to change this practice, and to stipulate that all purchases be made in the recipient country from manufacturers or suppliers who can demonstrate the necessary back-up capacity.

(3) Aid experts themselves may not be eminently suitable. The title suggests a group of people expert in the field of giving aid. Usually foreigners working in developing countries are chosen for a demonstrated ability in a project related field, rather than for the equally, or more important, demonstrated ability to transfer technology to, or work well with the local counterparts. Difficulties, particularly early on in aid programmes, could have been avoided if more attention had been paid to familiarisation of aid experts with the local language, social customs and relationships and the religious practices of the country of destination.

I should like to offer a final comment on the level of the technology which was deemed to be the most suitable for implementation in Indonesia to meet the aims of this particular aid project, namely FMD vaccine production. You have heard me describe the process as the simplified tissue culture method of production, basically a suspension culture virus production system performed in 10 litre bottles. While this is very easy to establish, and possibly consistent with the current level of technology, it is also very limited in potential for scale-up, or conversion to more modern production techniques. What has been achieved in Indonesia can be compared to a similar project sponsored by the Japanese in Thailand, where the aim is to establish FMD vaccine production by the more up-to-date roller-bottle culture and large vessel fermentation methodology. While after four years of direct aid and assistance the Japanese are still not at the stage of winding-up the project, they will eventually leave behind a plant and technology equal to that found in the developed countries. In contrast, for the Indonesians to reach the same stage will require a long process of self development or a further aid project in the future.

93

ISOLATION OF RECOMBINANT BLUETONGUE VIRUSES AND THEIR GENETIC ANALYSES

Polly Roy
Kazuo Sugiyama[1]
Ellen Collisson
Durga Rao
Jay Kahlon

The University of Alabama in Birmingham
School of Public Health
Birmingham, Alabama

Bluetongue virus, the prototype virus of the genus orbivirus, has a genome consisting of ten, double-stranded (ds) RNA species coding for at least seven different polypeptides. Virus neutralization tests have identified some 20 serotypes of BTV, four of which (10, 11, 13 and 17) are endemic in the U.S. Since BTV genome is segmented the question is therefore whether the segments can be reassorted *in vitro* or *in vivo* (as evidenced by analyses of natural isolates). The electrophoretic separation of the ten genome segments of BTV is distinct, but the electrophoretic patterns are very similar between and within the serotypes. Therefore, we use olibonucleotide fingerprint analysis of the genomes for detailed analysis of closely related viruses (2,3).

To measure the *in vitro* reassortment capability of representatives of two serotypes of BTV, we have used a 1973 Idaho isolate of BTV-11 (BTV73-27S) and the U.S. 1953 prototype BTV-10 strain (BTV CA8) (2). These virions were chosen since electrophoretic mobilities of their RNA segments 5 and 10 are distinguishable (see Figure 1). Procedures used to produce and recover reassortant virions by dual, wild-type virus infections have already been established (1,4). One

[1]*Present address: Hirosaki, Japan.*

VIRAL DISEASES IN SOUTH-EAST ASIA AND THE WESTERN PACIFIC
ISBN 0 12 484820 6

hundred cloned progeny virus stocks were grown in the presence of ^{32}P and viral RNA extracted from infected cells as described previously (2,3). The purified extracts of double-stranded RNA were resolved and compared with two parental virions in polyacrylamide gel electrophoresis as described previously (2,3). As shown in Figure 1, progeny reassortant virions were identified by this technique due to the segregation of the parental two RNA species (#5, #10). Approximately ten such reassortant progeny virions were screened by this procedure. Since this procedure does not really define the origin of their RNA segments, we have analyzed the oligonucleotide fingerprints of individual RNA segments of putative reassortant and compared each pattern with corresponding fingerprint patterns of two parental virus genomes. As shown in Figure 1A, it was found that for one such reassortant all the RNA segments were derived from BTV-10 other than segment #5; RNA segement #5 alone originated from BTV-11 (data not shown). Reassortant virions can be used to determine the coding assignments of the viral RNA

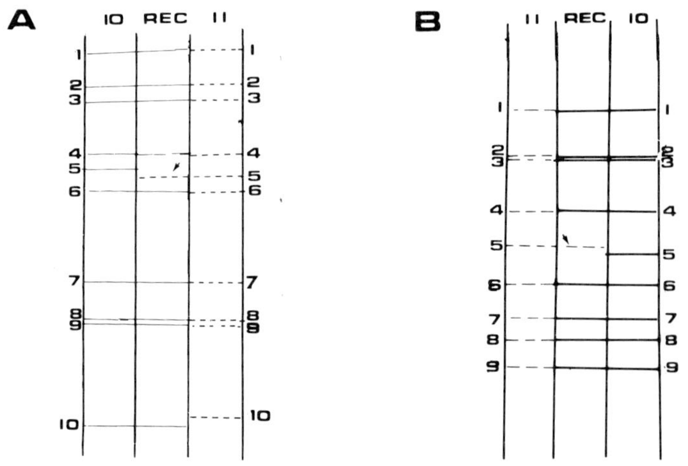

FIGURE 1. Diagrammatic resolution of the viral RNA (A) and proteins (B) of a progeny reassortant virus and the two-parent virus BTV-10 and BTV in PAGE. The RNA (A) and proteint (B) species are identified by numbers in order of increasing mobility.

species, therefore, polypeptides induced in cells infected with the reassortant BTV virions, as well as those of the two parental virions, were analyzed by polyacrylamide gel electrophoresis. Except for polypeptide 5, there were no detectable differences for the corresponding polypeptides of each of the three virions as shown in Figure 1B. Polypeptide 5 of BTV-10 exhibited a faster electrophoretic mobility by comparison to that of both BTV-11 and the reassortant virus. Since the only gene of the reassortant that was derived from BTV-11 virus was RNA segment #5, we conclude that it codes for the polypeptide designated 5 in Figure 1B. Each of these reassortants were serotyped and the above described reassortant was confirmed to be serotype 10 (not shown). We conclude from this study that the segment 5 gene product of the reassortant does not code for viral antigens recognized by the BTV specific antisera.

It has been shown previously by oligonucleotide fingerprint analyses that certain isolates of BTV (e.g., a BTV-11 isolate of Idaho) represents a naturally occurring intertyping reassortant virus (1). Although the RNA segment mobilities in gel electrophoresis are equivalent for both BTV-10, BTV-11 and the Idaho isolate of BTV-11, fingerprint patterns of each segment were distinct, indicating that each RNA species of BT virus contains unique RNA sequences. When each individual RNA species of serotype 10 was compared with the corresponding RNA species of prototype 11, some of the RNA species (e.g., 1, 4, 6 and 9) were sufficiently similar to be compared while by contrast segment 8 of two prototypes

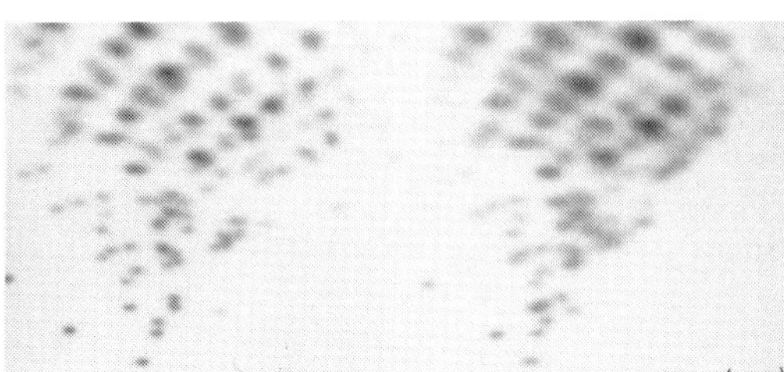

A B

FIGURE 2. Oligonucleotide fingerprints of Segment 1 of field isolate BTV-10 (A) and culicoides isolate of BTV-11 (B).

were almost identical. Similarly, when we compared fingerprints of the individual RNA species of an isolate BTV-11 (1973) with corresponding RNA segments of BTV-11 prototype, they were very similar except segment No. 3, which was completely dissimilar, but the variant being very similar to segment 3 of prototype 10 (not shown). We have recently fingerprinted the individual genome segments of a field isolate, isolated from a recent outbreak of BTV-10 in Washington State. The results indicated that some of the segments (2, 3, 5, 7 and 8) were closely related to prototype BTV-10 virus while some (e.g., #4, 9 and 10) were more comparable to prototype BTV-11. By contrast, segment 1 of this field isolate was almost identical to segment 1 of an isolate of BTV-11, isolated from culicoides, as shown in Figure 2. However, segment 6 of the isolate was observed to be unique when compared with corresponding segments of any of the U.S. BTV serotypes. It is evident that like *in vitro* system recombination involving RNA segment reassortment of BTV-10 and -11 demonstrated first *in vitro* system have also occurred in nature. The frequency with which such an event occurs depends upon the opportunity for simultaneous infection with genetically interactive viruses. Whether, and to what extent, other BTV serotypes present in the U.S. (BTV-13 and -17) can reassort with bluetongue virus serotypes not currently represented in the U.S. is not known. Nor is it known if other orbivirus also contribute to the bluetongue virus gene pool.

ACKNOWLEDGMENTS

This work was supported by a grant from the U.S. Department of Agriculture, grant CR 901-15-181. We would like to thank Dr. T.L. Barber and Dr. D.H.L. Bishop for their fruitful discussions.

REFERENCES

1. Gentsch, J., Wynne, L.R., Clewley, J.P., Shope, R.E., and Bishop, D.H.L., *J. Virol. 24,* 893 (1977).
2. Sugiyama, K., Bishop, D.H.L., and Roy, P., *Virology 114,* 210 (1981).

3. Sugiyama, K., Bishop, D.H.L., and Roy, P., *Amer. J. Epidemiol.*, In press (1982).
4. Walker, P.J., Mansbridge, J.N., and Gorman, B.M., *J. Virol. 34*, 583 (1980).

94

BLUETONGUE VIRUSES IN NORTHERN AUSTRALIA

A.J. Della-Porta
D.A. McPhee
I.M. Parsonson

CSIRO Division of Animal Health
Australian National Animal Health Laboratory
Geelong, Victoria

In 1975 bluetongue virus serotype 20 (BTV20; isolate CSIRO19) was isolated from a mixed pool of *Culicoides* spp. caught near Darwin (1). Subsequently, 2 further BTV serotypes were isolated from the blood of healthy cattle in Northern Australia: BTV 1 (CSIRO156) and CSIRO154 (not yet serotyped) (2). However no field cases of bluetongue disease have been reported in Australian cattle or sheep.

Studies of possible insect vectors revealed that *C.* (*Avaritia*) spp. No. 5 was efficient at transmitting virus but its range was limited to Northern Australia, whereas *C. brevitarsis* and other Culicoides were poor at transmitting virus (<1% of insects infected) but had a wider distribution in South East Asia and more temperate areas of Australia (3). Surveys revealed that BTV20 antibodies were restricted to cattle in the extreme north of Australia, whereas antibodies against other BTV group (agar gel diffusion precipitin - AGDP, and complement-fixing - CF) and serotype (neutralizing) antigens were present in cattle much further south. From recent surveys in South East Asia it would appear than many cattle in the region possess antibodies against BTV serotypes, especially BTV1 (4).

A number of Australian orbiviruses have been found to cross-react in serological tests with BTV. In particular, members in the epizootic haemorrhagic disease of deer-Ibaraki, Eubenangee and Palyam serogroups were most cross-reactive. These cross-reactions cause problems in interpretation of

VIRAL DISEASES IN SOUTH-EAST ASIA
AND THE WESTERN PACIFIC
ISBN 0 12 484820 6

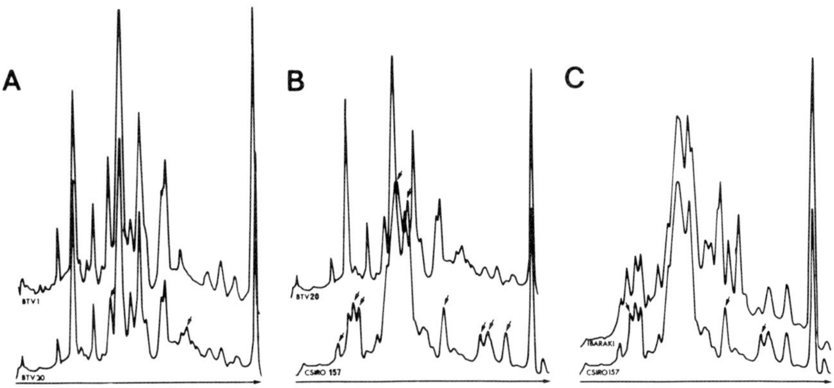

FIGURE 1. Densitometer tracings of autoradiographs from analysis of ^{35}S-methionine labelled orbivirus-infected cell protein profiles run in 10% SDS-Laemmli polyacrylamide gels. Differences in profiles arrowed. (A) BTV serogroup viruses, BTV1 and BTV20 (note similarities); (B) BTV20 and unknown CSIRO157 (note differences); and (C) Ibaraki and CSIRO157 (note similarities). In group serological tests (AGDP and CF), Ibaraki and CSIRO157 were indistinguishable and by neutralization tests they were distinct.

diagnostic tests and raise many questions about the origins and relationships of Australian orbiviruses. Other bio-chemical and immunochemical techniques, such as analysis of the virus-specified cytoplasmic proteins by polyacrylamide gel electrophoresis (figure 1), are being used to define these relationships.

REFERENCES

1. St. George, T.D., Standfast, H.A., Cybinski, D.H., Dyce, A.L., Muller, M.J., Doherty, R.L., Carley, J.G., Filippich, C. and Frazier, C.L. *Aust.Vet.J.*, *54*, 153, (1978).
2. Della-Porta, A.J., McPhee, D.A., Wark, M.C., St. George, T.D. and Cybinski, D.H. *Vet.Microbiol.*, *6*, 233, (1981).
3. Standfast, H.A., Dyce, A.L., St. George, T.D., Cybinski, D.H. and Muller, M.J. In: *Arbovirus Research in Australia*; Proc. 2nd Symp. (T.D. St. George and E.L. French, eds.) p.20. CSIRO Division of Animal Health and Queensland Institute of Medical Research, Brisbane, (1979).
4. Herniman, K.A.J., Gumm, I.D., Owen, L., Taylor, W.P. and Sellers, R.F. *Bull.Off.int.Epiz.*, *92*, 581, (1980).

95

PATHOGENESIS AND VIRULENCE STUDIES OF AUSTRALIAN SIMBU SEROGROUP BUNYAVIRUSES

I.M. Parsonson
A.J. Della-Porta
D.A. McPhee

Australian National Animal Health Laboratory
CSIRO Division of Animal Health
Geelong, Victoria

AKABANE VIRUS AND VIRULENCE STUDIES

Akabane (AKA) virus is known to cause sporadic epizootics of developmental deformities in cattle, sheep and goats (1). These epizootics have been observed in Australia, Japan, Israel and Turkey, with the presence of AKA virus being detected by serology in many South-East Asian countries, the Middle East and Africa. Epidemiological data, based on surveys for the presence of serum neutralizing (SN) antibodies, has helped define the distribution of seropositive cattle in Australia. This distribution was found to be similar to the ecological range of the probable insect vector, *Culicoides brevitarsis* (2). The virulence of AKA virus isolates and the effect of passage in laboratory systems and animals was studied (3). Experimental studies in pregnant sheep using different isolates of AKA virus with different passage histories, inoculated at a low multiplicity of infection (M.O.I. ; $10^{3.5}$ MLD_{50}/ewe), revealed striking differences in virulence. One isolate (CSIRO16 with mosquito/mouse passage) produced developmental defects in 100% of foetuses whereas the other two isolates (CSIRO16 cell culture passage and B8935 bovine/mouse passage) caused no foetal defects. AKA B8935 given at a high M.O.I. (10^6 MLD_{50}/ewe) had previously been shown to cause deformities in 31% of foetuses. Clones from the virulent pool (CSIRO16 mosquito/mouse) showed an apparently lower molecular weight

VIRAL DISEASES IN SOUTH-EAST ASIA AND THE WESTERN PACIFIC
ISBN 0 12 484820 6

G2 glycoprotein. The other AKA isolates, including 10 additional isolates made over an eleven year period, had protein profiles identical to AKAB8935. These studies suggested that the virion surface proteins (particularly G2) may be important in determining virulence.

PATHOGENICITY STUDIES OF OTHER AUSTRALIAN BUNYAVIRUSES

A number of the Australian Simbu serogroup bunyaviruses are known to produce SN antibodies in cattle and sheep and there is serological evidence that Aino virus may be a cause of congenital defects in cattle (4, 1, 5). AINO and Peaton (PEA) viruses have been isolated from *C. brevitarsis* and both have a similar antibody distribution in the cattle population to AKA virus (6). The Simbu serogroup viruses in Table 1 and the ungrouped Bunyaviridae member, Belmont virus, were assessed for their ability to produce deformities in the ovine foetus. Eight groups of eight ewes, pregnant 32 to 34 days, were inoculated intravenously with a 10% mouse brain suspension containing a high M.O.I. (>10^6PFU) of one of the viruses (Table 1). An additional group of eight pregnant ewes (controls) received a 10% suspension of uninfected mouse brain material. Clinical observations were carried out daily for 60 days after inoculation, up to slaughter when the ewes and the foetuses (90 days gestation) were examined. All the ewes remained clinically normal and the numbers in each group seroconverting are shown in Table 1. Ewes with foetuses with developmental abnormalities and SN antibody are shown in Table 1. Of the Simbu serogroup viruses Aino, Tinaroo, Douglas and CSIRO296 infected the ewes but did not cross the placenta to infect the foetus. Belmont virus did not appear to infect the ewes. AKA CSIRO16 and AKA B9835 produced similar percentages of abnormal foetuses as had previously been shown (7, 8), while the only other virus to cause developmental defects in one of twin foetuses was PEA. This is the first indication that this virus may be a cause of congenital defects. The AKA and PEA viruses elicited foetal IgG and SN antibody responses in the abnormal foetuses (Table 1). Twin foetuses from a ewe inoculated with CSIRO296 also developed IgG but had no SN antibodies to the virus. All foetuses produced IgM including the uninfected and control group and IgM may be produced to intrinsic antigenic stimuli (8). Neither IgG2 or IgA were detected in any foetal sera.

TABLE 1 Inoculation of Pregnant Ewes with Australian Bunyaviruses: Effect on the Foetus at 90 days Gestation

Inoculum		Ewes[a]		Foetuses		Number of foetal sera[b] with		
Virus	Isolate	No. Inoculated	No. with SN antibodies	Abnormal	Total	1gM	1gG1	SN antibodies
Aino	B7974	8	7	0	16	16	0	0
Akabane	B8935	8	8	5 (42%)	12	12	7	7
Akabane	CSIRO 16	8	8	10 (83%)	12	12	7	7[c]
Belmont	-	8	0	0	12	12	0	0
Douglas	CSIRO 150	8	8	0	11	11	0	0
Peaton	CSIRO 110	8	7	1 (17%)	14	14	1	1
Tinaroo	CSIRO 153	8	8	0	15	15	0	0
-	CSIRO 296	8	8	0	16	16	2	0
Controls	-	8	0	0	15	15	0	0

[a] Ewes inoculated intravenously at 32-34 days pregnant with 10^6 PFU of virus.

[b] We acknowledge the assistance of K.F. Fahey and P. McWaters for the foetal immunoglobulin estimations (8).

[c] Insufficient serum for testing for one foetus.
One serum positive by SN test.
One serum negative by both neutralization and immunoglobulin tests.

SUMMARY AND CONCLUSIONS

Both isolates of AKA virus (B8935 and CSIRO16) caused ovine foetal defects, but CSIRO16 was the more virulent causing deformities in 10 of 12 foetuses (83%), whereas B8935 caused deformities in 5 of 12 foetuses (42%). The presence of foetal IgG and SN antibodies to the virus responsible for deformities is of diagnostic importance. Peaton virus caused developmental defects in one twin foetus, the other foetus appeared grossly normal. This finding needs further experimental confirmation. The results of these experiments indicate that of the Australian Simbu serogroup viruses, AKA is the most important cause of developmental defects in sheep, however PEA and possibly other members may also be responsible for some losses in nature. There are a number of other Simbu serogroup bunyaviruses found in South-East Asia including Ingwavuma, Kailakur, and Sathuperi and the involvement of these and other viruses in producing congenital defects in domestic animals and in man has yet to be assessed (1). AKA virus produces no clinical signs of infection in the mother but its effects on the progeny including severe brain lesions and limb deformities can be most dramatic. The role of viruses as teratogens may be difficult to define but it is becoming evident that it is an explanation of many congenital defects which have previously been in search of a cause.

REFERENCES

1. Porterfield, J.S. and Della-Porta, A.J. (1981). *In "Comparative Diagnosis of Viral Diseases"* Vol. 4. (E. Kurstak and C. Kurstak, eds), p.479. Academic Press, New York.
2. Della-Porta, A.J., Murray, M.D. and Cybinski, D.H. (1976). *Aust.vet.J. 52,* 496.
3. Della-Porta, A.J., Parsonson, I.M., McPhee, D.A., Snowdon, W.A., Standfast, H.A., St. George, T.D. and Cybinski, D.H. (1981). *In "The Replication of Negative Strand Viruses"* (D.H.L. Bishop and R.W. Compans, eds.), p. 103. Elsevier/North-Holland, New York.
4. Bishop, D.H.L. and Shope, R.E. (1979). *Compr.Virol. 14,* 1.
5. Coverdale, O.R., Cybinski, D.H. and St. George, T.D. (1978). *Aust.vet.J. 54,* 151.
6. Cybinski, D.H. and St. George, T.D. (1978). *Aust.vet.J. 54,* 371.
7. Parsonson, I.M., Della-Porta, A.J., and Snowdon, W.A. (1977). *Infect.Immun. 15,* 254.
8. Parsonson, I.M., Della-Porta, A.J., O'Halloran, M.L., Snowdon, W.A., Fahey, K.J., and Standfast, H.A. (1981) *Vet.Microbiol. 6,* 197.

THE USE OF AUSTRALIAN STRAINS OF NEWCASTLE DISEASE VIRUS AS VACCINES[1]

P.B. Spradbrow

Department of Veterinary Pathology and Public Health,
University of Queensland
Brisbane

Clinical Newcastle disease does not occur in Australian poultry. None of the recognised velogenic, mesogenic or lentogenic strains is present and strict quarantine regulations forbid the introduction of such strains for experimental infections or for use as vaccines. However strains of Newcastle disease virus have been isolated in Australia. These viruses, which appear to cause no disease in chickens when they spread naturally, probably differ from lentogenic strains of Newcastle disease virus and might be better regarded as avirulent Newcastle disease viruses. The Australian poultry industry is interested in preparing for the possible introduction of pathogenic strains of Newcastle disease into Australia and the vaccine potential of the endemic, avirulent virus was investigated. Some aspects of these investigations, which would not have been possible without the excellent cooperation of colleagues in Malaysia, are discussed in the present paper.

The first of the avirulent Australian viruses, designated strain V_4 (or strain Queensland in some overseas literature) was isolated by Simmons in 1967 (3). Most studies have been undertaken with the V_4 strain although many other avirulent strains of Newcastle disease virus are now available in Australia. The Australian strains vary in some biological characters - heat stability of the haemagglutinin, haemagglutination and elution patterns,

1. *These studies were supported by grants from the Australian Chicken Meat Research Committee.*

VIRAL DISEASES IN SOUTH-EAST ASIA
AND THE WESTERN PACIFIC
ISBN 0 12 484820 6

ability to spread between infected chickens - but none has been shown to cause natural disease and all have low experimental pathogenicity. Kim and Spradbrow found that the V_4 strain produced insufficient mortality on inoculation of chicken embryos by the allantoic route to allow calculation of a mean death time, that the haemagglutinin was stable at 56°C and that the elution time at 4°C exceeded 96 hours (2). Strain V_4 had an intracerebral pathogenicity index of about 1.0 but mortalities were associated with hepatic lesions and not with neural lesions.

The vaccination experiments undertaken in Australia with Australian strains of Newcastle disease virus have been extensively reviewed (6). Challenge experiments have not been possible and the response to vaccination has been judged by the production of specific antibodies, usually measured by haemagglutinin-inhibition test. Chickens respond with the production of haemagglutinination -inhibition antibodies when vaccinated by several routes including application by aerosol and through the drinking water. No disease attributable to the vaccine virus has been reported and the V_4 strain spreads rapidly from vaccinated chickens to unvaccinated chickens placed in contact with them.

Some challenge experiments have been conducted in the U.S.A. and the U.K., using vaccines prepared from Australian strains of Newcastle disease virus. These have given promising results but the experimental chickens were bred in the host laboratories. Australian commercial chickens have not been selected, artificially or naturally, for resistance to Newcastle disease nor for responsiveness to Newcastle disease vaccines and they are the preferred experimental bird for such studies. Therefore arrangements were made to transport Australian poultry to the Veterinary School, Universiti Pertanian Malaysia and to conduct collaborative trials there.

The first Malaysian trial (4) involved one-day-old chickens that were air freighted to Malaysia and vaccinated orotracheally when two or three weeks of age with the V_4 strain of Newcastle disease virus. The vaccine virus was allowed to spread to other groups of chickens by direct or indirect contact. The chickens were challenged with a virulent strain of Newcastle disease virus when four weeks of age. Some chickens were infected by intra-muscular injection of the challenge virus and some by orotracheal instillation but most were challenged by contact. Only two of 150 vaccinated chickens died of Newcastle disease. There were no deaths in a group of

45 chickens to which the vaccine spread by direct contact and six of 43 chickens vaccinated by indirect contact died after challenge. All of 60 control chickens died when exposed to the virulent Newcastle disease virus. After challenge by contact, vaccinated chickens developed greatly enhanced levels of haemagglutination-inhibition antibody, indicating that there had been some replication in them of the challenge virus but insufficient to produce disease.

Further trials conducted in Malaysia on chickens bred in Malaysia or on chickens imported from Australia showed that other routes of vaccination were effective and that the period of protection following vaccination was several months (1).

Another question of interest to the Australian poultry industry was whether Australian poultry, acquiring antibodies as a result of natural infection with avirulent strains of Newcastle disease, would be resistant to infection with virulent strains of Newcastle disease virus. Breeders from flocks that had developed antibodies and broilers from flocks free of detectable antibodies to Newcastle disease virus were transported to Malaysia and challenged with virulent Newcastle disease virus. All of the 24 broilers died of Newcastle disease but only two of 68 breeders died. Virulent Newcastle disease virus was recovered from the two dead breeders and from a cloacal swab from one healthy breeder (5). Autopsy lesions typical of those expected with viscerotropic Newcastle disease were seen in the broilers but lesions were minimal in the breeders that died. It was not possible to record egg production in the breeders that were challenged but it was noted that eggs were produced throughout the experiment. The geometric mean titre of haemagglutination-inhibition antibody increased greatly in birds that survived challenge.

If poultry in Australian flocks reacted similarly to challenge with virulent Newcastle disease virus, flocks infected with avirulent virus similar to the V_4 strain might not suffer heavy mortalities and dead birds might not develop lesions typical of Newcastle disease. However birds would become infected with virulent virus and some would excrete virulent virus.

Thus the Australian poultry industry has gained valuable information as a result of these collaborative studies. The problems of diagnosing infection in partially protected flocks can be anticipated and the extreme susceptibility of unprotected chickens has been confirmed. The industry has been able to produce a stockpile of V_4 vaccine for possible use in the event of a serious outbreak of Newcastle disease. Because of the availability of this avirulent virus in Australia and because of the willing collaboration of colleagues in Malaysia, the poultry industry is better prepared than other animal industries to combat an important exotic disease.

ACKNOWLEDGMENTS

I am greatly indebted to Professor A. Mustaffa-Babjee and Dr. A.L. Ibrahim for providing facilities at the Universiti Pertanian Malaysia.

REFERENCES

1. Ibrahim, A.L., Chulan, U., and Mustaffa-Babjee, A., *Aust. vet. J. 57*, 277 (1981).
2. Kim, S.J., and Spradbrow, P.B., *Vet. Microbiol. 3*, 129 (1978).
3. Simmons, G.C. *Aust. vet. J. 43*, 29 (1967).
4. Spradbrow, P.B., Ibrahim, A.L., Mustaffa-Babjee, A. and Kim, S.J. *Avian Dis. 22*, 329 (1978).
5. Spradbrow, P.B., Ibrahim, A.L., Chulan, U., Millikin, G., Shapcott, R. and Kingston, D., *Aust. vet. J. 56*, 580 (1980).
6. Westbury, H.A. *Aust. vet. J. 57*, 292 (1981).

97

PARAMYXO- AND ORTHOMYXOVIRUSES OF POULTRY IN SOUTHEAST ASIA AND THEIR SIGNIFICANCE - A COMMENT

Kennedy F. Shortridge

Department of Microbiology
University of Hong Kong
Queen Mary Hospital Compound, Hong Kong

NEWCASTLE DISEASE

Disease attributable to orthomyxo- and paramyxoviruses almost exclusively concerns avian paramyxovirus type 1 (PMV-1) the causative agent of Newcastle disease (ND). Accurate statistics are not available, but the consensus of information indicates that ND is the most important of all poultry diseases in Southeast Asia. Considering that poultry meat is one of the main sources of protein in the diet of the people of the region, the significance of ND may be appreciated.

The disease is endemic. The factors that contribute to this situation are complex and poorly understood; two are noteworthy. Firstly, pathogenicity tests on avian PMV-1 isolates obtained in surveillance studies in Hong Kong on domestic poultry have shown that representative viruses from chickens are velogenic strains comparable with the most velogenic viruses isolated anywhere to date. However, in these studies, the isolates were derived from apparently healthy birds suggesting that local breeds may have an element of resistance to the virus. If this is so, then the outcome of the virus-host relationship may be dependent on a second factor, namely that poultry raising in the region is mainly carried out in "backyard farm" enterprises. Here, the poultry are subject to various kinds of stress, inadequate sanitary control and the lack of routine vaccination if it is practised at all. Under these conditions, the poultry are

VIRAL DISEASES IN SOUTH-EAST ASIA
AND THE WESTERN PACIFIC
ISBN 0 12 484820 6

readily exposed to other infected poultry and to wild birds which have been implicated in the spread of the disease. This situation arises in part from socioeconomic circumstances and the prevalence of backyard farms varies from area to area and country to country. There is now a trend in the region to more intensive units, a trend that is bound to increase. Although these units presently account for only a small percentage of poultry (chicken) production, the disease risk is, and will continue to be, unacceptably high in the face of ineffective vaccination programmes and the endemic occurrence of the disease.

The domestic duck is intensively raised in many parts of the region where there is suitable water and is probably the second most important type of poultry. In surveillance studies conducted on poultry originating from Hong Kong and southern China, ducks were found to have an incidence of avian PMV-1 slightly lower than that of chickens. As ducks generally do not appear to be adversely affected by the virus, the likelihood exists that they may be a major source of ND for chickens. The raising of ducks in or around the vicinity of chicken farms, particularly on small holdings, lends support to this view. Further, they may act as foci of infection for transmission by wild birds.

Geese, quail and pigeon are the other major poultry raised in the region but there is little evidence of their susceptibility to ND. The isolation rate of avian PMV-1 from apparently healthy geese was about half that from chickens; these poultry, too, may be a source of virus for chickens.

OTHER AVIAN PARAMYXOVIRUSES

The information on the occurrence of other avian PMVs in the region is sparse. Limited numbers of avian PMV-4 and -6 have been isolated from apparently healthy ducks and chickens. The pathogenicity indices of these isolates suggest that they have a low potential, if any, for causing disease. There is strong serological evidence for the occurrence of avian PMV-3 particularly in chickens; avian PMV-2 may also occur.

INFLUENZA VIRUSES

The information available on the influenza viruses of domestic poultry in the region stems mainly from the Hong Kong surveillance studies. The bulk of the isolations has been from ducks. As influenza viruses (like avian PMV-1) are faecally shed from the intestine into water, ducks would seem to be readily infected as a result of their aquatic preferences. The extensive waterways and innumerable ponds in the region support a large duck population with a high turnover for market. Consequently, the duck is able to act as a reservoir for a great range of influenza viruses. Infection appears to be asymptomatic; in the absence of information to the contrary, it seems unlikely that influenza is a problem in the region.

One interesting regional development has been the introduction of land based raising of ducks. Elsewhere, in the case of ducks raised on grass or stubble and of turkeys raised in the open, influenza viruses have assumed a hitherto unrecognised importance as disease producing entities in recent years. Although land based raising of ducks in the region is on a very small scale, it remains to be seen whether, in the absence of their exposure as ducklings to influenza viruses through contaminated water, such ducks will be subsequently susceptible to disease given the vast range of viruses in the region to which they might be exposed.

CONTROL

The major cause for concern in the poultry industry of Southeast Asia generally, lies in the lack of control of ND. Unless there is concerted effort at all levels of the industry, government and private, the prospects of bringing the disease under positive control are remote. The extension officer, acting as the link between veterinarian and farmer, has a cardinal role to play in disease prevention. There are simply not enough properly trained officers to cope with the situation, a difficulty that is compounded by the large number of small scale farmers. These farmers are not often easily accessible to the officers nor are they sufficiently informed to appreciate the value of routine vaccination programmes or the application of improved hygiene and management techniques.

In a region with a huge population that relies to a large extent on poultry meat for protein, the poultry industry is beset by many problems, notably ND. The establishment of an independent, regional diagnostic laboratory is seen as a positive approach to disease control. Such a centre might seek to:

(1) define the disease situation taking into account predisposing infections;
(2) characterise avian PMV-1 isolates, carry out ND vaccine potency testing and the production of reference antisera;
(3) be a training centre for veterinarians and extension officers alike;
(4) provide a regional network of information on all aspects of ND particularly vaccination and hygiene, other diseases and related aspects of poultry production.

While such a venture would require a capital input, the long-term benefits would be considerable. As there appears to be a deficiency in the training in avian medicine such a centre might be more appropriately located in conjunction with an established veterinary school. More substantial training in avian medicine is of paramount importance.

ACKNOWLEDGMENT

The surveillance studies which provided the background to aspects of this report were supported in part by Public Health Service Grants AI52524 and 02649 to K.F. Shortridge from the National Institute of Allergy and Infectious Diseases.

BIBLIOGRAPHY

1. Markwell, D.D., and Shortridge, K.F., *Applied and Environmental Microbiology 43,* 110 (1982).
2. Shortridge, K.F., Epidemiology of avian influenza and sources of infection in domestic species, *in* "Proceedings of the First International Symposium on Avian Influenza, April 22-24, 1981, Beltsville, Maryland", (R.A. Bankowski, ed.), pp.54-68. Carter Composition Corp., Richmond, Virginia, U.S.A. (1981).

3. Shortridge, K.F., Newcastle disease and its control in Southeast Asia, *in* "Proceedings of a UNESCO-sponsored Training Course and Workshop on Viral Vaccines in Poultry, July 27 - August 2, 1981, Hong Kong", (K.F. Shortridge, ed.), p.107. Hong Kong University Press, Hong Kong, (1982).

98

CANINE PARVOVIRUS IN AUSTRALIA

Margaret Sabine
Linda Herbert
Daria Love

Department of Veterinary Pathology
University of Sydney
N.S.W., Australia

The diseases canine parvovirus enteritis and myocarditis were first observed in Australia in September 1978 (1-3). The virus was first isolated from enteritis in Queensland (4) and from myocarditis in Western Australia (5). In a retrospective survey, antibody appeared for the first time in serum collected in N.S.W. in May, 1978 (6). A formalinized canine parvovirus vaccine was developed initially in 1979 (7) and such vaccines were manufactured by two companies in Australia. One vaccine was released for sale in July 1980.

This laboratory received a small but steady stream of specimens for viral diagnosis of both enteritis and myocarditis from October 1978 until mid-1980. On the release of a vaccine in Sydney publicity led to an increase in specimens but no increase in diagnoses of parvovirus. In October 1980 there was an explosive outbreak of canine parvovirus enteritis in Sydney with reports of serious outbreaks in some other places.

Because severe clinical manifestations of canine parvovirus infections have been difficult to reproduce experimentally, assessment of efficacy of vaccines has been a problem (7). In an attempt to determine the extent of morbidity and mortality due to canine parvovirus infections during 1980 as well as to evaluate vaccines, a questionnaire

VIRAL DISEASES IN SOUTH-EAST ASIA
AND THE WESTERN PACIFIC
ISBN 0 12 484820 6

was sent to all veterinary practitioners in Australia. Replies were received from 303 veterinary practices, an estimated 30% of the total.

The Questionnaire

The first part of the questionnaire was designed so that it could be completed readily by all veterinarians. The second part of the questionnaire asked for detailed information on numbers and age distribution of cases of enteritis with the vaccination history of the dogs concerned. There were overall 299 relevant replies, with 95 answering the second part. Numerical data were encoded and analysed by computer.

Analysis of Replies

Severe Outbreaks A severe outbreak was defined arbitrarily as one or more cases per day. While 4% of veterinarians had yet to see a single case of parvovirus enteritis 68% had experienced a severe outbreak. Some big practices recorded as many as 30 cases per day at the peak of an outbreak. On the east coast the disease appeared to spread from north to south beginning in September in North Queensland and finishing in Tasmania in December. However it was difficult to discern a pattern of spread over the whole continent.

Morbidity and Mortality 6824 cases of parvoviral enteritis were recorded with 1058 (16%) deaths. Table I gives the age distribution.

TABLE I. Age Distribution - Morbidity and Mortality

	Cases		Deaths	
Age	Number	% of Total	Number	% of age group
< 4 wks	127	2	93	73
4-16 wks	1749	26	481	28
17 wks-11 mths	2070	30	262	13
1-5 yrs	1762	26	148	8
> 5 yrs	1116	16	74	7
Total	6824	100	1058	16

TABLE II. Age Distribution of Cases in Vaccinated Dogs

Age	*Number*	*% of total*
< 4 wks	2	< 1
4-16 wks	206	45
17 wks-11 mths	158	34
1-5 yrs	84	18
> 5 yrs	12	3
Total	462	100

Cases in Vaccinated Dogs Over 230,000 dogs were vaccinated by the 265 respondents who supplied the figures. 462 of the 6824 cases of enteritis recorded occurred in dogs which had been vaccinated. The age distribution is given in Table II. It has now been established that maternal antibody against canine parvovirus may last for up to 16 weeks, which may have interfered with vaccination of pups under that age (8). When cases of disease occur within 14 days of vaccination veterinarians usually attribute them to infection either prior to vaccination or before sufficient time has elapsed to mount an adequate immune response. There were only 118 cases of disease, out of 6824 recorded, which occurred later than 14 days after vaccination in dogs older than 16 weeks. The vaccine appears to have been remarkably effective at least in the short term.

General Questions While unusual clinical features and reproductive failures were noted, on analysis the only significant finding was the observation of myocarditis. Correlation between onset of disease and visits to veterinary hospitals and clinics, dog shows and kennels was affirmed by 37% of respondents. Fluid replacement was the universally recommended therapy.

Canine Parvovirus in South-East Asia and the Western Pacific

While published reports of canine parvovirus in the area are as yet scanty, Australian canine parvovirus vaccines are exported to Hong Kong, Indonesia, Malaysia, New Caledonia, New Guinea, New Zealand, Singapore and Thailand.

REFERENCES

1. Kelly, R., *Australian Vet. J. 54*, 593 (1978)
2. Kelly, R. and Atwell, R.B., *Australian Vet. J. 55*, 37 (1979)
3. Huxtable, C.R., Howell, J. McC., Robinson, W.F., Wilcox, G.E. and Pass, D.A., *Australian Vet. J. 55*, 37 (1979)
4. Johnson, R.H. and Spradbrow, P.D., *Australian Vet. J. 55*, 151 (1979)
5. Robinson, W.F., Wilcox, G.E., Flower, R.L.P. and Smith, J.R., *Australian Vet. J. 55*, 294 (1979)
6. Walker, S.T., Feilen, C.P., Sabine, M., Love, D.N. and Jones, R.F., *Vet. Rec. 106*, 324 (1980)
7. Johnson, R.H. and Smith, J.R., *Australian Vet. Pract. 9*, 197 (1979)
8. Kramer, J.M., Meunier, P.C. and Pollock, R.V.H., *Vet. Med./Small Animal Clin. 75*, 1541 (1980).

99

CAPRINE SYNCYTIAL RETROVIRUS

V. W. Smith
W. Coackley
J. Dickson

Animal Health Laboratory
Department of Agriculture
South Perth, W. Australia

D. J. Houwers

Centraal Diergeneeskundig Instituut
Houtribweg, Lelystad, Holland

Robinson (1) described a chronic pneumonia associated with a granulomatous encephalitis in a goat in Western Australia and demonstrated that goats inoculated with tissue homogenates from the diseased goat developed antibodies to maedi-visna virus. The antibodies were demonstrated using an enzyme-linked immunosorbent assay (ELISA).

Coackley *et al.* (2) recorded the isolation of syncytial retroviruses from goats with progressive pneumonia or arthritis and Smith *et al.* (3) demonstrated that one of these viruses produced ELISA antibodies to maedi-visna virus when inoculated into goats but not in sheep.

It has been suggested that these viruses are essentially similar to viruses from cases of caprine leucoencephalomyelitis-arthritis (4) or the caprine arthritis-encephalitis syndrome (5). The latter viruses share a common antigen with maedi-visna virus but are claimed to be distinct antigenically.

VIRAL DISEASES IN SOUTH-EAST ASIA
AND THE WESTERN PACIFIC
ISBN 0 12 484820 6

Ten caprine viruses have been isolated in Western Australia by autoculture or explant culture of lung and synovial membrane or from leucocyte fractions sub-cultured onto synovial membrane monolayers prepared from healthy goats. These viruses produced syncytia and showed the characteristic morphology of members of the *Retroviridae* by electron microscopy.

Three groups of goats inoculated with any of three viruses have consistently developed ELISA antibodies to maedi-visna virus between 35 and 67 days following inoculation. A unilateral bursitis was the only common feature seen in the first group. No pathological changes were seen in the second group when they were killed nine and a half months after inoculation. The third group of goats is still under observation

Merino sheep inoculated with the same dose of one of the viruses remained serologically negative for 24 weeks.

Further investigations are in progress to determine whether these viruses can infect and produce disease in sheep.

REFERENCES

Robinson, W. F. *Aust. vet. J.* 57, 127 (1981)

Coackley, W., Smith, V. W., Maker, D. and Dickson, J. *Aust. vet. J.* 57. 480 (1981)

Smith, V. W., Dickson, J., Coackley, W. and Maker, D. *Aust. vet. J.* 57, 481 (1981)

Narayan, O., Clements, J. E., Strandberg, J. D., Cork, L. C. and Griffin, D.E. *J. gen. Virol.* 50, 69 (1980)

Crawford, T.B., Adams, D. S., Cheevers., W. F. and Cork, L. C. *Science.* 207, 997 (1980)

100

EQUINE HERPESVIRUS TYPE 1 (EHV1): DIFFERENTIATION OF RESPIRATORY AND FOETAL STRAINS USING PLAQUE SIZE, HOST CELL RANGE AND RESTRICTION ENDONUCLEASES

M. J. Studdert

School of Veterinary Science
University of Melbourne
Parkville, Victoria

From 1965 to 1977 EHV1 was regularly isolated from respiratory disease in young horses (R strains) in Australia, but not at all, until July 1977, from aborted equine foetuses (F strains). A comparison of 8 representative R strains with 11 F strains showed that, by plaque size in equine foetal kidney cells and host cell range R and F strains, with few exceptions, were distinguishable; R strains produced large plaques (≃1.5 mm diameter) and had a restricted host cell range whereas F strains produced small plaques (≃0.8 mm diameter) and had a wide host cell range (1).

Restriction endonuclease analysis of the DNA of 3 R strains and 6 F strains all of which were North American in origin, except 1 R strain which was isolated in Australia and 1 F strain which was isolated in Poland, showed that the patterns of R and F strains were entirely different. It was proposed that F and R strains be designated as separate species (= viruses) and called types 1 and 4 respectively (2).

We have now analysed, by restriction endonucleases, the DNA of 10 R strains and 34 F strains. All R strains produced a similar pattern which was entirely distinct from the pattern produced by 30 of the 34 F strains; 4 of the F strains produced R type patterns. These 4 exceptions were supposedly isolated from sporadic cf. epizootic abortion or abortion "storms".

VIRAL DISEASES IN SOUTH-EAST ASIA
AND THE WESTERN PACIFIC
ISBN 0 12 484820 6

Minor differences in the fingerprints of individual R and F viruses should allow specific identification of particular viruses associated with respiratory disease, abortion, perinatal mortality or encephalomyelitis as well as the monitoring of modified live virus vaccine strains.

REFERENCES

1. Studdert, M.J. and Blackney, M.H. *Aust. Vet. J. 55*, 488, (1979).
2. Studdert, M.J., Simpson, T. and Roizman, B. *Science 214*, 562 (1981).

101

BOVINE MUCOSAL DISEASE AND ITS FAMILIAL VIRUS.

Ian Littlejohns

N.S.W. Department of Agriculture,
Veterinary Research Station,
Glenfield, N.S.W. 2167

INTRODUCTION

1. The great majority of cattle infected by pestivirus develop no significant disease and a complete immune response occurs.

2. Persistent viraemic infection by the same virus is usually regarded as the cause of mucosal disease (MD). Antibody against the virus is minimal or not demonstrable. This may reflect immune tolerance from foetal infection.

3. Then, as a corollary, pre-clinical infections which persist from birth until disease develops, usually at 1-2 years of age, should be anticipated.

OBSERVATIONS

4. Clinically normal but persistently viraemic and overtly infective animals have been observed over many months during which many breed successfully. Unpredictably such animals may develop MD but ultimate death is not always attributable to MD.

5. Progeny are invariably viraemic and females may establish maternal viraemic families from which some individuals may similarly develop MD (Fig.1).

VIRAL DISEASES IN SOUTH-EAST ASIA
AND THE WESTERN PACIFIC
ISBN 0 12 484820 6

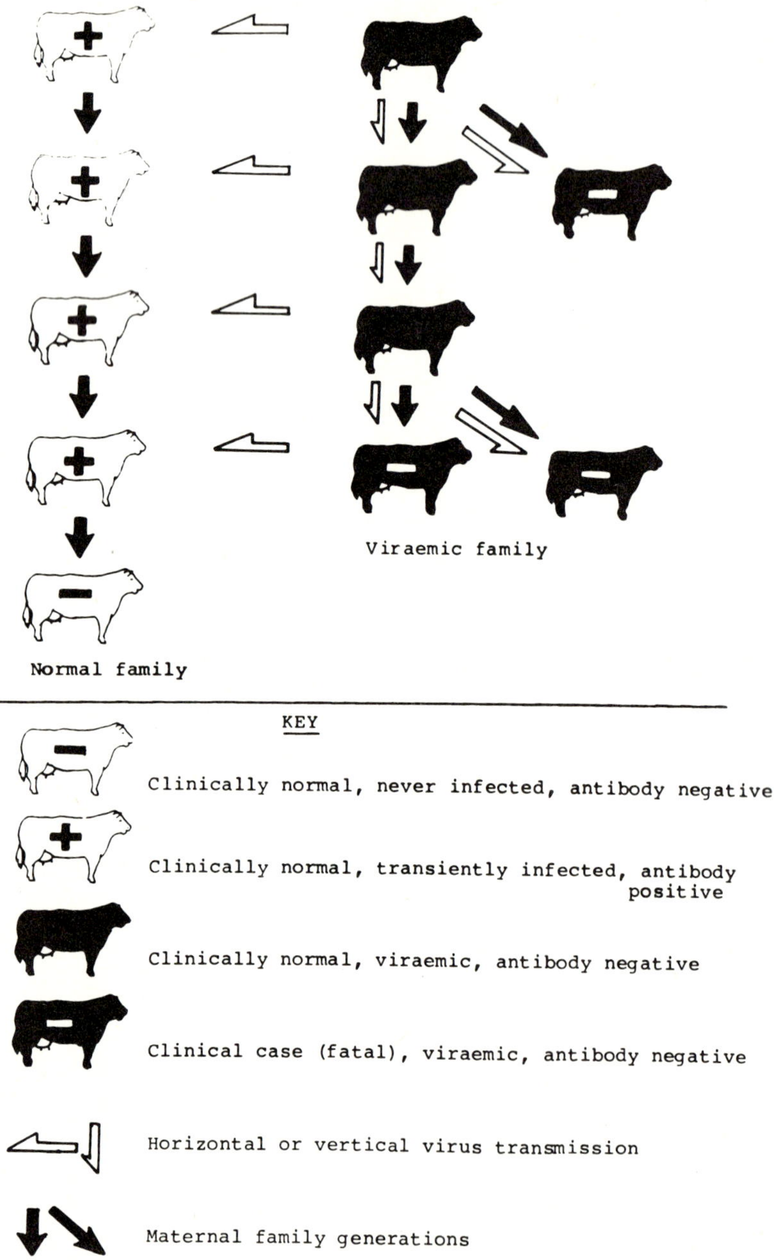

FIGURE 1. Enzootic familial distribution of mucosal disease.

6. A common epidemiological pattern of pestivirus infection and mucosal disease in a closed herd is for persistently infected maternal families to act as spreaders, infecting each generation of calves as they lose maternal antibody at 4-6 months of age (Fig. 1).

7. Consistent with these observations, a substantial proportion of dams of clinical cases of MD can be shown to be non-clinical viraemic carriers.

8. Paternal viraemic families may occur but are not proven. Virus may occur in the semen of infected bulls but the efficiency of transmission via semen is not known and may presumably be influenced by the immune status of the recipient cow.

9. Viraemic families tend to die out, either through classical MD or more subtle effects of the infection, so a mechanism for generating foundation members of new families must exist. Possibilities include providential infection of susceptible cows at a critical stage of pregnancy or genetic determination of immunological incompetence. In each case viraemia in subsequent generations may be guaranteed by mechanisms of immune tolerance.

10. Artificial breeding, either by artificial insemination or by embryo transfer after superovulation, presents opportunities to amplify the establishment of viraemic families, usually in valuable stock. Multiple cases in a litter resulting from embryo transfer have been demonstrated. In this context the high prevalence of pestivirus, and its thermal stability, in foetal calf serum deserves special attention.

CONCLUSION

The familial distribution of persistent pestivirus viraemia is relevant to consideration of the pathogenesis and epidemiology of mucosal disease in cattle. Immune tolerance and viraemia might be regarded as defining a sub-population of cattle within which mucosal disease occurs rather than as determining disease.

Artificial breeding techniques deserve special attention for their potential for introducing infection and disease susceptibility into elite families.

102

EMC VIRUS MYOCARDITIS IN PIGS

Ian Littlejohns

N.S.W. Dept. of Agriculture,
Veterinary Research Station,
Glenfield, N.S.W.

1. THE DISEASE

Disease in pigs due to encephaloymocarditis (EMC) virus infection is primarily a myocarditis. CNS lesions are minimal or absent. The myocarditis causes death due to heart failure, usually acute, in pigs from birth to 16 weeks with higher mortality rates in younger pigs. Virus has also been isolated from late abortions indicating that transplacental infection may occur.

The virus infection *per se* causes minimal malaise. After a brief viraemia it persists in tissues for about 10 days. The majority of deaths occur while infection persists but a substantial minority (~30%) result from residual heart disease when virus is no longer recoverable.

2. EPIDEMIOLOGY

Rodents, particularly rats, commonly carry the virus. They are assumed to be the source of virus infecting pigs but there is no direct proof of this. Pig to pig infection probably does not occur.

Geographically the disease in pigs is restricted. It is probably the major killer of young pigs on the north coast of N.S.W. but has never been diagnosed south of Sydney. There is no reason to believe that the virus in rodents is similarly restricted.

3. VIRUS STRAIN DIFFERENCES

EMC viruses are antigenically homogeneous but biologic-

VIRAL DISEASES IN SOUTH-EAST ASIA AND THE WESTERN PACIFIC
ISBN 0 12 484820 6

ally variable in many respects. Pathogenicity for pigs appears to be one of the variable biological properties.

Strains of pig (fatal disease) and rodent (enteric carrier) origin have been compared in experimental infections in pigs. Comparable doses of virus, as assayed in cell culture caused high mortality with the pig strain but none with the rodent strain. However in pigs sacrificed the gross cardiac lesions were roughly comparable for the two strains.

4. DIAGNOSIS AND EXCLUSION OF FOOT AND MOUTH DISEASE

Foot and mouth disease (FMD) virus may produce lesions of myocarditis which are morphologically indistinguishable from those induced by EMC. Specific confirmation of EMC virus infection, and exclusion of the FMD alternative, is therefore given high priority.

a) Inocula are prepared concurrently in phosphate buffered saline (pH ~7.2) and 0.1 M acid phosphate solution pH ~5.5). EMC virus is stable in the acid salt solution, which would be expected to inactivate FMD virus.

b) Inoculation of cell cultures is made concurrently into BHK and primary calf thyroid cells to provide preferred cells for either virus.

5. ALTERNATIVE DIAGNOSTIC METHODS

For circumstances where cell culture facilities are not available EMC virus may be recovered in mice from an EMC virus-free colony. Mice may be infected by inoculation but the simpler approach, with some advantages, is to feed diseased heart to mice.

From 45 cases diagnosed as EMC, virus was recovered from 35 via cells and from 32 by feeding tissue to mice. The 32 included 2 from which virus was not recovered, and 2 samples which were too decomposed to be successfully examined, in cell culture.

6. MODEL OF HUMAN DISEASE

EMC myocarditis in pigs has features in common with enterovirus myocarditis in man. It may provide a useful model for some aspects of human heart disease, both in acute form and possible long term sequelae.

103

IS SCRAPIE A ZOONOTIC DISEASE?

Colin L. Masters

Department of Pathology
University of Western Australia

Scrapie is a naturally occurring infectious disease of sheep and goats, and may also occur in certain captive species (mink, mule deer). The scrapie virus is unconventional in its physico-chemical and biological properties, most remarkable among which are its relative resistance to inactivation and long incubation period. A similar type of virus infects man to cause Creutzfeldt-Jakob disease (CJD) worldwide, and kuru which is restricted to the Eastern Highlands of Papua New Guinea.

In contrast to kuru, CJD occurs worldwide with an incidence of at least 1 per million. Up to 15% of cases occur within families, consistent with autosomal dominant transmission. Temporal, spatial or ethnic clustering of cases may rarely occur, the best documented example being the high incidence of CJD in Libyan-born Israelis (30 per million). There are three broad hypotheses to explain the occurrence of CJD: 1) Case-to-case transmission, including lateral contact transmission, vertical or familial transmission, and transmission resulting from iatrogenic contamination. The possibilities of asymptomatic subclinical infection and inherited susceptibility to infection must also be considered in this category. 2) Activation of an endogenous (latent) virus infection, through either some environmental trigger or genetically determined mechanism. 3) Zoonotic transmission of scrapie virus from sheep, goats, or other animals.

Of these three hypotheses, the available evidence favors case-to-case transmission: iatrogenic spread of CJD is the only mechanism that has been clearly demonstrated; the past medical and surgical histories of most cases of CJD present

VIRAL DISEASES IN SOUTH-EAST ASIA
AND THE WESTERN PACIFIC
ISBN 0 12 484820 6

frequent occasions where the potential for infection existed. Case-to-case transmission, invoking most mechanisms now demonstrated for the spread of hepatitis B virus, is consistent with the presumed mode of transmission of human kuru, and with the biological behaviour of CJD virus in experimental studies. There is little evidence to support the concept of activation of an endogenous virus.

The zoonotic transmission of scrapie is a difficult hypothesis to test. If it occurs, then the most likely mechanism would be through the ingestion of, or parenteral contamination with, scrapie infected sheep tissue. The dietary habits of the Libyan-born Israelis, the correlation between lamb consumption and the incidence of CJD in France, and the oral transmission of scrapie to experimental primates, are the only pieces of evidence which suggest the zoonotic hypothesis. The main argument against this hypothesis is that CJD occurs in countries where overt scrapie is absent. The best example of this is seen in Australia. Scrapie is not present in Australia, although a probable outbreak was recorded in British Suffolk ewes imported into Victoria in 1950/1952 (Bull and Murnane, 1958). Yet the annual incidence of CJD in Australia is 1-2 per million, and cases are readily identified where there is no history of travel outside Australia into scrapie infected countries (the areas closest to Australia known to have scrapie are the Indian subcontinent and North America). Other evidence against the zoonotic spread of scrapie comes from studies of the demography of CJD in the U.S., France and Japan. More recently, the occurrence of CJD in a vegetarian has been documented.

It seems likely, therefore, that scrapie in domesticated animals is not an important source of the zoonotic spread of CJD to man. Although the natural mechanism of spread and the resevoir of the CJD remain unknown at present, the evidence points to some form of case-to-case transmission, and provides hope that this disease of man can be controlled and eventually eliminated.

REFERENCE

Bull, L.B., and Murnane, D. (1958). An outbreak of scrapie in British sheep imported into Victoria. *Australian Veterinary Journal 34, 213.*

Part VI
Specific Viral Diseases
G.
Other Viruses

104

HERPESVIRUS INFECTIONS OF MAN

Marion R. Bucens

Virus Laboratory
State Health Laboratory Services
Queen Elizabeth II Medical Centre
Nedlands, Western Australia

J.S. Mackenzie
G.R. Shellam
N.F. Stanley

Department of Microbiology
University of Western Australia
Nedlands, Western Australia

Although more than 70 viruses of the herpes group are known to infect a wide range of animal species, there are only five distinct herpesviruses that commonly infect humans: herpes simplex virus (HSV) types 1 and 2, varicella-zoster virus (VZV), Epstein-Barr virus (EBV) and cytomegalovirus (CMV). These five ubiquitous viruses resemble each other structurally, being indistinguishable by electron microscopy, and share a number of biological properties, particularly latency and reactivation, but they exhibit a diverse spectrum of pathological and clinical effects. In developed countries virtually everyone is infected with HSV-1, VZV, EBV and CMV before middle age, whereas infection is usually much earlier in developing countries. Two other herpesviruses, herpes simiae and possibly simian cytomegalovirus, may occasionally infect humans.

VIRAL DISEASES IN SOUTH-EAST ASIA
AND THE WESTERN PACIFIC
ISBN 0 12 484820 6

STRUCTURE AND BIOLOGY

Herpesviruses are among the largest of viruses, with a diameter of 150-200 nm. The virus particles consist of a core or nucleoid composed of the DNA genome intertwined with protein and enclosed within an icosahedral protein capsid of 162 capsomers. The capsid is surrounded by a loose amorphous envelope derived from the nuclear membrane. There are at least 33 virus-coded polypeptides in the core, capsid and envelope.

The linear double-stranded DNA genomes range in molecular weight from 90 to 150 x 10^6 daltons, and for all except VZV which has still to be determined, display a variety of novel sequence arrangements with terminal and internal stretches of repeated sequences, the internal sequences separating a long and a short unique sequence. In addition, EBV can assume a closed circular genomic form within the nuclei of latently infected cells, but such forms have not yet been detected for the other human herpesviruses. The genomic sequences of the human herpesviruses have been found to be very different by cross-hybridization, except for HSV-1 and HSV-2 which share approximately 50 per cent of their genomic content. Furthermore, restriction enzyme analyses have shown that strain differences exist for HSV-1, HSV-2, EBV and CMV, with genomes isolated from various sources exhibiting great diversity. Indeed analyses of this sort provide exquisite sensitivity for epidemiological studies.

The herpesvirus genome contains sufficient genetic information to encode more than 50 different structural and non-structural proteins, many of which serve as efficient antigens. However, as might be expected from their genomic differences, there is little antigenic similarity between most members of the group. Only HSV-1 and HSV-2 share a significant degree of antigenic relatedness with cross-reacting antigens being identified among certain envelope, internal and non-structural proteins, and although HSV-1 and HSV-2 viruses are clearly separable by different serological techniques, "intermediate" strains have been recognised. Considerable antigenic diversity is found between different isolates of HSV-1, HSV-2, EBV and CMV, whereas VZV isolates are relatively homogeneous.

Aspects of the biology, epidemiology and clinical manifestations of human herpesviruses have recently been discussed in detail in the Proceedings of an International Conference on Human Herpesviruses (1).

HERPES SIMPLEX VIRUSES

HSV-1 and HSV-2 can be divided into distinct serotypes on the basis of serological, biological and biochemical differences (2). They have assumed major public health importance in recent years for the following reasons: there has been an alarming increase in the incidence of genital herpes; the proposed association between HSV-2 and carcinoma of the cervix; the risk to neonates born to mothers with genital herpes at the time of delivery; and the advent of new antiviral drugs.

The clinical manifestations of HSV infection vary widely from superficial infections of the skin, eye and mucous membranes to disseminated involvement of the internal organs and of the central nervous system in the form of meningitis (HSV-2) and encephalitis (HSV-1, HSV-2). Seroepidemiological studies show a wide variation in the incidence of infection according to socioeconomic conditions. In crowded communities with lower standards of hygiene the peak incidence of primary infection occurs between 1 and 3 years of age. HSV-2 is transmitted principally by sexual contact and antibody is not usually acquired before 15 years of age. Formerly HSV-1 and HSV-2 were broadly categorized as attacking above (HSV-1) and below (HSV-2) the waist, but this distinction no longer applies (3).

Clinically-apparent lesions may be either primary, initial or recurrent. A primary infection describes a patient's first encounter with the virus and results in seroconversion. Many primary infections are asymptomatic, but they may present as lesions associated with a systemic upset including fever, malaise and an associated painful lymphadenopathy. The illness resolves spontaneously in a week or two. An initial infection describes the first clinically apparent lesion occurring in the presence of antibody to either serotype of virus. Recurrent infections are usually due to reactivations, but in the case of HSV-2, have occasionally been shown to be due to exogenous reinfection. HSV persists in a latent form in sensory ganglia and in the ganglia of the autonomic nervous system. Infectious virus can only be recovered from the ganglia by explantation or co-cultivation. Latency in non-neural cells has been suggested but not yet substantiated in humans (4).

The vast majority of HSV infections are mild and cause mainly social and psychological trauma especially in relation to genital herpes, but there are three situations in which these infections are life-threatening; in the neonate, in the immunocompromised, and in cases of neurological involvement. HSV infection of the neonate has a 60% mortality rate and significant neurological and/or ocular sequelae occur in at least half of the survivors. Close monitoring of certain categories of women has been advocated in an attempt to reduce the risk to the newborn. Women with genital herpes at any time in pregnancy, those with a prior history of laboratory confirmed genital herpes and those whose sexual partners have herpes should be checked weekly from 36 weeks of gestation by virological methods. Caesarian section is recommended if HSV is present in the genital tract at the time of delivery.

Visceral dissemination of HSV is a particular risk in patients with eczema, severe burns or those who are immunocompromised either by disease (e.g., leukaemia), drug therapy or malnutrition (5). Diagnosis may be difficult in the absence of superficial lesions and the treatment is mainly supportive.

As stated above, neurological involvement may present either as meningitis, which is a rare but benign condition, or encephalitis, a very severe condition with a case fatality rate of 50-70% and with severe sequelae in the survivors.

Achievement of a definitive diagnosis should be mandatory in any form of HSV infection especially if antiviral therapy is contemplated. Virus isolation in tissue culture is still the most sensitive method. The newer rapid methods of immunofluorescent and immunoperoxidase staining are less sensitive, need to be well controlled for specificity, and require skillfully collected specimens early in the course of infection. Electron microscopy is rapid, but its sensitivity is dependent on the presence of virus in high titre and requires an experienced operator.

New antiviral agents active against HSV have been made available following large clinical trials (discussion by Dr. A.J. Beale in this seminar). Acyclovir has a very high therapeutic index and has been proven to be effective when administered topically (ocular and genital lesions) and systemically (encephalitis). It reduces the duration of viral shedding and accelerates healing of some genital infections, but does not prevent the establishment of latency and its potential for reactivation (6). Strains of HSV resistant to acyclovir have been reported.

VARICELLA-ZOSTER VIRUS

VZV causes two diseases: varicella (chickenpox) and zoster (shingles). Varicella is a widespread highly contagious disease characterized by a mild to moderate fever and by the development of maculo-papular and vesicular lesions following primary exposure, usually in childhood. Zoster is an endemic disease prevalent in elderly populations and characterized by painful, unilateral vesicular eruptions confined to dermatomes enervated by dorsal root or extramedullary cranial ganglions in which the virus has persisted since primary varicella infection.

Both varicella and zoster occur widely throughout the world. In temperate countries, varicella is usually a childhood disease, with less than 2% of cases in those over the age of 20, whereas in tropical countries, it is frequently seen in adults (7). Indeed, varicella is reported to be at least as common in adults as in children in Sri Lanka. On the other hand, there is no evidence to support geographic differences with zoster. Another difference between varicella and zoster is that of temporal distribution. Whereas zoster occurs sporadically throughout the year independently of the prevalence of varicella, varicella shows a marked seasonable distribution with peaks, in the U.S.A., from March to June (7). There is no strong evidence indicating different racial susceptibilities to VZV infection.

Varicella is more severe in adults than in children, with pneumonia a relatively common (16%) complication. The incidence of complications of both varicella and zoster is much higher in immunocompromised patients than in normal individuals. Progressive varicella is a life-threatening complication in children with underlying malignant disease or receiving high doses of steroids. Immunosuppressed children who have had varicella (with the exception of bone marrow transplant recipients) are not at risk of developing severe varicella from re-exposure. Adults undergoing treatment for cancer, particularly those with Hodgkin's disease and with bone marrow transplantation, are at a higher risk for developing zoster. Most cases result in cutaneous dissemination of virus, but only 10% of cases will have significant visceral involvement (8). The most successful approach in the management of varicella in immunocompromised children is the administration of zoster immune globulin. A more recent approach has been the development of a live attenuated VZV vaccine by Takahashi. The use of the vaccine has been recently reviewed by Gershon (9).

EPSTEIN-BARR VIRUS

EBV is the cause of infectious mononucleosis (IM) and is constantly associated with Burkitt's lymphoma (BL) and nasopharyngeal carcinoma (NPC). This section will concentrate on IM rather than the association of EBV with BL or NPC.

Although the Paul-Bunnell (heterophile antibody) test has been and still is a most useful test for diagnosis and surveillance, it is limited because it detects a non-specific IgM antibody which is transient. This test is now supplemented with immunofluorescence and other tests of IgG antibody to viral antigens, and of particular value in epidemiology is the presence of antibody to the viral capsid antigen (VCA). Antibodies to VCA and early antigen (EA) develop shortly after primary infection, but whereas antibodies to VCA persist for life, antibodies to EA fall to low or undetectable levels within a few months. Antibodies to the third major diagnositc antigen, the nuclear antigen (EBNA), appear 1 to 3 months after infection and then also persist for life. The most accurate marker of recent infection is IgM antibody to VCA.

Using these tests, it has now become clear that most EBV infections are inapparent except in the more affluent populations of developed nations where the peak incidence of clinical disease is in teenagers. The clinical disease is virtually unknown in developing nations or densely populated communities where the opportunity for virus transmission occurs in infants and young children (10). For example, in Indonesia, where IM is uncommon, the antibody prevalence (VCA) to EBV in children up to 6 years of age is 87% (10), whereas in Perth, Western Australia, where IM is a disease of adolescents, the antibody prevalence in the same age group is only 38%, and does not reach 90% until the 16-19 year age group (11). Particularly early infection within the first year of life has been reported in Papua New Guinea (12).

IM may vary in its severity from very mild to very severe. It is rarely fatal and complete recovery is usually expected after 4 weeks, although occasionally the illness may persist for months. The disease is characterised clinically by fever, sore throat and lymphadenopathy, often accompanied by hepatosplenomegaly. Haematologically, a relative as well as absolute lymphocytosis is seen with numerous atypical lymphocytes (13). Complications, when they occur, may affect any organ and include meningoencephalitis, Bell's palsy, Guillane-Barré syndrome, myocarditis, pneumonitis, renal failure and thrombocytopaenia. The clinical and haematological features are not specific for IM but are shared by other IM-like illnesses caused, among others, by cytomegalovirus, adenoviruses, rubella virus and *Toxoplasma gondii*. A persistent virus carrier state regularly follows primary infection with EBV. This may become activated by diseases that immunosuppress or alternatively by immunosuppressive therapy. Reactivation is usually associated with an increase in antibody to EA and VCA but not EBNA. It is probable that reactivation of EBV is not as serious in the immunocompromised as with the other herpesviruses, and this could relate to the presence of the virus in B lymphocytes, which are reduced by immunosuppression, rather than other sites (13).

Biopsy material from African BL patients and from NPC patients anywhere in the world have revealed the presence of EBV DNA at a high degree of frequency, and the tumour cells express EBNA. However there appears to be a difference between the lymphoblasts transformed by EBV in the peripheral circulation of patients with IM and those obtained from patients with BL. Although both express EBNA and have a permanent growth potential, the former are polyclonal and do not produce tumours in nude mice, whereas the latter have a monoclonal origin and may produce tumours following intraperitoneal inoculation of nude mice. It is likely that the emergence of BL or NPC is by no means a single event but that two or more events must occur successively. Despite extensive study, we are still far from understanding the basic mechanisms of induction of these two EBV-associated malignancies (14). Irrespective of the final outcome, the association, although not 100%, is sufficiently constant for the presence of EBV to be used for the early detection of NPC as outlined by Zeng Yi in this volume.

CYTOMEGALOVIRUS

The predominant features of CMV infection are that although infection is widespread in the community, infection is usually inapparent and symptomatic diseases induced by CMV are infrequent in normal individuals. Thus 40-60% of the population are seropositive after 35 years of age, although the prevalence of antibodies varies widely and may be 40-70% in western societies and 90-100% in less developed countries (15). Indeed these may be conservative estimates of the prevalence of infection because most seroepidemiologic data was obtained by the relatively insensitive complement-fixation test. Although symptomatic infection of the normal adult can occur, morbidity associated with CMV infection is usually restricted to individuals infected during the neonatal period or who are immunosuppressed or congenitally immunodeficient.

The diagnosis of CMV infections requires laboratory confirmation and cannot be made on clinical grounds alone. Laboratory diagnosis is based on either virus isolation or demonstration of a rise in antibody titre, or both. Specific IgM antibody is diagnostic of a recent infection but may also be present during reactivation. However, whilst the complement fixation test has been widely used it is less sensitive than immunofluorescent and Elisa tests. There are other difficulties in making a serological diagnosis of CMV infection; there may be no diagnostic antibody rise in the asymptomatically infected pregnant woman or severely immunosuppressed patient, and serologic diagnosis is even more difficult in the neonate.

Neonatal infection with CMV may result from virus acquired perinatally, either during birth from an infected cervix or after birth from the milk, urine or respiratory tract of the mother, or from blood transfusions. There appears to be an increase in the cervical infection rate during the third trimester of pregnancy (16) raising the possibility that pregnancy either activates latent infection or predisposes to primary infection of the cervix. The perinatal infection rate is probably 3-10% in various populations (16). The perinatally infected neonate does not usually become viruric for 4-8 weeks and virus replication is usually associated with a serologic response. These infants are usually asymptomatic and it is not yet known whether there are long-term effects.

In contrast, intrauterine infection is less frequent (0.5 - 2% of all live births) but may have more severe consequences. Most of these infections occur in infants of primiparous mothers who presumably have a primary infection during pregnancy. Primary infection at any stage of pregnancy presents a risk, but there is insufficient data available to ascribe a more precise risk to any particular trimester. Despite the fact that CMV is probably the most common infectious agent to reach the foetus, the majority of congenitally infected infants are asymptomatic at birth, although the risk of an infected infant exhibiting subsequent damage is about 10-20% (17). In contrast, the severely affected infant presenting with cytomegalic inclusion disease which may include microcephaly, intracerebral calcification, spasticity and severe retardation, is comparatively rare.

Although disease induced by CMV is infrequent in the normal adult, several distinct syndromes are discernible. CMV mononucleosis resembles EB virus mononucleosis but is distinguished from it by the absence of heterophile antibodies. It may result from a primary infection in normal subjects or from infection transmitted by transfused blood or in immunosuppressed patients. In addition, interstitial pneumonitis, hepatitis, the Guillain-Barré syndrome, meningoencephalitis, myocarditis, thrombocytopaenia and haemolytic anaemia have been reported.

In contrast, CMV infections often cause severe morbidity in patients following certain types of organ transplantation. Thus the rate of infection after renal transplantation, as determined by a rise in antibody titres or virus isolation, was found to vary from 52% to 100% in a study of 383 patients (18). Clinical illness in the first few months after transplantation occurs in almost all patients with primary infection and seldom in those with infection due to reactivation. Furthermore, primary CMV infection in transplant patients is usually accompanied by greater morbidity than reactivation infection. Most commonly, infected patients present with fever and mononucleosis followed by pneumonitis which can be rapidly fatal (19), hepatitis, infection of the gastrointestinal tract and retinitis.

Finally, cytomegalovirus has been found in association with certain malignancies such as adenocarcinoma of the colon, prostatic carcinoma and Kaposi's sarcoma (20,21) suggesting that CMV may have oncogenic potential in man and thus resemble other of the herpes viruses, especially EBV, for which strong circumstantial evidence of oncogenicity exists.

REFERENCES

1. Nahmias, A.J., Dowdle, W.R., and Schinazi, R.F. (eds). "The Human Herpesviruses". Elsevier, New York, (1981).
2. Nahmias, A.J., and Norrild, B., *Disease-a-Month 25 (10)*, (1979).
3. Editorial, *Lancet ii,* 1025 (1981).
4. Overall, J.C., *New Engl. J. Med. 305,* 95 (1981).
5. Templeton, A.C., *J. Clin. Path. 23,* 24 (1970).
6. Editorial, *Lancet ii,* 845 (1981).
7. Weller, T.H., *in* "Viral Infections of Humans: Epidemiology and Control", (A.S. Evans, ed.), p.457. Plenum, New York, (1976).

8. Zaia, J.A., *in* "The Human Herpesviruses", (A.J. Nahmias, W.R. Dowdle, and R.F. Schinazi, eds.), p.10. Elsevier, New York, (1981).
9. Gershon, A.A., *Rev. Infect. Dis. 2,* 393 (1980).
10. Evans, A.S., *in* "The Human Herpesviruses" (A.J. Nahmias, W.R. Dowdle, and R.F. Schinazi, eds.), p.172. Elsevier, New York, (1981).
11. Lai, P.K., Mackay-Scollay, E.M., and Alpers, M.P. *J. Hyg. Camb. 74,* 329 (1975).
12. Lang, D., Garruto, R.M., and Gajdusek, D.C., *Amer. J. Epidemiol. 105,* 480 (1977).
13. Henle, W., and Henle, G., *in* "The Human Herpesviruses", (A.J. Nahmias, W.R. Dowdle, and R.F. Schinazi, eds.), p.31. Elsevier, New York, (1981).
14. Miller, G., *in* "The Human Herpesviruses" (A.J. Nahmias, W.R. Dowdle, and R.F. Schinazi, eds.), p.228. Elsevier, New York, (1981).
15. Krech, U.H., *Bull. Wld Hlth Org. 49,* 103 (1973).
16. Ho, M., *Disease-a-Month 24,* 1 (1978).
17. Mellish, M.E., and Hanshaw, J.B., *Amer. J. Dis. Child. 126,* 190 (1973).
18. Ho, M., *Arch. Virol. 55,* 1 (1979).
19. Weller, T.H., *in* "The Human Herpesviruses", (A.J. Nahmias, W.R. Dowdle, and R.F. Schinazi, eds.), p.20. Elsevier, New York, (1981).
20. Giraldo, G., and Beth, E., *in* "The Role of Viruses in Human Cancer", Volume 1 (G. Giraldo, and E. Beth, eds.), p.57. Elsevier, New York, (1980).
21. Hanshaw, J.B., *in* "The Human Herpesviruses" (A.J. Nahmias, W.R. Dowdle, and R.F. Schinazi, eds.), p.38. Elsevier, New York, (1981).

105

EARLY DETECTION OF NPC

Zeng Yi

Institute of Virology
Chinese Academy of Medical Sciences
Beijing, China

Nasopharyngeal carcinoma (NPC) is a very common disease in southern China and in South-east Asia. The distribution of NPC showed very significant geographical variation (1,2). The central part of Guangdong and eastern part of Guangxi provinces formed geographically unique high risk areas with a decreasing rate tendency toward their periphery, and with a mortality rate up to 10/100,000. The mortality rate and the incidence of NPC has been quite stable. Viro-serological studies have shown that the EBV is closely related to NPC. We put our emphasis on the early detection of NPC by the combination of different viro-immunological tests with clinical, cytological and histological examination.

METHODS FOR DETECTION OF ANTIBODIES TO EB VIRUS AND EB VIRUS MARKERS

A. *Detection of IgA Antibody to EB Virus by Immuno-enzymatic Test*

The immunofluorescence test is commonly used for detection of antibodies to EB virus (3), but it needs a fluorescence microscope and is not convenient for NPC diagnosis and field study in China. So, we established a simpler and more sensitive immunoenzymatic test for serological diagnosis and mass survey of NPC (4). The preliminary results showed that the IgA/VCA antibody positive rate in NPC patients was 92%, but no such antibody was found in patients

VIRAL DISEASES IN SOUTH-EAST ASIA
AND THE WESTERN PACIFIC
ISBN 0 12 484820 6

with malignant tumors other than NPC and in normal persons. As compared to the immuno-fluorescence test, the immuno-enzymatic test is more sensitive. This test is now widely used for diagnosis of NPC in China. The positive rate of IgA/VCA antibody from NPC patients, patients with malignant tumors other than NPC, and normal individuals was 92.3-98.1% with a GMT of 1:35.7-1:84.4, 0-37% with a GMT of 1:1.25-1:17.13, and 0-6% with a GMT of 1:1.25-1:2.6 respectively (4-8). There is a striking difference between the NPC group and the other two groups. Thus detection of IgA/VCA antibody is valuable in the diagnosis of NPC, especially in its early stages or in NPC patients without notable tumor in the nasopharynx superficially, but with invasion beneath the mucosa or early metastases in the neck region.

B. Detection of EBNA by Anticomplement Immuno-enzymatic Test

NPC can be detected at an early stage by serological mass survey and follow up studies, but there remains a large number of IgA/VCA antibody-positive persons with no evidence of NPC. EBNA and EB virus DNA are regularly found in NPC cells. Detection of EBNA or EBV DNA in nasopharyngeal cells from IgA/VCA antibody-positive individuals and from NPC suspected persons might be of help in early diagnosis of NPC. The anticomplement immuno-fluorescence test requires a fluorescence microscope and the cell types can not be easily identified. We have established an anticomplement immuno-enzymatic test for detection of EBNA, which proved to be very sensitive (9). Exfoliated cells collected by negative pressure suction from the nasopharynx of patients with NPC, and of suspected patients, were examined for EBNA by this test (10). Among 79 NPC patients, all had EBNA-positive carcinoma cells, while the positive rate of cytological and histological examination was 87.3% and 91.1% respectively indicating the superiority of the anticomplement immuno-enzymatic test in detecting NPC patients, especially in stage I where the positive rate detected by the later two methods was only 86.4% and 80.0%. No EBNA was found in tumor cells from patients with malignant tumors other than NPC, nor was it found in nasopharyngeal epithelial cells from dead foetuses. The findings show that the anticomplement immuno-enzymatic test is specific and sensitive, and can be used for the early detection of NPC, especially in combination with the serological tests. The anticomplement immuno-enzymatic test was also applied to detect nasopharyngeal carcinoma cells with EBNA from IgA/VCA antibody-positive persons in the high risk area (11). Carcinoma cells with EBNA were found in 4 out of 64 antibody-positive individuals; cytological and histopathological examination also showed poorly differentiated carcinoma in these 4 cases at stage I. These results further established the value of anticomplement immuno-enzymatic test for the detection of early stages of NPC.

EBNA was not only found in nasopharyngeal carcinoma cells, but also in hyperplastic cells and normal epithelial cells from the nasopharynx of NPC patients or normal individuals. Follow-up studies of hyperplastic cells with EBNA in persons having IgA/VCA antibody may be important for early detection of NPC and for clarifying the role of EB virus in the development of NPC.

C. Detection of EB Virus DNA Repeats by Blot Hybridization

Blot hybridization was used for the detection of EBV DNA repeats by collaboration with Desgranges, Bornkamm and de Thé (12). Among 56 IgA/VCA antibody-positive persons, EBV DNA was detected in 3 out of 4 biopsies from NPC patients which had been confirmed histologically, and two of them were at a very early stage. In fourteen further individuals without clinical or histopathological evidence of tumors, EBV DNA was also detected, but not found in 7 biopsies from IgA antibody-negative individuals. Follow-up studies of IgA/VCA antibody-positive persons with EBV DNA marker may also be important for early detection of NPC. The spot hybridization technique is being assessed for analysing large numbers of samples necessary in field studies.

SEROLOGICAL MASS SURVEYS OF NPC

Approximately 150,000 persons aged 30 and over were screened in 1978-1980 in Zangwu county of Guangxi Autonomous Region by the immuno-enzymatic test. Of these, 3,539 were found to have IgA/VCA antibody to EB virus (13-15). Among them 54 cases were diagnosed histologically as NPC, 12 were in stage I, the majority of them with no subjective symptoms, 19 in stage II, 17 in stage III and 6 in stage IV. After 1-3 years in follow-up studies, 33 additional NPC cases were diagnosed. One was carcinoma in situ, 10 in stage I, 9 in stage II, 11 in stage III and 2 in stage IV. The IgA/VCA antibody was detected 8-30 months prior to the clinical diagnosis of NPC at stage I. These results were similar to those reported by Ho *et al* (16) and Lanier *et al* (17) in their retrospective studies. They found that IgA/VCA antibody was detectable 22 months-5 years before the clinical diagnosis was made. There was no difference in the GMT of IgA/VCA antibody in sera between the period before the onset of NPC and the diagnosis of stage I, but it was higher in stages II-IV, e.g. when the carcinoma cell metastasized to the cervical lymph node, the antibody titre increased. Some NPC patients were diagnosed at their late stage (III and IV), because they lived in the countryside far from the town and the clinical examinations were not carried out periodically or were missed in the early stage. Altogether 87 NPC cases were detected from 3,539 IgA/VCA antibody-positive persons; the detection rate was 2458.3/100,000. It was 82 times the annual incidence of NPC in the general population of the same age group (18).

In order to reduce the NPC mortality rate by early detection, a serological mass survey of NPC was carried out in Wuzhow city which is located in the center of Zangwu county (19). The mean annual incidence of NPC was 17/100,000 for 1975-1978. In the first-step study, sera were obtained from 12,932 persons of the 40-59 age group, and the positive rate of IgA/VCA antibody was 5.3%. Thirteen NPC cases were detected from 680 IgA/VCA antibody-positive persons by using a combination of tests including immuno-enzymatic tests for detection of IgA/VCA and IgA/EA antibodies, anticomplement immuno-enzymatic tests for detection of EBNA, clinical, cytological and histological examinations. Of 13 NPC patients, 9 were in stage I and 4 in stage II. No notable tumor was found in most of the patients at stage I. There were only some nonspecific lesions such as rough, pale and nodular mucosa. The frequency of early NPC (stage I) was 70% and was much higher than that in outpatients clinic where only 4.4-11.5% of NPC patients were at stage I (20-21). The detection rate of NPC from 680 IgA/VCA antibody-positive persons was 1,900/100,000 which was 38 times the annual incidence in the general population of the same age group for 1975-1978 in Wuzhow city.

CONCLUSION

The detection of IgA/VCA and IgA/EA antibody to EB virus and the EBV marker in combination with clinical, cytological and histopathological examination is valuable for the early diagnosis of NPC. Therefore application of serological tests in outpatient clinics, carrying out serological mass surveys and periodically follow-up studies of IgA-antibody and EBV-marker-positive persons, and education of public on the early signs of NPC are very essential in high NPC risk areas. The mortality rate can certainly be reduced through early detection and early treatment, even before the etiology of NPC has been clarified. The detection rate of NPC from IgA/VCA antibody-positive persons is much higher than the annual incidence of persons in the same age group, suggesting that the EB virus plays an important role in the development of NPC.

REFERENCES

1. Tumor Control Office of Ministry of Public Health, p.224, People's Health Press (1980).
2. Min, H.Q., Wu, Y.T., Pan, G.C., Huang, X.L., Wu, M.S. and Zeng, Y., *J. Prevention and Treatment of Cancer 3,* 24 (1978).
3. Henle, G., and Henle, W., *Int. J. Cancer 17,* 1 (1976).
4. Liu, Y.X., Zeng, Y., Dong, W.P. and Gao, G.R., *Chinese J. Oncol. 1,* 8 (1979).
5. Wei, J.N., Zhang, S., Tung, S.Z. and Huang, Z.L., *J. Guangxi Medicine 6,* 5 (1980).
6. Tang, Z.H., Wu, Y.T., Yang, J., Rong, B.P., Xu, Q.G., Zhao, C.N. and Meng, Q.G., *J. Shanghai Medicine 4,* 28 (1981).
7. Li, W.J., Ho, P.Y., Li, C.C., Liang, Y.R., Chen, A.M., Zhang, S.Q., Ye, Y.Z., Rong, B.P. and Xu, Q.G., Cancer Research Reports of Cancer Institute of Zhongshan Medical College 2, 95 (1981).
8. Jian, S.W., Li, Z.W., Luo, W.L., Li, M.C., Pan, W.X. and Zhang, X.H. Cancer Research Reports of Cancer Institute of Zhongshan Medical College 2, 23 (1981).
9. Pi, G.H., Zeng, Y., Zho, W.P. and Zhang, Q., *J. Immunol. Meth. 44,* 73 (1981).
10. Zeng, Y., Shen, S.J., Pi, G.H., Ma, J.L., Zhang, Q., Zhao, M.L. and Dong, H.J., *Cancer Campaign 5,* 237, Nasopharyngeal Carcinoma. Gustar Fischer Verlag, Stuttgart (1981).
11. Zeng, Y., Zhen, S.J., Dan, H., Ma, T.L., Zhang, Q., Zhu, J.S., Zheng, T.R. and Tan, B.F., *Acta. Acad. Med. Sin.,* in press (1981).

12. De Thé, G., Desgrange, C., Zeng, Y., Wang, P.C., Bornkamm, G.W., Zhu, J.S. and Shan, M., *Cancer Campaign* 5, 111, Nasopharyngeal Carcinoma. Gustar Fischer Verlag, Stuttgart (1981).
13. Zeng, Y., Liu, Z.Y., Zhen, S.W., Wei, J.N., Zhu, J.S. and Zai, H.J., *Chinese J. Oncol. 1,* 2 (1979).
14. Zeng, Y., Liu, Y.X., Wei, J.N., Zhu, J.S., Cai, S.L., Wang, P.Z., Zhong, J.M., Li, R.C., Pan, W.J., Li, E.J. and Tan, B.F., *Acta. Acad. Med. Sin. 1,* 123 (1979).
15. Zeng, Y., Liu, Y.X., Liu, Z.R., Zhen, S.W., Wei, J.N., Zhu, J.S. and Zai, H.S., *Intervirology 13,* 162 (1980).
16. Ho, J.H.C., Kwan, H.C., Ng, M.H. and De Thé, G., *Lancet 1,* 436 (1978).
17. Lanier, A.P., Henle, W., Bender, T.R., Henle, G. and Talbot, M.L., *Int. J. Cancer 26,* 133 (1980).
18. Zeng, Y., Wang, P.Z., Zhu, J.S., Zhong, J.M., Liu, Y.X., Wei, J.N., Li, E.J., Tan, B.F., unpublished data.
19. Zeng, Y., Zhang, L.G., Li, H.Y., Jan, M.C., Zhang, Q., Wu, Y.C., Wang, Y.S. and Su, G.R., *Int. J. Cancer,* in press (1982).
20. Zeng, Z.Y., Sun, Z.Z., Chen, S.Y., Li, D.Z., Zeng, S.Y. and Wang, N., Selected Papers of Cancer Hospital of Zhongshan Medical College, p. 51 (1981).
21. Pan, K.Y., Wong, K.Z., Zeng, C.S., Mao, Z.D. and Zhong, Z.A., *Chinese Med. J. 54,* 687 (1974).

MOUSE STRAIN VARIATION IN THE PROTECTIVE EFFECT OF INTERFERON DURING MCMV INFECTION[a]

J.E. Allan[1], *J.E. Grundy (Chalmer)*[2], *G.R.Shellam*[1], *J. Trapman*[3]

[1]Department of Microbiology, University of Western Australia, Nedlands, W.A.;[2]N.I.H., Bethesda, M.D., U.S.A.; [3]Erasmus University, Rotterdam, Holland.

Cytomegalovirus (CMV) infections are endemic in South East Asia where the frequency of seropositive individuals approaches 100% (1). Based on experience elsewhere, CMV is likely to be a significant cause of neonatal morbidity in Asia. In order to examine the factors which predispose to infection we have studied the resistance of inbred strains of mice to murine cytomegalovirus (MCMV) which is controlled by both H-2 associated and non-H-2 genes (2), whose influences include the replication of MCMV *in vitro* (3) and the activation of NK cells (4).

There was a good correlation between non-H-2 associated resistance and the production of pH 2 stable IFN at 6 hrs but not 48 hrs p.i. Titres were high in resistant CBA mice ($H\text{-}2^k$, 11.22 $\log_2$ international reference units/ml plasma), intermediate in resistant C3H ($H\text{-}2^k$ 7.31 $\log_2$ units) and C57BL/6 ($H\text{-}2^b$, 8.14 $\log_2$ units) and low in susceptible BALB/c ($H\text{-}2^d$, 5.72 $\log_2$ units), BALB.B ($H\text{-}2^b$, 5.56 $\log_2$ units), resistant BALB.K ($H\text{-}2^k$, 1.86 units) and resistant B10.BR ($H\text{-}2^k$ <5.18 $\log_2$ units) mice. This suggests that IFN production is controlled by non-H-2 rather than H-2 associated genes.

Treatment of C57BL/10 and C3H mice with anti-type I IFN antibody (sufficient to neutralise about 2×10^4 units) i.v. 2 hours before i.p. administration of MCMV, was found to

[a]*Supported by the Z.W.O., the TVW Telethon Foundation for Medical Research in W.A., and the NH&MRC.*

VIRAL DISEASES IN SOUTH-EAST ASIA AND THE WESTERN PACIFIC
ISBN 0 12 484820 6

decrease the LD_{50} as compared to control mice inoculated with normal rabbit serum. The resistance of C57BL/10 mice was reduced from 4.5 to 1.8 LD_{50} (χ^2 analysis, $P < 0.02$) and from 40.1 to 14.3 LD_{50} ($p < 0.01$) in C3H mice. The use of concentrated anti-IFN antibody further decreased resistance of C3H mice ($p < 0.001$). In contrast, the resistance of BALB/c mice was not significantly altered.

However, whilst IFN contributes to resistance in C3H and C57BL/10 mice it does not protect BALB/c or the more resistant BALB.K strain. Daily doses of 2×10^5 or 2×10^4 units of purified type I mouse IFN given i.p. beginning 4 hours after virus and thereafter at half-dose twice daily for 7 days did not protect these mice from challenge with 2 LD_{50} of MCMV appropriate to each strain.

Newborn mice are highly susceptible to MCMV and in preliminary experiments infection of newborn CBA but not BALB/c, was delayed by the administration of crude type I IFN. Mice received 7×10^2 units of IFN in 0.05 ml subcutaneously or the same volume of mock IFN at birth, on day 1 and day 2, in addition, to 5×10^3 MCMV i.p. on day 1. CBA mice were significantly protected (χ^2, $p < 0.01$) on day 10 with 10/25 mice dying in comparison to 18/23 animals treated with mock IFN. In contrast, 24/29 BALB/c mice treated with IFN and 25/26 control mice died giving no significant protection on day 10. By day 28 all mock IFN treated mice, 21/25 CBA mice and 28/29 BALB/c mice had died.

Thus type I IFN is important in resistance to MCMV in certain strains (C3H, CBA, C57BL/10) but not others (BALB/c, BALB/K). This may have implications for the treatment of CMV infections in man with IFN, the effectiveness of which may in part depend on the genetic constitution of the individual.

REFERENCES

1. Krech, U. (1973) *Bull. W.H.O. 49*, 103.
2. Grundy (Chalmer), J.E., Mackenzie, J.S. and Stanley, N.F. (1981) *Infec. Immun. 32*, 277.
3. Nedrud, J.G., Collier, A.M. and Pagano, J.S. (1979) *J. Gen. Virol. 45*, 737.
4. Bancroft, G.J., Shellam, G.R. and Chalmer, J.E. (1981) *J. Immunol. 126*, 988.

TORCHES (CONGENITAL DISEASES) PROGRAMME IN MALAYSIA

Dora S.K. Tan[1], *J.W. Mak*[1], *W. Cheah*[1]
K. Sukerman[1] *and H. Stern*[2]

1. Institute for Medical Research, Kuala Lumpur, Malaysia.
2. Department of Medical Microbiology, St. George's Hospital Medical School, London, U.K.

The "TORCHES" Programme is a collaborative antibody survey for TOxoplasmosis, Rubella, Cytomegalovirus infection, HErpes simplex and Syphilis in 3 parts: (i) in women of child-bearing age, 14-44 years old; (ii) in normal and defective (mentally and physically) children aged 0-4 years old; and (iii) in pregnant women, throughout their course of pregnancy and babies born to those who have undergone primary infection.

1. IN WOMEN OF CHILD-BEARING AGE

The antibody rates of the TORCHES diseases in this group of Malaysians were: Toxoplasmosis - 23% (84/365) by the FA test; Rubella - 64% (237/368) by the HI test; CMV infection - 83% (226/271) by the CF test; Herpes simplex - 79% (213/271) by the CF test and Syphilis - 5% (9/200) by the FTA-ABS test. These rates were almost similar to those of the general population (1-4). Toxoplasmosis infection was more highly prevalent among the Malays than the Chinese and Indians due probably to the greater affinity of the Malays for cats. Rubella infection was least common among the Malays maybe because of decreased transmission in their rural environment. Severe widespread epidemics of rubella were infrequent, despite the low immunity status (64%) and despite epidemics in Singapore which is closely adjacent to

VIRAL DISEASES IN SOUTH-EAST ASIA
AND THE WESTERN PACIFIC
ISBN 0 12 484820 6

Malaysia. The possible reasons were discussed by Tan *et al* (5). The 5% incidence of syphilis must be interpreted with caution as the FTA-ABS test employed also detects antibody to yaws which is still prevalent in Malaysia especially among the Malays.

2. IN NORMAL AND DEFECTIVE CHILDREN AGED 0-4 YEARS

Toxoplasmosis was not found to be a significant cause of congenital liver involvement or CNS defects as shown by the greater prevalence of specific IgM in normal children (3% or 8/278) compared to those with abnormalities (0.4% or 4/908).

In *rubella*, because the maternal HI antibodies are known to disappear by the 9th month of infancy and acquired rubella is rarely seen in children under 5 years of age, it may be presumed that any rubella HI antibody detected between 1 and 4 years of age is that synthesised by the infant itself from intra-uterine infection. Compared with 5.8% (7/120) in the normal children, aged 1 to 4 years, the rubella antibody rates in the defective children of the same age group were 71.4% (5/7) with "congenital rubella syndrome", 61.5% (8/13) with deafness, 50.0% (5/10) with congenital heart disease (mainly V.S.D.), 33.3% (6/18) with cataract (mainly bilateral) and 20% (10/49) with liver involvement. Only 2 of 49 (4.1%) mentally retarded children were positive. None of the 86 children with CNS defects (microcephaly, hydrocephalus, cerebral palsy) were positive. High GMTs were detected in children with congenital rubella (128), congenital heart disease (128), cataract (102) and mental retardation (128) indicating an active on-going infection even at this age group. The GMT in the normal group was 24. The study of rubella in children, aged 1 to 4 years, is being extended to include more cases.

Compared with the rubella antibody rate of normal infants, 1 day to 11 months old, (44.0% or 333/757), the rates of infants with the following defects were very much increased: cataract (83.9% or 47/56), congenital rubella syndrome (79.6% or 43/54), and congenital heart disease (64.7% or 44/68). Likewise, the GMTs in this group which ranged from 32 to 75 were higher than that in the normal infants which was 27. IgM estimation was not done.

CMV (CF) antibody rates were very high in normal neonates (99.1% or 229/231) but no specific IgM was detected in them. This indicates a high immune status of the mothers and warns against diagnosing CMV infection in infants based on serological evidence alone. At present, culture of the urine for the virus is the only reliable means for this purpose. CMV infection caused 11.6% (8/69) of congenital hepatomegaly (± jaundice) and 3.3% (2/60) of CNS defects as shown by the prevalence of specific IgM in infants less than 3 months old. No specific IgM was found in 60 infants with jaundice alone. One of the positive infants had microcephaly, hepatomegaly, a petechial rash and deafness.

Herpes simplex (CF) antibody was also highly prevalent in neonates. No specific IgM estimation was done, but typical lesions of congenital herpes simplex have so far not been encountered.

Syphilis antibodies were found in only 0.5% (8/1596) of normal neonates by the fluorescent treponemal antibody absorption (FTA-ABS) test. Although this test also detects antibody produced by yaws, the positive results in this study are not due to yaws which is never congenital and is rarely encountered under 1 year of age. Syphilis accounted for 4% (10/247) of hepatomegaly with or without jaundice, 1.3% (2/159) of jaundice alone, 47.1% (8/17) of rash and possibly 100% (3/3) of suspected "congenital syphilis syndrome". It does not seem to be an important cause of congenital CNS defects (0/181).

3. IN PREGNANT WOMEN DURING PREGNANCY AND BABIES BORN TO PRIMARY REACTORS

This prospective study was launched only recently and full results are not yet available. The plan of study is as follows: The mother's blood specimens are collected; (i) as soon as pregnancy is detected (before the 12th week); (ii) at the 12th week of pregnancy; and (iii) at the time of delivery; and examined for antibodies to the TORCHES diseases. The baby's (cord) blood is also taken at the time of delivery and examined for the same antibodies. Follow-up of babies of positive reactors allowed to proceed to full-term is done for a period of about 3 years to detect possible abnormalities apparent only later in childhood, e.g. deafness, mental retardation and congenital heart disease. It is hoped that early treatment and management of children with such defects can be given as a result of this study.

CONCLUSION

In Malaysia, of the 5 TORCHES diseases, rubella was most important especially as a cause of congenital heart disease, cataract, deafness, and liver involvement. CMV infection was not so important as a cause of congenital brain damage in Malaysia as in the west but could be significant as a cause of hepatomegaly in infants. Virus isolation studies are required to confirm this. Syphilis seems responsible for a high proportion of congenital rash, but more cases need to be studied.

REFERENCES

1. Jegethesan, M., Fan, Y.H. and Ong, K.J., *Southeast Asian J. Trop. Med. Pub. Hlth. 6,* 413 (1975).
2. Lam, S.K., *Bull. Wld. Hlth. Org. 47,* 127 (1972).
3. Tan, D.S.K. and Stern, H., *Bull. Wld. Hlth. Org.,* in press.
4. Tan, D.S.K. and Zaman, V., *Med. J. Malaysia 27,* 188 (1973).
5. Tan, D.S.K., Cheah, W., Sukumaran, K.D. and Stern, H., *Singapore Med. J. 17,* 207 (1976).

108

CONGENITAL RUBELLA VIRUS INFECTION AND DIABETES MELLITUS

Margaret A. Menser
Jill M. Forrest
Robyn D. Bransby
Judy R. Hudson

Children's Medical Research Foundation
University of Sydney
Sydney, Australia

Since diabetes mellitus (DM) was first induced in mice with the M variant of the encephalomyocarditis (EMC) virus, there has been increasing interest in the possibility that viral infection may play a part in the aetiology of diabetes in man (1). There have been reports of diabetes in humans following infection with mumps, infectious hepatitis, infectious mononucleosis, Coxsackie B_2, B_4 and B_5 viruses, and Coxsackie B_4 virus has been isolated from the pancreas of a boy dying of diabetes (2).

Among our group of 45 patients with congenital rubella (CR) born in Australia in 1941, 9 have diabetes. In a second group of 318 patients born in the 40's, 50's and 60's, 8 have diabetes. Nine of these 17 diabetics require insulin for control and 3 have diabetic retinopathy. The prevalence of diabetes in these subjects with congenital rubella is increased ten to twentyfold; there is no increase in diabetes among the patients' relatives (3). We know of 7 other subjects with CR and DM in Australia and 30 in other countries including 20 in U.S.A., 4 in Sweden, 2 in U.K., 2 in Japan and one each in New Zealand and France.

Clinically, it is not possible to know if the pathogenesis of the diabetes initiated by rubella virus is due solely to direct viral invasion of the β-cells of the

VIRAL DISEASES IN SOUTH-EAST ASIA AND THE WESTERN PACIFIC
ISBN 0 12 484820 6

islets of Langerhans, or whether the virus damages the islet cells by inducing an immunological reaction. It is likely that rubella virus persists postnatally in the congenitally infected human pancreas for months or even years, this may lead to progressive pancreatic damage. Lymphocytic infiltration in the pancreas similar to that described by Gepts at the onset of clinical diabetes (4) has been reported in 3 children with CR who died (5,6) one of whom had DM (7). Pancreatic islet cell antibodies have been demonstrated in a number of our patients with CR and DM (4 of 11 tested) and in two of our CR subjects who have not yet developed DM.

Experimental congenital rubella infection in rabbits in our laboratory resulted in changes in the β-cells of the pancreatic islets similar to those found in mice with EMC-induced diabetes (8), these changes included depletion of β granules, swelling of mitochondria and Golgi, distension of endoplasmic reticulum and disorganisation of cytoplasm by vacuolisation. When allowed to grow to maturity the animals showed poor insulin response to a glucose load but did not spontaneously develop diabetes (3).

While we do not think that CR is responsible for a large number of cases of diabetes in man, we believe that our studies show conclusively that the congenital infection can cause diabetes. Diabetes has also been reported in a patient with congenital cytomegalovirus infection (9). When reviewing the aetiology of insulin dependent diabetes recently, Cahill and McDevitt concluded that, although DM is a heterogeneous disorder, it is likely that most cases result from a virally initiated autoimmune destruction of β-cells (10). We suggest that some viral infections, such as rubella, are more likely to be diabetogenic when acquired transplacentally or in the neonatal period than in adult life.

REFERENCES

1. Gamble, D.R. *Epidemiologic Reviews*, *2*, 49 (1980).
2. Yoon, J.W. et al., *N. Engl. J. Med.*, *300*, 1173 (1979).
3. Menser, M.A. et al., *Lancet*, *i*, 57 (1978).
4. Gepts, W. *Diabetes*, *14*, 619 (1965).
5. Bunnell, C.E. et al., *J. Pediat.*, *80*, 465 (1972).
6. Jenson, A.B. et al., *Lancet*, *ii*, 354 (1980).
7. Patterson, K. et al., *Lancet*, *i*, 1048 (1981).
8. Craighead, J.E. et al., *Am. J. Path.*, *74*, 287 (1974).
9. Ward, K.P. et al., *Lancet*, *i*, 497 (1979).
10. Cahill, G.F. et al., *N. Engl. J. Med.*, *304*, 1454 (1981).

1980 RUBELLA OUTBREAK IN NEW ZEALAND

J.A. Miller
Y.E. Hermon
N.S. Kuttner

National Health Institute
Department of Health
Wellington, New Zealand

From late 1979 through to 1981 there was an epidemic of rubella in New Zealand. Most parts of the country were affected. This outbreak followed similar ones recorded in the United Kingdom, Canada and other parts of the world (1,2).

The Diagnostic Virus Laboratory at the National Health Institute (NHI), which offers a virus diagnostic service for approximately two-thirds of the country, examined 15,000 sera for rubella during the period of the epidemic; i.e. October 1979 to May 1981 inclusive. 186 positive cases (excluding babies) were diagnosed in this period. It is of concern that many of the positive cases were women of childbearing age (63% of total), and of these about half were in various stages of pregnancy at the time of infection. Thus rubella is still a significant problem for the group for which it has potentially the greatest significance.

The outbreak peaked in October 1980 and then gradually declined. In the months after this peak, increasing numbers of babies were diagnosed as having the congenital rubella syndrome. Diagnosis was made on laboratory and/or appropriate clinical evidence. At the time of this paper we had diagnosed three cases born in 1979, 18 in 1980 and 15 to date in 1981. We anticipate keeping these babies under surveillance for a period of three to five years. This would give a clearer picture of the aftermath of this rubella epidemic in the country.

VIRAL DISEASES IN SOUTH-EAST ASIA
AND THE WESTERN PACIFIC
ISBN 0 12 484820 6

REFERENCES

1. PHLS Communicable Disease Surveillance Centre, London. *Communicable Disease Report 79/20* (1979) (unpublished).
2. World Health Organization. Rubella surveillance. *Weekly Epidemiological Record 54*, 252 (1979).

Part VII
Final Discussion of Suggestions for the Future

Chairman F. J. Fenner

110

A SUMMARY OF THE DISCUSSION OF SUGGESTIONS FOR THE FUTURE

F. Fenner

Australian National University
Canberra

N.F. Stanley

University of Western Australia
Nedlands

The last session was devoted to a general discussion of suggestions for the future. Several participants had prepared written comments which had been seen by the Organizing Committee before the session began, but although several points raised therein were brought out in the discussion, the submitted comments were not circulated or discussed specifically.

The discussion was organized under four headings, which will be used in this report: follow-up of the seminar, communications, staff exchange and training, and the provision of laboratory materials and equipment.

FOLLOW-UP OF THE SEMINAR

The meeting agreed unanimously that the first International Seminar on Viral Diseases on South-East Asia and the Western Pacific had been a success and filled a real need of virologists in the region. It was also of considerable interest to virologists from Europe and North America. All participants supported the suggestion that there should be another meeting of the same general character in three or

VIRAL DISEASES IN SOUTH-EAST ASIA
AND THE WESTERN PACIFIC
ISBN 0 12 484820 6

four years time. They welcomed the statement by the Organizing Secretary that names and addresses of all participants would be circulated to all participants in the Seminar Proceedings. The Proceedings were being published as camera-ready copy by Academic Press.

COMMUNICATIONS

It was agreed that communications were of vital importance for ensuring that virologists in the Region were aware of what was happening elsewhere in the Region, as distinct from scientific advances reported in the international scientific literature. This was clearly essential for the control of viral diseases such as those due to arboviruses, some of which had recently circulated widely in the Region, poliovirus infections, influenza, epidemic viral conjunctivitis, and hepatitis.

Some specialists had established effective communication networks between themselves and other similar specialists in the Region. However, many laboratories which unavoidably could not carry out much research because of heavy diagnostic responsibilities, but which wished to be kept abreast of recent advances and of viral diseases in the Region, felt that they were left out of such networks. On the particular problem of dengue haemorrhagic fever/shock syndrome, Dr. D. Tarantola of WPRO of WHO stated that WHO could, if requested, organize a meeting of virologists and others to discuss this problem.

Attention was drawn to several information exchange mechanisms that were currently in operation and were not always adequately used: the Weekly Epidemiological Record of WHO and various newsletters associated with particular WHO programmes, such as Diarrhoeal Diseases, the Expanded Immunization Programme, and Respiratory Diseases. Such newsletters could be obtained by application to the Western Pacific or South-East Asian Regional Offices of WHO. There were also newsletters on communicable diseases produced by the South Pacific Commission (e.g., the Dengue Newsletter) and the Australian Department of Health (e.g., Communicable Diseases Intelligence). These organizations distributed Newsletters free on request and welcomed enquiries and information from all laboratories in the Region. The representative of the Australian Department of Health said that because of staff and financial constraints it would not be possible to expand the Communicable Diseases Intelligence

Bulletin produced by the Department to include information from other parts of the Region, but the existing bulletin would be regularly sent to anyone in the Region who asked for it. However, with the exception of the Communicable Diseases Intelligence Bulletin, the data presented in the other information exchange mechanisms are usually relatively old by the time they are disseminated.

Dr. S.K. Lam, of the University of Malaya in Kuala Lumpur, said he was trying to operate a Regional Newsletter among laboratories in the Region but only three laboratories sent in information. He emphasized that Newsletters were only as good as the inputs provided to them.

There was some discussion of the possibility of establishing a new SEARO-WPRO Newsletter for laboratory virologists in the Region, to provide monthly data on viral isolations and for circulating information on the availability of reagents, specific problems of particular laboratories, meetings and other relevant information. However, this would be expensive and would succeed only if many (hopefully all) laboratories in the Region supplied information *promptly*, as well as accepted and read the Newsletter. In this respect Dr. Lam's experience was not encouraging.

Attention was drawn to the availability of MEDLARS services through the Regional Offices of WHO (WPRO and SEARO) and the National Library of Australia.

STAFF EXCHANGE AND TRAINING

It was agreed that there were already considerable facilities available for the training of graduates in various countries - Australia, Japan, India and others. Attention was drawn to the Epidemiology course now being launched at the University of Newcastle Medical School under the sponsorship of the Rockefeller Foundation, which would be useful to scientists in developing countries. The Australian Institute of Health in Sydney was well placed to take graduates from the Region for a variety of appropriate Masters courses. Dr. Dora Tan from Kuala Lumpur pointed out that many laboratories in the Region were short-staffed and could not release staff to undertake such courses. It was suggested that some sort of exchange arrangement including the running of courses in the Region might help relieve this pressure and give graduates from developed countries useful experience. External supervision of degrees might also be possible, but this depended upon the rules applied by each University.

Dr. K. Pavri from Poona suggested that it would be helpful to have a listing of laboratories in the Region and the facilities that each offered; to some extent the attendance list of the seminar should provide some of this information, but in addition, a relatively frequent update of information would be necessary.

The meeting agreed that training of technicians was important but neglected. This should be carried out in laboratories in the developing countries, preferably the laboratory in which the technician was working, not in developed countries where facilities were usually better, but which might give a misleading impression to participants. One of the WHO representatives noted the need for training in the rapid diagnostic procedures for viral diseases which were now being developed. The possibility of regional "technical" courses was suggested.

LABORATORY MATERIALS

It was agreed that a necessary corollary to training programmes in, for example, rapid diagnostic methods was the availability of reagents. The problem here was largely one of cost. Commercial laboratories in Europe and North America produced a large range of such reagents and the Commonwealth Serum Laboratories in Australia was in the process of expanding its activities in diagnostic reagents. But cost was a factor; commercial distributors needed a large demand in order to undertake production of non-standard items, and the prices of standard items were often beyond the scope of laboratories in developing countries. A WHO representative said that WHO had no funds to provide reagents.

Dr. S.K. Lam suggested that various laboratories in the Region might be able to undertake the production of different diagnostic agents and circulate these by an exchange arrangement. Thus individual laboratories would be responsible for one specific reagent. Some form of quality control would be necessary; it was not clear how this could be organized, although if financial assistance was available, Commonwealth Serum Laboratories have offered to undertake quality control testing.

CONCLUSIONS

It was clear that within the Region covered by the seminar there was a great range of skills and facilities; very good in some countries and quite inadequate in others. To a large extent this reflected the variations in wealth in different countries. Some modern diagnostic methods offered possibilities of supplying much better service at no greater cost than at present; there was a need for training facilities and perhaps initial suppliers to be organized, perhaps with help from bilateral and multilateral aid agencies. Attention was also drawn to the problems of maintenance and repair of sophisticated laboratory equipment being experienced in a number of countries in the Region.

Exchange of views such as had occurred in the seminar was most valuable in giving many virologists in the Region a glimpse of the conditions prevailing in different parts of the Region, as well as information on modern views and techniques. Even if new initiatives were not possible at this time, many participants were now more aware of the facilities for the communication of information and for training that existed within the Region. Finally, it was generally felt that further efforts should be made towards better communication, increased bilateral aid programmes for training and for obtaining specific, quality controlled diagnostic reagents, and more encouragement for research between laboratories in the Region and between developed and developing countries.

Appendix

111

A SHORT BIBLIOGRAPHY OF RECENT PAPERS ON HUMAN VIRAL DISEASES IN SOUTH-EAST ASIA AND THE WESTERN PACIFIC

John S. Mackenzie

Department of Microbiology
University of Western Australia
Nedlands, Western Australia

This short bibliography has been prepared to provide additional background information on human viral diseases in the region. It cites many of the papers published between 1974 and 1981 which were written in English. It is *not* a comprehensive catalogue of all publications over the past eight years, but rather a guide to some of the valuable work being carried out in many regional laboratories and elsewhere, and as a reference source to expand the data presented by the contributors to this volume.

The bibliography includes only a few papers from the extensive literature on arboviruses; a full list of publications would have markedly increased the number of citations, and further information on arboviral diseases in the region is readily available from other sources such as the Arthropod-Borne Virus Information Exchange and the South Pacific Commission's Dengue Newsletter. Also, for the sake of brevity, only a few of the large number of excellent publications from India have been cited; they too would have substantially increased the length of the bibliography.

Further information on the incidence of viral diseases in the region and on vaccination programmes can be obtained from WHO publications such as the Weekly Epidemiological Record.

VIRAL DISEASES IN SOUTH-EAST ASIA
AND THE WESTERN PACIFIC
ISBN 0 12 484820 6

Enteroviruses

1. Wang, H.C., Hung, S.C., Tai, F.H., Studies on viral diarrhea in Taiwan. I. Viruses isolated from diarrheal cases and control subjects. *Chinese J. Microbiol. 6,* 63 (1973). (Echo 1, rotavirus, adenoviruses 1 and 2.)
2. Ming, C.K., *et al.*, Serologic survey for certain childhood viral infections in Rangoon in 1971. *J. Trop. Med. Hyg. 77,* 260 (1974). (Poliovirus, dengue, chikungunya, measles, rubella and Epstein-Barr virus.)
3. Chong, A.Y.H., Lee, L.H., Wong, H.B., Epidemic pleurodynia (Bornholm disease) outbreak in Singapore. *Trop. Geogr. Med. 27,* 151 (1975). (Coxsackie B2 and A9.)
4. Jayavasu, C., *et al.*, Characterization of a virus associated with epidemic conjunctivitis in Thailand. *Biken J. 18,* 249 (1975). (Echo 7.)
5. John, T.J., Oral polio vaccination of children in the tropics. II. Antibody response in relation to vaccine virus infection. *Am. J. Epidemiol. 102,* 414 (1975).
6. John, T.J., Christopher, S., Oral polio vaccination of children in the tropics. III. Intercurrent enterovirus infections, vaccine virus take and antibody response. *Am. J. Epidemiol. 102,* 422 (1975).
7. Sangkawibha, N., *et al.*, Surveillance of enterovirus infections in Bangkok. I. Isolation of enteroviruses from faecal specimens of healthy children. *S.E. Asian J. Trop. Med. Publ. Hlth 6,* 3 (1975). (Polioviruses, coxsackie A and B viruses, echoviruses.)
8. Bahrin, M.A., Joshi, N.D., Yin-Murphy, M., A Coxsackievirus type A 24 epidemic conjunctivitis in Brunei. *S.E. Asian J. Trop. Med. Publ. Hlth 7,* 355 (1976).
9. Goh, K.T., Doraisingham, S., An epidemiological study of five families in the 1975 conjunctivitis epidemic. *Singapore Med. J. 17,* 225 (1976). (Coxsackie A 24.)
10. John, T.J., Antibody response of infants in tropics to five doses of oral polio vaccine. *Brit. Med. J. 1,* 812 (1976).
11. John, T.J., *et al.*, Effect of breast-feeding on seroresponse of infants to oral poliovirus vaccination. *Pediatrics 57,* 47 (1976).
12. John, T.J., Devarajan, L.V., Balasubramanyan, A., Immunization in India with trivalent and monovalent oral poliovirus vaccines of enhanced potency. *Bull. Wld Hlth Org. 54,* 115 (1976).
13. Pongpanich, B., *et al.*, Coxsackie group B virus and acquired valvular heart disease in children. *J. Med. Ass. Thailand 59,* 452 (1976).
14. Yin-Murphy, M., Lim, K.H., Ho, Y.M., A Coxsackie type A 24 epidemic of acute conjunctivitis. *S.E. Asian J. Trop. Med. Publ. Hlth 7,* 1 (1976). (Coxsackie A 24, enterovirus 70.)
15. Arnow, P.M., *et al.*, Acute hemorrhagic conjunctivitis: a mixed virus outbreak among Vietnamese refugees on Guam. *Am. J. Epidemiol. 105,* 68 (1977). (Enterovirus 70, Adenovirus 11 and 8.)
16. Chang, W.K., *et al.*, Acute haemorrhagic conjunctivitis in Hong Kong, 1971-75. *S.E. Asian J. Trop. Med. Publ. Hlth 8,* 1 (1977). (Coxsackie A 24, enterovirus 70.)
17. Higgins, P.G., Chapman, T.E.D., Coxsackie-virus A 24 and acute haemorrhagic conjunctivitis in Sri Lanka. *Lancet 1,* 361 (1977).
18. Kono, R., *et al.*, Virological and serological studies of neurological complications of acute hemorrhagic conjunctivitis in Thailand. *J. Infect. Dis. 135,* 706 (1977). (Enterovirus 70.)
19. Lee, L.H., Lim, K.A., Eradication of poliomyelitis in Singapore. *Singapore Med. J. 18,* 34 (1977).
20. Lim, K.H., Yin-Murphy, M., The aetiologic agents of epidemic conjunctivitis. *Singapore Med. J. 18,* 41 (1977). (Coxsackie A 24, enterovirus 70, adenovirus.)
21. Baride, J.P., *et al.*, An epidemic of paralytic poliomyelitis in Aurangabad district. *Arch. Child Hlth 20,* 29 (1978).
22. Benfante, R.J., Gajdusek, D.C., Antibody studies in the Kuru region. Immunological epidemiology of population group in and adjacent to the Kuru region in Papua New Guinea. I. Enteroviruses. *Papua New Guinea Med. J. 21,* 124 (1978).
23. Limsuwan, A., *et al.*, Recurrent or persistent illness following acute Coxsackie B3 infections. *Asian J. Infect. Dis. 2,* 235 (1978).
24. Madhavan, H.N., Agarwal, S.C., Badrinath, S., Role of viruses in myocarditis during the years 1973-76 in Pondicherry area. *Indian J. Med. Res. 67,* 190 (1978). (Echo 9, Coxsackie A9, Coxsackie B1-B6, etc.)
25. Tan, D.S.K., Lam, S.K., Enterovirus survey before and after poliomyelitis vaccination in Kuala Lumpur, Malaysia. *S.E. Asian J. Trop. Med. Publ. Hlth 9,* 301 (1978).

26. Thongcharoen, P., *et al.*, Etiologic studies on acute hemorrhagic conjunctivitis in Thailand, 1971-75. *J. Med. Ass. Thailand 61*, 195 (1978).
27. John, T.J., The epidemiology of enterovirus infections and disease in India. *Bull. Haffkine Inst. 7*, 1 (1979).
28. Limson, B.M., *et al.*, Occurrence of infection with group B coxsackieviruses in rheumatic and nonrheumatic Filipino children. *J. Infect. Dis. 140*, 415 (1979).
29. Dizon, J.J., Epidemiological aspects of poliomyelitis in the Philippines, *in* "Potency and Efficacy of Vaccines," (F.E. André, ed.), pp.31-41. Smith Kline-RIT, Belgium, (1980).
30. Forbes, C.A.L., *et al.*, A survey to determine the immunity status and antibody creating effect of oral poliovaccine. *J. Trop. Med. Hyg. 83*, 109 (1980).
31. Idris, M.Z., *et al.*, Oral polio vaccination and factors affecting its efficacy. *Indian J. Med. Res. 71*, 671 (1980).
32. Tan, D.S.K., Yin-Murphy, M., Kandiah, S., An outbreak of acute conjunctivitis caused by coxsackievirus A 24 in Kuala Lumpur, Malaysia, 1978. *S.E. Asian J. Trop. Med. Publ. Hlth 11*, 24 (1980).
33. Nakao, J.C., *et al.*, A new candidate type of human enterovirus (Drilon strain) isolated in the Philippines. *Microbiol. Immunol. 25*, 163 (1981).
34. Snyder, J.D., *et al.*, Prevalence of residual paralysis from paralytic poliomyelitis in a rural population of Bangladesh. *Am. J. Trop. Med. Hyg. 30*, 426 (1981).
35. Ulfah, N.M., *et al.*, Polio and lameness in Yogyakarta, Indonesia. *Int. J. Epidemiol. 10*, 171 (1981).
36. Bernard, K.W., *et al.*, Acute hemorrhagic conjunctivitis in Southeast Asian refugees arriving in the United States. Isolation of enterovirus 70. *Am. J. Trop. Med. Hyg. 31*, 541 (1982).

Rotaviruses (see also reference 1)

37. Wyatt, G.B., *et al.*, Duovirus infection as a cause of infantile gastro-enteritis in Port Moresby. *Papua New Guinea Med. J. 19*, 134 (1976).
38. Echeverria, P., *et al.*, Age distribution of antibody to reovirus-like agent in children in Taiwan. *J. Pediat. 91*, 960 (1977).
39. Paniker, C.K.J., *et al.*, Epidemic gastroenteritis in children associated with rotavirus infection. *Indian J. Med. Res. 66*, 525 (1977).
40. Echeverria, P., *et al.*, Reovirus-like agent and enterotoxigenic *Escherichia coli* infections in pediatric diarrhea in the Philippines. *J. Infect. Dis. 138*, 326 (1978).
41. Black, R.E., *et al.*, A two-year study of bacterial, viral and parasitic agents associated with diarrhea in rural Bangladesh. *J. Infect. Dis. 142*, 660 (1980).
42. Qifang, P., *et al.*, Studies on the etiology of autumnal infantile acute gastroenteritis - rotavirus. *Chinese Med. J. 93*, 36 (1980).
43. Sack, D.A., *et al.*, Seroepidemiology of rotavirus infection in rural Bangladesh. *J. Clin. Micro. 11*, 530 (1980).
44. Shann, F.A., *et al.*, Rotavirus infection in young children in the Highlands of Papua New Guinea. *Med. J. Aust. 2*, 153 (1980).
45. Black, R.E., *et al.*, Incidence and severity of rotavirus and *Escherichia coli* diarrhoea in rural Bangladesh: implications for vaccine development. *Lancet 1*, 141 (1981).
46. Leksomboon, U., *et al.*, Viruses and bacteria in pediatric diarrhea in Thailand: a study of multiple antibiotic-resistant enteric pathogens. *Am. J. Trop. Med. Hyg. 30*, 1281 (1981).
47. Soenarto, Y., *et al.*, Acute diarrhea and rotavirus infection in newborn babies and children in Yogyakarta, Indonesia, from June 1978 to June 1979. *J. Clin. Micro. 14*, 123 (1981).
48. Williamson, H.G., *et al.*, Human rotavirus infection in Efate, Vanuatu. *Am. J. Trop. Med. Hyg. 31*, 136 (1982).

Norwalk agent

49. Kapikian, A.Z., *et al.*, Prevalence of antibody to the Norwalk agent by a newly developed immune adherence hemagglutination assay. *J. Med. Virol. 2*, 281 (1978).
50. Greenberg, H.B., *et al.*, Prevalence of antibody to the Norwalk virus in various countries. *Infect. Immun. 26*, 270 (1979).

Hepatitis A

51. Roberts, D.M., Differences between acute hepatitis A and B in Hong Kong. *Trans. Roy. Soc. Trop. Med. Hyg. 70*, 458 (1976).

52. Goh, K.T., Epidemiology of acute viral hepatitis in Singapore. *S.E. Asian J. Trop. Med. Publ. Hlth 8,* 289 (1977).
53. Santos-Ocampo, P.D., Caspellan, A.O., An overview of problems of children of the Philippines. *Indian Pediat. 14,* 779 (1977). (Also influenza and measles.)
54. Gust, I.D., Lehmann, N.I., Dimitrakakis, M., A seroepidemiologic study of infection with HAV and HBV in five Pacific islands. *Am. J. Epidemiol. 110,* 237 (1979).
55. Gust. I.D., *et al.,* Seroepidemiology of infection with hepatitis A and B viruses in an isolated Pacific population. *J. Infect. Dis. 139,* 559 (1979).
56. Moritsugu, Y., *et al.,* Prevalence of antibody to hepatitis A virus in Sri Lanka. *Asian J. Infect. Dis. 3,* 33 (1979).
57. Wong, D.C., Purcell, R.H., Rosen, L., Prevalence of antibody to hepatitis A and hepatitis B viruses in selected populations of the South Pacific. *Am. J. Epidemiol. 110,* 227 (1979).
58. Sung, J.L., *et al.,* Hepatitis A virus infection in Taiwan: a hospital-based study. *Trop. Geogr. Med. 32,* 324 (1980).
59. Wu, J-S., *et al.,* Hepatitis A virus infection in Taiwan. *J. Formosan Med. Assoc. 79,* 694 (1980).
60. Burke, D.S., *et al.,* Age-specific prevalence of hepatitis A virus antibody in Thailand. *Am. J. Epidemiol. 113,* 245 (1981).
61. Hawkes, R.A., Boughton, C.R., Ferguson, V., The seroepidemiology of hepatitis in Papua New Guinea. I. A long-term study of hepatitis A. *Am. J. Epidemiol. 114,* 554 (1981).

Hepatitis B (see also references 51, 52, 54, 55 and 57)

62. Blumberg, B.S., Australia antigen in the Solomon Islands. *Hum. Biol. 46,* 239 (1974).
63. Chiewslip, P., Vinyan, S., Bhamarapravati, N., HBAg and HBAb in Thai blood donors. *Trans. Roy. Soc. Trop. Med. Hyg. 68,* 339 (1974).
64. Anderson, K.E., *et al.,* Hepatitis B antigen in infants born to mothers with chronic hepatitis B antigenemia in Taiwan. *Am. J. Dis. Child. 129,* 1389 (1975).
65. Chainuvati, T., Viranuvatti, V., Pongpipat, D., Relationship of hepatitis B antigen in cirrhosis and hepatoma in Thailand. An etiological significance. *Gastroenterology 68,* 1261 (1975).
66. Clarke, C.W., Woodfield, D.G., Hepatitis B antigen, $Alpha_1$ fetoprotein and liver disease in the eastern highlands of Papua New Guinea. *Trop. Geogr. Med. 27,* 52 (1975).
67. Grossman, R.A., *et al.,* An epidemiologic study of hepatitis B virus in Bangkok, Thailand. *Am. J. Epidemiol. 101,* 144 (1975).
68. Lee, A.K.Y., Hepatitis B antigen and autoantibodies in chronic liver diseases in Hong Kong. *Aust. N.Z. J. Med. 5,* 235 (1975).
69. Lin-Kleiner, H.F.K., Lacson, P.S., Hepatitis B antigen in Filipino commercial donors. *J. Philipp. Med. Ass. 51,* 211 (1975).
70. Nishioka, K., Levin, A.G., Simons, M.J., Hepatitis B antigen, antigen subtypes, and hepatitis B antibody in normal subjects and patients with liver disease. *Bull. Wld Hlth Org. 52,* 293 (1975).
71. Snitbhan, R., *et al.,* Subtypes of hepatitis B surface antigen in Southeast Asia. *J. Infect. Dis. 131,* 708 (1975).
72. Stevens, C.E., *et al.,* Vertical transmission of hepatitis B antigen in Taiwan. *New Engl. J. Med. 292,* 771 (1975).
73. Woodfield, D.G., Acute viral hepatitis in Papua New Guinea: results of hepatitis B antigen and antibody studies. *Trop. Geogr. Med. 27,* 399 (1975).
74. Thongcharoen, P., *et al.,* The incidence of hepatitis B surface antigen in tropical infections and liver diseases in Thailand. *J. Med. Ass. Thailand 59,* 546 (1976).
75. Williams, H., Mazzur, S., Hepatitis B antigen subtypes in asymptomatic carriers in the Solomon Islands. *Aust. N.Z. J. Med. 6,* 210 (1976).
76. Chen, D.S., Sung, J.L., Hepatitis B virus infection on Taiwan. *New Engl. J. Med. 297,* 668 (1977).
77. Tan, A.Y.O., Law, C.H., Lee, Y.S., Hepatitis B antigen in the liver cells in cirrhosis and hepatocellular carcinoma. *Pathology 9,* 57 (1977).
78. Woodfield, D.G., Hepatitis B antigen - post-transfusion studies in Papua New Guinea. *Trop. Geogr. Med. 29,* 257 (1977).

79. Chen, D.S., Sung, J.L., Studies on the subtypes of hepatitis B surface antigen - demonstration of vertical and intrafamilial transmission of hepatitis B virus. *J. Formosan Med. Ass. 77,* 263 (1978).
80. Gaxotte, P., *et al.*, Hepatitis B antigenaemia on Wuvulu Island. *Am. J. Trop. Med. Hyg. 27,* 1037 (1978).
81. Gust, I.D., Dimitriakakis, M., Zimmet, P., Hepatitis B infection in Funafuti. *Asian J. Infect. Dis. 2,* 207 (1978).
82. Gust, I.D., Dimitrakakis, M., Zimmet, P., Studies on hepatitis B surface antigen and antibody in Nauru. I. Distribution amongst Nauruans. *Am. J. Trop. Med. Hyg. 27,* 1030 (1978).
83. Gust, I.D., *et al.*, Studies on hepatitis B surface antigen and antibody in Nauru. II. Distribution amongst Gilbert and Ellice (Tuvalu) islanders. *Am. J. Trop. Med. Hyg. 27,* 1206 (1978).
84. Makonkawkeyoon, S., Sanyanusin, P., Amastayakul, K., Partial purification of hepatitis B surface antigen and survey of this antigen in man and animals in Chiang Mai, Thailand. *S.E. Asian J. Trop. Med. Publ. Hlth 9,* 361 (1978).
85. Lee, Y.S., Hepatic cirrhosis in Singapore: differences between the Chinese and Indian ethnic groups. *Trop. Geogr. Med. 31,* 329 (1979).
86. Obata, H., Nishioka, K., Prevalence of hepatitis B virus and primary hepato-cellular carcinoma in Asia. *S.E. Asian J. Trop Med. Publ. Hlth 10,* 621 (1979).
87. Stevens, C.E., *et al.*, HBeAg and anti-HBe detection by radioimmunoassay: correlation with vertical transmission of hepatitis B virus in Taiwan. *J. Med. Virol. 3,* 237 (1979).
88. Ton, S.H., Lopez, C.G., Hasnah, H., Prevalence of anti-HBc in Malaysian male blood donors and its correlation with DNA polymerase activity. *S.E. Asian J. Trop. Med. Publ. Hlth 10,* 1 (1979).
89. Dingfeng, Z., *et al.*, Cell-mediated immune response in viral hepatitis B. *Chin. Med. J. 93,* 90 (1980).
90. Johnson, D.E., *et al.*, Hepatitis B in the rural tropics. *Int. J. Epidemiol. 9,* 123 (1980).
91. Lam, K.C., *et al.*, Etiological spectrum of liver cirrhosis in the Chinese. *J. Chron. Dis. 33,* 375 (1980).
92. Pongpipat, D., Suvatte, V., Assateerawatts, A., Vertical transmission of the hepatitis B surface antigen in Thailand. *S.E. Asian J. Trop. Med. Publ. Hlth 11,* 582 (1980).
93. Zhihua, G., *et al.*, Transfer of adoptive immunity of hepatitis B patient leukocytes with HBsAg specific immune RNA. *Chin. Med. J. 93,* 74 (1980).
94. Chien, M-C., Hepatitis B viral markers in patients with primary hepatocellular carcinoma in Taiwan. *J. Nat. Cancer Inst. 66,* 475 (1981).
95. Gust, I.D., *et al.*, The prevalence of hepatitis B infection amongst urban and rural populations in Western Samoa. *J. Hyg., Camb. 86,* 87 (1981).
96. Hawkes, R.A., *et al.*, The seroepidemiology of hepatitis in Papua New Guinea. II. A long-term study of hepatitis B. *Am. J. Epidemiol. 114,* 563 (1981).
97. Ho, J., Wu, P.C., Kung, T.M., An autopsy study of hepatocellular carcinoma in Hong Kong. *Pathology 13,* 409 (1981).
98. Ho, J.C.I., Wu, P-C., Mak, T-K., Liver cell dysplasia in association with hepatocellular carcinoma, cirrhosis and hepatitis B surface antigen in Hong Kong. *Int. J. Cancer 28,* 571 (1981).
99. Kuberski, T., *et al.*, Hepatitis B virus infections in Melanesians and Polynesians in New Caledonia. *Am. J. Epidemiol. 114,* 355 (1981).
100. Mazzur, S., Bastiaans, M.J.S., Nath, N., Hepatitis B virus (HBV) infection among children and adults in the Solomon Islands. *Am. J. Epidemiol. 113,* 510 (1981).

<u>Influenza</u> (see also references 24, 53)

101. Ming, C.K., *et al.*, Clinical and laboratory studies on haemorrhagic fever in Burma, 1970-72. *Bull. Wld Hlth Org. 51,* 227 (1974). (Also chikungunya, dengue, measles.)
102. Tan, D.S.K., Omar, M., Survey of influenza HI antibodies in peninsular Malaysian sera collected before and after the Hong Kong 'flu epidemic in 1968. *Med. J. Malaysia 29,* 17 (1974).
103. Ong, S.B., Lam, K.L., Lam, S.K., Respiratory virus disease in Malaysian children: a serological study. *Bull. Wld Hlth Org. 52,* 376 (1975). (Also respiratory syncytial virus, parainfluenza, adenovirus.)
104. Thein, S., *et al.*, Haemorrhagic manifestations of influenza A infection in children. *J. Trop. Med. Hyg. 78,* 78 (1975).

105. Olson, J.G., Epidemic appearance of a new influenza strain in Asia. *S.E. Asian J. Trop. Med. Publ. Hlth 7,* 6 (1976).
106. Scott, R.M., *et al.*, Epidemic influenza in a hill tribe of northwest Thailand. *Am. J. Trop. Med. Hyg. 25,* 718 (1976).
107. Olson, J.G., Epizootic swine influenza with evidence of a low rate of human infection associated with occupational exposure to swine. *S.E. Asian J. Trop. Med. Publ. Hlth 8,* 368 (1977).
108. Ong, S.B., Thong, M.L., Tay, L.K., Viruses and bacteria associated with acute respiratory illnesses in young children in general practice. *S.E. Asian J. Trop. Med. Publ. Hlth 9,* 98 (1978). (Also parainfluenza and adenoviruses.)
109. Retaillian, H.F., *et al.*, Excess mortality and influenza surveillance in Taiwan. *Int. J. Epidemiol. 7,* 223 (1978).
110. Shortridge, K.F., Osmund, I., H1N1 influenza in Hong Kong. *Lancet 1,* 322 (1978).
111. Austin, F.J., Mataika, J.U., Influenza virus A (H1N1) in Fiji. *N.Z. Med. J. 90,* 242 (1979).
112. Tan, D.S.K., Omar, M., Yap, T.C., Influenza HI antibodies in pig and man in Malaysia (with special reference to swine influenza). *Med. J. Malaysia 34,* 159 (1979).

<u>Measles, mumps and other paramyxoviruses</u> (see also references 2, 24, 53, 101, 103, 108)

113. Willis, M.F., Warburton, M.F., Measles susceptibility in two Pacific atoll populations. Epidemiological factors and response to live attenuated measles virus. *Med. J. Aust.,* 789 (1974).
114. Agarwal, D.K., *et al.*, Natural history of measles in rural and urban communities of Varanasi. *J. Comp. Dis. 8,* 289 (1976).
115. Fernandez, V.L., A clinical study of epidemic parotitis (mumps) as seen in a general practice. *Singapore Med. J. 17,* 233 (1976).
116. Wyatt, J.L., Wyatt, G.B., Measles in Port Moresby. *Papua New Guinea Med. J. 19,* 205 (1976).
117. Chen, S.T., Measles in peninsular Malaysia. *Med. J. Malaysia 34,* 18 (1979).
118. John, T.J., *et al.*, Epidemiology and prevention of measles in rural south India. *Indian J. Med. Res. 72,* 153 (1980).
119. Krishnamurthy, K.A., The epidemiology of measles in India, *in* "Potency and Efficacy of Vaccines", (F.E. André, ed.), pp.157-166. Smith Kline-RIT, Rixensart, Belgium, (1980).

<u>Adenoviruses</u> (see also references 1, 15, 20, 108)

120. Tai, F.H., *et al.*, A new form of acute conjunctivitis epidemic in Taiwan. A simultaneous outbreak of adenovirus type 11 and "acute hemorrhagic conjunctivitis" virus infections. *Chinese J. Microbiol. 7,* 79 (1974).
121. Tai, F.H., *et al.*, Epidemic haemorrhagic conjunctivitis associated with adenovirus type 11 in Taiwan. *S.E. Asian J. Trop. Med. Publ. Hlth 5,* 342 (1974).
122. Yin-Murphy, M., Lim, K-H., Chun, P.H., Adenovirus type 11 epidemic conjunctivitis in Singapore. *S.E. Asian J. Trop. Med. Publ. Hlth 5,* 333 (1974).
123. Chiu, F.H., *et al.*, Direct fluorescent antibody technique in early and rapid diagnosis of adenovirus pneumonia in children. *Chin. Med. J. 3,* 227 (1977). (Adenovirus types 3 and 7.)

<u>Rubella</u> (see also reference 2)

124. Silva, D.G., *et al.*, Infantile glaucoma associated with neonatal rubella - a case report. *Ceylon Med. J. 21,* 204 (1976).
125. Desudchit, P., Chatiyanonda, K., Bhamornsathit, S., Rubella antibody among Thai women of child bearing age. *S.E. Asian J. Trop. Med. Publ. Hlth 9,* 312 (1978).
126. Shortridge, K.F., Osmund, I.F., Seroepidemiology of rubella infection in Chinese and Caucasians in Hong Kong. *J. Hyg., Camb. 83,* 397 (1979).
127. André, F.E., Epidemiology of rubella: incidence in Asia, *in* "Potency and Efficacy of Vaccines", (F.E. André, ed.), pp.197-215. Smith Kline-RIT, Rixensart, Belgium, (1980).
128. Tantivanich, S., *et al.*, Serological studies on possible causes of intrauterine infections in Thai infants. *S.E. Asian J. Trop. Med. Publ. Hlth 11,* 387 (1980). (Also herpes simplex and cytomegalovirus.)

Rabies

129. Thongcharoen, P., The problems of rabies control in Thailand. *J. Med. Ass. Thailand 56,* 295 (1973).
130. Anderson, R.D., Parker, J.G., Progress in rabies is possible: a civic action program. *Milit. Med. 139,* 705 (1974).
131. Arambulo, P.V., *et al.*, Rabies in the Republic of the Philippines: with notes on its field control and possible eradication. *Acta Med. Philipp. 10,* Ser. 2, No. 1, 20 (1974).
132. Thongcharoen, P., *et al.*, Rabies: a study at Siriraj Hospital, Bangkok. *J. Med. Ass. Thailand 61,* 99 (1978).
133. Sinhaseni, A., Current status of rabies problems in Thailand. *Jap. J. Med. Sci. Biol. 32,* 367 (1979).
134. Trivedi, C.R., Profile of dog bites, rabies and default in antirabic immunization at V.S.G. Hospital, Ahmedabad. *J. Indian Med. Ass. 76,* 134 (1981).

Arboviruses (see also references 2, 101)

135. Bowen, E.T.W., *et al.*, Arbovirus infections in Sarawak, October 1968 - February 1970: human serological studies in a Land Dyak village. *Trans. Roy. Soc. Trop. Med. Hyg. 69,* 182 (1975). (Semliki Forest, chikungunya, getah, sindbis, tembusu, kunjin, West Nile, dengue 1 and 2, Bunyamwera.)
136. Srichaikul, T., *et al.*, Disseminated intravascular coagulation in adult dengue haemorrhagic fever: report of three cases. *S.E. Asian J. Trop. Med. Publ. Hlth. 6,* 106 (1975).
137. Sumarmo, Widya, M.S., Puranto, L., Observations on hospitalized patients with dengue hemorrhagic fever. *Pediat. Indones. 15,* (5/6), 125 (1975).
138. Tesh, R.B., *et al.*, The distribution and prevalence of group A arbovirus neutralizing antibodies among human populations in Southeast Asia and the Pacific Islands. *Am. J. Trop. Med. Hyg. 24,* 664 (1975). (Chikungunya, Ross River, getah, bebaru, sindbis.)
139. Thaung, U., *et al.*, Epidemiological features of dengue and chikungunya infections in Burma. *S.E. Asian J. Trop. Med. Publ. Hlth 6,* 276 (1975).
140. Gupta, S.N.S., *et al.*, Clinical profile of the epidemic of Japanese encephalitis at Bankura. *Indian J. Med. Res. 64,* 1393 (1976).
141. Maheswaran, K., *et al.*, Serological survey of arbovirus infection in Sri Lanka. *Ceylon Med. J. 21,* 105 (1976).
142. Pavri, K.M., *et al.*, Isolation of Wanowrie virus from brain of a fatal human case from Sri Lanka. *Indian J. Med. Res. 64,* 557 (1976).
143. Scott, R.M., *et al.*, Shock syndrome in primary dengue infections. *Am. J. Trop. Med. Hyg. 25,* 866 (1976).
144. Shanmugam, J., Smirnova, S.E., Chumakov, M.P., Presence of antibody to arboviruses of the Crimean haemorrhagic fever - Congo (CHF-Congo) group in human beings and domestic animals in India. *Indian J. Med. Res. 64,* 1403 (1976).
145. Chan, K.L., Ng, S.K., Chew, L.M., The 1973 dengue haemorrhagic fever outbreak in Singapore and its control. *Singapore Med. J. 18,* 81 (1977).
146. Khai Ming, C., *et al.*, Recent outbreaks of Japanese encephalitis in Burma. *S.E. Asian J. Trop. Med. Publ. Hlth 8,* 113 (1977).
147. Reed, D., Maguire, T., Mataika, J.U., Type 1 dengue with hemorrhagic disease in Fiji: epidemiologic findings. *Am. J. Trop. Med. Hyg. 26,* 784 (1977).
148. Bunnag, T., Disease ecology and control: a nidal base approach to arthropod-borne virus infection. *J. Med. Ass. Thailand 61,* 555 (1978).
149. Conference on dengue haemorrhagic fever: new developments and future research. Papers presented. *Asian J. Infect. Dis. 2,* 1-192 (1978).
150. Farrell, K.T., An epidemic of dengue fever in Wewak. *Papua New Guinea Med. J. 21,* 191 (1978).
151. Gubler, D.J., *et al.*, Epidemiologic, clinical and virologic observations on dengue in the Kingdom of Tonga. *Am. J. Trop. Med. Hyg. 27,* 581 (1978).
152. Shaikh, B.H., *et al.*, Antibodies to arboviruses in humans of Rajasthan. *Indian J. Med. Res. 67,* 175 (1978). (Chikungunya, sindbis, Japanese encephalitis, West Nile, dengue 1-4, Kyasanur forest disease.)
153. Sumarmo, *et al.*, Encephalopathy associated with dengue infection. *Lancet 1,* 449 (1978).
154. Van Tongeren, H.A.E., Van Kammen, A., Arthropod-borne virus infections in Western New Guinea (Irian Jaya). A serological retrospection. *Trop. Geogr. Med. 30,* 413 (1978). (Semliki forest, chikungunya, Ross River, alfuy, dengue 1 and 2, kokobera, Kunjun, Murray Valley encephalitis, trubanaman, corriparta.)

155. Kanamitsu, M., *et al.*, Geographic distribution of arbovirus antibodies in indigenous human populations in the Indo-Australian archipelago. *Am. J. Trop. Med. Hyg. 28,* 351 (1979). (Sindbis, getah, chikungunya, Ross River, dengue 2-3, Japanese encephalitis, Murray Valley encephalitis, Kunjin, Edge Hill.)
156. Self, L.S., Vectors of dengue fever/dengue haemorrhagic fever with advances in their control. *Asian J. Infect. Dis. 3,* 77 (1979).
157. Surharyono, W., *et al.*, Dengue virus infection in Indonesia, 1975-1978. *Asian J. Infect. Dis. 3,* 27 (1979).
158. Halstead, S.B., Dengue haemorrhagic fever - a public health problem and a field for research. *Bull. Wld Hlth Org. 58,* 1 (1980).
159. Johnson, D.E., *et al.*, Togavirus infection in rural Thailand. *S.E. Asian J. Trop. Med. Publ. Hlth 11,* 184 (1980). (Chikungunya, dengue 1-4.)
160. Khan, A.Q., *et al.*, An outbreak of Japanese encephalitis in Bangladesh. *Bangladesh Med. J. 8,* 71 (1980).
161. Marchette, N.J., Rudnick, A., Garcia, R., Alphaviruses in peninsular Malaysia. II. Serological evidence of human infection. *S.E. Asian J. Trop. Med. Publ. Hlth 11,* 14 (1980). (Chikungunya, sindbis, getah.)
162. Wallace, H.G., *et al.*, Dengue hemorrhagic fever in Malaysia: the 1973 epidemic. *S.E. Asian J. Trop. Med. Publ. Hlth 11,* 1 (1980).
163. Aaskov, J.G., *et al.*, An epidemic of Ross River virus infection in Fiji, 1979. *Am. J. Trop. Med. Hyg. 30,* 1053 (1981).
164. Gubler, D.J., *et al.*, Epidemic dengue 3 in Central Java, associated with low viraemia in man. *Am. J. Trop. Med. Hyg. 30,* 1094 (1981).
165. Gunakasem, P., *et al.*, Surveillance of Japanese encephalitis cases in Thailand. *S.E. Asian J. Trop. Med. Publ. Hlth 12,* 333 (1981).
166. Gunakasem, P., *et al.*, Surveillance of dengue haemorrhagic fever cases in Thailand. *S.E. Asian J. Trop. Med. Publ. Hlth 12,* 338 (1981).
167. Khan, A.M., *et al.*, A Japanese encephalitis focus in Bangladesh. *J. Trop. Med. Hyg. 84,* 41 (1981).
168. Nimmannitya, S., Nisalak, A., Burke, D.S., Passively acquired antibody to flavivirus in Thai infants. *S.E. Asian J. Trop. Med. Publ. Hlth 12,* 344 (1981).
169. Olson, J.G., *et al.*, Zika virus, a cause of fever in Central Java, Indonesia. *Trans. Roy. Soc. Trop. Med. Hyg. 75,* 389 (1981).
170. Rosen, L., Gubler, D.J., Bennett, P.H., Epidemic polyarthritis (Ross River) virus infection in the Cook Islands. *Am. J. Trop. Med. Hyg. 30,* 1294 (1981).

Herpesviruses (see also references 2, 24, 128)

171. Huda, Q., Islam, M.M., Nuruzzaman, M., Joint manifestation in chickenpox. *Bangladesh Med. J. 3,* 95 (1975).
172. Sinha, D.P., Chickenpox - a disease predominantly affecting adults in rural West Bengal, India. *Int. J. Epidemiol. 5,* 367 (1976).
173. Lang, D.J., Garruto, R.M., Gajdusek, D.C., Early acquisition of cytomegalovirus and Epstein-Barr virus antibody in several Melanesian populations. *Am. J. Epidemiol. 105,* 480 (1977).
174. Mukundan, P., Jadhav, M., John, T.J., Prevalence of cytomegalovirus antibody in young children in Vellore. *Indian J. Med. Res. 65,* 589 (1977).
175. Ho, H.C., *et al.*, Epstein-Barr virus infection in staff treating patients with nasopharyngeal carcinoma. *Lancet 1,* 710 (1978).
176. Vardthananusara, C., *et al.*, Herpes simplex virus type 2 and carcinoma of cervix uteri. *J. Med. Ass. Thailand 61,* 14 (1978).
177. Chantarakul, N., Angkustsiri, K., Thakerngpol, K., Cytomegalic inclusion disease. A study of fifty-five autopsies. *J. Med. Ass. Thailand 62,* 403 (1979).
178. Puthavathana, P., *et al.*, Presence of herpes simplex virus type 2 (HSV-2) antibodies and antigens in patients with cervical carcinoma in Thailand. *J. Med. Ass. Thailand 63,* 560 (1980).
179. Tantivanich, S., Tharavanij, S., Prevalence of genital herpesvirus infection in Thai women. *S.E. Asian J. Trop. Med. Hyg. 11,* 126 (1980).
180. Wang, T.R., Seroepidemiological survey of cytomegalovirus infections in the urban and suburban areas of Taipei City. *J. Formosan Med. Ass. 79,* 753 (1980).
181. Zeng, Y., *et al.*, Anticomplement immunoenzymatic method of detecting Epstein-Barr nuclear antigen in nasopharyngeal carcinoma cells and normal epithelial cells. *Chinese Med. J. 94,* 663 (1981).

Miscellaneous

182. Kim, K.H., Shin, H.K., Song, J.S., Recent epidemiological features of Korean hemorrhagic fever in the Republic of Korea. *Int. J. Zoonoses 4,* 87 (1977).
183. Jiang, Y., Li, Z., Song, G., Seroepidemiologic study of epidemic hemorrhagic fever with renal syndrome in China. *Chinese Med. J. 94,* 221 (1981).
184. Alpers, M.P., Gajdusek, D.C., Ono, S.G., Bibliography of Kuru. National Institute of Health, U.S.A., Department of Health, Education and Welfare Publication No. (NIH)76-800 (1975).
185. Gajdusek, D.C., Alpers, M.P., Recent data on the properties of the viruses of Kuru transmissible virus dementias. *Papua New Guinea Med. J. 18,* 207 (1975).
186. King, H.O.M., Kuru. Epidemiological developments. *Lancet 2,* 761 (1975).
187. Wong, D.C., *et al.*, Epidemic and endemic hepatitis in India: evidence for non-A, non-B hepatitis virus aetiology. *Lancet 2,* 876 (1980).

TABLE. CITATIONS BY COUNTRY

Country	Citation Numbers
Bangladesh	34, 41, 43, 45, 49, 50, 160, 167, 171
Burma	2, 101, 104, 139, 146, 149
Caroline Islands	57, 138, 149
China (People's Republic)	42, 89, 93, 123, 181, 183
China (Taiwan)	1, 38, 58, 59, 64, 72, 76, 79, 87, 94, 105, 107, 109, 120, 121, 127, 138, 180
Cook Islands	54, 149, 170
Fiji	54, 111, 147, 149, 163
French Polynesia	57, 149
Guam	15, 149
Hong Kong	16, 51, 68, 97, 98, 110, 126, 127, 175
India	5, 6, 10-12, 21, 24, 27, 31, 39, 114, 118, 119, 127, 134, 140, 144, 149, 152, 172, 174, 187
Indonesia	35, 47, 137, 138, 149, 153-155, 157, 164, 169
Kampuchea	71
Kirribati (Gilbert Islands)	149
Korea (South)	182
Laos	149, 155
Malaysia	8, 25, 32, 88, 102, 103, 108, 112, 117, 127, 135, 138, 149, 161, 162
Mariana Islands	149
Nauru	82, 83, 149
New Caledonia	57, 99, 138, 149
Niue	54, 149
Papua New Guinea	22, 37, 44, 57, 61, 66, 73, 78, 80, 96, 116, 138, 149, 150, (154), 155, 173, 184-186
Philippines	28, 29, 33, 40, 53, 69, 127, 131, 138, 149
Samoa	54, 57, 95, 138, 149
Singapore	3, 9, 14, 19, 20, 52, 70, 77, 85, 115, 122, 145, 149
Solomon Islands	62, 75, 100, 113, 138, 149, 173
Sri Lanka	17, 30, 56, 124, 141, 142
Thailand	4, 7, 13, 18, 23, 26, 46, 60, 63, 65, 67, 71, 74, 84, 90, 92, 106, 125, 127-130, 132, 133, 143, 148, 149, 155, 159, 165, 166, 168, 176, 177-179.
Tokelau Islands	149
Tonga	149, 151
Tuvalu (Ellice Islands)	54, 55, 81, 83, 149
Vanuatu (New Hebrides)	48, 138, 149, 173
Vietnam	71, 127, 138, 149
Wallis and Futuna	149

Participants

ADA, Prof. G.L.
Dept. of Microbiology
John Curtin Sch. Med. Res.
P.O. Box 334
Canberra City, ACT 2601
AUSTRALIA

ALBERT, Dr. M.J.
Dept. of Gastroenterology
Royal Children's Hospital
Parkville, Vic 3052
AUSTRALIA

ALLAN, Mrs. J.E.
Dept. of Microbiology
Univ. of Western Australia
Nedlands, WA 6009
AUSTRALIA

ALPERS, Dr. M.P.
Papua New Guinea Inst.
of Medical Res.
P.O. Box 60
Goroka, EHP
PAPUA NEW GUINEA

AUSTIN, Dr. F.J.
Virus Research Unit
University of Otago
P.O. Box 56
Dunedin
NEW ZEALAND

BALAYAN, Dr. M.S.
Inst. of Poliomyelitis
& Viral Encephalitides
USSR Acad. of Medical Sci.
Moscow Oblast
P.O.Inst.Poliomyel.142782
Moscow
USSR

BARNES, Dr. G.L.
Dept. of Gastroenterology
Royal Children's Hospital
Parkville, Vic 3052
AUSTRALIA

BARNETT, Dr. G.R.
Dept. of Microbiology
Newcastle Mater Hospital
Waratah, NSW 2298
AUSTRALIA

BARRY, A/Prof. R.D.
Faculty of Medicine
Royal Newcastle Hospital
Univ. of Newcastle
NSW 2308
AUSTRALIA

BEALE, Dr. A.J.
Wellcome Research Labs.
Langley Court
Beckenham
Kent BR3 3BS
ENGLAND

Bellamy, A/Prof. A.R.
Cell Biology Dept.
University of Auckland
Private Bag
Auckland
NEW ZEALAND

BEVERIDGE, Dr. W.I.B.
University House
P.O. Box 1535
Canberra City, ACT 2601
AUSTRALIA

BHAMARAPRAVATI, Prof. Natth
Dept. of Pathology
Faculty of Medicine
Mahidol University
Ramathibodi Hospital
Rama VI Road
Bangkok 4
THAILAND

BISHOP, Dr. R.
Dept. of Gastroenterology
Royal Children's Hospital
Parkville, Vic 3052
AUSTRALIA

BLACK, Prof. F.L.
Dept. of Epidemiology and
Public Health
Yale Univ. School of Med.
P.O. Box 3333
New Haven, Conn 06510
U.S.A.

BLANDEN, Dr. R.V.
Dept. of Microbiology
John Curtin Sch. Med. Res.
P.O. Box 334
Canberra City, ACT 2601
AUSTRALIA

BOOTH, Dr. D.
Department of Health
P.O. Box 100
Woden, ACT 2606
AUSTRALIA

BOUGHTON, A/Prof. C.R.
Div. of Infect. Diseases
Prince Henry Hospital
Little Bay, NSW 2036
AUSTRALIA

BOVEINGTON, Ms. C.
South Pacific Commission
Post Box D5
Noumea CEDEX
NEW CALEDONIA

BOWDEN, Dr. D.K.
P.O. Box 55
Port Vila
VANUATU
South-West Pacific

BRANSBY, Ms R.D.
Smith Kline & French Labs
(Aust.) Ltd
P.O. Box 90
Brookvale, NSW 2100
AUSTRALIA

BRESCHKIN, Dr. A.M.
Viral Products Section
Natl. Biological Standards
Laboratory
Private Bag No. 7
Parkville, Vic 3052
AUSTRALIA

BROWN, Dr. F.
Animal Virus Res. Inst.
Pirbright, Woking
Surrey GU24 ONF
ENGLAND

BUCENS, Dr. M.
Virus Laboratory
State Health Lab. Services
G.P.O. Box F312
Perth, WA 6001
AUSTRALIA

BURKE, Dr. D.S.
U.S. Component
Armed Forces Research
Inst. of Medical Sci.
Pramongkutklao Hospital
Rajvithi Road
Bangkok 4
THAILAND

BURNET, Sir Macfarlane
'Kenilworth'
48 Monomeath Avenue
Canterbury, Vic 3126
AUSTRALIA

BURRELL, Dr. C.J.
Div. of Medical Virology
Inst. of Medical and
Veterinary Science
Box 14, Rundle St. P.O.
Adelaide, SA 5000
AUSTRALIA

CAMERON, Dr. A.S.
C/- South Australian
Health Commission
Box 1313, G.P.O.
Adelaide, SA 5001
AUSTRALIA

CARTER, Mr. I.W.J.
Dept. of Microbiology
The Prince Henry Hospital
P.O. Box 233
Matraville, NSW 2036
AUSTRALIA

CHAN, Prof. Veronica F.
Dept. of Med. Microbiology
Inst. of Public Health
Univ. of Philippines Syst.
P.O. Box EA-460
Manila
PHILIPPINES

CHANG, Dr. W.K.
Virus Unit
Queen Mary Hospital
Pok Fu Lam Road
HONG KONG

CHANOCK, Dr. R.M.
Lab. of Infectious Dis.
National Inst. of Allergy
& Infect. Diseases
Building 7 Room 100
National Inst. of Health
Bethesda, MD 20205
U.S.A.

CHARLICK, Mr. P.J.
Dept. of Microbiology
Univ. of Western Australia
Nedlands, WA 6009
AUSTRALIA

CHATIYANONDA, Dr. Kanai
Virus Research Institute
Dept. of Medical Sciences
Yod-se, Bangkok 1
THAILAND

CHU, Prof. C.M.
(see under
ZHU, Prof. J.M.)

CHUBB, Dr. R.C.
Dept. of Microbiology
Univ. of New England
Armidale, NSW 2351
AUSTRALIA

COLE, Prof. G.A.
Microbiology Department
Univ. of Maryland Med. Sch.
660 West Redwood St.
BALTIMORE, MD 21201
U.S.A.

COOPER, Dr. M.G.
Aust. Bureau of Animal Hlth
Dept. of Primary Industry
Canberra, ACT 2600
AUSTRALIA

COSSART, A/Prof. Y.
Dept. of Bacteriology
School of Medicine
University of Sydney
NSW 2006
AUSTRALIA

COWLEY, Dr. J.A.
8/48 Selwyn Street
Merewether, NSW 2291
AUSTRALIA

CROUCH, Dr. A.A.
20 Kirkley Street
Acacia Ridge, Qld 4110
AUSTRALIA

CROXSON, Dr. M.C.
18 Montrose Terrace
Mairangi Bay
Auckland 10
NEW ZEALAND

DAVEY, Mr. V.F.
Commonwealth Serum Labs
45 Poplar Road
Parkville, Vic 3052
AUSTRALIA

DELLA-PORTA, Dr. A.J.
CSIRO Div. of Animal Hlth
Private Bag No. 1, P.O.
Parkville, Vic 3052
AUSTRALIA

DE SILVA, Dr. L.M.
Department of Virology
Institute of Pathology
P.O. Box 34
Camperdown, NSW 2050
AUSTRALIA

DIWAN, A/Prof. A.R.
Dept. of Tropical Med. and
Med. Microbiology
John A. Burns Sch. Med.
University of Hawaii
Leahi Hospital
3675 Kilauea Avenue
Honolulu, Hawaii 96816
U.S.A.

DIZON, Dr. J.J.
Bureau of Health Services
Ministry of Health
San Lazaro Comp., Sta. Cruz
Manila
PHILIPPINES

DOHERTY, Prof. P.C.
Dept. of Exp. Pathology
John Curtin Sch. Med. Res.
P.O. Box 334
Canberra City, ACT 2601
AUSTRALIA

DOHERTY, Prof. R.L.
Dean
Faculty of Medicine
Univ. of Queensland
Medical School
Herston, Qld 4006
AUSTRALIA

DORAISINGHAM, Dr. S.
Dept. of Pathology
Ministry of Health
Outram Road
SINGAPORE 0316

DOWNIE, Dr. J.C.
Natl. Biol. Standards
Laboratory
Private Bag No. 7
Parkville, Vic 3052
AUSTRALIA

DWYER, Lt. Col. M.
4 Forest Court
30 Eungella Street
DUFFY, ACT 2611
AUSTRALIA

DYCE, Dr. A.L.
CSIRO Div. of Trop.
Anim. Sci.
McMaster Laboratory
Private Bag No.1, P.O.
Glebe, NSW 2037
AUSTRALIA

EDWARDS, Ms E.
42 Horace Street
St. Ives, NSW 2075
AUSTRALIA

FAURAN, Dr. P.A.R.
Institut Pasteur
B.P. 61, Noumea
NEW CALEDONIA

FEERY, Dr. B.J.
Commonwealth Serum Labs
45 Poplar Road
Parkville, Vic 3052
AUSTRALIA

FENNER, Prof. F.J.
John Curtin Sch. Med. Res.
P.O. Box 334
Canberra City, ACT 2601
AUSTRALIA

FERGUSON, Dr. K.A.
Inst. of Animal and Food
Sciences, CSIRO
P.O. Box 225
Dickson, ACT 2602
AUSTRALIA

FRANCIS, Mrs. B.H.
Pathology Department
Mercy Maternity Hospital
Clarendon Street
E. Melbourne, Vic 3002
AUSTRALIA

FRANCIS, Prof. J.
Dept. of Vet. Pathology
Univ. of Queensland
St. Lucia, Qld 4067
AUSTRALIA

FRASER, Dr. J.R.E.
Dept. of Medicine
Univ. of Melbourne
Royal Melbourne Hosp. P.O.
Vic 3050
AUSTRALIA

FRENCH, Dr. E.L.
P.O. Box 141
Mt. Eliza, Vic 3930
AUSTRALIA

GAJDUSEK, Dr. D.C.
Natl. Inst. of Neurological
& Comm. Disorders & Stroke
Natl. Inst. of Health
Bethesda, MD 20205
U.S.A.

GARD, Dr. G.
P.O. Box 4160
Darwin, NT 5794
AUSTRALIA

GEERING, Dr. W.A.
Aust. Bur. of Animal Hlth
Dept. of Primary Industry
Canberra, ACT 2600
AUSTRALIA

GEIZER, Dr. I.
WHO Regional Office for
Western Pacific
P.O. Box 2932
12115 Manila
PHILIPPINES

GEYSEN, Dr. M.
Commonwealth Serum Labs
45 Poplar Road
Parkville, Vic 3052
AUSTRALIA

GIBBS, Dr. A.J.
Virus Ecology Res. Group
Res. Sch. of Biological Sci.
P.O. Box 475
Canberra City, ACT 2601
AUSTRALIA

GOLDWATER, Dr. P.N.
Dept. of Pathology
Univ. of Auckland
Private Bag
Auckland
NEW ZEALAND

GOODWIN, A/Prof. C.S.
Dept. of Microbiology
Royal Perth Hospital
Perth, WA 6000
AUSTRALIA

GORMAN, Dr. B.
Qld. Inst. of Medical Res.
Bramston Terrace
Herston, Qld 4006
AUSTRALIA

GRACEY, Dr. M.
Gastroenterology Unit
Princess Margaret Hosp.
Subiaco, WA 6008
AUSTRALIA

GRAHAM, Dr. D.M.
Dept. of Microbiology
Univ. of Melbourne
PARKVILLE, Vic 3052
AUSTRALIA

GRAY, Mr. D.G.
Commonwealth Serum Labs
45 Poplar Road
Parkville, Vic 3052
AUSTRALIA

GREWAL, Dr. A.S.
Vet. Res. Station
Roy Watts Road
Glenfield, NSW 2167
AUSTRALIA

GRICE, Mr. R.G.
State Hlth. Lab. of
Microbiology
63-79 George Street
Brisbane, Qld 4000
AUSTRALIA

GU, A/Prof. P.W.
Beijing Vaccine and Serum
Institute
Beijing
CHINA

GUBLER, Dr. D.J.
Chief Dengue Branch
CDC San Juan Labs.
G.P.O. Box 4532
San Juan PR00936
U.S.A.

GUST, Dr. I.D.
Fairfield Hospital
Yarra Bend Road
Fairfield, Vic 3078
AUSTRALIA

HALLETT, Dr. P.
P.O. Box 66
Garran, ACT 2605
AUSTRALIA

HALLSWORTH, Dr. P.G.
Dept. of Clin. Microbiology
Flinders Medical Centre
Bedford Park, SA 5042
AUSTRALIA

HALONEN, Prof. P.
Dept. of Virology
University of Turku
Kiinamyllynkatu 10
SF-20520 Turku
FINLAND

HARNETT, Mr. G.B.
Virology Section
State Health Lab. Services
G.P.O. Box F312
Perth, WA 6001
AUSTRALIA

HAWKES, Dr. R.A.
School of Microbiology
Univ. of New South Wales
P.O. Box 1
Kensington, NSW 2033
AUSTRALIA

HERMON, Dr. Y.E.
National Health Inst.
P.O. Box 50-348
Kenepuru Drive
Porirua
Wellington
NEW ZEALAND

HILEY, Mr. L.A.
Virology Lab.
2nd Floor
63-79 George Street
Brisbane, Qld 4000
AUSTRALIA

HOBBS, Dr. K.
Esso House
G.P.O. Box 4047
Sydney, NSW 2001
AUSTRALIA

HOFFMANN, Dr. P.J.
Dept. of Microbiology
John Curtin Sch. Med. Res.
P.O. Box 334
Canberra City, ACT 2601
AUSTRALIA

HOLMES, Dr. I.H.
Dept. of Microbiology
Univ. of Melbourne
Parkville, Vic 3052
AUSTRALIA

HSU, Dr. S.T.
P.O. Box 81-95
6th Floor
201 Tun-hua N. Road
Formosa Plastic Building
Taipei City
Taiwan,
CHINA

HUDSON, Dr. B.J.
35 Bellevue Parade
North Curl Curl
NSW 2099
AUSTRALIA

HULME, Mr. A.
C/- Flow Labs
P.O. Box 132
North Ryde, NSW 2113
AUSTRALIA

HUYGELEN, Dr. C.
Smith Kline-RIT
Rue de l'Institut 89
B-1330 Rixensart
BELGIUM

IGO, Dr. J.D.
Dean, Medical Faculty
Univ. of Papua New Guinea
P.O. Box 5623
Boroko, NCD
PAPUA NEW GUINEA

IKEGAMI, Dr. N.
Osaka Prefectural Inst. of Public Hlth
3-69 Nakamichi 1-Chrome
Hikashinari-ku
Osaka 537
JAPAN

IRVING, Dr. L.G.
Virus Laboratory
Fairfield Hospital
Yarra Bend Road
Fairfield, Vic 3078
AUSTRALIA

ISLAM, A/Prof. M.N.
Inst. of Postgrad. Medicine and Research
Shahabagh Avenue
Dacca
BANGLADESH

JACK, Mr. I.
Dept. of Pathology
Royal Children's Hosp.
Parkville, Vic 3052
AUSTRALIA

JAYAVASU, Dr. C.
Virus Research Inst.
Dept. of Medical Sciences
Yod-se
Bangkok 1
THAILAND

JENNINGS, Dr. L.C.
Microbiology Dept.
Christchurch Hospital
Private Bag
Christchurch
NEW ZEALAND

JOHN, Prof. T.J.
Dept. of Virology
Christian Medical College & Hospital
Vellore 632004
Tamil Nadu
INDIA

JOHNSON, Dr. K.M.
U.S. Army Medical Res. Inst. of Infect. Diseases
Fort Detrick
Frederick, MD 21701
U.S.A.

JOKLIK, Prof. W.K.
Dept. of Microbiology and Immunology
Duke Univ. Med. Center
P.O. Box 3020
Durham, NC 27710
U.S.A.

JONES, Dr. M.A.S.
Aust. Meat. Res. Committee
P.O. Box 4129
Sydney, NSW 2001
AUSTRALIA

KAPPAGODA, Dr. N.
Microbiology Dept.
Royal Prince Alfred Hosp.
Camperdown, NSW 2050
AUSTRALIA

KAY, Dr. B.H.
Qld. Inst. of Medical Res.
Bramston Terrace
Herston, Qld 4006
AUSTRALIA

KENNETT, Dr. M.L.
Virus Laboratory
Fairfield Hospital
Yarra Bend Road
Fairfield, Vic 3078
AUSTRALIA

KENRICK, Dr. K.G.
Red Cross Blood Trans. Service
153 Clarence Street
Sydney, NSW 2000
AUSTRALIA

KHIN, Dr. M.M.
Virology Res. Division
Dept. of Medical Research
No. 5 Zafar Shah Road
Rangoon
BURMA

KIRKLAND, Dr. P.D.
82 Alhambra Avenue
Cardiff, NSW 2285
AUSTRALIA

KIRSCH, Ms. S.
Biochemistry Dept.
Red Cross Blood Trans. Service
153 Clarence Street
Sydney, NSW 2000
AUSTRALIA

KITCHEN, Dr. R.G.
Wellcome Aust. Ltd.
P.O. Box 12
Concord, NSW 2137
AUSTRALIA

KONNO, Dr. T.
Dept. of Pediatrics
Tohoku University
School of Medicine
Sendai 980
JAPAN

LAKE, Dr. J.R.
Dept. of Health
P.O. Box 100
Woden, ACT 2606
AUSTRALIA

LAM, A/Prof. S.K.
Div. Communicable Diseases
World Health Organization
1211 Geneva 27
SWITZERLAND

LANSER, Dr. J.A.
Dept. of Clin. Microbiology
Flinders Medical Centre
Bedford Park, SA 5042
AUSTRALIA

LAU, Mr. R.C.H.
National Hlth Inst.
P.O. Box 50348
Porirua, Wellington
NEW ZEALAND

LAVER, Dr. W.G.
Dept. of Microbiology
John Curtin Sch. Med. Res.
P.O. Box 334
Canberra City, ACT 2601
AUSTRALIA

LEE, Prof. H.W.
Inst. for Viral Diseases
Korea Univ. Med. Coll.
4 Myungyun-Dong 2 Ga
Chongro-Ku
Seoul 110
KOREA

LEE, Dr. W.Y.
Dept. of Microbiology
Yonsei University
College of Medicine
Seoul 120
KOREA

LEHMANN-GRUBE, Prof. F.
Heinrich-Pette-Inst. Exp.
Virologie Immunologie
un der Univ. Hamburg
Martinstrasse 52
2000 Hamburg 20
WEST GERMANY

LITTLEJOHNS, Dr. I.R.
Veterinary Res. Station
Roy Watts Road
Glenfield, NSW 2167
AUSTRALIA

LIU, A/Prof. C.B.
Institute of Virology
Chinese Acad. Med. Sciences
100 Ying Xing Jie
Xuan Wu Qu
Beijing 100052
CHINA

LUCET, Dr. P.
Institut Pasteur
B.P. 61, Noumea
NEW CALEDONIA

LUNT, Dr. R.
Virus Laboratory
Fairfield Hospital
Yarra Bend Road
Fairfield, Vic 3078
AUSTRALIA

MACKENZIE, A/Prof. J.S.
Dept. of Microbiology
Univ. of Western Australia
Nedlands, WA 6009
AUSTRALIA

MACKERELL, Dr. J.R.
256 Ross River Road
Aitkenvale, Qld 4814
AUSTRALIA

MAHON, Dr. R.J.
CSIRO Div. Entomology
P.O. Box 1700
Canberra City, ACT 2601
AUSTRALIA

MALONEY, Dr. M.B.
22 Leslie Road
Essendon, Vic 3040
AUSTRALIA

MARMION, Prof. B.P.
Inst. of Medical & Vet. Sci.
Box 14 Rundle St. P.O.
Adelaide, SA 5000
AUSTRALIA

MARSHALL, Dr. I.D.
Dept. of Microbiology
John Curtin Sch. Med. Res.
P.O. Box 334
Canberra City, ACT 2601
AUSTRALIA

MARTIN, Prof. E.M.
Sch. of Biological Sci.
Flinders University
Bedford Park, SA 5042
AUSTRALIA

MASTERS, Dr. C.
Dept. of Neuropathology
Royal Perth Hospital
Perth, WA 6000
AUSTRALIA

MATA, Dr. L.
INISA
Univ. de Costa Rica
Ciudad Universitaria
Rodrigo Facio
COSTA RICA

MATAIKA, Dr. J.U.
Wellcome Virus Lab.
Tamavua Hospital
Suva
FIJI ISLANDS

McCARTHY, Dr. N.J.
Commonwealth Serum Labs
45 Poplar Road
Parkville, Vic 3052
AUSTRALIA

McDONALD, Mr. C.R.
Dept. Med. Lab. Science
Qld. Inst. of Technology
G.P.O. Box 2434
Brisbane, Qld 4001
AUSTRALIA

McINTOSH, Dr. B.M.
Natl. Inst. for Virology
Private Bag X4
Sandringham, 2131
SOUTH AFRICA

McKELLAR, Dr. P.
Medical Centre
Opunake
Taranaki
NEW ZEALAND

McLEAN, Dr. B.
C/- Dr. I. Holmes
Dept. of Microbiology
Univ. of Melbourne
Parkville, Vic 3052
AUSTRALIA

McPHEE, Dr. D.A.
CSIRO Division of
Animal Hlth
C/- Private Bag No. 1
Parkville, Vic 3052
AUSTRALIA

MEIER-EWERT, Prof. H.
Virologische Abteilung
Inst. Med. Mikrobiologie
Technischen Universitat
Biedersteiner Str. 29
8 Munich 40
WEST GERMANY

MENSER, Dr. M.A.
Children's Med. Res. Found.
Royal Alexandra Hosp.
P.O. Box 61
Camperdown, NSW 2050
AUSTRALIA

MILES, Prof. J.A.R.
C/- P.O., Lake Hawea
NEW ZEALAND

MIMS, Prof. C.A.
Dept. of Microbiology
Guy's Hospital Med. School
London Bridge SE1 9RT
ENGLAND

MOORE, Mr. B.W.
Div. of Med. Virology
Inst. of Medical Vet. Sci.
Box 14, Rundle St. P.O.
Adelaide, SA 5000
AUSTRALIA

MURPHY, Mr. A.M.
Inst. Clin. Path. Med. Res.
P.O. Box 60
Wentworthville, NSW 2145
AUSTRALIA

MURPHY, Prof. F.A.
College of Vet. Medicine
& Biomed. Sciences
Colorado State Univ.
Fort Collins
Colorado 80523
U.S.A.

MURRAY, Dr. M.D.
CSIRO Div. of Trop.
Anim. Sci.
McMaster Laboratory
Private Bag No. 1
Glebe, NSW 2037
AUSTRALIA

NISALAK, Dr. Ananda
Armed Forces Res. Inst. of
Medical Sciences
Pramongkutklao Hospital
Rajvithi Road
Bangkok 4
THAILAND

O'CONNOR, Mr. G.P.
16 Harborne Street
Wembley, WA 6014
AUSTRALIA

OTT, Dr. K.
Microbiology Dept.
Royal Hobart Hospital
G.P.O. Box 1061L
Hobart, Tas 7001
AUSTRALIA

PANG, Dr. T.
Dept. of Med. Microbiology
Faculty of Medicine
University of Malaya
Kuala Lumpur
MALAYSIA

PANIKER, Prof. C.K.J.
Dept. of Microbiology
Medical College
Calicut
Kerala 673008
INDIA

PANON, Ms. G.
Institut Pasteur
B.P. 61, Noumea
NEW CALEDONIA

PARSONSON, Dr. I.M.
CSIRO Div. of Animal Hlth
Aust. Nat. Animal Hlth Lab
Private Bag No. 1
Parkville, Vic 3052
AUSTRALIA

PATHMANATHAN, Dr. R.
Dept. of Pathology
Faculty of Medicine
University of Malaya
Kuala Lumpur
MALAYSIA

PAVRI, Dr. K.
Natl. Inst. of Virology
20-A Dr. Ambedkar Rd
P.O. Box 11
Pune 411001
INDIA

PAXTON, Mr. D.W.
Aust. Bureau Animal Hlth
Dept. of Primary Industry
Canberra, ACT 2600
AUSTRALIA

PEARSON, Dr. L.
Dept. of Immunology
John Curtin Sch. Med. Res.
P.O. Box 334
Canberra City, ACT 2601
AUSTRALIA

PHILLIPS, Ms. M.
Aust. Development Assist.
Bureau
P.O. Box 887
Canberra City, ACT 2601
AUSTRALIA

POOLE, Ms. E.S.
Virology
Dunedin Public Hospital
P.O. Box 946
Dunedin
NEW ZEALAND

POPE, Dr. J.H.
Qld Inst. of Medical Res.
Bramston Terrace
Herston, Qld 4006
AUSTRALIA

PORTERFIELD, Dr. J.S.
Sir William Dunn School
of Pathology
University of Oxford
South Parks Road
Oxford OX1 3RE
ENGLAND

REEVES, Prof. W.C.
Dept. of Biomedical and
Envir. Hlth Sciences
School of Public Hlth
Univ. of California
Berkeley, CA 94720
U.S.A.

ROBBINS, Dr. S.J.
Qld. Inst. Medical Res.
Bramston Terrace
Herston, Qld 4006
AUSTRALIA

RODGERS, Brig. W.O.
Directorate of Army Health
Services
Campbell Park Offices
Campbell, ACT 2601
AUSTRALIA

ROSEN, Prof. L.
Arbovirus Program
Pacific Biomed. Res. Cent.
University of Hawaii
P.O. Box 1680
Honolulu
Hawaii 96806
U.S.A.

ROUCH, Dr. G.J.
12 Gore Street
Fitzroy, Vic 3065
AUSTRALIA

ROY, Dr. P.
Dept. Environmental Hlth
Sch. of Public Health
Univ. of Alabama
Birmingham
Alabama 35294
U.S.A.

SABINE, A/Prof. J.M.
Dept. of Vet. Pathology
University of Sydney
Sydney, NSW 2006
AUSTRALIA

SANGKAWIBHA, Dr. Nadhirat
Deputy Director-General
Dept. of Medical Sciences
Yod-se
Bangkok 1
THAILAND

SANYAKORN, Dr. C.K.
Director, Disease Control
and Prevention
WHO Regional Office for
South-East Asia
World Health House
New Delhi 110002
INDIA

SAROSO, Prof. J. Sulianti
Jalan Hang Jebat 1
No. 1, Kebayoran Baru
Jakarta Selatan
INDONESIA

SAWERI, Dr. A.
Dept. of Clinical Sciences
Faculty of Medicine
Univ. of Papua New Guinea
P.O. Box 5623
Boroko, NCD
PAPUA NEW GUINEA

SELF, Dr. L.S.
Vector Biology & Control
WHO Regional Office for
the Western Pacific
P.O. Box 2932
Manila
PHILIPPINES

SERGIEV, Dr. V.P.
Chief, The Main Board of
Quarantine Diseases
3 Rakhmanovsky per.
Ministry of Health, USSR
Moscow
USSR

SEVILLE, Dr. P.R.
Smith Kline & French Labs
(Australia) Ltd
P.O. Box 90
Brookvale, NSW 2100
AUSTRALIA

SHELLAM, Dr. G.R.
Dept. of Microbiology
Univ. of Western Australia
Nedlands, WA 6009
AUSTRALIA

SIMASATHIEN, Dr. Phinit
Dept. of Microbiology
Pramongkutklao College
of Medicine
315 Rajvithi Road
Bangkok 4
THAILAND

SLOAN, Dr. W.N.
5 Inverness Way
North Balwyn, Vic 3105
AUSTRALIA

SMALLRIDGE, Mr. G.J.
Vickers Medical
Priestley Road
Basingstoke
Hampshire
ENGLAND

SMITH, Dr. H.V.
10 Manica Street
West Brunswick, Vic 3055
AUSTRALIA

SMITH, Dr. V.W.
Animal Health Lab.
Dept. of Agriculture
Jarrah Road
South Perth, WA 6151
AUSTRALIA

SNOWDON, Dr. W.A.
CSIRO Div. Anim. Hlth
Australian National
Animal Hlth Lab.
P.O. Box 679
Geelong, Vic 3320
AUSTRALIA

SONZA, Dr. S.
Dept. of Microbiology
Univ. of Melbourne
Parkville, Vic 3052
AUSTRALIA

SPRADBROW, Dr. P.R.
Veterinary Virus Lab.
Univ. of Queensland
P.O. Box 125
Kenmore, Qld 4069
AUSTRALIA

ST. GEORGE, Dr. T.D.
CSIRO Dvision of Trop.
Anim. Sci.
Private Bag No. 3, P.O.
Indooroopilly, Qld 4068
AUSTRALIA

STANDFAST, Dr. H.A.
CSIRO Divison of Trop.
Anim. Sci.
Private Bag No. 3, P.O.
Indooroopilly, Qld 4068
AUSTRALIA

STANLEY, Prof. N.F.
Dept. of Microbiology
Univ. of Western Australia
Nedlands, WA 6009
AUSTRALIA

STOUT, Ms. M.
Flow Laboratories
P.O. Box 132
North Ryde, NSW 2113
AUSTRALIA

STUDDERT, Dr. M.J.
School of Veterinary Sci.
Univ. of Melbourne
Parkville, Vic 3052
AUSTRALIA

SU, A/Prof. Cheng-qin
Chief, Dept of Enteroviruses
Inst. of Medical Biology
Chinese Academy of
Medical Sciences
Kunming, Yunnan,
CHINA

SURHARYONO, Dr. W.
Virology Department
Biomedical Research Cent.
Jln.Percetakan Negara No.1
Jakarta
INDONESIA

SUWARDJI, Dr. H.
Virus Laboratory
Microbiology Dept.
Medical Faculty
Univ. of Gadjah Mada
Yogyakarta
INDONESIA

TAN, Dr. Dora
Snr Virus Res. Officer
Inst. for Medical Research
Jalan Pahang
Kuala Lumpur 02-14
MALAYSIA

TANNOCK, Dr. G.A.
Dept. of Pathology
Medical Faculty
Univ. of Newcastle
Royal Newcastle Hosp.
NSW 2308
AUSTRALIA

TARANTOLA, Dr. D.J.M.
Regional Adviser in
Communicable Diseases
WHO Regional Office for
the Western Pacific
P.O. Box 2932
Manila
PHILIPPINES

TEH, Major J.
Directorate of Army Hlth
Services
Campbell Park Offices,
Campbell, ACT 2601
AUSTRALIA

THAIB, Dr. Soeprapti
Virus Department
Perum. Bio Farma
(Pasteur Institute)
Jln. Pasteur 28
Bandung
INDONESIA

THONGCHAROEN, Prof. Prasert
Dean, Faculty of Medical
Technology
Mahidol University
Siriraj Hospital
Bangkok 7
THAILAND

TZIPORI, Dr. S.
Attwood Vet. Res. Lab.
Westmeadows, Vic 3076
AUSTRALIA

UREN, Mr. E.C.
Virus Laboratory
Royal Children's Hospital
Parkville, Vic 3052
AUSTRALIA

VINEY, Mr. R.L.
Commonwealth Serum Labs
45 Poplar Road
Parkville, Vic 3052
AUSTRALIA

VITARANA, Dr. Tissa
Dept. of Virology
Medical Research Inst.
P.O. Box 527
Baseline Road
Colombo 8
SRI LANKA

WADE, Mrs. S.M.
Microbiology Dept.
Royal Prince Alfred Hosp.
Missenden Road
Camperdown, NSW 2050
AUSTRALIA

WALKER, Dr. P.J.
Qld. Inst. Medical Research
Bramston Terrace
Herston, Qld 4006
AUSTRALIA

WANG, Dr. A.X.
Virology Dept.
Fairfield Hospital
Yarra Bend Road
Fairfield, Vic 3078
AUSTRALIA

WARK, Ms. M.C.
Commonwealth Serum Labs
45 Poplar Road
Parkville, Vic 3052
AUSTRALIA

WAUGH, Ms. M.
Dept. of Health Sciences
Royal Melbourne Inst. Tech.
80 Victoria Street
Carlton, Vic 3053
AUSTRALIA

WESTAWAY, Dr. E.G.
Dept. of Microbiology
Monash University
Clayton, Vic 3168
AUSTRALIA

WHALLEY, Dr. J.M.
Sch. of Biological Sci.
MacQuarie University
NSW 2113
AUSTRALIA

WHITE, Prof. D.O.
Dept. of Microbiology
Univ. of Melbourne
Parkville, Vic 3052
AUSTRALIA

WILLIAMSON, Dr. G.
Regional Virus Lab.
Ruchill Hospital
Glasgow G20 9NB
SCOTLAND

WOODROOFE, Dr. G.M.
138 La Perouse St
Red Hill, ACT 2603
AUSTRALIA

YAMAZI, Prof. Y.
Dept. of Microbiology and
Immunology
Nippon Medical School
1-1 Sendagi, Bunkyo-ku
Tokyo 113,
JAPAN

YIN-MURPHY, A/Prof. M.
Dept. of Microbiology
Faculty of Medicine
National Univ. of Singapore
Sepoy Lines
SINGAPORE 0316

ZENG, A/Prof. Y.
Institute of Virology
Chinese Acad. Med. Sciences
100 Ying Xing Jie
Xuan Wu Qu
Beijing 100052
CHINA

ZHU, Prof. J.M.
Director, Inst. of Virology
Chinese Acad. Med. Sciences
100 Ying Xing Jie
Xuan Wu Qu
Beijing 100052
CHINA

ZHUANG, Dr. H.
Virology Dept.
Fairfield Hospital
Yarra Bend Road
Fairfield, Vic 3078
AUSTRALIA

Index

2 3 4 5 6 7 8 9 0 1
A B C D E F G H I J